Type II Diabetes Mellitus: A Multidisciplinary Approach

Editorial Advisor

JOEL J. HEIDELBAUGH

ELSEVIER

1600 John F. Kennedy Boulevard • Suite 1800 • Philadelphia, Pennsylvania, 19103-2899

http://www.theclinics.com

CLINICS COLLECTIONS
ISSN 2352-7986, ISBN-13: 978-0-323-35956-6

Editor: John Vassallo (j.vassallo@elsevier.com)
Developmental Editor: Patrick Manley

Clinics Collections (ISSN 2352-7986) is published by Elsevier Inc., 360 Park Avenue South, New York, NY 10010-1710. Business and editorial offices: 1600 John F. Kennedy Boulevard, Suite 1800, Philadelphia, PA 19103-2899. **POSTMASTER:** Send address changes to *Clinics Collections*, Elsevier Health Sciences Division, Subscription Customer Service, 3251 Riverport Lane, Maryland Heights, MO 63043. **Customer Service: Telephone: 1-800-654-2452** (U.S. and Canada); **1-314-447-8871** (outside U.S. and Canada). **Fax: 314-447-8029. E-mail: journalscustomerserviceusa@elsevier.com** (for print support); **journalsonlinesupport-usa@elsevier.com** (for online support).

Reprints. For copies of 100 or more of articles in this publication, please contact the Commercial Reprints Department, Elsevier Inc., 360 Park Avenue South, New York, NY 10010-1710. Tel.: 212-633-3874; Fax: 212-633-3820; E-mail: reprints@elsevier.com.

Contributors

EDITORIAL ADVISOR

JOEL J. HEIDELBAUGH, MD, FAAFP, FACG
Clinical Associate Professor, Departments of Family Medicine and Urology; Clerkship Director, Department of Family Medicine, University of Michigan Medical School, Ann Arbor, Michigan; Ypsilanti Health Center, Ypsilanti, Michigan

AUTHORS

BRIGID S. BOLAND, MD
Gastroenterology Fellow, Division of Gastroenterology, Department of Medicine, University of California, San Diego, La Jolla, California

W. KLINE BOLTON, MD
Division of Nephrology, Department of Medicine, University of Virginia Health System, Charlottesville, Virginia

BRENDAN T. BOWMAN, MD
Division of Nephrology, Department of Medicine, University of Virginia Health System, Charlottesville, Virginia

CAROLINA CASELLINI, MD
Research Associate, Internal Medicine, Strelitz Diabetes Center, Eastern Virginia Medical School, Norfolk, Virginia

JOSE M. CASTELLANO, MD, PhD
Zena and Michael A. Wiener Cardiovascular Institute and Marie-Josée and Henry R. Kravis Cardiovascular Health Center, Mount Sinai School of Medicine, New York, New York

STEVEN R. COHEN, MD, MPH
Division of Dermatology, Albert Einstein College of Medicine, Montefiore Medical Center, Bronx, New York

SARAH D. CORATHERS, MD
Assistant Professor of Pediatrics, Division of Endocrinology, Cincinnati Children's Hospital Medical Center; Assistant Professor of Internal Medicine, Division of Endocrinology, University of Cincinnati Medical Center, Cincinnati, Ohio

KATE CRAWFORD, RN, MSN, ANP-C, BC-ADM
Department of Endocrine Neoplasia and Hormonal Disorders, The University of Texas MD Anderson Cancer Center, Houston, Texas

JAIME A. DAVIDSON, MD, FACP, MACE
Clinical Professor of Medicine, Division of Endocrinology, Diabetes and Metabolism, Touchstone Diabetes Center, University of Texas Southwestern Medical Center, Dallas, Texas

SUZANNE M. DE LA MONTE, MD, MPH
Departments of Medicine, Pathology (Neuropathology), Neurology and Neurosurgery, Rhode Island Hospital, The Warren Alpert Medical School of Brown University, Providence, Rhode Island

CHAO DENG, PhD
Associate Professor and Head, Antipsychotic Research Laboratory, School of Health Sciences, Illawarra Health and Medical Research Institute, University of Wollongong, Wollongong, New South Wales, Australia

JOHN A. DIPRETA, MD
Clinical Associate Professor, Division of Orthopaedic Surgery, Capital Region Orthopaedics, Albany Medical Center, Albany Medical College, Albany, New York

ANDREW DREXLER, MD
Department of Endocrinology, Gonda Diabetes Center, University of California, Los Angeles School of Medicine, Los Angeles, California

STEVEN V. EDELMAN, MD
Professor of Medicine, Division of Endocrinology and Metabolism, University of California, San Diego, La Jolla; Director, Division of Endocrinology and Metabolism, Diabetes Care Clinic, Veterans Affairs Medical Center, San Diego, California

JOSEPHINE M. EGAN, MD
Chief, Diabetes Section, Laboratory of Clinical Investigation, National Institute on Aging/National Institutes of Health, Baltimore, Maryland

ANN E. EVENSEN, MD, FAAFP
Associate Professor, Department of Family Medicine, University of Wisconsin School of Medicine and Public Health, Madison, Wisconsin

MICHAEL E. FARKOUH, MD
Associate Clinical Professor, Zena and Michael A. Wiener Cardiovascular Institute and Marie-Josée and Henry R. Kravis Cardiovascular Health Center, Mount Sinai School of Medicine, New York, New York; Peter Munk Cardiac Centre and Heart and Stroke Richard Lewar Centre of Excellence in Cardiovascular Research, University of Toronto, Toronto, Ontario, Canada

DOROTHY A. FINK, MD
Fellow, Division of Endocrinology, Department of Medicine, Columbia University Medical Center, New York, New York

VALENTIN FUSTER, MD, PhD
Physician-in-Chief, Zena and Michael A. Wiener Cardiovascular Institute and Marie-Josée and Henry R. Kravis Cardiovascular Health Center, Mount Sinai School of Medicine, New York, New York; The Centro Nacional de Investigaciones Cardiovasculares (CNIC), Madrid, Spain

EMILY JANE GALLAGHER, MD
Assistant Professor of Medicine, Division of Endocrinology, Diabetes and Bone Diseases, Icahn School of Medicine at Mount Sinai, New York, New York

FRANCES L. GAME, FRCP
Consultant Diabetologist and Honorary Associate Professor, Department of Diabetes and Endocrinology, Derby Hospitals NHS Trust, Derby, United Kingdom

MARIANA GARCIA-TOUZA, MD
Assistant Professor of Medicine, Diabetes and Cardiovascular Research Center; Division of Endocrinology, Diabetes and Metabolism, Department of Internal Medicine, University of Missouri Columbia School of Medicine, Columbia, Missouri

GEORGE HAN, MD, PhD
Albert Einstein College of Medicine, Bronx, New York

ANKUR JINDAL, MD
Assistant Professor of Clinical Medicine, Hospital Medicine, Department of Internal Medicine; Diabetes and Cardiovascular Research Center, University of Missouri, Columbia, Missouri

NIDHI JINDAL, MD
Nephrology Fellow, Division of Nephrology and Hypertension, Department of Internal Medicine, University of Missouri Columbia School of Medicine, Columbia, Missouri

RITA RASTOGI KALYANI, MD, MHS
Assistant Professor, Division of Endocrinology and Metabolism, Department of Medicine, Johns Hopkins University School of Medicine, The Johns Hopkins University, Baltimore, Maryland

AMANDA KLEINER, MD
Division of Endocrinology, Department of Medicine, University of Virginia Health System, Charlottesville, Virginia

JASON C. KOVACIC, MD, PhD
Assistant Professor, Zena and Michael A. Wiener Cardiovascular Institute and Marie-Josée and Henry R. Kravis Cardiovascular Health Center, Mount Sinai School of Medicine, New York, New York

SALILA KURRA, MD
Assistant Professor of Medicine, Columbia University Medical Center; Department of Medicine, Metabolic Bone Diseases Unit, Toni Stabile Osteoporosis Center, Columbia University Medical Center, New York, New York

L. ROMAYNE KURUKULASURIYA, MD
Associate Professor of Medicine, Division of Endocrinology, Diabetes and Metabolism, Department of Internal Medicine, University of Missouri Columbia School of Medicine, Columbia, Missouri

GUIDO LASTRA, MD
Assistant Professor of Medicine, Division of Endocrinology, Diabetes and Metabolism, Department of Internal Medicine, University of Missouri Columbia School of Medicine; Diabetes and Cardiovascular Research Center, University of Missouri; Harry S Truman Memorial Veterans Hospital, Columbia, Missouri

JELENA MALETKOVIC, MD
Department of Endocrinology, Gonda Diabetes Center, University of California, Los Angeles School of Medicine, Los Angeles, California

CAMILA MANRIQUE, MD
Assistant Professor of Medicine, Division of Endocrinology, Diabetes and Metabolism, Department of Internal Medicine, University of Missouri Columbia School of Medicine; Diabetes and Cardiovascular Research Center, University of Missouri; Harry S Truman Memorial Veterans Hospital, Columbia, Missouri

CHRISTINE MARIC-BILKAN, PhD, FASN, FAHA
Associate Professor, Department of Physiology and Biophysics, University of Mississippi Medical Center, Jackson, Mississippi

BRANT L. MCCARTAN, DPM, MBA, MS
Chief Resident, Division of Podiatry, Beth Israel Deaconess Medical Center, Harvard Medical School, Boston, Massachusetts; Private Practice, Milwaukee Foot Specialists, New Berlin, Wisconsin

BLAIR MURPHY-CHUTORIAN, BA, MSIV
University of California, Irvine, Irvine, California

MARIE-LAURE NEVORET, MD
Clinical Research Coordinator, Internal Medicine, Strelitz Diabetes Center, Eastern Virginia Medical School, Norfolk, Virginia

HENRI PARSON, PhD
Director, Microvascular Biology; Assistant Professor, Internal Medicine, Strelitz Diabetes Center, Eastern Virginia Medical School, Norfolk, Virginia

SHAWN PEAVIE, DO
Fellow, Division of Endocrinology, University of Cincinnati Medical Center, Cincinnati, Ohio

DANIEL F. ROSBERGER, MD, PhD, MPH
Clinical Assistant Professor of Ophthalmology, Weill-Cornell Medical College of Cornell University; Medical and Surgical Director, MaculaCare, PLLC, New York, New York

BARRY I. ROSENBLUM, DPM, FACFAS
Assistant Clinical Professor, Surgery, Harvard Medical School, Beth Israel Deaconess Medical Center, Harvard Medical Center, Boston, Massachusetts

MARZIEH SALEHI, MD, MS
Associate Professor of Internal Medicine, Division of Endocrinology, University of Cincinnati Medical Center, Cincinnati, Ohio

ETHEL S. SIRIS, MD
Madeline C. Stabile Professor of Medicine, Columbia University Medical Center; Director, Toni Stabile Osteoporosis Center, Metabolic Bone Diseases Unit, Columbia University Medical Center, New York-Presbyterian Hospital, New York, New York

JAMES R. SOWERS, MD
Professor of Medicine, and Medical Pharmacology and Physiology; Diabetes and Cardiovascular Research Center, University of Missouri; Division of Endocrinology, Diabetes and Metabolism, Department of Internal Medicine, University of Missouri Columbia School of Medicine; Department of Internal Medicine, Harry S Truman Memorial Veterans Hospital; Department of Medical Physiology and Pharmacology, University of Missouri, Columbia, Missouri

SOFIA SYED, MD
Endocrine Fellow, Division of Endocrinology, Diabetes and Metabolism, Department of Internal Medicine, University of Missouri Columbia School of Medicine; Diabetes and Cardiovascular Research Center, University of Missouri, Columbia, Missouri

MAGDALENE M. SZUSZKIEWICZ-GARCIA, MD
Assistant Professor, Division of Endocrinology and Metabolism, Department of Medicine, Center for Human Nutrition, University of Texas Southwestern Medical Center, Dallas, Texas

AARON I. VINIK, MD, PhD
Professor of Medicine/Pathology/Neurobiology, Director of Research and Neuroendocrine Unit, Internal Medicine, Strelitz Diabetes Center, Eastern Virginia Medical School, Norfolk, Virginia

ADAM WHALEY-CONNELL, DO, MSPH
Associate Professor of Medicine, Diabetes and Cardiovascular Research Center, University of Missouri; Division of Endocrinology, Diabetes and Metabolism, Department of Internal Medicine; Division of Nephrology and Hypertension, Department of Internal Medicine, University of Missouri Columbia School of Medicine; Associate Chief of Staff for Research and Development, Harry S Truman Memorial Veterans Hospital, Columbia, Missouri

JAMES D. WOLOSIN, MD
Chief, Division of Gastroenterology, Sharp Rees-Stealy Medical Group, San Diego, California

ZARA ZELENKO, BA, PhD(c)
Division of Endocrinology, Diabetes and Bone Diseases, Icahn School of Medicine at Mount Sinai, New York, New York

Contents

> Diabetic ketoacidosis (DKA) and the hyperglycemic hyperosmolar state
> (HHS) are potentially fatal hyperglycemic crises that occur as acute com-
> plications of uncontrolled diabetes mellitus. The authors provide a review
> of the current epidemiology, precipitating factors, pathogenesis, clinical
> presentation, evaluation, and treatment of DKA and HHS. The discovery
> of insulin in 1921 changed the life expectancy of patients with diabetes
> mellitus dramatically. Today, almost a century later, DKA and HHS remain
> significant causes of morbidity and mortality across different countries,
> ages, races, and socioeconomic groups and a significant economic
> burden for society.

> Diabetes and impaired glucose tolerance affect a substantial proportion of
> older adults. Abnormal glucose metabolism is not a necessary component
> of aging. Older adults with diabetes and altered glucose status likely repre-
> sent a subset of the population at high risk for complications and adverse
> geriatric syndromes. Goals for treatment of diabetes in the elderly include
> control of hyperglycemia, prevention and treatment of diabetic compli-
> cations, avoidance of hypoglycemia, and preservation of quality of life.
> Research exploring associations of dysglycemia and insulin resistance
> with the development of adverse outcomes in the elderly may ultimately
> inform use of future glucose-lowering therapies in this population.

> Current strategies for the treatment of type 2 diabetes mellitus promote
> individualized plans to achieve target glucose levels on a patient-by-
> patient basis while minimizing treatment related risks. Maintaining glyce-
> mic control over time is a significant challenge because of the progressive
> nature of diabetes as a result of declining β-cell function. This article iden-
> tifies complications of non-insulin treatments for diabetes. The major clas-
> ses of medications are reviewed with special focus on target population,
> mechanism of action, effect on weight, cardiovascular outcomes and
> additional class-specific side effects including effects on bone. Effects
> on β-cell function are also highlighted.

Podiatric Complications

Patients with diabetes and peripheral neuropathy are at risk for foot deformities and mechanical imbalance of the lower extremity. Peripheral neuropathy leads to an insensate foot that puts the patient at risk for injury. When combined with deformity due to neuropathic arthropathy, or Charcot foot, the risks of impending ulceration, infection, and amputation are significant to the diabetic patient. Education of proper foot care and shoe wear cannot be overemphasized. For those with significant malalignment or deformity of the foot and ankle, referral should be made immediately to an orthopedic foot and ankle specialist.

The diabetic foot is more susceptible than the non-diabetic foot to collapse. This frequently leads to bony prominences followed by ulceration. Offloading of areas of increased pressure is paramount to ulcer prevention and healing. Several devices and accommodations can aid practitioners in saving patients' extremities and allow them to ambulate. A team approach works best, and patient education is a must. Regular assessment and modifications are required for longevity of each device. In this article, different therapeutic options are detailed. A variety of presentations and situations are discussed and the authors' best tips for avoiding complications are offered.

Osteomyelitis of the foot in diabetes is common and frequently undiagnosed. Diagnosis should be clinical and based on signs of infection, the size of the lesion, and the visibility of bone in the first instance but supported by the results of radiologic examination. The gold standard for diagnosis is histologic and microbiological examination of bone, which is not possible or necessary in all patients. There is no consensus as to whether management should be primarily medical or surgical; the pros and cons of each approach must be taken into account on an individual basis and after discussion with patients.

Cardiovascular Complications

There is a looming global epidemic of obesity and diabetes. Of all the end-organ effects caused by diabetes, the cardiovascular system is particularly susceptible to the biologic perturbations caused by this disease, and many patients may die from diabetes-related cardiovascular complications. Substantial progress has been made in understanding the pathobiology of the diabetic vasculature and heart. Clinical studies have illuminated the optimal way to treat patients with cardiovascular manifestations of this disease. This article reviews these aspects of diabetes and the cardiovascular system, broadly classified into diabetic vascular disease, diabetic cardiomyopathy, and the clinical management of the diabetic cardiovascular disease patient.

Cardiovascular disease is a serious complication of diabetes mellitus. In the last 2 decades, great strides have been made in reducing microvascular complications in patients with diabetes through improving glycemic control. Decreasing rates of cardiovascular events have proved to be more difficult than simply intensifying the management of hyperglycemia. A tremendous effort has been made to deepen understanding of cardiovascular disease in diabetes and to formulate the best treatment approach. This review summarizes the current state of knowledge and discusses areas of uncertainty in the care of patients with diabetes who are at risk for cardiovascular disease.

Patients with hypertension and type 2 diabetes are at increased risk of cardiovascular and chronic renal disease. Factors involved in the pathogenesis of both hypertension and type 2 diabetes include inappropriate activation of the renin-angiotensin-aldosterone system, oxidative stress, inflammation, impaired insulin-mediated vasodilatation, augmented sympathetic nervous system activation, altered innate and adaptive immunity, and abnormal sodium processing by the kidney. The renin-angiotensin-aldosterone system blockade is a key therapeutic strategy in the treatment of hypertension in type 2 diabetes. Emerging therapies for resistant hypertension as often exists in patients with diabetes, include renal denervation and carotid body denervation.

Renal Complications

Diabetic kidney disease (DKD) is a common disorder, and few patients achieve current therapeutic targets. Careful collaboration between all health care providers and the creation of disorder-specific health care systems seem to offer the best opportunity for improving the management and clinical outcomes of these patients. This article explores the barriers to effective collaboration between physicians in the management of patients with DKD, attitudes and perceptions of physicians toward collaborative management, and the physiologic challenges in patients with DKD that would warrant specialist involvement in their care. A model for collaborative DKD care delivery is also proposed.

> In this article, the literature is reviewed regarding the role of blood pressure variability and nocturnal nondipping of blood pressure as well as the presence of diabetic kidney disease (DKD), in the absence of albuminuria, as risk predictors for progressive DKD. The importance of glycemic and blood pressure control in patients with diabetes and chronic kidney disease, and the use of oral hypoglycemic agents and antihypertensive agents in this patient cohort, are also discussed.

> Obesity and diabetes are major health concerns worldwide. Along with other elements of the metabolic syndrome, including hypertension, they contribute to the development and progression of renal disease, which, if not treated, may lead to end-stage renal disease (ESRD). Although early intervention and management of body weight, hyperglycemia, and hypertension are imperative, novel therapeutic approaches are also necessary to reduce the high morbidity and mortality associated with renal disease. This review provides perspectives regarding the mechanisms by which obesity may lead to ESRD and discusses prevention strategies and treatment of obesity-related renal disease.

Gastrointestinal Complications

> This review provides an overview of the vast gastrointestinal tract complications of diabetes that can occur from the mouth to the anus. The presentation, diagnosis, and management of gastrointestinal disorders, ranging from gastroparesis, celiac disease, and bacterial overgrowth to nonalcoholic fatty liver disease, are reviewed to heighten awareness. When managing care of patients with diabetes, one should keep in mind the potential gastrointestinal complications, as well as the frequent disorders that are not related to diabetes.

Ophthalmologic Complications

> More Americans become blind each year from microvascular complications of diabetes than from any other cause. Several studies have indicated that tight glucose control and lifestyle modification can dramatically reduce the incidence and prevalence of diabetic retinopathy. Research over the past several years has yielded a tremendous increase in our knowledge of the pathogenesis of the damage to the retina that occurs in diabetes and has facilitated our ability to intervene and control the damage. New intravitreal medical therapies supported by government- and

industry-supported research are gradually replacing standard laser photo-coagulation for the treatment of all forms of retinopathy.

Dermatologic Complications

Diabetes mellitus affects every organ of the body including the skin. Certain skin manifestations of diabetes are considered cutaneous markers of the disease, whereas others are nonspecific conditions that occur more frequently among individuals with diabetes compared with the general population. Diabetic patients have an increased susceptibility to some bacterial and fungal skin infections, which account, in part, for poor healing. Skin complications of diabetes provide clues to current and past metabolic status. Recognition of cutaneous markers may slow disease progression and ultimately improve the overall prognosis by enabling earlier diagnosis and treatment.

Neurological and Psychological Complications

Diabetic neuropathy (DN) is the most common and troublesome complication of diabetes mellitus, leading to the greatest morbidity and mortality and resulting in a huge economic burden for diabetes care. The clinical assessment of diabetic peripheral neuropathy and its treatment options are multifactorial. Patients with DN should be screened for autonomic neuropathy, as there is a high degree of coexistence of the two complications. A review of the clinical assessment and treatment algorithms for diabetic neuropathy, painful neuropathy, and autonomic dysfunction is provided.

Epidemics of obesity, diabetes, nonalcoholic fatty liver disease, and cognitive impairment/Alzheimer disease have emerged over the past 3 to 4 decades. These diseases share in common target-organ insulin resistance with a constellation of molecular and biochemical abnormalities that lead to organ/tissue degeneration over time. This article discusses the fundamental links among these diseases and how peripheral organ insulin resistance diseases contribute to cognitive impairment and neurodegeneration. A future role of endocrinologists and diabetologists could be to provide integrative diagnostic and treatment approaches for this collection of diseases that seem to share pathophysiological and pathogenetic bases.

Although clozapine, olanzapine, and other atypical antipsychotic drugs (APDs) have fewer extrapyramidal side effects, they have serious metabolic side effects such as substantial weight gain, intra-abdominal obesity, and type 2 diabetes mellitus. Given that most patients with mental disorders face chronic, even life-long, treatment with APDs, the risks of weight gain/obesity and other metabolic symptoms are major considerations for APD maintenance treatment. This review focuses on the effects of APDs on weight gain, appetite, insulin resistance, and glucose dysregulation, and the relevant underlying mechanisms that may be help to prevent and treat metabolic side effects caused by APD therapy.

Special Considerations

antibiotic use, and lengthened hospitalization. Identification and proper treatment of hyperglycemia and diabetes are therefore essential for prevention of significant morbidity and mortality to the patient and to conserve ever-shrinking health care resources. The author discusses standards for the identification of diabetes and hyperglycemia, provides recommendations for target blood glucose values, and discusses current consensus guidelines on inpatient glycemic management in non–critically ill hospitalized patients.

Preface

Each year, Elsevier's prestigious *Clinics Review Articles* series publishes more than 250 issues (3000 plus articles) encompassing nearly 60 medical and surgical disciplines. This curated collection of articles, devoted to Type II Diabetes Mellitus, draws from the robust *Clinics'* database to provide multidisciplinary teams with practical clinical advice on comorbidities and complications of this highly prevalent disease.

Featured articles from the *Endocrinology and Metabolism Clinics of North America*, *Medical Clinics of North America*, *Primary Care: Clinics in Office Practice*, *Clinics in Podiatric Medicine and Surgery*, and *Critical Care Nursing Clinics of North America* reflect the wide range of clinicians who manage the diabetic patient. This multidisciplinary perspective is essential to successful team-based management.

I hope you share this volume with your colleagues and that it spurs more collaboration, deeper understanding, and safer, more effective care for your patients.

Joel J. Heidelbaugh, MD, FAAFP, FACG
Ypsilanti, MI
September 2014

Clinics Collections 1 (2014) xvii
http://dx.doi.org/10.1016/j.ccol.2014.08.001
2352-7986/14/$ – see front matter © 2014 Published by Elsevier Inc.

Diabetic Ketoacidosis and Hyperglycemic Hyperosmolar State

Jelena Maletkovic, MD*, Andrew Drexler, MD

KEYWORDS

- Diabetes mellitus • Ketoacidosis • Hyperosmolar state • Hyperglycemic crisis

KEY POINTS

- Diabetic ketoacidosis and the hyperglycemic hyperosmolar state are potentially fatal hyperglycemic crises that occur as acute complications of uncontrolled diabetes mellitus.
- The discovery of insulin in 1921 changed the life expectancy of patients with diabetes.

BACKGROUND AND EPIDEMIOLOGY

Diabetic ketoacidosis (DKA) and the hyperglycemic hyperosmolar state (HHS) are potentially fatal hyperglycemic crises that occur as acute complications of uncontrolled diabetes mellitus.

Because of the improved awareness, prevention, and treatment guidelines, the age-adjusted death rate for hyperglycemic crises in 2009 was less than half the rate in 1980 (7.5 vs 15.3 per 1,000,000 population); however, hyperglycemic crises still caused 2417 deaths in 2009 in the United States.[1] The mortality rate from HHS is much higher than that of DKA and approaches 20%.[2] On the other hand, the incidence of HHS is less than 1 case per 1000 person-years. The annual incidence of DKA varies in different reports and is related to the geographic location.[3-7] It has been reported to be as low as 12.9 per 100,000 in the general population in Denmark[3]; in Malaysia the rate of DKA is high, with 26.3 per 100 patient-years.[4]

The incidence of DKA is increasing in the United States (**Fig. 1**). The National Diabetes Surveillance Program of the Centers for Disease Control and Prevention estimated that from 1988 to 2009, the age-adjusted hospital discharge rate for DKA per 10,000 population consistently increased by 43.8%, so the number of hospital discharges with DKA as the first-listed diagnosis increased from about 80,000 in 1988 to about 140,000 in 2009.[1]

This article originally appeared in Endocrinology and Metabolism Clinics of North America, Volume 42, Issue 4, December 2013.

Disclosures: The authors have no conflict of interest regarding this article.

Department of Endocrinology, UCLA School of Medicine, Gonda Diabetes Center, 200 UCLA Medical Plaza, Suite 530, Los Angeles, CA 90095, USA

* Corresponding author.

E-mail address: jmaletkovic@mednet.ucla.edu

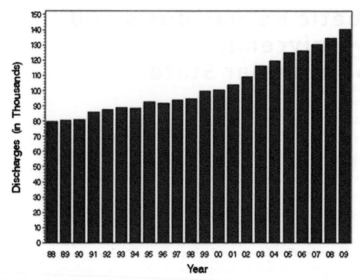

Fig. 1. Number (in thousands) of hospital discharges with DKA as first-listed diagnosis, United States, 1988 to 2009. The number of hospital discharges with DKA as the first-listed diagnosis increased from about 80,000 discharges in 1988 to about 140,000 in 2009. (*From* Centers for Disease Control and Prevention. National hospital discharge survey. Available at: http://www.cdc.gov/nchs/nhds.htm. Accessed April 25, 2013.)

DEFINITION AND DIAGNOSIS

Both DKA and HHS are severe complications of diabetes mellitus and are found to occur simultaneously in about one-third of cases.[8] Although both represent acute hyperglycemic states, DKA is more characterized by ketonemia and anion-gap acidosis and HHS by hyperosmolarity and dehydration.

HHS used to be named *hyperglycemic hyperosmolar nonketotic coma*, but it was found that it frequently presents without coma. It was also named *hyperglycemic hyperosmolar nonketotic state*, but findings of moderate ketonemia in several patients lead to the acceptance of its current term *HHS*. Laboratory findings differ, but some features overlap and are given in **Table 1**:

1. Anion-gap acidosis: Although this is the most important feature of DKA, with serum pH less than 7.3, serum bicarbonate less than 15 mEq/L, and anion gap greater than 10, it is not the finding typical for HHS.

Table 1 Laboratory findings in DKA and HHS		
	DKA	**HHS**
Anion-gap acidosis	pH <7.3 Bicarbonate <18 Anion gap >10	pH >7.3 Bicarbonate >18 Anion-gap variable
Osmolality	<320	>320
Hyperglycemia	>250	>600
Ketonemia/ketonuria	Present	Rare

2. Ketonemia and ketonuria are more pronounced in DKA but can be present in HHS.
3. Hyperglycemia is elevated in both conditions but more pronounced in HHS, with glucose concentrations frequently greater than 600 mg/dL. Cases of euglycemic DKA have been reported and occur more frequently in pregnancy.[9,10]
4. Osmolality is usually normal in DKA, but may be elevated, and is invariably elevated in hyperosmolar state to above 320 mOsm/kg.

DKA most commonly occurs in patients with type 1 diabetes mellitus although it can occur with type 2 diabetes after serious medical or surgical illness.[11] On the other hand, HHS is more frequently associated with type 2 diabetes, however it has also been reported in type 1 diabetes as a simultaneous occurrence with DKA.[12–14] Many investigators report ketosis-prone type 2 diabetes,[15–17] which is also called Flatbush diabetes after the area in the city of Brooklyn, New York where this type of diabetes was first described and is most frequently diagnosed. These patients are commonly African American and obese with acute defects in insulin secretion and no islet cell autoantibodies.[18–20] Following treatment, some insulin secretory capacity is recovered, and many of them do not require insulin therapy in the future.[21,22]

PRECIPITATING FACTORS

Newly diagnosed individuals with type 1 diabetes mellitus account for 15% of cases of DKA. The frequency of DKA at the diagnosis of type 1 diabetes also varies across different countries,[23] with some extremes, such as United Arab Emirates where it has been reported to be 80%[4] or Sweden where it is 12.8%.[7] Data from Europe reported an inverse correlation between the background incidence of type1 diabetes and the frequency of DKA.[24,25] Most DKA events occur in patients with known diabetes at times of extreme stress, especially infection, such as pneumonia or urinary tract infection, but also myocardial ischemia or any other medical or surgical illness. These cases account for about 40% of all DKA events. The second most important contributor to development of DKA is inadequate insulin treatment, commonly seen as a result of noncompliance, especially in the young population.[26,27] DKA has also been reported with the mismanagement of insulin pumps and undetected leakage of the infusion system or[28] at the time of religious fasting.[29,30] In some cases, medications, such as corticosteroids, pentamidine, and terbutaline, have been identified as triggers for DKA.[31–33] Recent reports from the United States and Canada point to a significant role of atypical antipsychotic medications in the development of fatal cases of DKA.[34–37] Cocaine use is associated with frequent omissions of insulin administration, but it also has significant effects on counter-regulatory hormones. It was found to be an important contributor in the development of DKA and HHS together with alcohol and other abused substances.[27,38–41] In a small number of cases, the workup does not identify any precipitating factor. A rough estimate of most common precipitating factors in development of DKA is given in **Fig. 2**.

In HHS, the most common precipitating events are also inadequate insulin therapy and underlying illness, such as infection, ischemia, or surgery. Because HHS develops more slowly and in a more subtle way, the important contributor to this complication is decreased water intake, especially in elderly patients, that leads to gradual but severe dehydration.[8,42] These patients have either a reduced thirst mechanism or they are unable to access water because of physical or neurologic limitations.

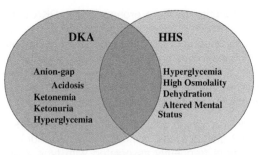

Fig. 2. Major characteristics of DKA and HHS and their estimated overlap.

PATHOGENESIS

The pathogenesis of HHS results from disturbances in glucose metabolism and fluid balance. In DKA, a third component, ketogenesis also contributes to the condition. Both conditions present with hyperglycemia and dehydration.

HORMONES

Both DKA and HHS result from diminished or absent insulin levels and elevated counter-regulatory hormone levels. Insulin deficiency causes glycogenolysis, gluconeogenesis, lipolysis, and protein catabolism. The counter-regulatory hormones present in both of these conditions are glucagon, norepinephrine, epinephrine, cortisol, and growth hormone. Glucagon is the most important of these, whereas growth hormone is probably the least important. DKA is much less likely to occur in the absence of glucagon, but cases of DKA have been reported in patients with complete pancreatectomy. Norepinephrine increases ketogenesis not only by stimulating lipolysis but also by increasing intrahepatic ketogenesis. Catecholamines stimulate lipolysis and fatty acid release even in the presence of insulin. Growth hormone has little effect in the presence of insulin but can enhance ketogenesis in insulin deficiency. The difference between DKA and HHS is that in the latter, the insulin levels do not decrease to a level whereby unrestrained ketogenesis occurs.

Hyperglycemia results from increases in glucose levels obtained from 4 sources:

- Intestinal absorption
- Gluconeogenesis (from carbohydrate, protein, fat)
- Glycogenolysis
- Decreased utilization of glucose by cells, primarily muscle and fat cells

The fate of glucose in the cell can be different depending of the current metabolic needs of the body. It can be stored or it can enter glycolysis and form pyruvate. Pyruvate can be reduced to lactate, transaminated to alanine, or converted to acetyl coenzyme A (CoA). Acetyl CoA can be oxidized to carbon dioxide and water, converted to fatty acids, or used for ketone body or cholesterol synthesis.

Insulin deficiency, absolute or relative, is present in both conditions and results in increased gluconeogenesis and glycogenolysis. Insulin deficiency prevents glucose from entering cells and being metabolized. One of the consequences of insulin deficiency is protein, primarily muscle, breakdown with the provision of precursors for gluconeogenesis. Gluconeogenesis is the crucial action in the development of severe hyperglycemia that is found in DKA and HHS.

Gluconeogenic enzymes are stimulated by the actions of glucagon, catecholamines, and cortisol.[43] The lack of inhibitory action of insulin further drives gluconeogenesis and glycogenolysis and causes increased glucagon activity.[43–45] The end result of insulin deficiency is impairment in carbohydrate utilization, and energy must be obtained from an alternative source, namely, fatty acid metabolism.

Lipid

Lipid mobilization and metabolism are affected by insulin deficiency. In normal subjects, insulin affects fat metabolism by different mechanisms.[46–48] Insulin increases the clearance of triglyceride-rich chylomicrons from the circulation, stimulates creation of triglycerides from free fatty acids (FFA), and inhibits lipolysis of triglycerides.[49–51] In insulin deficiency, fat mobilization is accelerated, resulting in an abundant supply of FFA to the liver. An increase in FFA availability increases ketone production not only by a mass effect but also by a diversion of hepatic fatty acid metabolism toward ketogenesis.[52] FFA levels may be as high in HHS as in DKA.

Ketogenesis

Ketogenesis depends on the amount of FFA supplied to the liver and on the hepatic metabolic fate of fatty acids in the direction of either oxidation and ketogenesis or reesterification.[52] Ketogenesis occurs inside hepatic mitochondria. The glucagon/insulin ratio activates carnitine palmitoyltransferase I, the enzyme that allows FFA in the form of CoA to cross mitochondrial membranes after their esterification with carnitine. In HHS, this ratio does not reach a level whereby unrestrained ketoacidosis occurs. This increase in carnitine palmitoyltransferase I occurs associated with a decrease in malonyl CoA. Fatty acids that are in the mitochondria are converted to acetyl CoA. Most of the acetyl CoA is used in the synthesis of beta-hydroxybutyric acid and acetoacetic acid.[53] Acetoacetate is converted to acetone through nonenzymatic decarboxylation in linear relation to its concentration. Ketones are filtered by the kidney and partially excreted in urine. Progressive volume depletion leads to a reduced glomerular filtration and the shift of acetoacetate to beta-hydroxybutyrate.[54]

Hyperosmolar

Hyperosmolar state develops as a result of osmotic diuresis caused by hyperglycemia, which then creates severe fluid loss. The total body deficit of water is usually about 7 to 12 L in HHS, which represents a loss of about 10% to 15% of body weight. Although mild ketosis can be seen with HHS, it is generally absent in this state. It is considered that patients with HHS who are usually older patients with type 2 diabetes still do have enough insulin to be protected from exaggerated lipolysis and the consequent abundance of FFA.[55] They do not, however, have enough insulin to prevent hyperglycemia.[56]

CLINICAL PRESENTATION

DKA and HHS can have similar clinical presentations. There are usually signs and symptoms of hyperglycemia and a general unwell feeling with malaise, fatigue, and anorexia. Patients can present with symptoms of the preceding illness, such as infection (pneumonia, urinary tract infection, and so forth) or myocardial ischemia. DKA will usually develop faster than HHS, sometimes in less than 24 hours. HHS takes days to weeks to develop in most patients.

Some of the differences in the clinical presentations result from the state of metabolic acidosis in DKA. Patients with DKA will frequently have hyperventilation (Kussmaul ventilation) as a compensatory mechanism for acidosis that is rarely seen with HHS. DKA will also present with abdominal pain that is associated with the level of acidosis.[57] Sometimes the presentation with significant abdominal pain is associated with an underlying abdominal process, such as acute pancreatitis.[58] Abdominal pain is frequently associated with acidosis only and no underlying pathological condition can be identified; however, it always requires a workup for acute abdominal process.

Most patients with HHS will have some degree of neurologic disturbance, whereas only patients with more advanced DKA will be comatose. If they present early in the course of the disease, patients with DKA will frequently have a normal neurologic examination. This difference is caused by greater hyperosmolality in HHS caused by osmotic diuresis and free water loss.[59–62] Hyperosmolar state causes cellular dehydration produced by osmotic shifts of water from the intracellular fluid space to the extracellular space.[63,64] If osmolality is normal and patients show severe neurologic deficit, further workup is indicated to rule out underlying neurologic pathologic condition. Elderly patients are particularly susceptible to these disturbances. Some possible neurologic presentations include irritability, restlessness, stupor, muscular twitching, hyperreflexia, spasticity, seizures, and coma.[65–68] The clinical signs and symptoms reflect both the severity of the hyperosmolality and the rate at which it develops.[69]

Free water deficit is more pronounced in HHS, as compared with DKA; patients with HHS will have more evidence of severe dehydration. An additional source of dehydration is impaired water intake, particularly in elderly patients with ongoing lethargy and confusion.[70] Evaluation of volume status is one of the initial assessments of patients with DKA or HHS. **Table 2** shows some of the important clinical features of DKA and HHS.

INITIAL EVALUATION

Both DKA and HHS are medical emergencies with improved, but high, mortality rates that require careful evaluation. As a first step in evaluating patients who present with a hyperglycemic emergency, the physician should secure the airway and ensure adequate ventilation and oxygenation. Patients should also have secure intravenous (IV) access, with at least 2 ports, and continuous cardiac monitoring. A Foley catheter should be placed for strict monitoring of intake and output.

The initial laboratory investigation should include the following: serum glucose, metabolic panel, serum phosphate and magnesium, arterial blood gas analysis, complete blood count (CBC) with differential, hepatic enzymes, serum ketones, urinalysis, cardiac enzymes, hemoglobin A1C, and coagulation profile. Additional laboratory values that should be considered are infectious workup with urine and blood cultures,

Table 2		
Clinical features of DKA and HHS		
Clinical Presentation	**DKA**	**HHS**
Development of Symptoms	**Hours to Days**	**Days to Weeks**
Polydipsia/polyuria	+	+
Nausea/vomiting	+	+
Abdominal pain	+	−
Anorexia	+	+
Fatigue/malaise	+	+
Neurologic abnormalities	±	+ +
Hyperventilation	+	−
Dehydration	+	+ +

lumbar puncture in selected cases, serum lipase, and amylase. Other investigations should include electrocardiogram and chest radiograph, and selected cases will require additional chest/abdomen/brain or other imaging depending on the clinical presentation. Serum glucose and electrolytes should be repeated every 1 to 2 hours until patients are stable and then every 4 to 6 hours. The most important points in the initial evaluation of DKA and HHS are given in **Table 3**. The initial calculations include serum sodium correction, serum osmolality, anion gap, and free water deficit.

Basic considerations in the evaluation of DKA and HHS laboratory values are given in the following text.

Serum Glucose

Serum glucose is usually more elevated in HHS than in DKA. This elevation is partly caused by the acidosis of DKA leading to an earlier diagnosis of the condition before glucoses levels have increased as high. Also contributing is the fact that about a half of the patients with type 1 diabetes mellitus have glomerular hyperfiltration in the first years in the course of their disease. Patients with type 2 diabetes mellitus also initially have an increased glomerular filtration rate of about 2 standard deviations more than their age-matched nondiabetic and obese controls, but the degree of hyperfiltration is less than that of patients with type 1 diabetes. These differences allow for an increased glucose excretion degree in DKA and less hyperglycemia as compared with HHS.[71] In

Table 3 Initial evaluation of patients with hyperglycemic emergency (DKA/HHS)	
First steps	IV line (at least 2 ports, consider central access) Airway and adequate ventilation/oxygenation Cardiac monitor In and out monitoring (Foley catheter)
Initial laboratory test results	Serum glucose Basic metabolic panel with electrolytes Arterial blood gas analysis BUN/creatinine CBC with differential Serum phosphate Liver enzymes Urinalysis Cardiac enzymes Coagulation profile Serum ketones Hemoglobin A1C
Additional laboratory test results (case-by-case basis)	Blood and urine culture Lumbar puncture Amylase and lipase Other laboratory tests based on clinical presentation
Initial imaging	CXR Optional imaging based on clinical presentation (CT head/chest/abdomen)
Initial calculations	Anion gap Corrected serum sodium Free water deficit Serum osmolality

Abbreviations: BUN, serum urea nitrogen; CT, computed tomography; CXR, chest X-ray.

HHS, the glucose level is more than 600 mg/dL and can frequently be more than 1000 mg/dL.[72] The degree of hyperglycemia reflects the degree of dehydration and hyperosmolality.[73] Cases of normoglycemic DKA have been described in pregnant patients.[74,75] Patients with renal failure usually have severe hyperglycemia because of poor renal clearance of glucose. These patients, however, usually do not develop hyperosmolality because of the lack of osmotic diuresis, and their mental status with HHS tends to be less affected than with patients who have preserved renal function.[76–79]

Serum Sodium

Serum sodium levels are affected in both DKA and HHS. In the setting of hyperglycemia, osmotic forces drive water into the vascular space and cause dilution with resulting hyponatremia. Each 100 mg/dL of the glucose level more than normal lowers the serum sodium level by about 1.6 mEq/L. The treatment of DKA and HHS with insulin causes reversal of this process and drives water back into the extravascular space with a subsequent increase in serum sodium level. Corrected serum sodium is calculated with the following formula:

Corrected sodium = serum sodium (mEq/L) + (1.6 mEq/L for each 100 mg/dL of glucose more than 100 mg/dL)

One study suggested that a more accurate correction factor in extreme hyperglycemic states is 2.4 mEq/L for each 100 mg/dL because of the nonlinear relationship between the glucose and sodium concentration.[80] An additional decrease in serum sodium is present with confounding pseudohyponatremia that occurs with hyperlipidemia or hyperproteinemia with some laboratory assays.[81,82] Thus, most patients will present with hyponatremia. In some cases of HHS, patients may present with hypernatremia secondary to osmotic diuresis and more severe dehydration.[83,84] Hypernatremia indicates a profound degree of water loss. The measured, and not the calculated, serum sodium level should be used to calculate the anion gap.[85]

Serum Potassium

Serum potassium is frequently paradoxically elevated despite the total body deficit in DKA and HHS. This elevation is caused by the extracellular shift of potassium in exchange for the hydrogen ions accumulated in acidosis, reduced renal function, release of potassium from cells caused by glycogenolysis, insulin deficiency, and hyperosmolality.[86,87] It is thought that the water deficit from the cells creates passive potassium flux to the extracellular space leading to relative hyperkalemia without having significant acidosis in HHS.[88] The body deficit of potassium occurs with diuresis but also with gastrointestinal losses.[89] Treatment with insulin shifts potassium into the cell and causes a rapid decrease of the serum potassium levels. Hypokalemia is frequently encountered after starting insulin treatment. Careful monitoring and potassium supplementing are required in patients with DKA and HHS, especially if they initially present with a normal or low potassium level.[90–93]

Serum Phosphate

Serum phosphate is lost by diuresis in DKA and HHS, and its typical deficit is usually up to 7 mmol/kg.[94,95] Similarly, as in the case of potassium deficit, patients may present with normal or even high levels of phosphate because insulin deficiency drives phosphate out of the cells. The level of serum phosphate will start decreasing as soon as insulin treatment is established. Hyperphosphatemia, on the first presentation, also reflects volume depletion. Acidosis is another mechanism that causes falsely normal or high phosphate levels. Patients who present with profound acidosis are at higher risk of developing hypophosphatemia when insulin administration is started. The severity of subsequent hypophosphatemia can be predicted by the degree of metabolic acidosis on presentation.[38] Untreated hypophosphatemia can lead to serious complications, including cardiac arrest.[39–41]

Serum Bicarbonate

Serum bicarbonate is typically more than 18 mEq/L in HHS. Because DKA is characterized by acidosis, the serum bicarbonate is lower than 18 mEq/L and frequently lower than 15 mEq/L. A decrease of bicarbonate to less than 10 mEq/L indicates severe DKA.[96,97]

Serum Ketones

Serum ketones are used as an energy source when glucose is not readily available and are increased in DKA, as a response to low insulin levels and high levels of counter-regulatory hormones.[98] Acetoacetate is a ketoacid, whereas beta-hydroxybutyrate represents a hydroxy acid that is formed by the reduction of acetoacetate. The third ketone body, acetone, is the least abundant of all and is formed by decarboxylation of acetic acid. Although ketones are always present, their levels increase in certain conditions, such as starvation, pregnancy, and exercise. DKA causes the most prominent increase in ketone body levels compared with the other common conditions. Serum ketone testing is performed when a urinary dipstick tests positive for urine ketones. The most commonly used test for serum ketones is nitroprusside. However, it detects only acetoacetate and acetone and not hydroxybutyrate. Because beta-hydroxybutyrate is the most prominent ketone body and is disproportionally so in DKA, it is possible to have a negative testing for serum ketones in the presence of severe ketoacidosis.[99] Cases of children who developed DKA, that could have potentially been prevented, as a consequence of false-negative home ketone test-strip readings with nitroprusside have been described.[100]

The initiation of treatment with insulin causes a conversion of beta-hydroxybutyrate to acetoacetate while the overall levels of ketone bodies are decreasing.[101] This effect can potentially create a false observation that DKA is worsening, although, in fact, it is improving; subsequent unnecessary increases in insulin treatment could lead to other complications.[102] Quantitative enzymatic tests have been developed and can be used as point-of-care tests that identify beta-hydroxybutyrate.[99,103,104] On the other hand, false-positive results for serum ketone bodies have been identified in patients using drugs with sulfhydryl groups.[105–109] The risk of inappropriate therapy with insulin caused by false-positive ketones in serum is low but existing.

Anion Gap

Anion gap represents unmeasured anions in serum (ketones) after subtracting the major measured anions from the major measured cation.

AG = (serum sodium) − (chloride + bicarbonate)

where *AG* is anion gap

Measured, not corrected, serum sodium levels should be used to estimate the anion gap.[110] The anion gap is usually more than 20 mEq/L in DKA, and it reflects the production and accumulation of acetoacetate and beta-hydroxybutyrate in the serum. It inversely reflects the rate of excretion of acids that will be impaired with renal failure.[112] Patients admitted with diabetic ketoacidosis have a mean bicarbonate deficit that is approximately equal to the excess anion gap.

Arterial Blood

Arterial blood gas measurement is recommended in all cases of hyperglycemic complications of diabetes mellitus. Acidosis is one of the main features of DKA and is included in the diagnostic criteria, with arterial pH of less than 7.3. Arterial pH in HHS is usually more than 7.3. In order to avoid the painful and more difficult procedure of arterial blood drawing, in patients with normal oxygen saturation on room air, venous blood gas is sometimes used to estimate acidosis. It has been found that there is a high degree of correlation and agreement with the arterial value, with acceptably narrow 95% limits of agreement.[111] Arterial blood gas analysis can, on the other hand, indicate an underlying disease associated with DKA or HHS. Hypoxemia may be found with cardiac or pulmonary trigger diseases, and low carbon dioxide may represent hyperventilation as a compensatory mechanism for metabolic acidosis.

Serum Osmolality

The serum osmolality elevation correlates with the degree of neurologic disturbance.[112] The serum osmolality is determined by the concentrations of the different solutes in the plasma. In normal subjects, sodium salts, glucose, and urea are the primary circulating solutes. Increased serum osmolality to more than 320 mosmol/kg is seen in patients with neurologic abnormalities and is typical for HHS. Rarely, serum osmolality can be more than 400 mOsm/kg. Neurologic deficits ranging from confusion to coma can be seen with DKA, with a less significant increase in serum osmolality, which then reflect the degree of acidosis.[113] The formula for the calculation of serum osmolality is given next[114–116]:

$$\text{Serum osmolality} = (2 \times \text{serum [Na]}) + (\text{glucose, in mg/dL})/18 + (\text{BUN in mg/dL})/2.8$$

where *BUN* is serum urea nitrogen

The formula with all units in millimoles per liter is the following:

$$\text{Serum osmolality} = (2 \times \text{serum [Na]}) + (\text{glucose}) + (\text{urea})$$

The serum osmolal gap represents the difference between the measured and calculated serum osmolality. In normal individuals, the osmolal gap was not significant and was found to be 1.9 ± 3.7 mosmol/kg and -1.7 ± 1.7 mosmol/kg in 2 studies.[117] The measured serum osmolality can be significantly higher than the calculated value in the presence of an additional solute, such as ethylene glycol, methanol, ethanol, formaldehyde, isopropyl alcohol, diethyl ether, glycine, sorbitol, or mannitol, or in presence of significant pseudohyponatremia caused by severe hyperproteinemia or hyperlipidemia.[118–120]

Leukocytosis

Leukocytosis is present in hyperglycemic emergencies even in the absence of infection. This presence is explained by elevated stress hormones, such as cortisol and catecholamines, and cytokines and is proportional to the degree of ketonemia.[121–123] True leukocytosis is also frequent, and a source of infection should be investigated in all cases. White blood cell counts of greater than 25,000/μL were independently associated with altered sensorium in one study.[124]

Amylase and Lipase

Amylase and lipase can be elevated with DKA in the absence of pancreatitis. An increase in lipase correlates with plasma osmolality, and an increase in amylase correlates with plasma osmolality and pH.[125] True pancreatitis is also a frequent precipitating factor for hyperglycemic emergencies and can be confirmed with other clinical characteristics and imaging **Fig. 3**.[59]

TREATMENT

The management of DKA and HHS consists of fluid and electrolyte repletion, insulin administration, and the treatment of the precipitating cause if one can be identified. Patients should be admitted to a monitored unit where close observation of mental status, blood pressure, heart rate and rhythm, and urine output can be done.

Fluid Replacement

Fluid replacement should be the initial therapy in DKA and HHS, with the goal of correcting a fluid deficit in the first 24 hours. The initial fluid should be normal saline. The rate in the first hours should be 10 to 15 mL/kg. Once patients are euvolemic, switching to half-normal saline is appropriate for those with normal sodium or hypernatremia. This change allows for more efficient replacement of the free water deficit induced by the glucose osmotic diuresis. Half-normal saline should be administered at a rate of 4 to 14 mL/kg. Five percent dextrose with half-normal saline should be started when the blood glucose level decreases less than 250 mg/dL in DKA and 300 mg/dL in HHS.[56]

Cerebral edema is a serious complication of DKA treatment with a high mortality of 21% to 24% that is primarily seen in children when hyperosmolality was corrected too rapidly.[126] Symptomatic cerebral edema occurs in 0.5% to 1.0% of pediatric DKA episodes, and 15% to 26% of children remain with permanent neurologic sequelae.[127] Children who presented with higher osmolality and higher serum urea nitrogen (BUN) demonstrated a more severe clinical picture, with the most profound acidosis and hypocapnia.[128]

Treating patients with renal or cardiac compromise is challenging because a fine balance needs to be established between the volume deficit and the volume overload. These patients require frequent monitoring of volume status and parameters of fluid

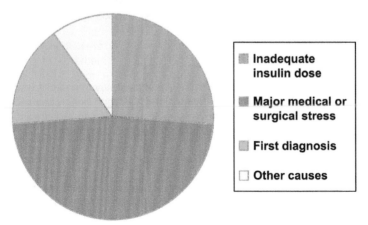

Fig. 3. Estimated prevalence of precipitating factors in development of DKA.

Legend:
- Inadequate insulin dose
- Major medical or surgical stress
- First diagnosis
- Other causes

homeostasis, such as osmolality, serum sodium, BUN and creatinine, blood glucose, and urine output, as well as frequent clinical monitoring for signs of respiratory compromise caused by volume overload.

Potassium

Potassium may initially be elevated because of the extracellular shift caused by insulin deficiency, acidosis, and proteolysis.[129] This elevation will rapidly correct with the administration of fluids that create dilution and insulin treatment that will allow for potassium to be shifted back to the cell. Urinary and gastrointestinal loss of potassium also causes an overall deficit in potassium concentration. Glucosuria results in the loss of 70 mEq of sodium and potassium for each liter of fluid lost. The correction of actual deficit of potassium should be started when the potassium level is less than 5.3 mEq/L. The potassium level should be maintained between 4 and 5 mEq/L.

Insulin

Insulin at a low dose should be started approximately 1 hour after the initiation of fluid replacement therapy, with regular insulin as a treatment of choice. This treatment should be further delayed if serum potassium is less than 3.3 mEq/L because of the risk of hypokalemia. The administration of an initial bolus dose of insulin is not associated with a significant benefit to patients with DKA.[130] As an alternative to IV regular insulin, an intramuscular regimen with rapid-acting analogues has been reported to decrease the cost of DKA treatment.[131] When the plasma glucose level is less than 250 mg/dL in DKA or 300 mg/dL in HHS, the insulin rate should be decreased and maintained to keep blood glucose between 150 to 200 mg/dL in DKA and 250 to 300 mg/dL in HHS, until the ketoacidosis and/or hyperosmolar states are resolved.[129,132] It is critical that insulin therapy be based on the correction of the anion gap and not the serum glucose level. In some cases, it may be necessary to give IV 50% dextrose solution to allow adequate insulin therapy.

Bicarbonate therapy is controversial given the potential problems, such as hypokalemia, acidosis, hypoxia, hypernatremia, and the lack of a therapeutic effect.[133,134] There is insufficient data to confirm a benefit of treatment. It should be reserved only for severe cases of ketoacidosis with a very low bicarbonate of less than 10 and severe acidosis. In similar fashion, phosphate repletion is not recommended in all patients. Studies do not show a clear benefit of this treatment, and it may only be of some use in patients who are symptomatic for hypophosphatemia with heart or skeletal muscle involvement.[135–137] The main risk of phosphate therapy is hypocalcemia, especially as the pH normalizes.

SUMMARY

The discovery of insulin in 1921 changed the life expectancy of patients with diabetes mellitus dramatically. Today, almost a century later, DKA and HHS remain a significant economic burden and, most importantly, a significant cause of morbidity and mortality across different countries, ages, races, and socioeconomic groups.

REFERENCES

1. Centers for Disease Control and Prevention. National hospital discharge survey. Available at: www.cdc.gov/nchs/nhds.htm. Accessed April 25, 2013.
2. Wachtel TJ, Tctu-Mouradjian LM, Goldman DL, et al. Hyperosmolarity and acidosis in diabetes mobility. J Gen Intern Med 1991;6:495–502.

3. Henriksen OM, Roder ME, Prahl JB, et al. Diabetic ketoacidosis in Denmark incidence and mortality estimated from public health registries. Diabetes Res Clin
   Pract 2007;76(1):51–6.
4. Craig ME, Jones TW, Silink M, et al. Diabetes care, glycemic control, and complications in children with type 1 diabetes from Asia and the Western Pacific region. J Diabetes Complications 2007;21(5):280–7.
5. Campbell-Stokes PL, Taylor BJ. Prospective incidence study of diabetes mellitus in New Zealand children aged 0 to 14 years. Diabetologia 2005;48(4):
   643–8.
6. Pronina EA, Petraikina EE, Antsiferov MB, et al. A 10-year (1996–2005) prospective study of the incidence of type 1 diabetes. Diabet Med 2008;25(8):956–9.
7. Samuelsson U, Stenhammar L. Clinical characteristics at onset of type 1 diabetes in children diagnosed between 1977 and 2001 in the south-east region
   of Sweden. Diabetes Res Clin Pract 2005;68:49–55.
8. Wachtel TJ. The diabetic hyperosmolar state. Clin Geriatr Med 1990;6(4):797.
9. John R, Yadav H, John M. Euglycemic ketoacidosis as a cause of a metabolic
   acidosis in the intensive care unit. Acute Med 2012;11(4):219–21.
10. Guo RX, Yang LZ, Li LX, et al. Diabetic ketoacidosis in pregnancy tends to occur
    at lower blood glucose levels: case-control study and a case report of euglyce-
    mic diabetic ketoacidosis in pregnancy. J Obstet Gynaecol Res 2008;34(3):
    324–30.
11. Bowden SA, Duck MM, Hoffman RP. Young children (<5 yr) and adolescents
    (>12 yr) with type 1 diabetes mellitus have low rate of partial remission: diabetic
    ketoacidosis is an important risk factor. Pediatr Diabetes 2008;9(3 Pt 1):
    197–201.
12. DeFronzo R, Matsuda M, Barrett E. Diabetic ketoacidosis: a combined meta-
    bolic nephrologic approach to therapy. Diabetes Rev 1994;2:209–38.
13. Rosenbloom A. Hyperglycemic hyperosmolar state: an emerging pediatric
    problem. J Pediatr 2010;156:180–4.
14. Lotz M, Geraghty M. Hyperglycemic, hyperosmolar, nonketotic coma in a
    ketosis-prone juvenile diabetic. Ann Intern Med 1968;69(6):1245–6 No abstract
    available.
15. Umpierrez GE, Casals MM, Gebhart SP, et al. Diabetic ketoacidosis in obese Af-
    rican-Americans. Diabetes 1995;44:790–5.
16. Kitabchi AE. Ketosis-prone diabetes-A new subgroup of patients with atypical
    type 1 and type 2 diabetes? J Clin Endocrinol Metab 2003;88:5087–9.
17. Mauvais-Jarvis F, Sobngwi E, Porcher R, et al. Ketosis-prone type 2 diabetes in
    patients of sub-Saharan African origin: clinical pathophysiology and natural his-
    tory of beta-cell dysfunction and insulin resistance. Diabetes 2004;53:645–53.
18. Banerji MA. Diabetes in African Americans: unique pathophysiologic features.
    Curr Diab Rep 2004;4(3):219–23.
19. Banerji MA. Impaired beta-cell and alpha-cell function in African-American chil-
    dren with type 2 diabetes mellitus-"Flatbush diabetes". J Pediatr Endocrinol
    Metab 2002;15(Suppl 1):493–501.
20. Banerji MA, Chaiken RL, Huey H, et al. GAD antibody negative NIDDM in adult
    black subjects with diabetic ketoacidosis and increased frequency of human
    leukocyte antigen DR3 and DR4. Flatbush diabetes. Diabetes 1994;43(6):
    741–5.
21. Rodacki M, Zajdenverg L, Lima GA, et al. Case report: diabetes Flatbush - from
    ketoacidosis to non pharmacological treatment. Arq Bras Endocrinol Metabol
    2007;51(1):131–5 [in Portuguese].

22. Maldonado M, Hampe CS, Gaur LK, et al. Ketosis-prone diabetes: dissection of a heterogeneous syndrome using an immunogenetic and beta-cell functional classification, prospective analysis, and clinical outcomes. J Clin Endocrinol Metab 2003;88:5090–8.
23. Kitabchi AE, Umpierrez GE, Murphy MB, et al. Management of hyperglycemic crises in patients with diabetes. Diabetes Care 2001;24(1):131–53.
24. Lévy-Marchal C, Patterson CC, Green A. Geographical variation of presentation at diagnosis of type I diabetes in children: the EURODIAB study. European and Diabetes. Diabetologia 2001;44(Suppl 3):B75–80.
25. Ellis D, Naar-King S, Templin T, et al. Multisystemic therapy for adolescents with poorly controlled type 1 diabetes: reduced diabetic ketoacidosis admissions and related costs over 24 months. Diabetes Care 2008;31(9):1746–7.
26. Umpierrez GE, Kelly JP, Navarrete JE, et al. Hyperglycemic crises in urban blacks. Arch Intern Med 1997;157(6):669–75.
27. Walter H, Günther A, Timmler R, et al. Ketoacidosis in long-term therapy with insulin pumps. Incidence, causes, circumstances. Med Klin 1989;84(12):565–8.
28. Hanas R, Lindgren F, Lindblad B. A 2-yr national population study of pediatric ketoacidosis in Sweden: predisposing conditions and insulin pump use. Pediatr Diabetes 2009;10(1):33–7.
29. Friedrich I, Levy Y. Diabetic ketoacidosis during the Ramadan fast. Harefuah 2000;138(1):19–21, 86.
30. Ahmedani MY, Haque MS, Basit A, et al. Ramadan Prospective Diabetes Study: the role of drug dosage and timing alteration, active glucose monitoring and patient education. Diabet Med 2012;29(6):709–15.
31. Herchline TE, Plouffe JF, Para MF. Diabetes mellitus presenting with ketoacidosis following pentamidine therapy in patients with acquired immunodeficiency syndrome. J Infect 1991;22(1):41–4.
32. Ramaswamy K, Kozma CM, Nasrallah H. Risk of diabetic ketoacidosis after exposure to risperidone or olanzapine. Drug Saf 2007;30(7):589–99.
33. Tibaldi JM, Lorber DL, Nerenberg A. Diabetic ketoacidosis and insulin resistance with subcutaneous terbutaline infusion: a case report. Am J Obstet Gynecol 1990;163(2):509–10.
34. Ely SF, Neitzel AR, Gill JR. Fatal diabetic ketoacidosis and antipsychotic medication. J Forensic Sci 2012 [Epub ahead of print]. Available at: http://www.ncbi.nlm.nih.gov/pubmed/23278567.
35. Guenette MD, Giacca A, Hahn M, et al. Atypical antipsychotics and effects of adrenergic and serotonergic receptor binding on insulin secretion in-vivo: an animal model. Schizophr Res 2013;146(1–3):162–9.
36. Bobo WV, Cooper WO, Epstein RA Jr, et al. Positive predictive value of automated database records for diabetic ketoacidosis (DKA) in children and youth exposed to antipsychotic drugs or control medications: a Tennessee Medicaid study. BMC Med Res Methodol 2011;11:157.
37. Makhzoumi ZH, McLean LP, Lee JH, et al. Diabetic ketoacidosis associated with aripiprazole. Pharmacotherapy 2008;28(9):1198–202.
38. Warner EA, Greene GS, Buchsbaum MS, et al. Diabetic ketoacidosis associated with cocaine use. Arch Intern Med 1998;158(16):1799–802.
39. Ng RS, Darko DA, Hillson RM. Street drug use among young patients with type 1 diabetes in the UK. Diabet Med 2004;21(3):295–6.
40. Nyenwe EA, Loganathan RS, Blum S, et al. Active use of cocaine: an independent risk factor for recurrent diabetic ketoacidosis in a city hospital. Endocr Pract 2007;13(1):22–9.

41. Isidro ML, Jorge S. Recreational drug abuse in patients hospitalized for diabetic ketosis or diabetic ketoacidosis. Acta Diabetol 2013;50(2):183–7.
42. Wachtel TJ, Silliman RA, Lamberton P. Predisposing factors for the diabetic hyperosmolar state. Arch Intern Med 1987;147(3):499–501.
43. Taborsky GJ Jr. The physiology of glucagon. J Diabetes Sci Technol 2010;4(6): 1338–44.
44. Miles JM, Gerich JE. Glucose and ketone body kinetics in diabetic ketoacidosis. Clin Endocrinol Metab 1983;12(2):303–19.
45. Fanelli CG, Porcellati F, Rossetti P, et al. Glucagon: the effects of its excess and deficiency on insulin action. Nutr Metab Cardiovasc Dis 2006;16(Suppl 1): S28–34.
46. Farese RV Jr, Yost TJ, Eckel RH. Tissue-specific regulation of lipoprotein lipase activity by insulin/glucose in normal-weight humans. Metabolism 1991;40(2): 214.
47. Fielding BA, Frayn KN. Lipoprotein lipase and the disposition of dietary fatty acids. Br J Nutr 1998;80(6):495.
48. Zimmermann R, Lass A, Haemmerle G. Fate of fat: the role of adipose triglyceride lipase in lipolysis. Biochim Biophys Acta 2009;1791(6):494.
49. Lass A, Zimmermann R, Oberer M, et al. Lipolysis - a highly regulated multienzyme complex mediates the catabolism of cellular fat stores. Prog Lipid Res 2011;50(1):14.
50. Enoksson S, Degerman E, Hagström-Toft E, et al. Various phosphodiesterase subtypes mediate the in vivo antilipolytic effect of insulin on adipose tissue and skeletal muscle in man. Diabetologia 1998;41(5):560.
51. Strålfors P, Honnor RC. Insulin-induced dephosphorylation of hormone-sensitive lipase. Correlation with lipolysis and cAMP-dependent protein kinase activity. Eur J Biochem 1989;182(2):379.
52. Beylot M. Regulation of in vivo ketogenesis: role of free fatty acids and control by epinephrine, thyroid hormones, insulin and glucagon. Diabetes Metab 1996; 22(5):299–304.
53. Chiasson JL, Aris-Jilwan N, Bélanger R, et al. Diagnosis and treatment of diabetic ketoacidosis and the hyperglycemic hyperosmolar state. CMAJ 2003; 168(7):859–66.
54. Adrogue HJ, Eknoyan G, Suki WK. Diabetic ketoacidosis: role of the kidney in the acid-base homeostasis re-evaluated. Kidney Int 1984;25:591–8.
55. Kitabchi AE, Umpierrez GE, Miles JM, et al. Hyperglycemic crises in adult patients with diabetes. Diabetes Care 2009;32(7):1335–43.
56. Smiley D, Chandra P, Umpierrez G. Update on diagnosis, pathogenesis and management of ketosis-prone type 2 diabetes mellitus. Diabetes Manag (Lond) 2011;1(6):589–600.
57. Umpierrez G, Freire AX. Abdominal pain in patients with hyperglycemic crises. J Crit Care 2002;17(1):63.
58. Pant N, Kadaria D, Murillo LC, et al. Abdominal pathology in patients with diabetes ketoacidosis. Am J Med Sci 2012;344(5):341–4.
59. Park BE, Meacham WF, Netsky MG. Nonketotic hyperglycemic hyperosmolar coma. Report of neurosurgical cases with a review of mechanisms and treatment. J Neurosurg 1976;44(4):409–17.
60. Braaten JT. Hyperosmolar nonketotic diabetic coma: diagnosis and management. Geriatrics 1987;42(11):83–8, 92.
61. Lorber D. Nonketotic hypertonicity in diabetes mellitus. Med Clin North Am 1995;79(1):39.

62. Gaglia JL, Wyckoff J, Abrahamson MJ. Acute hyperglycemic crisis in the elderly. Med Clin North Am 2004;88(4):1063–84, xii.
63. Verbalis JG. Control of brain volume during hypoosmolality and hyperosmolality. Adv Exp Med Biol 2006;576:113–29.
64. Derr RF, Zieve L. Weakness, neuropathy, and coma following total parenteral nutrition in underfed or starved rats: relationship to blood hyperosmolarity and brain water loss. J Lab Clin Med 1978;92(4):521–8.
65. Arieff AI. Central nervous system manifestations of disordered sodium metabolism. Clin Endocrinol Metab 1984;13:269–94.
66. Star RA. Hyperosmolar states. Am J Med Sci 1990;300(6):402–12.
67. Butts DE. Fluid and electrolyte disorders associated with diabetic ketoacidosis and hyperglycemic hyperosmolar nonketotic coma. Nurs Clin North Am 1987; 22(4):827–36.
68. Ellis EN. Concepts of fluid therapy in diabetic ketoacidosis and hyperosmolar hyperglycemic nonketotic coma. Pediatr Clin North Am 1990;37(2):313–21.
69. Palevsky PM. Hypernatremia. Semin Nephrol 1998;18(1):20–30.
70. Levine SN, Sanson TH. Treatment of hyperglycaemic hyperosmolar non-ketotic syndrome. Drugs 1989;38(3):462–72.
71. Jerums G, Premaratne E, Panagiotopoulos S, et al. The clinical significance of hyperfiltration in diabetes. Diabetologia 2010;53(10):2093–104.
72. Delaney MF, Zisman A, Kettyle WM. Diabetic ketoacidosis and hyperglycemic hyperosmolar nonketotic syndrome. Endocrinol Metab Clin North Am 2000;29: 683–705.
73. Nugent BW. Hyperosmolar hyperglycemic state. Emerg Med Clin North Am 2005;23(3):629–48, vii.
74. Chico M, Levine SN, Lewis DF. Normoglycemic diabetic ketoacidosis in pregnancy. J Perinatol 2008;28(4):310–2.
75. Cullen MT, Reece EA, Homko CJ, et al. The changing presentations of diabetic ketoacidosis during pregnancy. Am J Perinatol 1996;13(7):449–51.
76. Al-Kudsi RR, Daugirdas JT, Ing TS, et al. Extreme hyperglycemia in dialysis patients. Clin Nephrol 1982;17(5):228.
77. Popli S, Sun Y, Tang HL, et al. Acidosis and coma in adult diabetic maintenance dialysis patients with extreme hyperglycemia. Int Urol Nephrol 2013. [Epub ahead of print].
78. Tzamaloukas AH, Ing TS, Elisaf MS, et al. Abnormalities of serum potassium concentration in dialysis-associated hyperglycemia and their correction with insulin: review of published reports. Int Urol Nephrol 2011;43(2):451–9.
79. Tzamaloukas AH, Ing TS, Siamopoulos KC, et al. Body fluid abnormalities in severe hyperglycemia in patients on chronic dialysis: review of published reports. J Diabetes Complications 2008;22(1):29–37.
80. Hiler TA, Abbott D, Barrett EJ. Hyponatremia: evaluating the correction factor for hyperglycemia. Am J Med 1999;106:399–403.
81. Weisberg LS. Pseudohyponatremia: a reappraisal. Am J Med 1989;86(3): 315–8.
82. Dhatt G, Talor Z, Kazory A. Direct ion-selective electrode method is useful in diagnosis of pseudohyponatremia. J Emerg Med 2012;43(2):348–9.
83. Liamis G, Gianoutsos C, Elisaf MS. Hyperosmolar nonketotic syndrome with hypernatremia: how can we monitor treatment? Diabetes Metab 2000;26(5):403–5.
84. Milionis HJ, Liamis G, Elisaf MS. Appropriate treatment of hypernatraemia in diabetic hyperglycaemic hyperosmolar syndrome. J Intern Med 2001;249(3): 273–6.

85. Beck LH. Should the actual or the corrected serum sodium be used to calculate the anion gap in diabetic ketoacidosis? Cleve Clin J Med 2001;68(8):673–4.
86. Uribarri J, Oh MS, Carroll HJ. Hyperkalemia in diabetes mellitus. J Diabet Complications 1990;4(1):3–7.
87. Adrogué HJ, Lederer ED, Suki WM, et al. Determinants of plasma potassium levels in diabetic ketoacidosis. Medicine (Baltimore) 1986;65(3):163.
88. Arieff AI, Carroll HJ. Nonketotic hyperosmolar coma with hyperglycemia: clinical features, pathophysiology, renal function, acid-base balance, plasma-cerebrospinal fluid equilibria and the effects of therapy in 37 cases. Medicine (Baltimore) 1972;51(2):73.
89. Schultze RG. Recent advances in the physiology and pathophysiology of potassium excretion. Arch Intern Med 1973;131(6):885–97.
90. Abramson E, Arky R. Diabetic acidosis with initial hypokalemia. Therapeutic implications. JAMA 1966;196(5):401.
91. Greenberg A. Hyperkalemia: treatment options. Semin Nephrol 1998;18(1):46–57.
92. Kim HJ, Han SW. Therapeutic approach to hyperkalemia. Nephron 2002;92(Suppl 1):33–40.
93. Unwin RJ, Luft FC, Shirley DG. Pathophysiology and management of hypokalemia: a clinical perspective. Nat Rev Nephrol 2011;7(2):75–84.
94. Ennis ED, Stahl EJ, Kreisberg RA. The hyperosmolar hyperglycemic syndrome. Diabetes Rev 1994;2:115–26.
95. Ennis ED, Kreisberg RA. Diabetic ketoacidosis and hyperosmolar syndrome. In: Leroith D, Taylor SI, Olefsky JM, editors. Diabetes mellitus. A fundamental and clinical text. 3rd edition. Philadelphia: Lippincott Williams & Wilkins; 2004. p. 627–42.
96. Kitabchi AE, Fisher JN, Murphy MB, et al. Diabetic ketoacidosis and the hyperglycemic hyperosmolar nonketotic state. In: Kahn CR, Weir GC, editors. Joslin's diabetes mellitus. 13th edition. Philadelphia: Lea & Febiger; 1994. p. 738–70.
97. Kitabchi AE, Murphy MB. Hyperglycemic crises in adult patients with diabetes mellitus. In: Wass JA, Shalet SM, Amiel SA, editors. Oxford textbook of endocrinology. New York: Oxford University Press; 2002. p. 1734–47.
98. Laffel L. Ketone bodies: a review of physiology, pathophysiology and application of monitoring to diabetes. Diabetes Metab Res Rev 1999;15(6):412–26.
99. Meas T, Taboulet P, Sobngwi E, et al. Is capillary ketone determination useful in clinical practice? In which circumstances? Diabetes Metab 2005;31(3 Pt 1):299–303.
100. Rosenbloom AL, Malone JI. Recognition of impending ketoacidosis delayed by ketone reagent strip failure. JAMA 1978;240(22):2462–4.
101. Davidson M. Diabetic ketoacidosis and hyperosmolar nonketotic syndrome. In: Davidson M, editor. Diabetes mellitus: diagnosis and treatment. 4th edition. Philadelphia: W.B Saunders Co; 1998. p. 159–94.
102. Kitabchi AE, Young R, Sacks H, et al. Diabetic ketoacidosis: reappraisal of therapeutic approach. Annu Rev Med 1979;30:339–57.
103. Arora S, Henderson SO, Long T, et al. Diagnostic accuracy of point-of-care testing for diabetic ketoacidosis at emergency-department triage: {beta}-hydroxybutyrate versus the urine dipstick. Diabetes Care 2011;34(4):852–4.
104. Naunheim R, Jang TJ, Banet G, et al. Point-of-care test identifies diabetic ketoacidosis at triage. Acad Emerg Med 2006;13(6):683–5.
105. Csako G. False-positive results for ketone with the drug mesna and other free-sulfhydryl compounds. Clin Chem 1987;33:289–92.

106. Csako G. Causes, consequences, and recognition of false-positive reactions for ketones. Clin Chem 1990;36:1388–9.

107. Viar M, Wright R. Spurious ketonemia after mesna therapy. Clin Chem 1987;33: 913.

108. Csako G, Elin RJ. Spurious ketonuria due to captopril and other free sulfhydryl drugs. Diabetes Care 1996;19:673–4.

109. Csako G, Benson CC, Elin RJ. False-positive ketone reactions in CAP surveys. Clin Chem 1993;39:915–7.

110. Adrogué HJ, Wilson H, Boyd AE 3rd. Plasma acid-base patterns in diabetic ketoacidosis. N Engl J Med 1982;307(26):1603–10.

111. Kelly AM, McAlpine R, Kyle E. Venous pH can safely replace arterial pH in the initial evaluation of patients in the emergency department. Emerg Med J 2001; 18(5):340–2.

112. Kitabchi AE, Wall BM. Diabetic ketoacidosis. Med Clin North Am 1995;79(1): 9–37.

113. Nyenwe EA, Razavi LN, Kitabchi AE, et al. Acidosis: the prime determinant of depressed sensorium in diabetic ketoacidosis. Diabetes Care 2010;33(8): 1837.

114. Rasouli M, Kalantari KR. Comparison of methods for calculating serum osmolality: multivariate linear regression analysis. Clin Chem Lab Med 2005;43(6): 635.

115. Worthley LI, Guerin M, Pain RW. For calculating osmolality, the simplest formula is the best. Anaesth Intensive Care 1987;15(2):199.

116. Lynd LD, Richardson KJ, Purssell RA, et al. An evaluation of the osmole gap as a screening test for toxic alcohol poisoning. BMC Emerg Med 2008;8:5.

117. Schelling JR, Howard RL, Winter SD, et al. Increased osmolal gap in alcoholic ketoacidosis and lactic acidosis. Ann Intern Med 1990;113(8):580.

118. Glasser L, Sternglanz PD, Combie J, et al. Serum osmolality and its applicability to drug overdose. Am J Clin Pathol 1973;60(5):695.

119. Gennari FJ. Current concepts. Serum osmolality. Uses and limitations. N Engl J Med 1984;310(2):102.

120. Robinson AG, Loeb JN. Ethanol ingestion–commonest cause of elevated plasma osmolality? N Engl J Med 1971;284(22):1253.

121. Razavi L, Taheri E, Larijani B, et al. Catecholamine-induced leukocytosis in acute hypoglycemic stress. J Investig Med 2007;55:S262.

122. Karavanaki K, Kakleas K, Georga S, et al. Plasma high sensitivity C-reactive protein and its relationship with cytokine levels in children with newly diagnosed type 1 diabetes and ketoacidosis. Clin Biochem 2012;45(16–17):1383–8.

123. Stentz FB, Umpierrez GE, Cuervo R. Proinflammatory cytokines, markers of cardiovascular risks, oxidative stress, and lipid peroxidation in patients with hyperglycemic crises. Diabetes 2004;53(8):2079.

124. Ekpebegh C, Longo-Mbenza B. Determinants of altered sensorium at presentation with diabetic ketoacidosis. Minerva Endocrinol 2011;36(4):267–72.

125. Yadav D, Nair S, Norkus EP, et al. Nonspecific hyperamylasemia and hyperlipasemia in diabetic ketoacidosis: incidence and correlation with biochemical abnormalities. Am J Gastroenterol 2000;95(11):3123.

126. Orlowski JP, Cramer CL, Fiallos MR. Diabetic ketoacidosis in the pediatric ICU. Pediatr Clin North Am 2008;55(3):577–87.

127. Wolfsdorf J, Glaser N, Sperling MA. Diabetic ketoacidosis in infants, children, and adolescents. A consensus statement from the American Diabetes Association. Diabetes Care 2006;29:1150–9.

128. Glaser NS, Wootton-Gorges SL, Marcin JP, et al. Mechanism of cerebral edema in children with diabetic ketoacidosis. J Pediatr 2004;145:164–71.
129. Kitabchi AE, Nyenwe EA. Hyperglycemic crises in diabetes mellitus: diabetic ketoacidosis and hyperglycemic hyperosmolar state. Endocrinol Metab Clin North Am 2006;35(4):725–51, viii.
130. Goyal N, Miller JB, Sankey SS, et al. Utility of initial bolus insulin in the treatment of diabetic ketoacidosis. J Emerg Med 2010;38(4):422–7.
131. Kaiserman K, Rodriguez H, Stephenson A. Continuous subcutaneous infusion of insulin lispro in children and adolescents with type 1 diabetes mellitus. Endocr Pract 2012;18(3):418–24.
132. Tridgell DM, Tridgell AH, Hirsch IB. Inpatient management of adults and children with type 1 diabetes. Endocrinol Metab Clin North Am 2010;39(3):595–608.
133. White NH. Diabetic ketoacidosis in children. Endocrinol Metab Clin North Am 2000;29(4):657–82.
134. Bureau MA, Begin R, Berthiaume Y, et al. Cerebral hypoxia from bicarbonate infusion in diabetic acidosis. J Pediatr 1980;96:968–73.
135. Fisher JN, Kitabchi AE. A randomized study of phosphate therapy in the treatment of diabetic ketoacidosis. J Clin Endocrinol Metab 1983;57:177–80.
136. Amanzadeh J, Reilly RF Jr. Hypophosphatemia: an evidence-based approach to its clinical consequences and management. Nat Clin Pract Nephrol 2006;2(3):136–48.
137. Shiber JR, Mattu A. Serum phosphate abnormalities in the emergency department. J Emerg Med 2002;23(4):395–400.

Diabetes and Altered Glucose Metabolism with Aging

Rita Rastogi Kalyani, MD, MHS[a],*, Josephine M. Egan, MD[b]

KEYWORDS

- Diabetes • Aging • Insulin resistance • Beta-cell dysfunction

KEY POINTS

- Adults aged 60 and over have more than twice the prevalence of diabetes compared with younger age groups. The number of older persons with diabetes will continue to grow as the population ages.
- Abnormal glucose metabolism is associated with aging but is not a necessary component.
- Older persons with diabetes and/or abnormal glucose metabolism may be at higher risk of developing adverse geriatric syndromes, such as accelerated muscle loss, functional disability, and frailty.
- Goals of care for older persons with diabetes need to be individualized and consider treatment of symptomatic hyperglycemia, prevention of long-term complications, avoidance of hypoglycemia, and preservation of quality of life.
- Lifestyle modifications, in particular, regular exercise as tolerated, and pharmacologic therapies that account for the presence of comorbid renal and hepatic impairments or physical and cognitive limitations are important components of diabetes management in older adults.

EPIDEMIOLOGY OF DIABETES AND IMPAIRED GLUCOSE STATES WITH AGING

Diabetes in older adults is a growing public health concern, with almost one-third of US adults over the age of 60 years having diabetes, of whom approximately half are

This article originally appeared in Endocrinology and Metabolism Clinics of North America, Volume 42, Issue 2, June 2013.

Funding Sources: This work is supported in part by the National Institute of Diabetes and Digestive and Kidney Diseases (R.R. Kalyani; K23DK093583) and the Intramural Research Program/National Institutes of Health, and the National Institute on Aging (J.M. Egan).

Conflict of Interest: None.

[a] Division of Endocrinology and Metabolism, Department of Medicine, Johns Hopkins University School of Medicine, The Johns Hopkins University, 1830 East Monument Street, Suite 333, Baltimore, MD 21287, USA; [b] National Institute on Aging/National Institutes of Health, Suite 100, Room 8C222, 251 Bayview Boulevard, Baltimore, MD 21224, USA

* Corresponding author.

E-mail address: rrastogi@jhmi.edu

http://dx.doi.org/10.1016/j.ccol.2014.08.003
2352-7986/14/$ – see front matter

undiagnosed; an additional one-third of older adults have prediabetes.[1] Diabetes prevalence in older adults is more than twice that of middle-aged adults.[1] It is projected that the numbers of elderly persons will approximately double by the year 2030.[2,3] In addition, the number of people in nursing homes with diabetes continues to increase.[4] Consequently, the burden of diabetes in the elderly is significant and growing.

Glucose intolerance is associated with aging.[1,5–7] Aging has been associated with elevated levels of both glucose and insulin after oral glucose challenge testing.[8] The 2-hour plasma glucose during an oral glucose tolerance test (OGTT) rises much more steeply than fasting glucose levels with aging.[8–10] As a result, elderly individuals are more likely to be classified as having abnormal glucose status compared with younger adults using similar diagnostic criteria for diabetes.[11] Some investigators have suggested that the diagnosis of diabetes can be made many years earlier using OGTT versus fasting glucose levels alone in older persons.[12] Data from the Baltimore Longitudinal Study of Aging demonstrate an age-related increase in progression rate from normal glucose status to impaired glucose tolerance that is almost twice the progression rate from normal to impaired fasting glucose after 20 years of follow-up.[12] These findings suggest that OGTT, in particular, is important to consider when characterizing abnormal glucose status in the elderly.

ALTERED GLUCOSE METABOLISM WITH AGING

Using hyperinsulinemic-euglycemic clamp methodology as a method for quantification of insulin effectiveness in regulating glucose transport into tissues, whole-body insulin sensitivity is demonstrably reduced in older versus younger adults.[13,14] Impaired intracellular whole-body rates of glucose oxidation in elderly versus young adults have also been reported.[15] Potential explanations for reduced insulin effectiveness with aging include (1) increased abdominal fat mass, (2) decreased physical activity, (3) sarcopenia, (4) mitochondrial dysfunction, (5) hormonal changes (ie, lower insulinlike growth factor 1 and dehydroepiandrosterone), and (6) increased oxidative stress and inflammation.[16] Nonetheless, insulin sensitivity decreases with age even after adjustment for differences in adiposity, fat distribution, and physical activity.[17]

Beta-cell dysfunction with aging is also a significant contributing factor to abnormal glucose metabolism. Insulin secretion is most commonly tested using an OGTT; it is standardized, simple to administer, and widely used in longitudinal studies. An oral load of 75 g of glucose is delivered as a rapid bolus to the gut and can trigger neural and incretin responses, over and beyond stimulus by the glucose per se, to the insulin-secreting β-cells. Responses to physiologic stimuli, such as a meal containing complex carbohydrates, fat, and protein, may be different from that of a glucose load. With those limitations in mind, there is a gradual decline with aging in insulin secretion during the first hour in response to an oral glucose load, despite older adults having higher glucose levels after the glucose challenge.[18,19] Once plasma glucose levels reach the diabetic range, however, insulin secretion is severely compromised.[20]

β-Cell function has also been evaluated using the hyperglycemic clamp, in which plasma glucose levels are increased in a square wave fashion and maintained at this level for a fixed duration of time in a controlled manner. The final attained stable (or clamped) plasma glucose level can be varied and insulin secretion studied with clamped plasma glucose levels as high as 450 mg/dL.[13] The β-cell response to a hyperglycemic clamp is stereotypical in that there is a first-phase insulin secretion that occurs within 2 to 3 minutes of the initiation of the square wave of infused glucose, followed by a slower plateau phase that reaches stability in approximately 100 to 120 minutes. In general, among older adults with normal glucose tolerance based on the OGTT, deficits in insulin secretion are seen only when high plasma glucose levels are achieved when compared with the young. But, as with all patients with type 2 diabetes mellitus, once an elderly patient has developed diabetes, the first-phase insulin secretion in response to the square wave of a hyperglycemic clamp is defective to absent,[13] and the plateau-phase insulin secretion is less than in nondiabetic subjects.

Insulin secretion falls under 2 types: constitutive (sometimes called basal) and stimulated (such as occurs after a meal, an OGTT, or hyperglycemic clamp), with constitutive insulin accounting for approximately 50% of the total 24-hour insulin output. Insulin secretion is pulsatile in nature. Using 1-minute blood sampling and highly sensitive insulin assays, rapid, low-amplitude insulin pulses occurring approximately every 8 to 14 minutes and larger-amplitude ultradian pulses occurring every 60 to 140 minutes can be elucidated.[21] The rapid pulses persist even in isolated islets and are independent of circulating glucose levels whereas the ultradian pulses are tightly coupled to glucose, by which they are entrained. In the fasting state, elderly subjects without diabetes have disorderly pulsatile insulin secretion, with reduced amplitude and mass of the rapid pulses and decreased frequency of the ultradian pulses. Scheen and colleagues[22] and Meneilly and colleagues[23] studied pulsatile insulin secretion in young and elderly subjects under conditions of sustained experimentally induced hyperglycemia. Overall, the findings were similar to the fasting state; specifically, older subjects displayed reduced amplitude and mass of the rapid insulin pulses, and the ultradian pulses were more irregular with lower amplitude compared to younger subjects. The investigators also found that glucose infusion for up to 53 hours[22] was not capable of normalizing pulsatile insulin secretion in older individuals. Pulsatile insulin secretion is important for regulating glucose output from the liver and may be involved in maintaining skeletal muscle in a state of metabolic readiness, such as maintaining insulin receptors and glucose transporters in a primed state. The disordered pulsatile insulin secretion seen in the elderly may play a role in the previously described decrease in insulin sensitivity observed with aging. In type 2 diabetes mellitus, severe disorderliness is found because the oscillatory pattern of insulin secretion is almost totally disrupted. The rapid pulses are replaced by irregular pulses of short duration, and the ultradian pulses are disrupted, chaotic, and uncoupled from glucose, because glucose fails to control the periodicity of the ultradian pulses.[24]

Rising plasma glucose accounts for approximately 50% of the secreted insulin after a meal or OGTT; the remaining 50% is due to incretin hormones released from the enteroendocrine cells lining the gut.[25] Incretins are peptide hormones, of which there are 2 main types: gastric inhibitory polypeptide (GIP) and glucagon-like peptide 1 (GLP-1). Their effect on β-cells is to increase glucose-dependent insulin secretion. There is no evidence that secretion of incretins, as measured by plasma levels after OGTT, is defective in aging per se, although the β-cell may be less responsive to their stimulatory effects. In an elegant study, Elahi and colleagues[26] combined the hyperglycemic clamp with oral glucose (to stimulate endogenous GIP secretion) and found that, in older individuals, GIP secretion in response to the oral glucose was increased compared with that in younger participants but led to slightly lower insulin secretion in response to the endogenous GIP. Hyperglycemic clamps at 100 mg/dL and 230 mg/dL above basal have been performed in young and elderly subjects[27] with combined GIP infusions. At the lower clamped plasma glucose level, the potentiation of glucose-induced insulin secretion by GIP was reduced by half in the elderly compared with the young, whereas at the higher clamped plasma glucose level, insulin response to GIP was similar in both age groups. Becuase the lower clamped plasma glucose level is more physiologic, however, this probably reflects a true decline in GIP effectiveness with aging. In type 2 diabetes mellitus, GIP no longer potentiates glucose-induced insulin secretion and also increases glucagon secretion, which exacerbates hyperglycemia[28]; however, GIP secretion is not lower in type 2 diabetes mellitus compared with nondiabetic subjects.[25] The data on GLP-1 secretion with increasing age and onset of type 2 diabetes mellitus are similar to those of GIP in that secretion of GLP-1 is not necessarily decreased with older age or the presence of diabetes but, unlike GIP, GLP-1 is still a powerful stimulus to insulin secretion—hence, the robust development of several agents for treating type 2 diabetes mellitus that activate the GLP-1 receptor on β-cells (ie, exenatide and liragulatide). Also, unlike GIP, use of GLP-1 receptor agonists leads to a decrease in glucagon secretion.[25]

The enzyme, dipeptidyl-peptidase 4 (DPP 4), inactivates both GIP and GLP-1 and has decreasing activity with older age,[29] which may explain the higher GIP levels observed in the elderly.[26] The recent development of DPP 4 inhibitors (ie, sitagliptin, saxagliptin, and linagliptin) as therapeutic agents may also have a role for treatment of diabetes in the elderly.

COMPLICATIONS OF DIABETES IN THE ELDERLY

Microvascular and macrovascular complications of diabetes occur in older patients, similar to younger persons, although the absolute risk of cardiovascular disease is much higher in older adults.[30] Diabetes in the older adult population, however, is heterogeneous and includes individuals with both middle age–onset and elderly-onset diabetes,[31] with the latter group accounting for up to one-third of older adults with diabetes. Middle age–onset adults may have worse glycemic control and are more likely to be taking glucose-lowering medications. Whereas the prevalence of macrovascular diseases (stroke, coronary heart disease, and peripheral arterial disease) may be similar between the middle age–onset and elderly-onset diabetes groups, the burden of microvascular disease (particularly retinopathy) may be greater in the former.[31,32] Thus, the age of diabetes onset may have an impact on the burden of disease and diabetic complications present in elderly patients with diabetes, but more studies need to be done.

GERIATRIC SYNDROMES ASSOCIATED WITH DIABETES

Descriptions of otherwise healthy centenarians without impaired glucose uptake suggest that insulin resistance is not a necessary component of the aging process.[33,34] Instead, older adults with abnormal glucose status and diabetes likely represent a vulnerable subset at high risk for adverse outcomes. Geriatric syndromes that have been described to occur more frequently in persons with diabetes include loss of muscle function, functional limitations and disability, and frailty—all of which can have a significant impact on quality of life in older patients—in addition to early mortality (**Fig. 1**). Diabetes also increases the risk of other common geriatric syndromes, such as depression, cognitive dysfunction, chronic pain, injurious falls, urinary incontinence, and polypharmacy,[30] but is not specifically discussed in this article.

Loss of Muscle Function

Previous studies of older adults with diabetes have demonstrated decreased muscle strength and mass, especially in the lower extremities.[35] Older adults with type 2 diabetes mellitus have approximately 50% more rapid decline in knee extensor strength than those without diabetes over a 3-year period,[36] suggesting that decreased muscle strength is a consequence of type 2 diabetes mellitus, with similar findings for muscle mass.[37] Disease duration and severity may have a role in the decreased muscle strength observed among persons with diabetes. Park and colleagues[35] reported

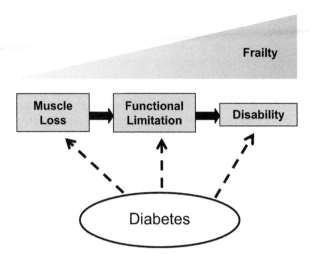

Fig. 1. Diabetes and the pathway to disability. Proposed associations of diabetes with each step in the pathway to disability are depicted. Accelerated loss of muscle mass and strength, particularly in the lower extremities, may lead to functional limitations in routine tasks of daily living, which may ultimately result in physical disability among older persons with diabetes. Frailty is a geriatric syndrome that encompasses the full spectrum of the disability process and is also more common with impaired glucose states and diabetes.

that leg muscle quality was lowest in older adults with diabetes (mean age 74 years) who had the longest diabetes duration ($\geq$6 years) or most severe hyperglycemia (hemoglobin A_{1c} [HbA_{1c}] >8%). Even among persons without diabetes, associations between hyperglycemia and insulin resistance with decreased muscle mass and strength, have been described.[38–40]

In older adults, skeletal muscle protein synthesis may be resistant to the anabolic action of insulin.[41,42] Insulin resistance is also associated with activation of muscle proteolysis pathways,[43] which may further lead to muscle loss. In turn, muscle is the primary site for insulin-dependent glucose uptake, and reduced muscle surface area for insulin-mediated glucose uptake may aggravate peripheral insulin resistance, leading to a vicious cycle. Oral insulin sensitizers have been reported to preserve muscle mass[44] although similar associations for muscle strength have yet to be investigated. Skeletal muscle mitochondrial function is reduced in type 2 diabetes mellitus and may be improved with peripheral insulin sensitization.[45,46]

Potential pathways underlying the association of diabetes with reduced muscle function include the presence of comorbidities, such as peripheral neuropathy, which may mediate these associations[47,48]; however, decreased leg muscle strength is present even after accounting for lower extremity nerve dysfunction in diabetes.[49] Diabetes is associated with inflammatory markers, which in turn may also lead to impaired muscle function.[50,51]

Functional Limitations and Physical Disability

In the general population, muscle strength is a predictor of functional limitations and disability.[52] Persons with diabetes perform worse on objective measures of lower extremity physical performance, such as walking, chair stands, and tandem stand.[53] Slower walking speed in persons with type 2 diabetes mellitus has been demonstrated.[53,54] The greatest differences have been observed, however, at maximal walking speeds.[55] There is some evidence that impaired muscle function mediates the association of diabetes with lower gait speed in older adults.[54] Severe hyperglycemia and insulin resistance have also been associated, however, with walking difficulties and poorer performance-based measures of lower extremity function both in persons with and without diabetes.[53,56,57]

Similarly, diabetes can have a significant impact on physical functioning, such as lower extremity mobility, potentially mediated through effects on muscle function.[58] Functional disability or difficulty in performing routine physical tasks is more common in older adults with diabetes compared with those without diabetes.[57–64] Older adults with diabetes have significantly greater difficulty in a range of routine physical activities, including walking a quarter mile, climbing stairs, reaching overhead, doing housework, bathing, eating, and participating in leisure activities compared with their counterparts. Up to 70% of adults with diabetes have difficulties performing these tasks of everyday living.[64]

The higher prevalence of functional disability in older adults with diabetes may be related to the presence of comorbidities, such as cardiovascular disease, vision loss, obesity, and arthritis.[59,63,64] These comorbidities may be associated with decreased cardiopulmonary reserve or restricted physical movement, which contributes to physical disability. These factors, however, do not consistently explain the association of diabetes with disability; the degree of glycemic control is also related to disability among older adults with diabetes.[57,64,65] Support for an association between hyperglycemia and disability comes from previous studies reporting a significant correlation between higher HbA_{1c} levels and disability.[57,65] Alternatively, physical and cognitive impairment may affect ability to self-manage diabetes and lead to poorer glycemic control; thus, the relationship between hyperglycemia and disability is likely bidirectional and requires further investigation.

Frailty Syndrome

Diabetes has been associated with the presence of frailty, a geriatric condition of physiologic vulnerability to stressors associated with adverse outcomes, such as disability and mortality.[66–69] Frailty increases with age and is distinguished by a characteristic phenotype. A common definition includes the presence of 3 or more of the following criteria: unintentional weight loss, self-reported exhaustion, muscle weakness (poor grip strength), slow walking speed, or low physical activity.[67]

Recent literature has suggested an association between insulin resistance and frailty[16,70] in cross-sectional studies of persons with and without diabetes. Altered glucose-insulin dynamics has also been reported in frail women compared with their counterparts with 120-minute post-OGTT levels of both glucose and insulin discriminating frailty status better compared with fasting values.[71,72] Similar alterations in glucose dynamics have also been described in frail older adults who underwent a mixed meal test and had a more exaggerated and prolonged glucose response after 2 hours compared with nonfrail older adults.[73] These studies suggest relative insulin resistance in frail older adults compared with nonfrail older adults.

The presence of hyperglycemia and insulin resistance is also temporally related to the subsequent development of frailty in longitudinal cohort studies.[53,74] In the Cardiovascular Health Study, homeostasis model–insulin resistance was calculated based on fasting glucose and insulin levels. For every standard deviation increment in homeostasis model–insulin resistance, the adjusted hazard ratio for frailty was 1.15 (95% CI, 1.02–1.31).[74] Individuals who eventually developed frailty were also more likely, in parallel, to develop diabetes compared with older adults who never developed frailty (8.6% vs 4.2%). Thus, the association between frailty and abnormal glucose status is likely bidirectional. In the Women's Health and Aging Study, older women in the highest HbA_{1c} category ($\geq$8%) compared with lowest HbA_{1c} category (<5.5%) had a significant 3-fold increased risk for the development of frailty, with most events occurring in the highest HbA_{1c} category.[53] These findings suggest that hyperglycemia, particularly in the diabetic range, can predict the onset of incident frailty less than a decade later.[53]

The underlying physiologic mechanisms relating insulin resistance to the development of frailty remain unclear. Frail older adults have a higher burden of inflammatory markers that may also affect glucose metabolism.[71,75,76] Hyperglycemia may further activate inflammatory pathways that subsequently cause muscle catabolism and disability as part of the frailty process.[77] Frail women on average are also more likely to be obese, which may be associated with chronic inflammation.[72,78] One study found that only frail obese adults, but not frail lean adults, had reduced insulin sensitivity versus nonfrail counterparts.[16] Another study found, however, that associations of insulin resistance and frailty are independent of obesity.[72] In addition, chronic hyperglycemia may be a risk factor for cardiovascular disease, which, in turn, has been associated with frailty[79]; however, the presence of cardiovascular disease does not fully explain these associations. Thus, underlying mechanisms linking hyperglycemia with frailty remain unclear but are likely multifactorial.[80]

Early Mortality

Diabetes in older adults is associated with increased disability, frailty, and accelerated muscle loss. These adverse geriatric syndromes can be associated with both increased health care expenditures[81,82] and early mortality.[66,69,83] On average, persons with diabetes have an almost 2-fold increased risk of death from any cause, with 40% of this difference in survival due to nonvascular deaths.[84] Results from the Baltimore Longitudinal Study of Aging demonstrate higher total and cardiovascular mortality even in older adults with impaired glucose tolerance compared with those with normal glucose metabolism.[85,86] A J-shaped association of HbA_{1c} with mortality has also been described, with increased mortality rates seen at higher levels of HbA_{1c} but also, to a lesser degree, at lower HbA_{1c} levels.[87,88] Reduced length and activity of the telomerase enzyme, which maintains stability of chromosomes with aging, has been linked to impaired glucose-stimulated insulin islet secretion and may also underlie these epidemiologic associations but is currently still an area of active investigation.[89]

TREATMENT OF DIABETES IN THE ELDERLY
Guidelines

The goals of diabetes care in older patients with diabetes include (1) control of hyperglycemia, (2) prevention and treatment of macrovascular and microvascular complications of diabetes, (3) avoidance of hypoglycemia, and (4) preservation of quality of life. Although the goals are similar to those in younger adults, older adults with diabetes are heterogeneous in their physical and cognitive functioning capacity, multiple comorbidities, and life expectancy. Otherwise robust older adults with expected life expectancy over 10 years might benefit from similar glycemic goals as younger adults (ie, HbA_{1c} <7%) to prevent diabetic complications. For frail older adults with multiple comorbidities and limited life expectancy, however, avoidance of hypoglycemia and symptomatic hyperglycemia and preservation of quality of life are arguably just as important, and less stringent targets (ie, HbA_{1c} <8%) may be more appropriate. Furthermore, patient preferences must also be recognized in decisions related to diabetes management. Thus, treatment often requires an individualized approach for older patients with diabetes.

Current glycemic targets of HbA$_{1c}$ less than 7% are based on older studies (eg, United Kingdom Prospective Diabetes Study) that showed a significantly reduced risk of developing diabetic microvascular complications with intensive versus standard glucose control.[90] Long-term follow-up of the United Kingdom Prospective Diabetes Study demonstrated further benefits of early and intensive glucose control in reducing long-term risk of developing macrovascular disease.[90] Elderly individuals were excluded from the United Kingdom Prospective Diabetes Study, however, and there have been few other clinical trials examining the benefits of intensive glycemic control in older individuals; thus, extrapolation of previous results of clinical trials to elderly patients is challenging.[91] Recent clinical trials studying the effect of intensive glucose control that included older patients with diabetes failed to show a clear benefit of intensive glucose control on mortality and demonstrated potential harm with too aggressive glucose lowering (ie, HbA$_{1c}$ <6%).[92–94] As a result, recent recommendations from the American Diabetes Association and the American Geriatrics Society recognize that a patient-centered approach may be more appropriate for older adults with diabetes.[11,95,96] Cardiovascular risk factor control (ie, lowering blood pressure, treating dyslipidemia, smoking cessation, and aspirin therapy) is also recommended for the majority of adults with diabetes based on health status.

Management of older patients with diabetes is complex and often individualized. Avoiding hypoglycemia and preserving functional independence are additional considerations for older patients with diabetes. Alternatively, an evolving area of research is exploring the degree to which hyperglycemia may be associated with the presence of adverse geriatric syndromes, such as physical disability, accelerated muscle loss, and frailty, and may ultimately have an impact on glycemic goals in the elderly. Current guidelines recognize the need to account for the presence of limited life expectancy and/or multiple comorbidities in treatment decisions for this vulnerable and growing population of individuals with diabetes.

Treatment

Lifestyle recommendations for older adults with prediabetes or diabetes can be tailored to physical function ability and are more appropriate for obese elderly individuals than those who are underweight. Encouragingly, the oldest age group in the Diabetes Prevention Program (>60 years at of age at baseline) had the most dramatic improvement in glycemic control over time with lifestyle modification programs and was associated with better adherence to lifestyle programs compared with younger age groups.[97,98] In prescribing dietary modification, additional factors to consider in elderly patients with diabetes include social factors, such as whether patients are eating alone (easier to eat precooked meals) and the presence of depression. Impaired perception of sweet and salty occurs with age, so using potassium chloride for saltiness and using sucralose or stevia for sweetness may be preferred because they are perceived as saltier and sweeter than sodium chloride or sucrose.[99] A sedentary lifestyle in older patients might signify the need for a reduced intake of total calories. Alcohol consumption is also associated with a significant number of calories and should be ascertained when formulating a lifestyle modification program.

Daily exercise, as part of activities of daily living, is necessary for older patients with diabetes. Weight-bearing exercises can improve insulin sensitivity. In older patients with diabetes, usual recommendations for aerobic and resistance exercise can be prescribed as tolerated in the context of other medical conditions (ie, arthritis and heart disease) that may otherwise limit exercise tolerance or participation in physical activities.[100]

The choice of pharmacologic therapy for older patients with diabetes may be affected by changes in renal and hepatic functions with aging and the physical and cognitive abilities of each patient, in addition to other coexisting comorbidities. **Fig. 2** outlines the sites of action for common glucose-lowering therapies used in diabetes management. Special considerations in the elderly include the need to monitor renal function using both creatinine and glomerular filtration rate when prescribing metformin due to risk of lactic acidosis; hypoglycemia with sulfonylureas, which work by increasing endogenous insulin secretion, and often require dose reductions when used with insulin and in patients with renal insufficiency (short-acting glimepiride and glipizide may be preferred); and the use of weight-neutral agents, such as DPP 4 inhibitors, which increase endogenous levels of incretins, and may be appropriate in cachetic older adults. Thiazolidenediones, which are *peroxisome proliferator-activated receptor γ*-activators, may exacerbate underlying heart failure and are associated with increased risk of bone fractures, so they should be avoided in persons with underlying bone disease, but they are less likely to result in hypoglycemia. GLP-1 receptor agonists are injectable agents that can slow gastric motility and lead to weight loss. Thus, these agents may be useful for obese older patients with diabetes but not in those with complications, such as gastroparesis. Endogenous insulin clearance may also be decreased with aging[101,102] and, perhaps, exogenous insulin clearance as well, although this has not been consistently described.[103] Insulin clearance is particularly affected by changes in renal function, which may affect dosing.

Monitoring of blood glucose in older patients with diabetes is similar to that in younger adults. HbA_{1c} may rise by approximately 0.1% with each decade of age independent of changes in blood glucose and potentially affect the interpretability of HbA_{1c}

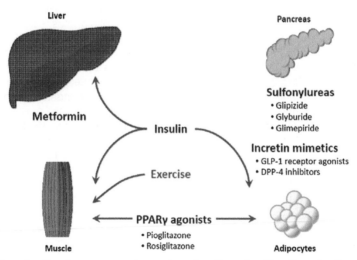

Fig. 2. Sites of action for common glucose-lowering therapies. The sites of action for common glucose-lowering therapies used in persons with type 2 diabetes mellitus are illustrated. The different mechanisms by which these drugs improve blood glucose, along with potential benefits and side effects, are important considerations in the management of older patients with diabetes. Exercise, in particular, muscle-strengthening or resistance activities, can have additional benefits on glucose uptake by skeletal muscle. PPARγ, *peroxisome proliferator-activated receptor* γ.

in older patients.[104] Self-monitoring of blood glucose can be considered based on a patient's cognitive ability, functional status, and risk of hypoglycemia.

SUMMARY

Diabetes and altered glucose metabolism commonly occur with aging. OGTT may help characterize abnormal glucose status in the elderly population. Diabetes in this population is heterogeneous, with middle age–onset versus elderly-onset individuals possibly representing groups at different risks for the development of microvascular complications. Geriatric syndromes, such as muscle loss, disability, and frailty, are more prevalent in older patients with diabetes and may be related to the presence of hyperglycemia or insulin resistance but more research is needed. Treatment of diabetes in the elderly includes lifestyle recommendations, when appropriate, and the use of pharmacologic therapies that account for the presence of comorbidities, especially renal and hepatic impairment, as well as the physical and cognitive abilities of patients, while seeking to minimize hypoglycemia. Ultimately, goals of care need to be individualized for elderly patients with diabetes.

ACKNOWLEDGMENTS

We thank David Liu (National Institute on Aging) for help with **Fig. 2** illustration.

REFERENCES

1. Cowie CC, Rust KF, Ford ES, et al. Full accounting of diabetes and pre-diabetes in the U.S. population in 1988-1994 and 2005-2006. Diabetes Care 2009;32: 287–94.
2. Centers for Disease Control and Prevention (CDC). Public health and aging: trends in aging—United States and worldwide. JAMA 2003;289:1371–3.
3. Wild S, Roglic G, Green A, et al. Global prevalence of diabetes: estimates for the year 2000 and projections for 2030. Diabetes Care 2004;27:1047–53.
4. Zhang X, Decker FH, Luo H, et al. Trends in the prevalence and comorbidities of diabetes mellitus in nursing home residents in the United States: 1995-2004. J Am Geriatr Soc 2010;58:724–30.
5. Shimokata H, Muller DC, Fleg JL, et al. Age as an independent determinant of glucose tolerance. Diabetes 1991;40:44–51.
6. DeFronzo RA. Glucose intolerance and aging. Diabetes Care 1981;4:493–501.
7. Ferrannini E, Vichi S, Beck-Nielsen H, et al. Insulin action and age. European Group for the Study of Insulin Resistance (EGIR). Diabetes 1996;45:947–53.
8. Davidson MB. The effect of aging on carbohydrate metabolism. Metabolism 1979;28:688–705.
9. Elahi D, Muller DC, Egan JM, et al. Glucose tolerance, glucose utilization and insulin secretion in ageing. Novartis Found Symp 2002;242:222–42.
10. Elahi D, Muller DC. Carbohydrate metabolism in the elderly. Eur J Clin Nutr 2000;54(Suppl 3):S112–20.
11. American Diabetes Association. Standards of medical care in diabetes—2012. Diabetes Care 2012;35(Suppl 1):S11–63.
12. Meigs JB, Muller DC, Nathan DM, et al. The natural history of progression from normal glucose tolerance to type 2 diabetes in the Baltimore Longitudinal Study of Aging. Diabetes 2003;52:1475–84.
13. DeFronzo RA, Tobin JD, Andres R. Glucose clamp technique: a method for quantifying insulin secretion and resistance. Am J Physiol 1979;237:E214–23.

14. Defronzo RA. Glucose intolerance and aging: evidence for tissue insensitivity to insulin. Diabetes 1979;28:1095–101.
15. Gumbiner B, Thorburn AW, Ditzler TM, et al. Role of impaired intracellular glucose metabolism in the insulin resistance of aging. Metabolism 1992;41: 1115–21.
16. Goulet ED, Hassaine A, Dionne IJ, et al. Frailty in the elderly is associated with insulin resistance of glucose metabolism in the postabsorptive state only in the presence of increased abdominal fat. Exp Gerontol 2009;44:740–4.
17. Elahi D, Muller DC, McAloon-Dyke M, et al. The effect of age on insulin response and glucose utilization during four hyperglycemic plateaus. Exp Gerontol 1993; 28:393–409.
18. Chen M, Halter JB, Porte D Jr. The role of dietary carbohydrate in the decreased glucose tolerance of the elderly. J Am Geriatr Soc 1987;35:417–24.
19. Muller DC, Elahi D, Tobin JD, et al. The effect of age on insulin resistance and secretion: a review. Semin Nephrol 1996;16:289–98.
20. Tabák AG, Jokela M, Akbaraly TN, et al. Trajectories of glycaemia, insulin sensitivity, and insulin secretion before diagnosis of type 2 diabetes: an analysis from the Whitehall II study. Lancet 2009;373:2215–21.
21. Polonsky KS, Given BD, Van Cauter E. Twenty-four-hour profiles and pulsatile patterns of insulin secretion in normal and obese subjects. J Clin Invest 1988; 81:442–8.
22. Scheen AJ, Sturis J, Polonsky KS, et al. Alterations in the ultradian oscillations of insulin secretion and plasma glucose in aging. Diabetologia 1996;39:564–72.
23. Meneilly GS, Veldhuis JD, Elahi D. Disruption of the pulsatile and entropic modes of insulin release during an unvarying glucose stimulus in elderly individuals. J Clin Endocrinol Metab 1999;84:1938–43.
24. O'Meara NM, Sturis J, Van Cauter E, et al. Lack of control by glucose of ultradian insulin secretory oscillations in impaired glucose tolerance and in non-insulin-dependent diabetes mellitus. J Clin Invest 1993;92:262–71.
25. Kim W, Egan JM. The role of incretins in glucose homeostasis and diabetes treatment. Pharmacol Rev 2008;60:470–512.
26. Elahi D, Andersen DK, Muller DC, et al. The enteric enhancement of glucose-stimulated insulin release. The role of GIP in aging, obesity, and non-insulin-dependent diabetes mellitus. Diabetes 1984;33:950–7.
27. Meneilly GS, Ryan AS, Minaker KL, et al. The effect of age and glycemic level on the response of the beta-cell to glucose-dependent insulinotropic polypeptide and peripheral tissue sensitivity to endogenously released insulin. J Clin Endocrinol Metab 1998;83:2925–32.
28. Chia CW, Carlson OD, Kim W, et al. Exogenous glucose-dependent insulinotropic polypeptide worsens post prandial hyperglycemia in type 2 diabetes. Diabetes 2009;58:1342–9.
29. Meneilly GS, Demuth HU, McIntosh CH, et al. Effect of ageing and diabetes on glucose-dependent insulinotropic polypeptide and dipeptidyl peptidase IV responses to oral glucose. Diabet Med 2000;17:346–50.
30. Chiniwala N, Jabbour S. Management of diabetes mellitus in the elderly. Curr Opin Endocrinol Diabetes Obes 2011;18:148–52.
31. Selvin E, Coresh J, Brancati FL. The burden and treatment of diabetes in elderly individuals in the U.S. Diabetes Care 2006;29:2415–9.
32. Wang Y, Qin MZ, Liu Q, et al. Clinical analysis of elderly patients with elderly-onset type 2 diabetes mellitus in China: assessment of appropriate therapy. J Int Med Res 2010;38:1134–41.

33. Barbieri M, Rizzo MR, Manzella D, et al. Age-related insulin resistance: is it an obligatory finding? The lesson from healthy centenarians. Diabetes Metab Res Rev 2001;17:19–26.

34. Paolisso G, Gambardella A, Ammendola S, et al. Glucose tolerance and insulin action in healty centenarians. Am J Physiol 1996;270:E890–4.

35. Park SW, Goodpaster BH, Strotmeyer ES, et al. Decreased muscle strength and quality in older adults with type 2 diabetes: the health, aging, and body composition study. Diabetes 2006;55:1813–8.

36. Park SW, Goodpaster BH, Strotmeyer ES, et al. Health, aging, and body composition study. Accelerated loss of skeletal muscle strength in older adults with type 2 diabetes: the health, aging, and body composition study. Diabetes Care 2007;30:1507–12.

37. Park SW, Goodpaster BH, Lee JS, et al. Health, aging, and body composition study. Excessive loss of skeletal muscle mass in older adults with type 2 diabetes. Diabetes Care 2009;32:1993–7.

38. Barzilay JI, Cotsonis GA, Walston J, et al, Health ABC Study. Insulin resistance is associated with decreased quadriceps muscle strength in nondiabetic adults aged ≥70 years. Diabetes Care 2009;32:736–8.

39. Lazarus R, Sparrow D, Weiss ST. Handgrip strength and insulin levels: cross-sectional and prospective associations in the Normative Aging Study. Metabolism 1997;46:1266–9.

40. Kalyani RR, Metter EJ, Ramachandran R, et al. Glucose and insulin measurements from the oral glucose tolerance test and relationship to muscle mass. J Gerontol A Biol Sci Med Sci 2012;67:74–81.

41. Rasmussen BB, Fujita S, Wolfe RR, et al. Insulin resistance of muscle protein metabolism in aging. FASEB J 2006;20:768–9.

42. Volpi E, Mittendorfer B, Rasmussen BB, et al. The response of muscle protein anabolism to combined hyperaminoacidemia and glucose-induced hyperinsulinemia is impaired in the elderly. J Clin Endocrinol Metab 2000;85:4481–90.

43. Wang X, Hu Z, Hu J, et al. Insulin resistance accelerates muscle protein degradation: activation of the ubiquitin-proteasome pathway by defects in muscle cell signaling. Endocrinology 2006;147:4160–8.

44. Lee CG, Boyko EJ, Barrett-Connor E, et al, Osteoporotic Fractures in Men (MrOS) Study Research Group. Insulin sensitizers may attenuate lean mass loss in older men with diabetes. Diabetes Care 2011;34:2381–6.

45. Phielix E, Schrauwen-Hinderling VB, Mensink M, et al. Lower intrinsic ADP-stimulated mitochondrial respiration underlies in vivo mitochondrial dysfunction in muscle of male type 2 diabetic patients. Diabetes 2008;57:2943–9.

46. Rabøl R, Boushel R, Almdal T, et al. Opposite effects of pioglitazone and rosiglitazone on mitochondrial respiration in skeletal muscle of patients with type 2 diabetes. Diabetes Obes Metab 2010;12:806–14.

47. Strotmeyer ES, de Rekeneire N, Schwartz AV, et al, Health ABC Study. Sensory and motor peripheral nerve function and lower-extremity quadriceps strength: the health, aging and body composition study. J Am Geriatr Soc 2009;57:2004–10.

48. Andersen H, Nielsen S, Mogensen CE, et al. Muscle strength in type 2 diabetes. Diabetes 2004;53:1543–8.

49. Volpato S, Bianchi L, Lauretani F, et al. Role of muscle mass and muscle quality in the association between diabetes and gait speed. Diabetes Care 2012;35:1672–9.

50. Van Hall G, Steensberg A, Fischer C, et al. Interleukin-6 markedly decreases skeletal muscle protein turnover and increases nonmuscle amino acid utilization in healthy individuals. J Clin Endocrinol Metab 2008;7:2851–8.

51. Duncan BB, Schmidt MI, Pankow JS, et al. Low-grade systemic inflammation and the development of type 2 diabetes: the atherosclerosis risk in communities study. Diabetes 2003;52:1799–805.
52. Visser M, Kritchevsky SB, Goodpaster BH, et al. Leg muscle mass and composition in relation to lower extremity performance in men and women aged 70 to 79: the health, aging and body composition study. J Am Geriatr Soc 2002;50: 897–904.
53. Kalyani RR, Tian J, Xue QL, et al. Hyperglycemia and incidence of frailty and lower extremity mobility limitations in older women. J Am Geriatr Soc 2012;60: 1701–7.
54. Volpato S, Blaum C, Resnick H, et al, Women's Health and Aging Study. Comorbidities and impairments explaining the association between diabetes and lower extremity disability: the Women's Health and Aging Study. Diabetes Care 2002;25:678–83.
55. Ko SU, Stenholm S, Chia CW, et al. Gait pattern alterations in older adults associated with type 2 diabetes in the absence of peripheral neuropathy—results from the Baltimore Longitudinal Study of Aging. Gait Posture 2011;34:548–52.
56. Kuo HK, Leveille SG, Yen CJ, et al. Exploring how peak leg power and usual gait speed are linked to late-life disability: data from the National Health and Nutrition Examination Survey (NHANES), 1999-2002. Am J Phys Med Rehabil 2006;85: 650–8.
57. De Rekeneire N, Resnick HE, Schwartz AV, et al, Health, Aging, and Body Composition Study. Diabetes is associated with subclinical functional limitation in nondisabled older individuals: the Health, Aging, and Body Composition study. Diabetes Care 2003;26:3257–63.
58. Sinclair AJ, Conroy SP, Bayer AJ. Impact of diabetes on physical function in older people. Diabetes Care 2008;31:233–5.
59. Gregg EW, Beckles GL, Williamson DF, et al. Diabetes and physical disability among older U.S. adults. Diabetes Care 2000;23:1272–7.
60. Volpato S, Ferrucci L, Blaum C, et al. Progression of lower-extremity disability in older women with diabetes: the Women's Health and Aging Study. Diabetes Care 2003;26:70–5.
61. Ryerson B, Tierney EF, Thompson TJ, et al. Excess physical limitations among adults with diabetes in the U.S. population, 1997-1999. Diabetes Care 2003; 26:206–10.
62. Egede LE. Diabetes, major depression, and functional disability among U.S. adults. Diabetes Care 2004;27:421–8.
63. Maty SC, Fried LP, Volpato S, et al. Patterns of disability related to diabetes mellitus in older women. J Gerontol A Biol Sci Med Sci 2004;59:148–53.
64. Kalyani RR, Saudek CD, Brancati FL, et al. The Association of Diabetes, Comorbidities, and Hemoglobin A1c with Functional Disability in Older Adults: results from the National Health and Nutrition Examination Survey (NHANES), 1999-2006. Diabetes Care 2010;33:1055–60.
65. Bossoni S, Mazziotti G, Gazzaruso C, et al. Relationship between instrumental activities of daily living and blood glucose control in elderly subjects with type 2 diabetes. Age Ageing 2008;37:222–5.
66. Boyd CM, Xue QL, Simpson CF, et al. Frailty, hospitalization, and progression of disability in a cohort of disabled older women. Am J Med 2005;118:1225–31.
67. Fried LP, Tangen CM, Walston J, et al, Cardiovascular Health Study. Frailty in older adults: evidence for a phenotype. J Gerontol A Biol Sci Med Sci 2001; 56:M146–56.

68. Bandeen-Roche K, Xue QL, Ferrucci L, et al. Phenotype of frailty: characterization in the women's health and aging studies. J Gerontol A Biol Sci Med Sci 2006;61:262–6.
69. Wolinsky FD, Callahan CM, Fitzgerald JF, et al. Changes in functional status and the risks of subsequent nursing home placement and death. J Gerontol 1993; 48:S94–101.
70. Blaum CS, Xue QL, Tian J, et al. Is hyperglycemia associated with frailty status in older women? J Am Geriatr Soc 2009;57:840–7.
71. Walston J, McBurnie MA, Newman A, et al, Cardiovascular Health Study. Frailty and activation of the inflammation and coagulation systems with and without clinical comorbidities: results from the Cardiovascular Health Study. Arch Intern Med 2002;162:2333–41.
72. Kalyani RR, Varadhan R, Weiss CO, et al. Frailty status and altered glucose-insulin dynamics. J Gerontol A Biol Sci Med Sci 2012;67:1300–6.
73. Serra-Prat M, Palomera E, Clave P, et al. Effect of age and frailty on ghrelin and cholecystokinin responses to a meal test. Am J Clin Nutr 2009;89:1410–7.
74. Barzilay JI, Blaum C, Moore T, et al. Insulin resistance and inflammation as precursors of frailty: the Cardiovascular Health Study. Arch Intern Med 2007;167: 635–41.
75. Senn JJ, Klover PJ, Nowak IA, et al. IL-6 induces cellular insulin resistance in hepatocytes. Diabetes 2002;51:3391–9.
76. Lee CC, Adler AI, Sandhu MS, et al. Association of C-reactive protein with type 2 diabetes: prospective analysis and meta-analysis. Diabetologia 2009;52:1040–7.
77. Barbieri M, Ferrucci L, Ragno E, et al. Chronic inflammation and the effect of IGF-I on muscle strength and power in older persons. Am J Physiol Endocrinol Metab 2003;284:E481–7.
78. Hubbard RE, Lang IA, Llewellyn DJ, et al. Frailty, body mass index, and abdominal obesity in older people. J Gerontol A Biol Sci Med Sci 2010;65:377–81.
79. Newman AB, Gottdiener JS, Mcburnie MA, et al, Cardiovascular Health Study Research Group. Associations of subclinical cardiovascular disease with frailty. J Gerontol A Biol Sci Med Sci 2001;56:M158–66.
80. Fried LP, Xue QL, Cappola AR, et al. Nonlinear multisystem physiological dysregulation associated with frailty in older women: implications for etiology and treatment. J Gerontol A Biol Sci Med Sci 2009;64:1049–57.
81. Fried TR, Bradley EH, Williams CS, et al. Functional disability and health care expenditures for older persons. Arch Intern Med 2001;161:2602–7.
82. Janssen I, Shepard DS, Katzmarzyk PT, et al. The healthcare costs of sarcopenia in the United States. J Am Geriatr Soc 2004;52:80–5.
83. Newman AB, Kupelian V, Visser M, et al. Strength, but not muscle mass, is associated with mortality in the health, aging and body composition study cohort. J Gerontol A Biol Sci Med Sci 2006;61:72–7.
84. Emerging Risk Factors Collaboration, Seshasai SR, Kaptoge S, Thompson A, et al. Diabetes mellitus, fasting glucose, and risk of cause-specific death. N Engl J Med 2011;364:829–41.
85. Metter EJ, Windham BG, Maggio M, et al. Glucose and insulin measurements from the oral glucose tolerance test and mortality prediction. Diabetes Care 2008;31:1026–30.
86. Sorkin JD, Muller DC, Fleg JL, et al. The relation of fasting and 2-h postchallenge plasma glucose concentrations to mortality: data from the Baltimore Longitudinal Study of Aging with a critical review of the literature. Diabetes Care 2005;28:2626–32.

87. Selvin E, Steffes MW, Zhu H, et al. Glycated hemoglobin, diabetes, and cardiovascular risk in nondiabetic adults. N Engl J Med 2010;362:800–11.
88. Huang ES, Liu JY, Moffet HH, et al. Glycemic control, complications, and death in older diabetic patients: the diabetes and aging study. Diabetes Care 2011;34: 1329–36.
89. Kuhlow D, Florian S, von Figura G, et al. Telomerase deficiency impairs glucose metabolism and insulin secretion. Aging (Albany NY) 2010;2:650–8.
90. UK Prospective Diabetes Study (UKPDS) Group. Intensive blood-glucose control with sulphonylureas or insulin compared with conventional treatment and risk of complications in patients with type 2 diabetes (UKPDS 33). Lancet 1998;352:837–53.
91. Finucane TE. "Tight control" in geriatrics: the emperor wears a thong. J Am Geriatr Soc 2012;60:1571–5.
92. Action to Control Cardiovascular Risk in Diabetes Study Group, Gerstein HC, Miller ME, et al. Effects of intensive glucose lowering in type 2 diabetes. N Engl J Med 2008;358:2545–59.
93. Patel A, MacMahon S, Chalmers J, et al, ADVANCE Collaborative Group. Intensive blood glucose control and vascular outcomes in patients with type 2 diabetes. N Engl J Med 2008;358:2560–72.
94. Duckworth W, Abraira C, Moritz T, et al. Glucose control and vascular complications in veterans with type 2 diabetes. N Engl J Med 2009;360:129–39.
95. Durso SC. Using clinical guidelines designed for older adults with diabetes mellitus and complex health status. JAMA 2006;295:1935–40.
96. Brown AF, Mangione CM, Saliba D, et al. Guidelines for improving the care of the older person with diabetes mellitus. J Am Geriatr Soc 2003;51:S265–80.
97. Knowler WC, Barrett-Connor E, Fowler SE, et al, Diabetes Prevention Program Research Group. Reduction in the incidence of type 2 diabetes with lifestyle intervention or metformin. N Engl J Med 2002;346:393–403.
98. Wing RR, Hamman RF, Bray GA, et al, Diabetes Prevention Program Research Group. Achieving weight and activity goals among diabetes prevention program lifestyle participants. Obes Res 2004;12:1426–34.
99. Shin YK, Cong WN, Cai H, et al. Age-related changes in mouse taste bud morphology, hormone expression, and taste responsivity. J Gerontol A Biol Sci Med Sci 2012;67:336–44.
100. Colberg SR, Sigal RJ, Fernhall B, et al, American College of Sports Medicine, American Diabetes Association. Exercise and type 2 diabetes: the American College of Sports Medicine and the American Diabetes Association: joint position statement executive summary. Diabetes Care 2010;33:2692–6.
101. McGuire EA, Tobin JD, Berman M, et al. Kinetics of native insulin in diabetic, obese, and aged men. Diabetes 1979;28:110–20.
102. Fink RI, Revers RR, Kolterman OG, et al. The metabolic clearance of insulin and the feedback inhibition of insulin secretion are altered with aging. Diabetes 1985;34:275–80.
103. Mooradian AD. Special considerations with insulin therapy in older adults with diabetes mellitus. Drugs Aging 2011;28:429–38.
104. Pani LN, Korenda L, Meigs JB, et al. Effect of aging on A1C levels in individuals without diabetes: evidence from the Framingham Offspring Study and the National Health and Nutrition Examination Survey 2001-2004. Diabetes Care 2008;31:1991–6.

Complications of Diabetes Therapy

Sarah D. Corathers, MD[a,b],*, Shawn Peavie, DO[b], Marzieh Salehi, MD, MS[b]

KEYWORDS

- Diabetes • Treatment complications • Cardiovascular outcomes • β-cell function

KEY POINTS

- The increasing incidence of diabetes over the last few decades, along with the increased pace of new antidiabetic drug development, calls for a better understanding of the efficacy, mechanism of action, and safety of these drugs.
- Current strategies for the treatment of type 2 diabetes mellitus promote the achievement of target glucose levels to minimize microvascular and macrovascular complications.
- Maintaining the glycemic control over time is a significant challenge, owing to the progressive nature of diabetes as a result of declining β-cell function.
- Given the chronic nature of diabetes management, efficacy must be balanced against side effects to achieve a tolerable long-term regimen.
- Individualized therapy started at an earlier stage of disease guided by the principle of "do not harm" seems to be essential in the patient-centric, shared decision-making model of diabetes care.

INTRODUCTION AND BACKGROUND

Type 2 diabetes mellitus (T2DM) is increasingly prevalent in the United States population and is associated with significant morbidity, mortality, and rising health care costs. Microvascular[1,2] and, to a lesser extent, macrovascular[3,4] complications are recognized to result from uncontrolled hyperglycemia. However, intensive therapy to achieve normal glucose levels is not without risk, as demonstrated by increased rates of hypoglycemia, weight gain, and all-cause mortality rates in the intensive treatment arm of the ACCORD (Action to Control Cardiovascular Risk in Diabetes)

This article originally appeared in Endocrinology and Metabolism Clinics of North America, Volume 42, Issue 4, December 2013.

Conflict of Interest: The authors do not have any conflict of interest to disclose.

[a] Division of Endocrinology, Cincinnati Children's Hospital Medical Center, 3333 Burnet Avenue, MLC 7012, Cincinnati, OH 45229, USA; [b] Division of Endocrinology, University of Cincinnati Medical Center, 260 Stetson, Suite 4200, Cincinnati, OH 45229, USA

* Corresponding author. Division of Endocrinology, Cincinnati Children's Hospital Medical Center, 3333 Burnet Avenue, MLC 7012, Cincinnati, OH 45229.

E-mail address: Sarah.corathers@cchmc.org

trial.[5] In addition, observational studies indicate that the presence of diabetes increases the risk of other comorbidities such as fracture[6] and certain cancers,[7,8] and treatment choice may affect risk. Thus, in an effort to maintain glucose control, the clinician encounters a complex interplay of primary disease management while simultaneously seeking to avoid complications associated with glucose lowering. Given the chronic nature of diabetes management, efficacy must be balanced against side effects to achieve a tolerable long-term regimen. The goal of this review is to identify complications of non-insulin treatment of diabetes. The major classes of medication are reviewed with special attention given to patient considerations, mechanism of action, effect on weight, and cardiovascular outcomes, and additional class-specific side effects including effects on bone. In addition, effects on β-cell function are highlighted. Hypoglycemia is a recognized feature of many diabetes treatment modalities, and is not covered in depth in this article.

INSULIN SENSITIZERS

The 2 classes of drugs categorized as insulin sensitizers are biguanides (metformin) and thiazolidinediones (rosiglitazone and pioglitazone).

Biguanides

Indications and patient considerations

Metformin remains the primary drug within the class of biguanides in current use, and remains the preferred initial agent for T2DM based on a recent joint statement by the American Diabetes Association (ADA) and the European Association for the Study of Diabetes (EASD) as well as the American Association of Clinical Endocrinologists (AACE).[9–11] Metformin was approved by the Food and Drug Administration (FDA) for use in the United States in 1994 for the treatment of T2DM in adults, with a pediatric indication for children older than 10 years. Concern about risk for lactic acidosis potentiated by decreased clearance of drug led to a black-box warning for use within specific populations including those with renal or hepatic impairment, acute congestive heart failure, sepsis, dehydration, and excessive alcohol intake. In addition, it is recommended that therapy be temporarily discontinued before the administration of intravascular radiocontrast agents or surgical procedures, because of the potential for dehydration and/or kidney injury.

Mechanism of action, efficacy, and kinetics

Metformin (Glucophage) reduces fasting plasma glucose and decreases hemoglobin A_{1c} (HbA1c) by approximately 1.0%.[12,13] Although the precise mechanism of action remains uncertain, the glycemic reducing effect of metformin is primarily attributed to inhibition of hepatic glucose production and, possibly, to improved peripheral insulin sensitivity.[12,14,15] Theories for the antihyperglycemic action of metformin include inhibition of key enzymes in gluconeogenesis,[15–18] direct action on the insulin receptor,[19] or modulation of components of the incretin axis.[20] The mean $t_{1/2}$ of the standard formulation is 5 hours; a sustained-release once-daily formulation is also available. Metformin is excreted unchanged in the urine, and renal clearance is the primary form of elimination of the drug.[21]

Effects on weight, cardiovascular outcomes, and risk of lactic acidosis

In the DPP (Diabetes Prevention Program) study, 3234 participants from 27 clinics in the United States were enrolled between 1996 and 1999 and randomly assigned to metformin (n = 1073) or placebo (n = 1082) treatment. Participants randomized to metformin experienced an average weight loss of 2 kg[22] that was maintained following a 7- to 8-year open-label extension.[23] Among patients with established T2DM, reported weight benefits of metformin monotherapy ranged from a 0.6- to 2.9-kg reduction in treatment-naïve patients followed for up to 5 years.[24] Combination treatment with metformin has been also observed to mitigate weight gain associated with other agents such as sulfonylurea or thiazolidinediones.[12,24,25]

In the 1970s phenformin, an older member of the biguanide class, was removed from the market after 306 case reports of severe lactic acidosis in patients with congestive heart failure (CHF).[26] Subsequently, CHF was labeled as a contraindication to biguanide therapy in general, although the reported incidence with metformin therapy remained extremely low.[27,28] In fact, among a nested case-control series of more than 50,000 patients with T2DM, overall incidence of lactic acidosis was rare, but occurred more often in those treated with sulfonylurea (4.8 cases per 100,000 patient-years of treatment) than those in the metformin group (3.3 cases per 100,000 patient-years of treatment).[29] In several large observational studies in the United States and United Kingdom of patients with CHF, treatment with metformin had no documented events of lactic acidosis.[26,28,30] A recent meta-analysis of more than 30 clinical trials confirmed the reduction of cardiovascular mortality by metformin in comparison with any other oral diabetes agent or placebo,[31,32] suggesting that not only is metformin safe in this population, it is likely beneficial. In 2005, the FDA removed the CHF contraindication from the product labeling, although a cautionary black-box warning remains for the increased risk of lactic acidosis among patients with concurrent CHF.[26] Following the recent benefit-risk analysis there are calls for urgent reassessment of the relative contraindications of metformin use, given the paucity of data supporting the incidence of lactic acidosis and the likelihood of benefit on glucose control and mortality.[33]

Effects on bone and other side effects
Animal studies indicate that metformin may have a positive effect on osteoblast differentiation and a negative effect on osteoclast differentiation and bone loss.[6] Studies of the safety and efficacy of metformin monotherapy versus a rosiglitazone/metformin combination demonstrated improved glycemic control in the combination group but a significant reduction in lumbar bone mineral density (BMD) in comparison with the metformin monotherapy group.[34] Moreover, studies in rodent models have shown that coadministration of metformin and rosiglitazone mitigates the adverse effects of rosiglitazone on bone.[35] However, data on reduction of fracture risk in patients with T2DM treated with metformin have been inconsistent.[6]

In United States clinical trials approximately 4% of patients were unable to continue metformin because of adverse effects. The most common side effect of metformin is gastrointestinal (GI), which may be transient in nature and can often be avoided with gradual dose titration and taking the drug with meals.[14] In the DPP trial, through year 4 of analysis GI symptoms were significantly more common among the metformin-treated than the placebo participants (28% vs 16%). Nonserious adverse events during the DPP were uncommon and similar in the treatment and placebo groups. There were no reported serious adverse events of lactic acidosis during the nearly 18,000 patient-years of follow-up.[36] Additional documented side effects of metformin are rare, but include taste disturbance, decreased absorption of vitamin B_{12} (<1 in 10,000) and rashes.[14,26] A favorable association between metformin and a lower risk of cancer among patients with T2DM has been observed. Investigation into the anticancer properties and underlying mechanism of this effect is an area of active ongoing research.[37–40]

Thiazolidinediones

Indications and patient considerations

Pioglitazone (Actos) and rosiglitazone (Avandia) are thiazolidinedione (TZD) drugs approved by the FDA for the treatment of T2DM. Caution is advised for use with CHF (New York Heart Association [NYHA] class I or II), and both drugs are contraindicated in advanced CHF (NYHA class III or IV). Despite demonstrated glycemic efficacy and improved insulin sensitivity, because of troublesome side effects including weight gain and fluid retention, the ADA consensus statement favors metformin over TZD for first-line treatment of impaired glucose tolerance (IGT) or impaired fasting glucose (IFG).[41]

Mechanism of action, efficacy, and kinetics

The TZDs are synthetic ligands for peroxisome proliferative-activated receptor gamma (PPARγ), and are potent insulin sensitizers in muscle, liver, and adipocytes.[42–44] Rosiglitazone and pioglitazone bind to PPARγ, modulate the transcription of insulin-sensitive genes involved in the control of glucose and lipid metabolism,[26] and may have important effects on β cells. Because TZDs both improve insulin sensitivity and preserve β-cell function, they are very effective at preventing progression of IGT to T2DM and maintaining durable HbA1c reduction.[45] TZDs are extensively metabolized in the liver by the cytochrome P450 enzyme CYP2C8 and are eliminated through the feces.[46,47] Dose adjustment of TZDs is not required for geriatric patients, or those with renal or mild hepatic impairment. However, monitoring is recommended for patients with known hepatic toxicity (alanine aminotransferase 3 time the upper limit of the reference range) or those taking concurrent strong CYP2C8 inhibitors such as gemfibrozil.

Effects on weight and cardiovascular outcomes

Weight gain and fluid retention with associated edema are well-recognized side effects of TZDs.[24,26,48–50] Initiation of TZD in the intensive treatment arm of the ACCORD trial has been described as a predominant medication-related determinant of weight gain. Patients who received combination therapy of TZD with insulin had a weight gain of 4.6 to 5.3 kg at 2 years.[51] TZD-associated weight gain has been attributed to increased uptake of fatty acids and enhanced adipogenic capacity elicited by PPARγ activation of white adipose tissue.[48]

Within 2 years of approval by the FDA, reports of increased risk of heart failure associated with rosiglitazone began surfacing[52] and by 2002, the FDA added a precaution regarding rosiglitazone-induced heart failure followed by a more stringent "restricted access program" designation in 2011 after a meta-analysis of 42 clinical trials that compared rosiglitazone with placebo, which found a statistically significant increased risk of myocardial infarction in the rosiglitazone-treated group.[53,54] The FDA is scheduled to review a readjudication of the RECORD (Rosiglitazone Evaluated for Cardiovascular Outcomes and Regulation of Diabetes) trial findings in June 2013.

Evidence for a strong association with heart failure appears to be a class effect of TZDs.[55–57] However, in contrast to rosiglitazone, meta-analyses of pioglitazone suggest the possibility of ischemic cardiovascular benefit and overall reduction in mortality despite an increase in serious heart failure.[57] Systemic review and meta-analysis of 16 observational studies representing more than 800,000 TZD users reports that compared with pioglitazone, rosiglitazone is associated with a significantly increased risk of myocardial infarction (pooled odds ratio 1.2, 95% confidence interval [CI] 1.07–1.24), CHF (odds ratio 1.2, 95% CI 1.14–1.31) and overall mortality (odds ratio 1.1, 95% CI 1.09–1.20). The investigators calculate that the use of rosiglitazone would result in an annual number needed to harm (NNH) of 587 or an excess of 170 myocardial infarctions for every 100,000 patients who received rosiglitazone over pioglitazone. Use of rosiglitazone would result in an NNH of 154 for CHF, which equates to 649 excess cases for every 100,000 patients.[55]

Effects on bone and other side effects

PPARγ expression and the mechanism by which TZDs affect bone are complex and include antiosteoblastic, proadipocytic, and proosteoclastic activities. Multiple clinical studies in patients with T2DM and polycystic ovarian syndrome, and in postmenopausal nondiabetic women indicate that both rosiglitazone and pioglitazone decrease BMD and change bone markers.[6] Increased risk of fracture was demonstrated in posttrial analysis from ADOPT (A Diabetes Outcome Progression Trial).[58] The study was a randomized, double-blind controlled trial of 4600 individuals, designed to compare time to failure of monotherapy (defined as fasting plasma glucose >180 mg/dL) in prediabetic individuals randomly assigned to treatment with either rosiglitazone, metformin, or glyburide. Posttrial analysis of fracture rates, time to first fracture, and fracture location were analyzed after a median of 4 years of treatment. In men, there was no increased risk of fracture. However, among both premenopausal and postmenopausal women treated with rosiglitazone, the cumulative incidence of fractures was 15.1% (95% CI 11.2–19.1), whereas it was only 7.3% (95% CI 4.4–10.1) in the metformin group and 7.7% (95% CI 3.7–11.7) in the glyburide group, representing a hazard ratio of 1.8 versus 2.1 for rosiglitazone versus other therapies.[59] Subsequent meta-analysis of 10 randomized controlled trials and 2 observational studies, reflecting more than 40,000 participants, confirmed a 2-fold increased risk of fractures in women exposed to long-term TZD use, but not in men.[60] Other large-scale studies conducted in Canada, the United Kingdom, and the United States support that fracture risk is strongly associated with age and duration of TZD treatment, independent of gender. In summary, there is evidence that TZDs exert a negative effect on bone with increased risk of fracture in the following subpopulations: those with a history of prior fracture, longer duration of TZD treatment, older age, and, possibly, female predominance.[6]

Following conflicting reports, in 2012 a systematic review and meta-analysis was performed on the available studies that reported bladder cancer among adults taking either pioglitazone or rosiglitazone. In sum, a total of 3643 patients had newly diagnosed bladder cancer, for an overall incidence of 53.1 per 100,000 patient-years. All 5 studies assessing pioglitazone demonstrated an elevated risk of bladder cancer associated with pioglitazone use, whereas in the 3 studies reporting incidence of bladder cancer among rosiglitazone users, no association was found. The investigators concluded that based on a pooled estimate of 1.7 million individuals there is evidence of an increased risk of bladder cancer with pioglitazone but not with rosiglitazone.[61]

SECRETAGOGUES

Sulfonylureas and meglitinides, lower glucose levels by stimulating insulin secretion.

Sulfonylureas

Indications and patient considerations

Sulfonylureas are approved by the FDA for the treatment of T2DM in adults. In addition, clinical efficacy has been demonstrated in single-gene diabetes (HNF1A MODY) and permanent neonatal diabetes associated with the KCNJ11 and ABCC9 genes.[62] Because of the risk for hypoglycemia, sulfonylureas should be used with caution in elderly, debilitated, or malnourished patients, or in patients with renal or hepatic insufficiency. In these patients the initial dosing, dose increments, and maintenance dosage should be conservative.

Mechanism of action, efficacy, and kinetics

Sulfonylureas stimulate the release of insulin secretion by binding to the sulfonylurea receptor (SUR-1), a component of the adenosine triphosphate (ATP)-sensitive potassium channel (K_{ATP}) expressed in the pancreatic β cells,[63] leading to calcium influx and increased responsiveness of β cells to glucose and nonglucose stimuli. These drugs lower HbA1c levels by 1% to 2%,[64] and their glycemic effect is dependent on residual β-cell function. Although the therapeutic mechanism of all sulfonylureas is similar, first-generation sulfonylureas, for example, tolbutamide (Oranase) and chlorpropamide (Diabinase), have significantly lower affinity for the SUR receptor than do second-generation sulfonylureas such as glyburide (Micronase), glipizide (Glucotrol), and glimepiride (Amaryl). This difference accounts for the greater potency and efficacy of the second-generation drugs. Most sulfonylureas are transformed by cytochrome P450 in the liver to inactive metabolites; thus, their circulatory levels can be affected by any factors modifying the cytochrome P450 system.[65] Renal excretion is important for 2 drugs in this category, glyburide and chlorpropamide, therefore they should be used with caution in patients with renal impairment.[66]

Effects on weight and cardiovascular outcomes

Weight gain of 1.5 to 2.0 kg is common in the first year following initiation of sulfonylurea therapy, and typically levels off thereafter.[2,67,68] At present, all sulfonylureas carry an FDA-required warning about the increased risk of cardiovascular death. This decision was based in part on findings from the UGDP (University Group Diabetes Program) trial, in which diabetic patients treated with tolbutamide, a first-generation sulfonylurea, experienced higher cardiovascular mortality compared with insulin or placebo.[69] However, findings from the UKPDS (United Kingdom Prospective Diabetes Study) did not reveal an increased risk of cardiovascular complications over 10 years of follow-up in patients with T2DM treated with sulfonylurea.[2,70,71] Experimentally, sulfonylureas that bind to myocardial K_{ATP} channels have been shown to block the beneficial effects of ischemic preconditioning, which refers to a cardioprotective phenomenon recognized to reduce infarct size, augment postischemic function, and prevent arrhythmias.[71,72] Newer sulfonylureas, such as gliclazide (Diamicron) or glimepiride, are exclusively pancreatic β-cell specific and might offer advantages over older agents. Among sulfonylurea-treated patients in a French registry of acute myocardial infarction, in-hospital mortality was significantly lower in patients receiving pancreatic cell–specific sulfonylureas (gliclazide or glimepiride) (2.7%), compared with glyburide (7.5%). Arrhythmias and ischemic complications were also markedly less frequent in patients receiving gliclazide/glimepiride (11% vs 18%).[73] Thus, tissue-specific effects of sulfonylureas may account for the apparent conflict of beneficial and deleterious cardiovascular outcomes reported in previous studies.

Effects on bone and other adverse effects

Results from ADOPT did not indicate adverse effects of these compounds on bone mass or fracture risk.[59] Beyond the most common side effects of hypoglycemia, other adverse effects include nausea, abdominal discomfort, headache, hypersensitivity, skin reactions (including photosensitivity), and abnormal liver function tests. Differential tissue specificity of particular sulfonylureas outside the pancreas could account for variability in complications related to these drugs. Unique to chlorpropamide is water retention and potential for hyponatremia mediated through secretion of antidiuretic hormone.[66,74] In addition, chlorpropamide can cause an unpleasant flushing reaction after alcohol ingestion by inhibiting the metabolism of acetaldehyde.[75]

Meglitinides

Indications and patient considerations
Meglitinide analogues, nateglinide (Starlix) and repaglinide (Prandin), are approved for the treatment of T2DM in adults. Caution is recommended for moderate to severe hepatic impairment, and dose adjustment is indicated for creatinine clearance of less than 20 to 40 mL/min for repaglinide.

Mechanism of action, efficacy, and kinetics
Similar to sulfonylureas, meglitinides stimulate insulin release by inhibiting K_{ATP} channels, causing membrane depolarization, increased intracellular calcium, and insulin exocytosis. However, meglitinides have a distinct binding site of the β-cell membrane.[76] Although both drugs are rapid acting,[77] nateglinide dissociates from the receptor 90 times faster than repaglinide, indicating a very short on-and-off effect on insulin release. Nateglinide is hepatically cleared, with approximately 65% excreted in the bile and feces and 35% in the urine.[78] Repaglinide is metabolized by cytochrome P450 CYP3A4, with 90% excreted in bile and less than 10% in urine. Substances that inhibit CYP3A4 (eg, ketoconazole, steroids) may reduce repaglinide clearance, whereas drugs that induce CYP3A4 (eg, rifampin, carbamazepine) may accelerate repaglinide metabolism.[76] The efficacy of meglitinide monotherapy is similar to that of the sulfonylureas.[79–81] Repaglinide reduces HbA1c values by 0.1% to 2.1%, and nateglinide reduces HbA1c values by 0.2% to 0.6%.[82]

Effects on weight and cardiovascular outcomes
A Cochrane review of meglitinide analogues reports a range of weight gain from 0.7 to 2.1 kg across several trials.[82] To date, there have been no reported significant differences in blood pressure or lipid profiles among patients treated with meglitinide.[83] Because the mechanism of action of meglitinides affects the ATP-dependent potassium channels, it is possible that meglitinide analogues may have an association with poorer outcomes following a myocardial infarction, similar to sulfonylureas[73]; however, studies of long-term cardiovascular outcomes of meglitinides are lacking.

Other side effects or known complications of treatment
Similar to sulfonylureas, the most common side effect of meglitinides is mild hypoglycemia. Meglitinides have been associated with several other nonspecific side effects including dizziness, diarrhea, constipation, arthralgias, headache, and cough.[82,84,85]

α-GLUCOSIDASE INHIBITORS
Indications and Patient Considerations

The α-glucosidase inhibitors (AGI), acarbose (Precose), miglitol (Glyset), and voglibose (Voglib), are indicated for treatment of adults with T2DM. The class is contraindicated in patients with cirrhosis, inflammatory bowel disease, colonic ulceration, intestinal obstruction, or predisposition to obstruction and diabetic ketoacidosis.

Mechanism of Action, Efficacy, and Kinetics

Relative to placebo, both acarbose and miglitol have demonstrated reduction of HbA1c to 0.5% to 0.8%.[86] AGIs lower glucose levels through reversible, competitive inhibition of pancreatic α-amylase and membrane-bound intestinal α-glucoside hydrolyases. These enzymes inhibit the conversion of complex polysaccharide carbohydrates into monosaccharides, which slows the absorption of glucose and improves postprandial glucose levels.[87] In addition, following treatment with voglibose there is a measureable increase of endogenous glucagon-like peptide[88] that may further facilitate glucose-lowering effects. Acarbose has a short $t_{1/2}$ of 2 hours; thus, to be effective it must be dosed at least 3 times daily with meals. Acarbose is metabolized within the GI tract by digestive enzymes and intestinal bacteria. The fraction that is absorbed intact is excreted by the kidneys. Therefore, use with renal impairment (creatinine clearance <25 mL/min) is not recommended for acarbose or miglitol because of the risk for increased plasma concentrations of the drug; however, voglibose is minimally excreted in the urine and therefore dose adjustment is not required. Elevated liver transaminases have been reported, and the package insert recommends reduced doses or withdrawal of treatment if abnormalities of liver enzymes develop.

Effects on Body Weight and Cardiovascular Outcomes

Meta-analysis of 41 randomized controlled trials and systematic review confirm that acarbose and miglitol are weight neutral.[24] The mode of action of acarbose is to diminish glucose and insulin response to meal ingestion; and lower insulin levels are proposed to explain weight neutrality.[89]

Acarbose therapy has been shown to have a beneficial effect in comparison with placebo in preventing progression of an increase in carotid intimal wall thickness in patients with established coronary artery disease and either IGT or established T2DM,[90] as well as favorable effect on the level of low-density lipoprotein (LDL) and triglyceride.[91] Cardiovascular outcomes were the primary end point of the multicenter, international, double-blind, randomized controlled STOP-NIDDM (Study to Prevent Non Insulin Dependent Diabetes Mellitus) trial, in which 1429 patients with IGT were randomized to either placebo or acarbose 100 mg 3 times daily, and followed for a mean of 3.3 years. At the end of the study, acarbose use was associated with 49% relative risk reduction in combined cardiovascular events (coronary heart disease, cardiovascular death, CHF, cerebrovascular event, peripheral vascular disease, and hypertension >140/90 mm Hg; hazard ratio [HR] 0.51, 95% CI 0.28%–0.95%; 2.5% absolute risk reduction). The major reduction was in the risk of myocardial infarction and development of hypertension.[92]

Other Side Effects

Fermentation of an increased amount of undigested carbohydrate by bacteria in the colon accounts for the common observed side effects of abdominal pain, diarrhea, and flatulence.[91] Incidence of GI side effects varies widely across international trials. In a surveillance study of 6142 patients in the United States, intolerance was 37%, compared with 13.4% of 27,803 patients from Germany and just 2% of 14,418 patients in China and other Asian countries enrolled in postmarketing studies. The difference may in part be due to dose and titration schedules; however, given the mechanism of action it is likely that nutritional factors contribute as well. Diets higher in fiber are associated with a lower incidence of side effects. Incidence of side effects has been shown to be dose dependent, and slow titration of dose is recommended to limit the onset of unpleasant side effects.[89] Elevation of hepatic enzymes has been reported, as has one case of fulminant hepatitis with a fatal outcome. It is recommended to monitor patients with liver disease and to adjust dose or discontinue the dosing if necessary.

GLUCAGON-LIKE PEPTIDE 1–BASED DRUGS

Glucagon-like peptide 1 (GLP-1) is a gut hormone secreted in response to nutrient ingestion, which regulates postprandial glucose homeostasis. Once secreted into the circulation, GLP-1 is metabolized rapidly to inactive compounds by the action of ubiquitous enzyme dipeptidyl-peptidase 4 (DPP-4), leading to a plasma $t_{1/2}$ of 1 to 2 minutes.[93] Two classes of drugs in this category, GLP-1 receptor (GLP-1r) agonists and DPP-4 inhibitors, have been developed using strategies to bypass or block DPP-4 action, leading to compounds with half-lives longer than native GLP-1 or causing higher concentrations of native GLP-1 levels, respectively.

Indications and Patient Considerations

Exenatide (Byetta) was the first GLP-1r agonist to be approved in the United States in 2005, and sitagliptin (Januvia) the first DPP-4 inhibitor approved a year later. To date, liraglutide (Victoza) and exenatide long-acting release (LAR; Bydureon) from the class of GLP-1r agonists, and saxagliptin (Onglyza), linagliptin (Tradjenta), and alogliptin (Nesina) from the class of DPP-4 inhibitors, have been approved for the treatment of T2DM as an add-on to metformin, thiazolidinediones, sulfonylureas, and basal insulin, or a combination of these drugs. These drugs were recommended as second-line agents after metformin in the recent joint statement by the ADA/ESD[9] because of the weight neutrality with DPP-4 inhibitors or weight loss with GLP-1r agonist therapy, as well as the lack of hypoglycemia with both classes of drugs. DPP-4 inhibitors, unlike the injectable GLP-1r agonists, are administered orally, which might be preferred by patients. Caution is advised for use with concurrent renal or hepatic impairment. GLP-1r agonists are contraindicated in patients with prior history of or current pancreatitis, and individual or family history of medullary thyroid cancer.

Mechanism of Action, Efficacy, and Kinetics

GLP-1 actions are mediated by binding to a specific GLP-1 receptor that is expressed on β cells, along with many other cells such as gastric and small intestinal mucosal cells, cardiac myocytes, neurons in some brain regions, and the vagus nerve.[94,95] Administration of GLP-1 or GLP-1r agonists improves glycemia by enhancing insulin response,[96,97] inhibiting glucagon release from pancreatic α cells,[96] delaying gastric emptying,[98–100] inducing satiety,[101] and lowering hepatic glucose production.[102] The noninsulin effects of GLP-1 are equally essential in glycemic control, as GLP-1 infusion has been shown to normalize hyperglycemia in patients with type 1 diabetes mellitus (T1DM) and no residual β-cell function,[103,104] even though the use of these compounds in T1DM has not been approved. Although DPP-4 inhibitors share the insulin and glucagon effect of GLP-1r agonists, they have a trivial effect on gastric emptying.[105]

Treatment with GLP-1r agonists leads to HbA1c reduction of 1.1% to 1.6% compared with 0.6% to 1.1% with DPP-4 inhibitors; the greatest efficacy on HbA1c and fasting plasma glucose among GLP-1r agonists was reported with long-acting agents, liraglutide (once a day) and exenatide LAR once weekly, in comparison with short-acting drugs (twice a day). Available GLP-1r agonists are excreted by the kidney; therefore, their use is not recommended in the setting of severe renal impairment. In patients with moderate renal impairment, short-acting exenatide can be used with careful optimization of the dose, but there are not enough data to support the use of long-acting GLP-1r agonists. In hepatic impairment, lack of data for the use of liraglutide limits its utility, but dose adjustment is not necessary for exenatide therapy. DPP-4 inhibitors and their metabolites have distinctive pharmacokinetic properties leading to drug-specific adverse effects in this class of drugs. Saxagliptin is excreted through renal and hepatic clearance mechanisms, whereas sitagliptin is excreted mainly through renal excretion. Therefore, dose adjustment is necessary in the setting of both moderate and severe renal impairment.[106,107] By contrast, linagliptin is excreted mostly in feces through enterohepatic circulation, and requires no dose adjustment for renal impairment.[106,108] Evidence regarding the use of DPP-4 inhibitors in severe hepatic failure is lacking.

Effects of Treatment on Weight and Cardiovascular Outcomes

GLP-1r agonist therapy results in a weight reduction of greater than 2 kg, whereas DPP-4 inhibitors are weight neutral.[109] Data on long-term effects of GLP-1 based drugs on cardiovascular outcomes are lacking, although these drugs may have beneficial effects on surrogate markers of cardiovascular disease. The evidence suggests that GLP-1r agonists improve systolic blood pressure[110–112] as early as 2 weeks from initiation of treatment,[113] indicating the weight-loss independence of this effect. Moreover, comparative studies of sitagliptin versus liraglutide or exenatide LAR therapy for 26 weeks have shown a greater effect on systolic and diastolic blood pressure as a result of sitagliptin treatment, whereas the effect on weight loss was trivial in comparison with GLP-1r agonist therapy.[114] GLP-1r agonists also improve the levels of triglyceride and free fatty acid,[115] although it is not clear whether this effect is weight independent. The evidence for antilipid effects of DPP-4 inhibitors is mixed, with neutral[116] to favorable effects[117] being reported on lipid profile with sitagliptin therapy.

Other Side Effects or Known Complications of Treatment

Because of glucose dependence of GLP-1 action on insulin secretion and glucagon suppression,[118] hypoglycemia is not associated with treatment of GLP-1r agonists or DPP-4 inhibitors, unless these drugs are administered in combination with other insulin secretagogues or insulin without proper dose adjustment.[117,119–123]

GI side effects, mainly nausea and vomiting, are the most common adverse effects associated with GLP-1r agonist therapy (30%–60%) and are the main cause for early termination of treatment with these drugs. However, nausea is mostly mild and dose dependent, and wanes over time.[119,120,124] Whereas nausea is less frequently reported with long-acting GLP-1r agonists compared with short-acting exenatide,[115,125] diarrhea seems to be more frequent with long-acting agents.[125] DPP-4 inhibitors do not cause GI side effects seen with GLP-1r agonists.[117,121–123]

The FDA has issued a warning about the potential risk of acute pancreatitis with the use of GLP-1–based drugs, given early postmarketing reports[126,127] and findings from a recent population database study.[127] Although the causal relationship between pancreatitis and GLP-1–based drugs has not yet been established[128] and the number of cases reported with this condition is small, patients should be informed about the symptoms of acute pancreatitis, and therapy should be discontinued if these develop.

Long-acting GLP-1r agonists should also not be used in patients with any personal or family history of medullary thyroid cancer or multiple endocrine neoplasia type 2. Animal studies have suggested that liraglutide could increase the risk of C-cell hyperplasia and medullary thyroid cancer via activation of functional GLP-1rs that are expressed on thyroid C cells.[129,130] It is noteworthy that these results were not replicated in the studies of nonhuman primates,[131] nor did 2 years of treatment with liraglutide result in increased calcitonin levels.[131]

The wide expression of DPP-4 in different tissue cells, including T cells, has raised concerns about the potential adverse effects of DPP-4 inhibitors on immunomodulation and T-cell signaling, which need to be addressed in future studies.

AMYLIN ANALOGUES
Indications and Patient Considerations

Pramlintide (Symlin) is indicated for adjunctive use in both T1DM and T2DM in patients already taking prandial insulin. It is contraindicated in patients with a confirmed diagnosis of gastroparesis and hypoglycemia unawareness, owing to the increased risk of hypoglycemia. Dose titration is recommended, and prandial insulin doses should be reduced by 50% at the onset of therapy to limit the risk of hypoglycemia.

Mechanism of Action, Efficacy, and Kinetics

Amylin, also called islet amyloid polypeptide or diabetes-associated peptide, is produced by pancreatic β cells and is cosecreted with insulin in a 1:100 amylin/insulin ratio. Soluble amylin analogue, pramlintide acetate, is synergistic with insulin; that is, when given subcutaneously at mealtimes in combination with prandial insulin, pramlintide provides further reduction in postprandial hyperglycemia and concomitant reduction of glucagon levels in comparison with insulin monotherapy.[132] Multiple daily dosing is required, as the $t_{1/2}$ is 48 minutes; metabolism is primarily via the kidneys. Amylin may further contribute to improved glucose levels via central anorectic effects, inhibition of ghrelin release, delayed gastric emptying, and reduced insulin dose requirements.[133,134] A 1-year randomized controlled trial of pramlintide as adjunct to insulin therapy among patients with T1DM demonstrated reduction of HbA1c by 0.3% in the treated group compared with no change of HbA1c in the placebo group.[135]

Effects of Treatment on Weight and Cardiovascular Outcomes

When pramlintide is added to basal insulin, no weight gain is observed.[24] In a dose-finding study with pramlintide added to a variety of insulin regimens, weight loss (−1.4 kg) was observed across the active treatment groups.[136] Pramlintide decreases the insulin requirement, thus the weight-neutral or weight-beneficial effects may be a result of the decreased weight-promoting effects of insulin. A modest and dose-dependent beneficial effect on lipid profiles has been observed in short-term studies.[137] There are no data on long-term cardiovascular outcome.

Other Side Effects

When compared with placebo, frequently reported side effects (>10% of patients) include mild to moderate hypoglycemia, nausea, vomiting, and anorexia during the first month of therapy.[138]

SODIUM-GLUCOSE TRANSPORTER INHIBITORS
Indications and Patient Considerations

Sodium-glucose transporter 2 (SGLT2) inhibitors are a novel class of antidiabetes agents that exert glucose lowering primarily through effects on renal glucose handling. Several drugs in this class are in various stages of clinical development; canagliflozin (Invokana) is the first agent in this class to achieve a recent FDA approval for the treatment of T2DM. Use is contraindicated in severe renal impairment (glomerular filtration rate [GFR] <30 mL/min) or severe liver disease, and dose adjustment is advised for moderate renal impairment (GFR <45 mL/min). Monitoring for hypotension is recommended, particularly for elderly patients.

Mechanism of Action, Efficacy, and Kinetics

Under normal conditions, filtered glucose is actively reabsorbed by the sodium-glucose transporters SGLT1 and SGLT2 in the proximal tubule.[139] SGLT2 inhibitors

Table 1
Comparison of diabetes treatment complications and therapeutic considerations

Medication Class Drug Examples	Dose-Adjustment Considerations	Weight Effect	CV Effects	Bone Effect	Association with Cancer	Pregnancy Category
Biguanide Metformin	Renal insufficiency Hepatic insufficiency	Neutral or loss	Neutral or possible benefit on lipid profile and CV outcomes	Neutral or possible benefit	Possible beneficial effects	B
Thiazolidinedione Rosiglitazone Pioglitazone	Caution: CHF (class I and II) Contraindication: CHF (class III and IV); concurrent use of CYP2C8 inhibitors	Gain and edema	Increased risk of CHF; rosiglitazone associated with higher risk of ischemia and CV mortality	Negative impact on BMD; increased fracture risk in select populations	Pioglitazone associated with increased risk of bladder cancer	C
Sulfonylurea Chlorpropamide, tolbutamide Glyburide, glipizide, glimepiride	Renal insufficiency (chlorpropamide, glyburide) Hepatic insufficiency Elderly or malnourished	Neutral or gain	Increased risk of CV death following myocardial infarction	No effect	Unknown	C (glyburide, class B)
Meglitinide analogues Nateglinide Repaglinide	Renal insufficiency Hepatic insufficiency Concomitant use with gemfibrozil (repaglinide) Monitor with concurrent CYP3A4 metabolized medications	Neutral or gain	No change in lipids or blood pressure	Unknown	Unknown	C

α-Glucosidase inhibitors Acarbose Miglitol Voglibose	Renal insufficiency (acarbose, miglitol) Hepatic insufficiency Contraindication: cirrhosis, inflammatory bowel disease, colonic ulceration or obstruction	Neutral	Risk reduction for myocardial infarction and hypertension	Unknown	Unknown	B
GLP-1r agonist Exenatide Liraglutide	Renal insufficiency (long-acting exenatide) Hepatic insufficiency (liraglutide) Contraindicated with prior pancreatitis	Loss or neutral	Beneficial, improves blood pressure and lipid profiles	No effect	Black-box warning for personal or family history of medullary thyroid cancer or MEN 2	C
DPP-4 analogues Saxagliptin Linagliptin Alogliptin	Renal insufficiency (saxagliptin, alogliptin) Hepatic insufficiency	Neutral	Neutral, possible beneficial effects on lipid profiles	Decreased fractures	Unknown	B
Amylin analogues Pramlintide	Reduce prandial insulin	Neutral or loss	Possible beneficial effect on lipid profiles	Unknown	Unknown	C
SGLT2 inhibitors Canagliflozin	Renal insufficiency Hepatic insufficiency	Loss or neutral	Beneficial effects on systolic blood pressure	Unknown	Unknown	C

Abbreviations: BMD, bone mineral density; CHF, congestive heart failure; CV, cardiovascular; MEN 2, multiple endocrine neoplasia type 2.

reduce renal glucose reabsorption, resulting in increased excretion of urinary glucose and corresponding osmotic diuresis.[140] Completed trials of canagliflozin, dapagliflozin, and empagliflozin have demonstrated a mean reduction in HbA1c ranging from 0.6% to 0.9%.[141] Patients treated for 26 weeks with canagliflozin demonstrated decreases in proinsulin/insulin and proinsulin/C-peptide ratios compared with placebo,[139] suggestive of some improvement in β-cell function. Canagliflozin is converted to inactive metabolites via O-glucuronidation in the liver, and excreted via feces and urine.

Effects of Treatment on Weight and Cardiovascular Outcomes

SGLT2 inhibitors have demonstrated a 2- to 3-kg weight loss in short-term (12 weeks' duration) trials.[140–142] Fluid loss secondary to osmotic diuresis may account for early weight reduction; however, the glucose excreted in the urine as a result of SGLT2 inhibition equates to a loss of 200 to 300 calories daily,[140] which may provide ongoing beneficial effects on weight. A trial of dapagliflozin demonstrated a reduction in waist circumference[143] and sustained weight loss over 102 weeks when used in combination with metformin.[144] Reductions in systolic blood pressure up to 5 mm Hg have been described in trials of canagliflozin[139] and dapagliflozin,[140] likely attributable to glycosuria-induced diuresis. A statistically significant dose-related decrease in high-density lipoprotein cholesterol was observed in the 26-week randomized controlled trial of canagliflozin,[139] with a trend toward lower triglycerides and LDL cholesterol. Data regarding cardiovascular outcomes for SGLT2 inhibitors are limited; however, a series of ongoing safety trials and the CANVAS (Canagliflozin Cardiovascular Assessment Study) are anticipated to provide additional evidence in the upcoming years.[141]

Other Side Effects

The predominant reported side effect of SGLT2 inhibitors to date are increased rates of mycotic infections (vulvovaginitis, balanitis) and, less commonly, urinary tract infections,[139,141,144] presumably as a result of elevated urinary glucose levels.

EFFECTS ON β-CELL OUTCOMES

Once fasting hyperglycemia is detectable, β-cell function deteriorates progressively and contributes to further decline in the ability to maintain normal glycemic levels.[145,146] Thus, preservation of β-cell function in the prediabetes state (IGT, IFG) and prevention of further loss of β-cell function once diabetes occurs is a critical aim of therapy and is an important factor for selection of antidiabetic treatment.

Despite initial beneficial therapeutic effects, metformin may not have long-term beneficial effects on β-cell function based on disease progression (failure of monotherapy to maintain goal HbA1c).[45] Sulfonylureas may have a negative effect on β-cell function, based on some in vitro studies showing that the closure of the ATP-dependent potassium channels by tolbutamide and glibenclamide may induce calcium-dependent β-cell apoptosis in rodent and human islets.[79,81] TZDs and GLP-1–based drugs, on the other hand, may have a beneficial effect on β-cell function and may promote β-cell survival based on in vitro and animal studies.[44,147,148] However, it is not known how much of these preclinical data could be translated to clinical outcomes given the current ability to measure β-cell mass directly in humans.

Comparative studies on the durability of glycemic reduction effects of various drugs have been used to provide information about the chronic effects of these agents on islet preservation, considering that the progressive nature of β-cell dysfunction requires a continuous intensification of treatment to maintain target glycemia. ADOPT[149] is the first randomized trial to compare the long-term effect of 3 conventional oral agents, glyburide, metformin, and rosiglitazone, on glucose control for a 4-year follow-up. The findings from this trial indicated that patients with early-stage T2DM receiving glyburide had the fastest decline in glycemic control and those assigned to rosiglitazone the slowest, with patients treated with metformin being somewhere in between.

Recently, findings from a randomized trial comparing the long-term effect on glucose control of adding short-acting exenatide or glimepiride to metformin therapy in approximately 10,000 patients with uncontrolled T2DM (average basal HbA1c 7.5%) showed that more patients in the glimepiride group than in the exenatide group (54% vs 41%) experienced treatment failure. In this study, the median time to inadequate glucose control and the need for alternative treatment was markedly shorter in those treated with sulfonylurea than in patients treated with a GLP-1r agonist (140 vs 180 weeks).[150] However, the largest risk reduction as a result of GLP-1r agonist therapy was observed in patients with higher baseline HbA1c level (>7.3%), who had the highest risk of treatment failure in general. Moreover, patients in the exenatide group had an average weight loss of 3 kg, which could contribute to treatment outcome.

Although these studies are not able to prove the beneficial effects of GLP-1–based drugs or TZDs on β-cell survival and β-cell expansion based on preclinical data, they raise the question as to whether treatment with these agents should be considered for prevention purposes, or should be initiated at an earlier stage of diabetes.

SUMMARY

T2DM is a progressive disease characterized by the need for additional antidiabetic treatments over time to maintain glycemic control at the target. A large body of evidence now supports the maintenance of glycemic control as a means of eliminating the microvascular complications of diabetes. Therefore, individualized therapy started at an earlier stage of disease, guided by the principle of "do not harm," seems to be essential in the patient-centric, shared decision-making model of diabetes care. Long-term clinical outcome data are needed to address the differential disease-modifying effects of various antidiabetic drugs (**Table 1**).

REFERENCES

1. The effect of intensive treatment of diabetes on the development and progression of long-term complications in insulin-dependent diabetes mellitus. The Diabetes Control and Complications Trial Research Group. N Engl J Med 1993; 329(14):977–86.
2. Intensive blood-glucose control with sulphonylureas or insulin compared with conventional treatment and risk of complications in patients with type 2 diabetes (UKPDS 33). UK Prospective Diabetes Study (UKPDS) Group. Lancet 1998; 352(9131):837–53.
3. Stratton IM, Adler AI, Neil HA, et al. Association of glycaemia with macrovascular and microvascular complications of type 2 diabetes (UKPDS 35): prospective observational study. BMJ 2000;321(7258):405–12.
4. Holman RR, Paul SK, Bethel MA, et al. 10-year follow-up of intensive glucose control in type 2 diabetes. N Engl J Med 2008;359(15):1577–89.
5. Gerstein HC, Miller ME, Byington RP, et al. Effects of intensive glucose lowering in type 2 diabetes. N Engl J Med 2008;358(24):2545–59.

6. Lecka-Czernik B. Safety of anti-diabetic therapies on bone. Clin Rev Bone Miner Metab 2013;11(1):49–58.
7. Giovannucci E, Harlan DM, Archer MC, et al. Diabetes and cancer: a consensus report. Diabetes Care 2010;33(7):1674–85.
8. Larsson SC, Orsini N, Brismar K, et al. Diabetes mellitus and risk of bladder cancer: a meta-analysis. Diabetologia 2006;49(12):2819–23.
9. Nathan DM, Buse JB, Davidson MB, et al. Medical management of hyperglycemia in type 2 diabetes: a consensus algorithm for the initiation and adjustment of therapy: a consensus statement of the American Diabetes Association and the European Association for the Study of Diabetes. Diabetes Care 2009;32(1): 193–203.
10. Inzucchi SE, Bergenstal RM, Buse JB, et al. Management of hyperglycaemia in type 2 diabetes: a patient-centered approach. Position statement of the American Diabetes Association (ADA) and the European Association for the Study of Diabetes (EASD). Diabetologia 2012;55(6):1577–96.
11. Garber AJ, Abrahamson MJ, Barzilay JI, et al. AACE comprehensive diabetes management algorithm 2013. Endocr Pract 2013;19(2):327–36.
12. DeFronzo RA, Goodman AM. Efficacy of metformin in patients with non-insulin-dependent diabetes mellitus. The Multicenter Metformin Study Group. N Engl J Med 1995;333(9):541–9.
13. DeFronzo RA, Stonehouse AH, Han J, et al. Relationship of baseline HbA1c and efficacy of current glucose-lowering therapies: a meta-analysis of randomized clinical trials. Diabet Med 2010;27(3):309–17.
14. Kirpichnikov D, McFarlane SI, Sowers JR. Metformin: an update. Ann Intern Med 2002;137(1):25–33.
15. Cusi K, Consoli A, DeFronzo RA. Metabolic effects of metformin on glucose and lactate metabolism in noninsulin-dependent diabetes mellitus. J Clin Endocrinol Metab 1996;81(11):4059–67.
16. Dorella M, Giusto M, Da Tos V, et al. Improvement of insulin sensitivity by metformin treatment does not lower blood pressure of nonobese insulin-resistant hypertensive patients with normal glucose tolerance. J Clin Endocrinol Metab 1996;81(4):1568–74.
17. Hundal RS, Krssak M, Dufour S, et al. Mechanism by which metformin reduces glucose production in type 2 diabetes. Diabetes 2000;49(12):2063–9.
18. Natali A, Ferrannini E. Effects of metformin and thiazolidinediones on suppression of hepatic glucose production and stimulation of glucose uptake in type 2 diabetes: a systematic review. Diabetologia 2006;49(3):434–41.
19. Gunton JE, Delhanty PJ, Takahashi S, et al. Metformin rapidly increases insulin receptor activation in human liver and signals preferentially through insulin-receptor substrate-2. J Clin Endocrinol Metab 2003;88(3):1323–32.
20. Maida A, Lamont BJ, Cao X, et al. Metformin regulates the incretin receptor axis via a pathway dependent on peroxisome proliferator-activated receptor-alpha in mice. Diabetologia 2011;54(2):339–49.
21. Graham GG, Punt J, Arora M, et al. Clinical pharmacokinetics of metformin. Clin Pharmacokinet 2011;50(2):81–98.
22. Knowler WC, Barrett-Connor E, Fowler SE, et al. Reduction in the incidence of type 2 diabetes with lifestyle intervention or metformin. N Engl J Med 2002; 346(6):393–403.
23. Knowler WC, Fowler SE, Hamman RF, et al. 10-year follow-up of diabetes incidence and weight loss in the Diabetes Prevention Program Outcomes Study. Lancet 2009;374(9702):1677–86.

24. Meneghini LF, Orozco-Beltran D, Khunti K, et al. Weight beneficial treatments for type 2 diabetes. J Clin Endocrinol Metab 2011;96(11):3337-53.
25. Phung OJ, Scholle JM, Talwar M, et al. Effect of noninsulin antidiabetic drugs added to metformin therapy on glycemic control, weight gain, and hypoglycemia in type 2 diabetes. JAMA 2010;303(14):1410-8.
26. Wong AK, Struthers AD, Choy AM, et al. Insulin sensitization therapy and the heart: focus on metformin and thiazolidinediones. Heart Fail Clin 2012;8(4): 539-50.
27. Salpeter SR, Greyber E, Pasternak GA, et al. Risk of fatal and nonfatal lactic acidosis with metformin use in type 2 diabetes mellitus: systematic review and meta-analysis. Arch Intern Med 2003;163(21):2594-602.
28. Masoudi FA, Inzucchi SE, Wang Y, et al. Thiazolidinediones, metformin, and outcomes in older patients with diabetes and heart failure: an observational study. Circulation 2005;111(5):583-90.
29. Bodmer M, Meier C, Krahenbuhl S, et al. Metformin, sulfonylureas, or other antidiabetes drugs and the risk of lactic acidosis or hypoglycemia: a nested case-control analysis. Diabetes Care 2008;31(11):2086-91.
30. Eurich DT, McAlister FA, Blackburn DF, et al. Benefits and harms of antidiabetic agents in patients with diabetes and heart failure: systematic review. BMJ 2007; 335(7618):497.
31. Selvin E, Bolen S, Yeh HC, et al. Cardiovascular outcomes in trials of oral diabetes medications: a systematic review. Arch Intern Med 2008;168(19):2070-80.
32. Lamanna C, Monami M, Marchionni N, et al. Effect of metformin on cardiovascular events and mortality: a meta-analysis of randomized clinical trials. Diabetes Obes Metab 2011;13(3):221-8.
33. Scheen AJ, Paquot N. Metformin revisited: a critical review of the benefit-risk balance in at-risk patients with type 2 diabetes. Diabetes Metab 2013;39(3): 179-90.
34. Borges JL, Bilezikian JP, Jones-Leone AR, et al. A randomized, parallel group, double-blind, multicentre study comparing the efficacy and safety of Avandamet (rosiglitazone/metformin) and metformin on long-term glycaemic control and bone mineral density after 80 weeks of treatment in drug-naive type 2 diabetes mellitus patients. Diabetes Obes Metab 2011;13(11):1036-46.
35. Sedlinsky C, Molinuevo MS, Cortizo AM, et al. Metformin prevents anti-osteogenic in vivo and ex vivo effects of rosiglitazone in rats. Eur J Pharmacol 2011;668(3):477-85.
36. Diabetes Prevention Program Research Group. Long-term safety, tolerability, and weight loss associated with metformin in the Diabetes Prevention Program Outcomes Study. Diabetes Care 2012;35(4):731-7.
37. Chung HH, Moon JS, Yoon JS, et al. The relationship between metformin and cancer in patients with Type 2 diabetes. Diabetes Metab J 2013;37(2):125-31.
38. Bost F, Sahra IB, Le Marchand-Brustel Y, et al. Metformin and cancer therapy. Curr Opin Oncol 2012;24(1):103-8.
39. Ben Sahra I, Le Marchand-Brustel Y, Tanti JF, et al. Metformin in cancer therapy: a new perspective for an old antidiabetic drug? Mol Cancer Ther 2010;9(5): 1092-9.
40. Loubiere C, Dirat B, Tanti JF, et al. New perspectives for metformin in cancer therapy. Ann Endocrinol (Paris) 2013;74(2):130-6 [in French].
41. Nathan DM, Davidson MB, DeFronzo RA, et al. Impaired fasting glucose and impaired glucose tolerance: implications for care. Diabetes Care 2007;30(3): 753-9.

42. Molavi B, Rassouli N, Bagwe S, et al. A review of thiazolidinediones and metformin in the treatment of type 2 diabetes with focus on cardiovascular complications. Vasc Health Risk Manag 2007;3(6):967–73.
43. Yki-Jarvinen H. Thiazolidinediones. N Engl J Med 2004;351(11):1106–18.
44. Gastaldelli A, Ferrannini E, Miyazaki Y, et al. Thiazolidinediones improve beta-cell function in type 2 diabetic patients. Am J Physiol Endocrinol Metab 2007; 292(3):E871–83.
45. DeFronzo RA, Abdul-Ghani MA. Preservation of beta-cell function: the key to diabetes prevention. J Clin Endocrinol Metab 2011;96(8):2354–66.
46. Budde K, Neumayer HH, Fritsche L, et al. The pharmacokinetics of pioglitazone in patients with impaired renal function. Br J Clin Pharmacol 2003;55(4): 368–74.
47. Kirchheiner J, Thomas S, Bauer S, et al. Pharmacokinetics and pharmacodynamics of rosiglitazone in relation to CYP2C8 genotype. Clin Pharmacol Ther 2006;80(6):657–67.
48. Ahmadian M, Suh JM, Hah N, et al. PPARgamma signaling and metabolism: the good, the bad and the future. Nat Med 2013;19(5):557–66.
49. Tschope D, Hanefeld M, Meier JJ, et al. The role of co-morbidity in the selection of antidiabetic pharmacotherapy in type-2 diabetes. Cardiovasc Diabetol 2013; 12(1):62.
50. Kung J, Henry RR. Thiazolidinedione safety. Expert Opin Drug Saf 2012;11(4): 565–79.
51. Fonseca V, McDuffie R, Calles J, et al. Determinants of weight gain in the action to control cardiovascular risk in diabetes trial. Diabetes Care 2013. [Epub ahead of print].
52. Benbow A, Stewart M, Yeoman G. Thiazolidinediones for type 2 diabetes. All glitazones may exacerbate heart failure. BMJ 2001;322(7280):236.
53. Nissen SE, Wolski K. Effect of rosiglitazone on the risk of myocardial infarction and death from cardiovascular causes. N Engl J Med 2007;356(24):2457–71.
54. Khalaf KI, Taegtmeyer H. After avandia: the use of antidiabetic drugs in patients with heart failure. Tex Heart Inst J 2012;39(2):174–8.
55. Loke YK, Kwok CS, Singh S. Comparative cardiovascular effects of thiazolidinediones: systematic review and meta-analysis of observational studies. BMJ 2011;342:d1309.
56. Singh S, Loke YK, Furberg CD. Thiazolidinediones and heart failure: a teleoanalysis. Diabetes Care 2007;30(8):2148–53.
57. Lincoff AM, Wolski K, Nicholls SJ, et al. Pioglitazone and risk of cardiovascular events in patients with type 2 diabetes mellitus: a meta-analysis of randomized trials. JAMA 2007;298(10):1180–8.
58. Kahn SE, Haffner SM, Heise MA, et al. Glycemic durability of rosiglitazone, metformin, or glyburide monotherapy. N Engl J Med 2006;355(23):2427–43.
59. Kahn SE, Zinman B, Lachin JM, et al. Rosiglitazone-associated fractures in type 2 diabetes: an analysis from A Diabetes Outcome Progression Trial (ADOPT). Diabetes Care 2008;31(5):845–51.
60. Loke YK, Singh S, Furberg CD. Long-term use of thiazolidinediones and fractures in type 2 diabetes: a meta-analysis. CMAJ 2009;180(1):32–9.
61. Colmers IN, Bowker SL, Majumdar SR, et al. Use of thiazolidinediones and the risk of bladder cancer among people with type 2 diabetes: a meta-analysis. CMAJ 2012;184(12):E675–83.
62. Klupa T, Skupien J, Malecki MT. Monogenic models: what have the single gene disorders taught us? Curr Diab Rep 2012;12(6):659–66.

63. Aguilar-Bryan L, Nichols CG, Wechsler SW, et al. Cloning of the beta cell high-affinity sulfonylurea receptor: a regulator of insulin secretion. Science 1995; 268(5209):423–6.
64. Hermann LS, Schersten B, Bitzen PO, et al. Therapeutic comparison of metformin and sulfonylurea, alone and in various combinations. A double-blind controlled study. Diabetes Care 1994;17(10):1100–9.
65. Xu H, Murray M, McLachlan AJ. Influence of genetic polymorphisms on the pharmacokinetics and pharmaco-dynamics of sulfonylurea drugs. Curr Drug Metab 2009;10(6):643–58.
66. Melander A. Kinetics-effect relations of insulin-releasing drugs in patients with type 2 diabetes: brief overview. Diabetes 2004;53(Suppl 3):S151–5.
67. Nathan DM, Buse JB, Davidson MB, et al. Management of hyperglycemia in type 2 diabetes: a consensus algorithm for the initiation and adjustment of therapy: a consensus statement from the American Diabetes Association and the European Association for the Study of Diabetes. Diabetes Care 2006;29(8):1963–72.
68. Nichols GA, Gomez-Caminero A. Weight changes following the initiation of new anti-hyperglycaemic therapies. Diabetes Obes Metab 2007;9(1):96–102.
69. Feinglos MN, Bethel MA. Therapy of type 2 diabetes, cardiovascular death, and the UGDP. Am Heart J 1999;138(5 Pt 1):S346–52.
70. UKPDS 28: a randomized trial of efficacy of early addition of metformin in sulfonylurea-treated type 2 diabetes. U.K. Prospective Diabetes Study Group. Diabetes Care 1998;21(1):87–92.
71. Zarich SW. Does choice of antidiabetes therapy influence macrovascular outcomes? Curr Diab Rep 2010;10(1):24–31.
72. Cleveland JC Jr, Meldrum DR, Cain BS, et al. Oral sulfonylurea hypoglycemic agents prevent ischemic preconditioning in human myocardium. Two paradoxes revisited. Circulation 1997;96(1):29–32.
73. Zeller M, Danchin N, Simon D, et al. Impact of type of preadmission sulfonylureas on mortality and cardiovascular outcomes in diabetic patients with acute myocardial infarction. J Clin Endocrinol Metab 2010;95(11):4993–5002.
74. Kadowaki T, Hagura R, Kajinuma H, et al. Chlorpropamide-induced hyponatremia: incidence and risk factors. Diabetes Care 1983;6(5):468–71.
75. Groop L, Eriksson CJ, Huupponen R, et al. Roles of chlorpropamide, alcohol and acetaldehyde in determining the chlorpropamide-alcohol flush. Diabetologia 1984;26(1):34–8.
76. Landgraf R. Meglitinide analogues in the treatment of type 2 diabetes mellitus. Drugs Aging 2000;17(5):411–25.
77. Dunning BE. New non-sulfonylurea insulin secretagogues. Expert Opin Investig Drugs 1997;6(8):1041–8.
78. Karara AH, Dunning BE, McLeod JF. The effect of food on the oral bioavailability and the pharmacodynamic actions of the insulinotropic agent nateglinide in healthy subjects. J Clin Pharmacol 1999;39(2):172–9.
79. Wolffenbuttel BH, Landgraf R. A 1-year multicenter randomized double-blind comparison of repaglinide and glyburide for the treatment of type 2 diabetes. Dutch and German Repaglinide Study Group. Diabetes Care 1999;22(3):463–7.
80. Hollander PA, Schwartz SL, Gatlin MR, et al. Importance of early insulin secretion: comparison of nateglinide and glyburide in previously diet-treated patients with type 2 diabetes. Diabetes Care 2001;24(6):983–8.
81. Moses R, Slobodniuk R, Boyages S, et al. Effect of repaglinide addition to metformin monotherapy on glycemic control in patients with type 2 diabetes. Diabetes Care 1999;22(1):119–24.

82. Black C, Donnelly P, McIntyre L, et al. Meglitinide analogues for type 2 diabetes mellitus. Cochrane Database Syst Rev 2007;(2):CD004654.
83. Eleftheriadou I, Grigoropoulou P, Katsilambros N, et al. The effects of medications used for the management of diabetes and obesity on postprandial lipid metabolism. Curr Diabetes Rev 2008;4(4):340–56.
84. Horton ES, Foley JE, Shen SG, et al. Efficacy and tolerability of initial combination therapy with nateglinide and metformin in treatment-naive patients with type 2 diabetes. Curr Med Res Opin 2004;20(6):883–9.
85. Horton ES, Clinkingbeard C, Gatlin M, et al. Nateglinide alone and in combination with metformin improves glycemic control by reducing mealtime glucose levels in type 2 diabetes. Diabetes Care 2000;23(11):1660–5.
86. van de Laar FA, Lucassen PL, Akkermans RP, et al. Alpha-glucosidase inhibitors for patients with type 2 diabetes: results from a Cochrane systematic review and meta-analysis. Diabetes Care 2005;28(1):154–63.
87. Chiasson JL, Josse RG, Hunt JA, et al. The efficacy of acarbose in the treatment of patients with non-insulin-dependent diabetes mellitus. A multicenter controlled clinical trial. Ann Intern Med 1994;121(12):928–35.
88. Goke B, Fuder H, Wieckhorst G, et al. Voglibose (AO-128) is an efficient alpha-glucosidase inhibitor and mobilizes the endogenous GLP-1 reserve. Digestion 1995;56(6):493–501.
89. Rosak C, Mertes G. Critical evaluation of the role of acarbose in the treatment of diabetes: patient considerations. Diabetes Metab Syndr Obes 2012; 5:357–67.
90. Koyasu M, Ishii H, Watarai M, et al. Impact of acarbose on carotid intima-media thickness in patients with newly diagnosed impaired glucose tolerance or mild type 2 diabetes mellitus: a one-year, prospective, randomized, open-label, parallel-group study in Japanese adults with established coronary artery disease. Clin Ther 2010;32(9):1610–7.
91. Derosa G, Maffioli P. Efficacy and safety profile evaluation of acarbose alone and in association with other antidiabetic drugs: a systematic review. Clin Ther 2012;34(6):1221–36.
92. Chiasson JL, Josse RG, Gomis R, et al. Acarbose treatment and the risk of cardiovascular disease and hypertension in patients with impaired glucose tolerance: the STOP-NIDDM trial. JAMA 2003;290(4):486–94.
93. Hansen L, Deacon CF, Orskov C, et al. Glucagon-like peptide-1-(7-36)amide is transformed to glucagon-like peptide-1-(9-36)amide by dipeptidyl peptidase IV in the capillaries supplying the L cells of the porcine intestine. Endocrinology 1999;140(11):5356–63.
94. Bullock BP, Heller RS, Habener JF. Tissue distribution of messenger ribonucleic acid encoding the rat glucagon-like peptide-1 receptor. Endocrinology 1996; 137(7):2968–78.
95. Nakagawa A, Satake H, Nakabayashi H, et al. Receptor gene expression of glucagon-like peptide-1, but not glucose-dependent insulinotropic polypeptide, in rat nodose ganglion cells. Auton Neurosci 2004;110(1):36–43.
96. Schirra J, Nicolaus M, Roggel R, et al. Endogenous glucagon-like peptide 1 controls endocrine pancreatic secretion and antro-pyloro-duodenal motility in humans. Gut 2006;55(2):243–51.
97. Salehi M, Vahl TP, D'Alessio DA. Regulation of islet hormone release and gastric emptying by endogenous glucagon-like peptide 1 after glucose ingestion. J Clin Endocrinol Metab 2008;93(12):4909–16.

98. Nauck MA, Niedereichholz U, Ettler R, et al. Glucagon-like peptide 1 inhibition of gastric emptying outweighs its insulinotropic effects in healthy humans. Am J Physiol 1997;273(5 Pt 1):E981–8.

99. Wettergren A, Schjoldager B, Mortensen PE, et al. Truncated GLP-1 (proglucagon 78-107-amide) inhibits gastric and pancreatic functions in man. Dig Dis Sci 1993;38(4):665–73.

100. Meier JJ, Gallwitz B, Salmen S, et al. Normalization of glucose concentrations and deceleration of gastric emptying after solid meals during intravenous glucagon-like peptide 1 in patients with type 2 diabetes. J Clin Endocrinol Metab 2003;88(6):2719–25.

101. Flint A, Raben A, Astrup A, et al. Glucagon-like peptide 1 promotes satiety and suppresses energy intake in humans. J Clin Invest 1998;101(3):515–20.

102. Prigeon RL, Quddusi S, Paty B, et al. Suppression of glucose production by GLP-1 independent of islet hormones: a novel extrapancreatic effect. Am J Physiol Endocrinol Metab 2003;285(4):E701–7.

103. Kielgast U, Holst JJ, Madsbad S. Antidiabetic actions of endogenous and exogenous GLP-1 in type 1 diabetic patients with and without residual beta-cell function. Diabetes 2011;60(5):1599–607.

104. Creutzfeldt WO, Kleine N, Willms B, et al. Glucagonostatic actions and reduction of fasting hyperglycemia by exogenous glucagon-like peptide I(7-36) amide in type I diabetic patients. Diabetes Care 1996;19(6):580–6.

105. Vella A, Bock G, Giesler PD, et al. Effects of dipeptidyl peptidase-4 inhibition on gastrointestinal function, meal appearance, and glucose metabolism in type 2 diabetes. Diabetes 2007;56(5):1475–80.

106. Russell S. Incretin-based therapies for type 2 diabetes mellitus: a review of direct comparisons of efficacy, safety and patient satisfaction. Int J Clin Pharm 2013;35(2):159–72.

107. Bergman AJ, Cote J, Yi B, et al. Effect of renal insufficiency on the pharmacokinetics of sitagliptin, a dipeptidyl peptidase-4 inhibitor. Diabetes Care 2007; 30(7):1862–4.

108. Baetta R, Corsini A. Pharmacology of dipeptidyl peptidase-4 inhibitors: similarities and differences. Drugs 2011;71(11):1441–67.

109. Aroda VR, Henry RR, Han J, et al. Efficacy of GLP-1 receptor agonists and DPP-4 inhibitors: meta-analysis and systematic review. Clin Ther 2012;34(6): 1247–58.e22.

110. Nauck MA, Duran S, Kim D, et al. A comparison of twice-daily exenatide and biphasic insulin aspart in patients with type 2 diabetes who were suboptimally controlled with sulfonylurea and metformin: a non-inferiority study. Diabetologia 2007;50(2):259–67.

111. Diamant M, Van Gaal L, Stranks S, et al. Safety and efficacy of once-weekly exenatide compared with insulin glargine titrated to target in patients with type 2 diabetes over 84 weeks. Diabetes Care 2012;35(4):683–9.

112. Bergenstal RM, Wysham C, Macconell L, et al. Efficacy and safety of exenatide once weekly versus sitagliptin or pioglitazone as an adjunct to metformin for treatment of type 2 diabetes (DURATION-2): a randomised trial. Lancet 2010; 376(9739):431–9.

113. Gallwitz B, Vaag A, Falahati A, et al. Adding liraglutide to oral antidiabetic drug therapy: onset of treatment effects over time. Int J Clin Pract 2010;64(2):267–76.

114. Pratley RE, Nauck M, Bailey T, et al. Liraglutide versus sitagliptin for patients with type 2 diabetes who did not have adequate glycaemic control with

metformin: a 26-week, randomised, parallel-group, open-label trial. Lancet 2010;375(9724):1447–56.

115. Buse JB, Rosenstock J, Sesti G, et al. Liraglutide once a day versus exenatide twice a day for type 2 diabetes: a 26-week randomised, parallel-group, multinational, open-label trial (LEAD-6). Lancet 2009;374(9683):39–47.

116. Aschner P, Kipnes MS, Lunceford JK, et al. Effect of the dipeptidyl peptidase-4 inhibitor sitagliptin as monotherapy on glycemic control in patients with type 2 diabetes. Diabetes Care 2006;29(12):2632–7.

117. Charbonnel B, Karasik A, Liu J, et al. Efficacy and safety of the dipeptidyl peptidase-4 inhibitor sitagliptin added to ongoing metformin therapy in patients with type 2 diabetes inadequately controlled with metformin alone. Diabetes Care 2006;29(12):2638–43.

118. Nauck MA, Heimesaat MM, Behle K, et al. Effects of glucagon-like peptide 1 on counterregulatory hormone responses, cognitive functions, and insulin secretion during hyperinsulinemic, stepped hypoglycemic clamp experiments in healthy volunteers. J Clin Endocrinol Metab 2002;87(3):1239–46.

119. Buse JB, Henry RR, Han J, et al. Effects of exenatide (exendin-4) on glycemic control over 30 weeks in sulfonylurea-treated patients with type 2 diabetes. Diabetes Care 2004;27(11):2628–35.

120. Kendall DM, Riddle MC, Rosenstock J, et al. Effects of exenatide (exendin-4) on glycemic control over 30 weeks in patients with type 2 diabetes treated with metformin and a sulfonylurea. Diabetes Care 2005;28(5):1083–91.

121. Raz I, Hanefeld M, Xu L, et al. Efficacy and safety of the dipeptidyl peptidase-4 inhibitor sitagliptin as monotherapy in patients with type 2 diabetes mellitus. Diabetologia 2006;49(11):2564–71.

122. DeFronzo RA, Hissa MN, Garber AJ, et al. The efficacy and safety of saxagliptin when added to metformin therapy in patients with inadequately controlled type 2 diabetes with metformin alone. Diabetes Care 2009;32(9):1649–55.

123. Del Prato S, Barnett AH, Huisman H, et al. Effect of linagliptin monotherapy on glycaemic control and markers of beta-cell function in patients with inadequately controlled type 2 diabetes: a randomized controlled trial. Diabetes Obes Metab 2011;13(3):258–67.

124. DeFronzo RA, Ratner RE, Han J, et al. Effects of exenatide (exendin-4) on glycemic control and weight over 30 weeks in metformin-treated patients with type 2 diabetes. Diabetes Care 2005;28(5):1092–100.

125. Drucker DJ, Buse JB, Taylor K, et al. Exenatide once weekly versus twice daily for the treatment of type 2 diabetes: a randomised, open-label, non-inferiority study. Lancet 2008;372(9645):1240–50.

126. Elashoff M, Matveyenko AV, Gier B, et al. Pancreatitis, pancreatic, and thyroid cancer with glucagon-like peptide-1-based therapies. Gastroenterology 2011; 141(1):150–6.

127. Singh S, Chang HY, Richards TM, et al. Glucagonlike peptide 1-based therapies and risk of hospitalization for acute pancreatitis in type 2 diabetes mellitus: a population-based matched case-control study. JAMA Intern Med 2013;173(7):534–9.

128. Garg R, Chen W, Pendergrass M. Acute pancreatitis in type 2 diabetes treated with exenatide or sitagliptin: a retrospective observational pharmacy claims analysis. Diabetes Care 2010;33(11):2349–54.

129. Crespel A, De Boisvilliers F, Gros L, et al. Effects of glucagon and glucagon-like peptide-1-(7-36) amide on C cells from rat thyroid and medullary thyroid carcinoma CA-77 cell line. Endocrinology 1996;137(9):3674–80.

130. Butler PC, Elashoff M, Elashoff R, et al. A critical analysis of the clinical use of incretin-based therapies: are the GLP-1 therapies safe? Diabetes Care 2013; 36(7):2118–25.
131. Bjerre Knudsen L, Madsen LW, Andersen S, et al. Glucagon-like peptide-1 receptor agonists activate rodent thyroid C-cells causing calcitonin release and C-cell proliferation. Endocrinology 2010;151(4):1473–86.
132. Adeghate E, Kalasz H. Amylin analogues in the treatment of diabetes mellitus: medicinal chemistry and structural basis of its function. Open Med Chem J 2011;5(Suppl 2):78–81.
133. Young A. Inhibition of food intake. Adv Pharmacol 2005;52:79–98.
134. Fineman M, Weyer C, Maggs DG, et al. The human amylin analog, pramlintide, reduces postprandial hyperglucagonemia in patients with type 2 diabetes mellitus. Horm Metab Res 2002;34(9):504–8.
135. Ratner RE, Dickey R, Fineman M, et al. Amylin replacement with pramlintide as an adjunct to insulin therapy improves long-term glycaemic and weight control in type 1 diabetes mellitus: a 1-year, randomized controlled trial. Diabet Med 2004;21(11):1204–12.
136. Hollander PA, Levy P, Fineman MS, et al. Pramlintide as an adjunct to insulin therapy improves long-term glycemic and weight control in patients with type 2 diabetes: a 1-year randomized controlled trial. Diabetes Care 2003;26(3): 784–90.
137. Thompson RG, Pearson L, Schoenfeld SL, et al. Pramlintide, a synthetic analog of human amylin, improves the metabolic profile of patients with type 2 diabetes using insulin. The Pramlintide in Type 2 Diabetes Group. Diabetes Care 1998; 21(6):987–93.
138. Singh-Franco D, Robles G, Gazze D. Pramlintide acetate injection for the treatment of type 1 and type 2 diabetes mellitus. Clin Ther 2007;29(4):535–62.
139. Stenlof K, Cefalu WT, Kim KA, et al. Efficacy and safety of canagliflozin monotherapy in subjects with type 2 diabetes mellitus inadequately controlled with diet and exercise. Diabetes Obes Metab 2013;15(4):372–82.
140. List JF, Woo V, Morales E, et al. Sodium-glucose cotransport inhibition with dapagliflozin in type 2 diabetes. Diabetes Care 2009;32(4):650–7.
141. Foote C, Perkovic V, Neal B. Effects of SGLT2 inhibitors on cardiovascular outcomes. Diab Vasc Dis Res 2012;9(2):117–23.
142. Ferrannini E, Seman LJ, Seewaldt-Becker L, et al. The potent and highly selective sodium-glucose co-transporter (SGLT-2) inhibitor BI 10773 is safe and efficacious as monotherapy in patients with type 2 diabetes mellitus [abstract]. Diabetologia 2010;53(Suppl 2):877.
143. Bailey CJ, Gross JL, Pieters A, et al. Effect of dapagliflozin in patients with type 2 diabetes who have inadequate glycaemic control with metformin: a randomised, double-blind, placebo-controlled trial. Lancet 2010;375(9733):2223–33.
144. Bailey CJ, Gross JL, Hennicken D, et al. Dapagliflozin add-on to metformin in type 2 diabetes inadequately controlled with metformin: a randomized, double-blind, placebo-controlled 102-week trial. BMC Med 2013;11:43.
145. Turner RC, Cull CA, Frighi V, et al. Glycemic control with diet, sulfonylurea, metformin, or insulin in patients with type 2 diabetes mellitus: progressive requirement for multiple therapies (UKPDS 49). UK Prospective Diabetes Study (UKPDS) Group. JAMA 1999;281(21):2005–12.
146. Levy J, Atkinson AB, Bell PM, et al. Beta-cell deterioration determines the onset and rate of progression of secondary dietary failure in type 2 diabetes mellitus: the 10-year follow-up of the Belfast Diet Study. Diabet Med 1998;15(4):290–6.

147. Farilla L, Bulotta A, Hirshberg B, et al. Glucagon-like peptide 1 inhibits cell apoptosis and improves glucose responsiveness of freshly isolated human islets. Endocrinology 2003;144(12):5149–58.
148. Farilla L, Hui H, Bertolotto C, et al. Glucagon-like peptide-1 promotes islet cell growth and inhibits apoptosis in Zucker diabetic rats. Endocrinology 2002; 143(11):4397–408.
149. Viberti G, Kahn SE, Greene DA, et al. A diabetes outcome progression trial (ADOPT): an international multicenter study of the comparative efficacy of rosiglitazone, glyburide, and metformin in recently diagnosed type 2 diabetes. Diabetes Care 2002;25(10):1737–43.
150. Gallwitz B, Guzman J, Dotta F, et al. Exenatide twice daily versus glimepiride for prevention of glycaemic deterioration in patients with type 2 diabetes with metformin failure (EUREXA): an open-label, randomised controlled trial. Lancet 2012;379(9833):2270–8.

Outpatient Assessment and Management of the Diabetic Foot

John A. DiPreta, MD

KEYWORDS

- Diabetes mellitus • Peripheral neuropathy • Charcot arthropathy • Ulceration

KEY POINTS

- Patients with diabetes are at risk for the development of peripheral neuropathy.
- Peripheral neuropathy, when associated with a traumatic event, can lead to Charcot (neuropathic) arthropathy.
- Charcot arthropathy often leads to significant deformity of the ankle and hindfoot.
- Deformity due to neuropathic arthropathy when associated with the insensate foot puts the patient at significant risk for ulcer formation.
- Neuropathic changes in the foot and ankle are best initially managed with immobilization. This immobilization protects the foot from injury, allowing for the process to develop while minimizing further progression.
- For unstable deformities or neuropathic ulcers, surgical correction of these deformities may be required. Urgent referral should be made to the foot and ankle specialist for those individuals with an ulcer or in whom Charcot arthropathy is suspected.

INTRODUCTION

Diabetes is characterized by high blood glucose. Individuals with high blood sugars fall into one of 2 categories. Type I diabetes is characterized by an inability to manufacture insulin due to autoimmune destruction of the insulin-producing pancreatic beta cells.[1] It represents approximately 5% of all diagnosed cases of diabetes. Exogenous insulin is necessary for survival. It typically is first diagnosed in children and young adults. Risk factors included autoimmune, genetic, or environmental causes. Type II diabetes accounts for 95% of diagnosed diabetes in adults. A well-balanced diet along with exercise and certain prescription medications can help control complications. Diabetes is a major cause of heart disease, vision loss, kidney

This article originally appeared in Medical Clinics of North America, Volume 98, Issue 2, March 2014.

Division of Orthopaedic Surgery, Albany Medical Center, Albany Medical College, Capital Region Orthopaedics, 1367 Washington Avenue, Suite 200, Albany, NY 12206, USA

E-mail address: jamddipreta@netscape.net

failure, and lower extremity amputation. The final common pathway to limb loss is peripheral neuropathy, peripheral vascular disease, ulceration, and infection. Tight glucose control, as measured by A1C levels, can help prevent these complications.[2]

From 1990 through 2010, the number of new cases of diagnosed diabetes nearly tripled. This rise in incidence is attributed to increases in obesity, decreases in physical activity, and an aging US population.[3] The prevalence during this same time period also increased, and many people are unaware of their undiagnosed diabetes. It is thought that if trends continue, as many as 1 in 3 American adults will have diabetes by 2050.[4]

Medical expenses for a person with diabetes are more than twice as high as those without diabetes. In 2007, the estimated cost of diabetes in the United States was $174 billion. This included $116 billion in direct medical care costs and $58 billion in costs due to disability, productivity loss, and premature death.[5]

The ability to lead a functional life hinges on one's mobility. Managing the sequelae of diabetic foot disease (peripheral neuropathy, Charcot arthropathy, and peripheral vascular disease) is thus essential.

The focus of this review is to define the various manifestations of peripheral neuropathy, the pathophysiology of foot ulceration, neuropathic arthropathy (Charcot arthropathy), their assessment, and initial steps in management. Criteria for referral to an orthopedic foot and ankle surgeon are also discussed.

PATHOGENESIS OF INSULIN-DEPENDENT DIABETES MELLITUS

Insulin-dependent diabetes mellitus (IDDM) is most common in individuals of Northern European descent and less common in African American, Native American, and Asian individuals. These differences may be explained by varied genetic susceptibility in racially distinct populations; however, diet and environmental factors likely play a role.[6] Susceptibility is inherited, and the main gene associated with a predisposition to IDDM is the major histocompatibility complex (MHC) on chromosome 6 in the region associated with the genes encoding for HLA recognition molecules. The interaction to a cell bearing an HLA molecule associated with an antigenic peptide and a T lymphocyte bearing a receptor capable of recognizing the HLA peptide complex triggers the activation and proliferation of T lymphocytes. Susceptibility or resistance to IDDM is associated with different HLA-DR and HLA-DQ genotypes, and 95% of patients with IDDM has at least 1 of these HLA-DR antigens.[1]

IDDM is a chronic autoimmune disease that exists in a preclinical phase. The most consistent histologic finding of the pancreas is the lack of insulin-secreting beta cells. Associated with this is a chronic inflammatory infiltrate. Histologic studies have suggested that an 80% reduction in the volume of beta cells is necessary to induce symptomatic IDDM.[7]

The association of microvascular disease and neuropathy with diabetes and the relationship of these conditions to the duration of diabetes suggest that they are linked to hyperglycemia. The Diabetes Control and Complications Trial (DCCT) demonstrated that the incidence and development of retinopathy, nephropathy, and neuropathy could be reduced by intensive treatment.[2]

The retina, kidney, and nerves are freely permeable to glucose. Increases in blood glucose concentrations leads to increased intracellular concentration of both glucose and its metabolic by-products. The mechanism by which hyperglycemia leads to microvascular and neurologic complications includes the increased accumulation of polyols through the aldose reductase pathway and of advanced glycosylation end products.[8]

PERIPHERAL NEUROPATHY

Diabetic neuropathy is one of the most common complications of diabetes mellitus and has many clinical presentations. The intensity and the functional and anatomic abnormalities parallel the degree and duration of hyperglycemia. It is the chronic hyperglycemia that leads to the loss of myelinated and unmyelinated fibers, Wallerian degeneration, and blunted nerve fiber production. Proposed mechanisms for these changes include the formation of sorbitol by aldose reductase and the formation of advanced glycosylation end products. Thus, treatment is directed at optimization of blood glucose levels. In the DCCT, intensive treatment decreased the occurrence of clinical neuropathy by 60%.[2]

Peripheral neuropathy can be broadly classified in 3 ways: sensory, motor, and autonomic. Each type will manifest itself into distinct patterns, and it is these patterns that contribute to the complications that can occur in the diabetic patient. The practitioner must suspect that neuropathy will be present in all patients with type 2 diabetes and in patients with type 1 diabetes of more than 5 years' duration. A single type of neuropathy may exist in isolation or, more commonly, in combination with the other neuropathies.

Sensory neuropathy can be classified as distal symmetric polyneuropathy, focal neuropathy, and diabetic amyotrophy. Motor neuropathies may be defined by the muscles that are involved. Associated with motor neuropathy are predictable patterns of foot deformities that put the patient at risk for ulceration. Autonomic neuropathy is classified by the system that is affected. In particular, this relates to the sudomotor function that controls sweat production in the feet.

In sensory nerve involvement, the nerves with the longest axons are affected first. This leads to the classic "stocking-and-glove" distribution. Large fiber damage results in diminished vibratory sensation, position sense, muscle strength, sharp dull discrimination, and 2-point discrimination. Diabetic amyotrophy is an uncommon variant of somatic neuropathy that is predominantly motor in nature and affects the proximal muscles of the lower extremities. Its clinical presentation is similar to a muscular dystrophy. In sensorimotor neuropathy, it is important to ask about recent falls, balance problems, and gait disturbances. In addition, assessing for loss of Achilles tendon and patellar reflexes is important.

Distal symmetric polyneuropathy is the most common form of diabetic neuropathy. It is associated with variable pain, motor disturbance, nerve palsies, ulcerations, burns, gangrene, and Charcot arthropathy.[9]

Motor neuropathy can manifest itself by affecting the intrinsic musculature of the foot. This results in unopposed function of the extrinsic muscles, which leads to clawing of the toes. This clawing creates a significant mechanical imbalance that puts the diabetic foot at risk for ulceration.

Autonomic neuropathy affects both sympathetic and parasympathetic function. Sympathetic dysfunction can be seen with abnormal neurogenic blood flow. This is thought also to play a role in the development of neuropathic arthropathy. Sudomotor neuropathy may cause hyperhidrosis in the upper extremities and anhidrosis in the lower extremities. The skin of the lower extremities may feel pruritic and display thinning, hair loss, dryness, flaking, cracks, and increased callus formation. These skin changes put the patient at risk for ulceration and ultimately infection.

Neuropathy has a lifetime prevalence of approximately 25% to 50% in those with diabetes.[10] Complications from diabetic neuropathy account for 50% to 75% of nontraumatic amputations.[11] Although frequent screening of diabetic patients reduces the risk of lower extremity amputations, reversing existent diabetic neuropathy is difficult to achieve.[12]

Pathogenesis

Proposed mechanisms to the development of diabetic neuropathy include nonenzymatic glycosylation, increases in oxidative stress, neuroinflammation, and activation of the polyol and protein kinase C (PKC) pathways.[12]

Advanced glycosylation end products (AGEs) are formed in an irreversible fashion as glucose becomes incorporated into proteins. AGE receptors on macrophages induce monocytes and endothelial cells to increase production of inflammatory cytokines and adhesion molecules. This increased inflammatory response may lead to vascular permeability and procoagulant activity. Patients with this type of neuropathy complain of pain and stiffness throughout their bodies. The neuropathic pain may be diffuse and not localized to the hands and the feet.

The polyol pathway activates increasing intracellular levels of fructose and sorbitol. Neither of these products can easily exit cells, and thus create an osmotic gradient leading to water penetration of proteins, and in peripheral nerves this leads to axonal edema and alteration of nerve function. Peripheral nerves become increasing sensitive to light touch and patients will have hyperalgesia on examination.

The protein kinase C pathway activation affects renal blood flow as well as vascular contractility and permeability. Activation of this pathway has been most closely linked to retinopathy and neuropathy.

In response to hyperglycemia, cellular mitochondria activate superoxide production, amplifying the cytotoxic effects induced by other pathogenic pathways. Oxidative stress appears to be triggered more as a result of postprandial fluctuations of blood glucose than with sustained hyperglycemia.

The production of free radicals and superoxide leads to activation of microglial cells, which in turn produce inflammatory cytokines, further damaging neural structures and altering their activity. **Fig. 1** is a schematic representation of the effects of hyperglycemia on the biochemical pathways leading to diabetic neuropathy.

Assessment

The highest rates of neuropathy in patients with type 2 diabetes occur in those who have hyperglycemia for longer than 25 years. In these individuals, it is important to identify modifiable and nonmodifiable risk factors that contribute to the hyperglycemia and, thus, neuropathy. In doing so, there is an opportunity to intensify management or possibly eliminate an individual's progression toward long-term neuropathic complications. Examples of modifiable risk factors include obesity, smoking, hyperglycemia (elevated Hb A1C), and hypertension. Nonmodifiable risk factors include age, family history, and duration of diabetes.[12]

A routine history and neurologic examination are essential when screening diabetic patients thought to be at risk for neuropathy. This is a critical step, as it is neuropathy that leads to the devastating complications associated with it. The neuropathic pain experienced by the patient is chronic, progressive, and serves no protective function. Minimal stimuli may lead to hyperalgesic symptoms. In addition to the structural and mechanical imbalances it creates (Charcot arthropathy, ulceration), it also contributes to depression and sleep disturbances.[12] The clinical evaluation should include the following:

1. Careful inspection of the foot. It is important to assess for skin turgor, ulceration, and deformity. Dry skin in combination with deformity and neuropathy is a significant risk factor for ulceration.

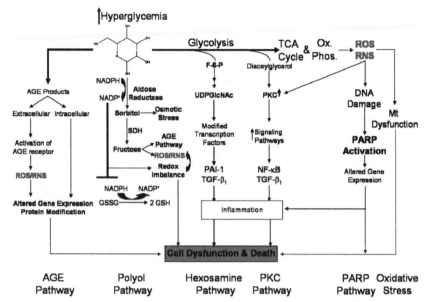

AGE   Polyol   Hexosamine   PKC   PARP   Oxidative
Pathway   Pathway   Pathway   Pathway   Pathway   Stress

Fig. 1. A schematic representation of the effects of hyperglycemia on the biochemical pathways leading to diabetic neuropathy. (*From* Edwards JL, Vincent AM, Cheng HT, et al. Diabetic neuropathy: mechanisms to management. Pharmacol Ther 2008;120:1–34; with permission.)

2. Evaluate ankle reflexes, as this indicates advanced peripheral neuropathy.
3. Check for proprioception. Move the hallux up or down with the patient's eyes closed and determine the patient's ability to determine direction.
4. Check for allodynia and hyperalgesia. Using a cold stimulus or a vibrating 128-Hz tuning fork may elicit allodynia.
5. Determine protective sensation. Using a Semmes-Weinstein 5.07 monofilament (Northcoast Medical, Gilroy, CA), check for sensation in areas of pressure, considered to be at risk for ulceration (**Fig. 2**).

Once it is established that an individual has diabetic neuropathy, follow-up is essential. In a patient with neuropathy but no mechanical deformities, visits with the primary care physician on a routine basis is appropriate. An individual with deformity or with a history of or a current ulcer needs more frequent follow-up, and an urgent referral to the appropriate foot and ankle specialist is critical.

The varied mechanisms for neuropathic changes in the diabetic patient pose potential targets for pharmacotherapeutic treatment. Although few options to reverse the root causes exist, the readers are referred to a review of therapeutic strategies in the medical management of diabetic neuropathy.[13]

The American Orthopedic Foot and Ankle Society has recommendations that can be viewed in the "Patient Section" at www.aofas.org. Suggested care for patients includes inspection of their feet on a daily basis for ulcers, blisters, and skin irritations. They should never walk barefoot or in flip-flops or sandals. They should call their physician for any injuries or disruptions in their skin. Shoes should be purchased at the end of the day and should not be "broken in." Patients should avoid paring or trimming calluses on their own, leaving it a medical professional. Nail and toe care should be focused on trimming nails straight across and avoiding chemical agents on corns and calluses.

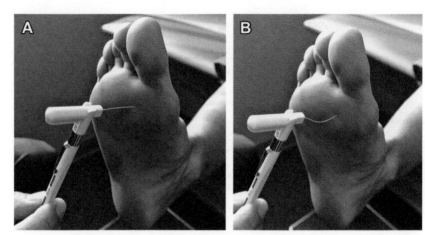

Fig. 2. Demonstration of the assessment of peripheral neuropathy using the Semmes-Weinstein monofilament: (*A*) depicts application of the monofilament, (*B*) demonstrates the bend in the filament when assessing for neuropathy.

CHARCOT ARTHROPATHY

Charcot arthropathy is a progressive deterioration of weight-bearing joints, typically in the foot and ankle in patients with diabetic peripheral neuropathy. In 1868, Jean Marie Charcot described this pattern of bone destruction in patients with tabes dorsalis. Involvement of the knee was commonly associated with syphilis. The first description of neuroarthropathy occurring in conjunction with diabetes was described in 1936.

There are believed to be 2 general causes of neuropathic arthropathy. One is termed the neurotraumatic theory, the other being the neurovascular theory. The neurotraumatic theory is based on the repetitive microtrauma and ensuing bony dissociation and destruction that occurs in the foot that is insensate and lacks proprioception. The neurovascular causes are believed to be due to autonomic dysfunction leading to hyperemia and osteopenia, which effectively weakens and allows progressive destruction in the setting of ongoing trauma. Muscle imbalance in combination with joint stiffness creates eccentric forces and high pressures on the foot, setting the stage for ulceration. The initial bony dissolution and dissociation leads to ligamentous laxity and the supporting structures of the foot become completely compromised. A common pattern seen is a rocker-bottom deformity, which is essentially a reversal of the normal foot architecture. Up to 50% of those individuals with a Charcot foot can recall an injury or an inciting event. Such events may include a twisting injury to the foot or the ankle, or it may occur subsequent to a procedure on the foot (**Fig. 3**).

Neuropathic arthropathy may be seen in up to 10% patients with neuropathy and up to 35% of those affected will have bilateral involvement. It is typically encountered in patients with poorly controlled diabetes and in those who have had the disease for more than 10 years.[14] **Fig. 3** represents the summary of events that lead to the Charcot foot.

The clinical appearance of the foot will vary based on the stage of presentation. Eichenholtz[15] was credited with the description of the clinical stages of the disease. Stage I is considered the fragmentation stage, and is what is typically seen in the acute stages. This is characterized by radiographic evidence of periarticular erosion and joint dislocation. Patients may present earlier with warmth, erythema, and swelling of the foot before the onset of deformity. It often has the appearance of an infection. Stage II represents the coalescence phase, whereby the bony changes begin to

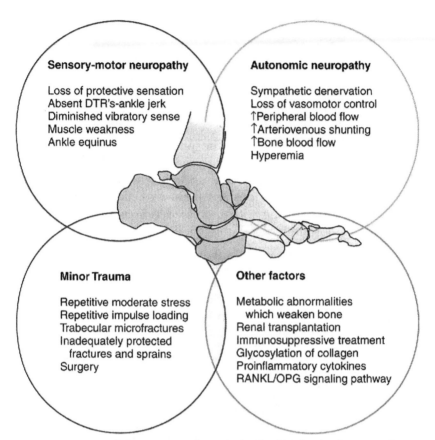

Sensory-motor neuropathy

Loss of protective sensation
Absent DTR's-ankle jerk
Diminished vibratory sense
Muscle weakness
Ankle equinus

Autonomic neuropathy

Sympathetic denervation
Loss of vasomotor control
↑Peripheral blood flow
↑Arteriovenous shunting
↑Bone blood flow
Hyperemia

Minor Trauma

Repetitive moderate stress
Repetitive impulse loading
Trabecular microfractures
Inadequately protected
   fractures and sprains
Surgery

Other factors

Metabolic abnormalities
   which weaken bone
Renal transplantation
Immunosuppressive treatment
Glycosylation of collagen
Proinflammatory cytokines
RANKL/OPG signaling pathway

Fig. 3. Representation of the summary of events that lead to the development of a neuro-pathic foot deformity. *Abbreviations:* DTR, deep tendon reflexes, OPG, osteoprotegerin. (*From* Sanders LJ, Frykberg RG. The Charcot foot. In: Bowker JH, Pfeifer MA, editors. Levin and O'Neal's the diabetic foot. 7th edition. Philadelphia: Elsevier; 2008. p. 257–83; with permission.)

stabilize and there is resorption of bony debris. Stage III is the consolidation or repar-ative phase and represents the stage at which the foot deformity becomes stable (**Fig. 4**). The foot is often deformed, but progression has ceased. Recognition of this process in its earliest stages is critical to optimize intervention and to prevent the long-term sequelae.

Radiographically and anatomically, Charcot arthropathy can be characterized. In its atrophic form, osteolysis occurs in the distal metatarsals, localizing it to the forefoot (**Fig. 5**). Hypertrophic Charcot is localized to the midfoot, hindfoot, or ankle, and it is this form that is classified by the Eichenholtz scheme.

Brodsky[16] described 3 types of Charcot arthropathy based on the involvement of the anatomic location of the foot. Type 1 involves the midfoot and leads to plantar and medial prominences. Type 2 involves the transverse tarsal joint and leads to the greatest instability of the hindfoot. Type 3 has 2 subparts: 3A involves the ankle joint, which also is characterized by instability and prolonged bone healing, and 3B is a pathologic fracture of the calcaneus creating a wide heel and a flat foot.[17] **Fig. 6** demonstrates the geographic radiographic appearance of the Charcot foot.

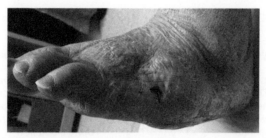

Fig. 4. Clinical appearance of a 49-year-old man with a midfoot neuropathic foot deformity.

The diagnosis of Charcot is largely a clinical one based on the physician's suspicion and the clinical presentation of the patient. When a neuropathic patient demonstrates bone and joint abnormalities, the diagnosis of Charcot arthropathy must be suspected. Distinguishing an acute Charcot process from osteomyelitis can be very challenging. The diagnosis hinges on a detailed history, thorough examination of the foot and ankle, and initial radiographic studies. Use of magnetic resonance imaging (MRI) can be equivocal when trying to distinguish Charcot arthropathy from osteomyelitis. Osteomyelitis should be presumed when there is chronic soft tissue ulceration and infection contiguous to bone. However, in the case of Charcot arthropathy, noninfectious soft tissue inflammation accompanies progressive bone and joint destruction in a well-vascularized, neuropathic, nonulcerated foot.[18] Bone biopsy should be reserved for those individuals in whom the diagnosis remains ambiguous.

Computed tomography, MRI, and technetium scans have limitations in distinguishing between Charcot arthropathy and osteomyelitis. Leukocyte scanning with

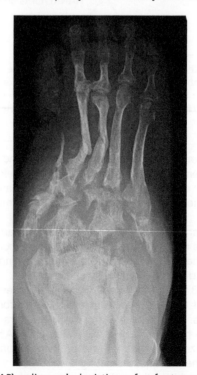

Fig. 5. Anteroposterior (AP) radiograph depicting a forefoot neuropathic deformity.

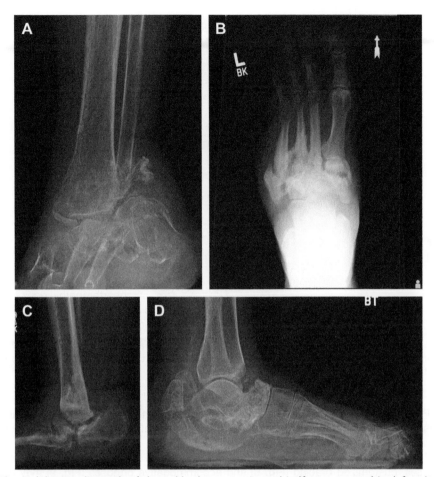

Fig. 6. (*A*) AP radiograph of the ankle demonstrating a hindfoot neuropathic deformity. There is dislocation of the calcaneus under the talus where it is resting under the fibula. (*B*) AP radiograph of a patient with neuropathic changes of the tarsometatarsal joints. (*C*) Lateral radiograph of the ankle demonstrating absence of the talus and dissolution of the hindfoot. (*D*) Lateral radiograph of the foot depicting neuropathic changes of the calcaneus demonstrating rocker bottom appearance.

Indium-111 has been shown to have high specificity and negative predictive value for osteomyelitis.[19] It has also been noted that 111-In labeled leukocytes do not accumulate in neuropathic bone.

When the diagnosis of Charcot arthropathy has been established, management is based on the stage of presentation to the practitioner and the presence or absence of infection. The goal of treatment is to maintain a stable, plantigrade foot so as to prevent ulceration. Optimal treatment for the Charcot foot is prevention. Risk assessment and stratification help identify those at risk: individuals in the sixth or seventh decade, patients who have had diabetes for more than 10 years, and those with loss of protective sensation. Physical manifestations include swelling, redness, increased skin temperature, and deformity.[20]

Initial management should include elevation to control limb edema, weight-bearing restriction, and, in select individuals, immobilization in a total contact cast (**Fig. 7**).

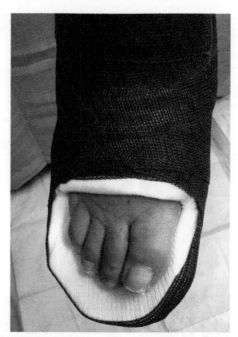

Fig. 7. A total contact cast (TCC). It extends from below the knee and extends past the plantar surface of the toes to provide support and protect the neuropathic foot from further deformity.

Patients who present acutely and are considered candidates for a total contact cast, or those with an ulcer, should be immediately referred to a foot and ankle specialist.

For those who present with deformity and who have passed through the acute phases, customized bracing (**Fig. 8**) and accommodative orthoses (**Fig. 9**) may be considered. Patients should be referred to a foot and ankle specialist or an orthotist experienced with the prescription and/or manufacturing of the appropriate devices. The goal of these devices is to offload prominent areas on the foot and distribute pressure within the shoe in such a way as to minimize risk of ulceration.

The role for use of antiresorptive agents in the management of acute Charcot osteoarthropathy is beginning to emerge; however, their role has yet to be defined.[21] Other emerging technologies include targeting the receptor activator for nuclear factor kappa B ligand (RANKL). RANK is thought to be a critical element in mechanisms controlling osteoclastogenesis and metabolic bone disease.[22]

Surgical intervention is necessary when conservative treatment at offloading and medical optimization have failed to create a stable, plantigrade, ulcer-free foot. Surgical correction is performed when the Charcot process has become quiescent. Surgical intervention typically requires realignment fusions (**Fig. 10**) or, in select cases, primary amputation.

FOOT ULCERATION

The pathophysiology of the development of the diabetic foot ulcer is multifactorial. In combination with the loss of protective sensation that these patients possess, there is

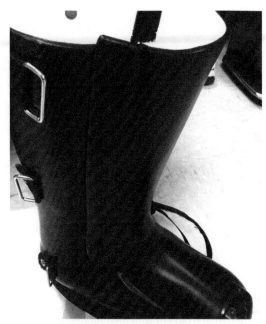

Fig. 8. An accommodative Charcot Restraining Orthotic Walker. It is designed to support the neuropathic foot and can be used when transitioning from a TCC.

a mechanical coupling that increases the risk of development and progression of ulcer formation. Deformity created by Charcot arthropathy, soft tissue contractures, clawing of the toes, and gait abnormality contribute to the mechanical milieu that causes ulceration.

Clawing of the toes is a manifestation of the motor neuropathy that selectively targets the intrinsic muscles of the foot. The deformity created makes the toes vulnerable to ulceration with shoe wear, affecting the plantar and dorsal surfaces of the foot.

Soft tissue contractures, particularly involving the gastrocsoleus complex, are an end result of the advanced glycosylation products causing collagen crosslinking along the length of the entire molecule, causing stiffening of its construct.[23] Altered proprioception and postural instability have been reported in patients with diabetic neuropathy.[24] The loss of afferent feedback during the gait cycle causes increased variability

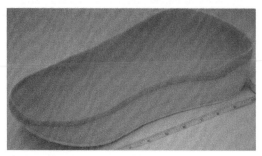

Fig. 9. An accommodative trilayer custom-molded foot insert for a neuropathic foot deformity. The multilayer foam allows for conformity and protection from shear.

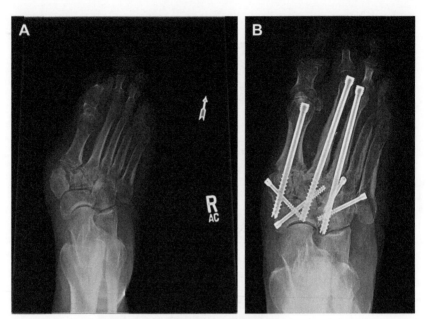

Fig. 10. (*A*) An AP radiograph of a patient with midfoot neuropathic deformity with abduction of the foot that lead to an ulceration. (*B*) Postoperative radiograph of the same patient after undergoing midfoot corrective osteotomy.

of gait kinematics. Additionally, increased plantar flexor moments contribute to abnormal forces contributing to ulcer formation.

The integrity of the skin and the effects of parasympathetic dysfunction compromise the sweat production of the skin. As a result, the skin becomes dry and scaly, and fissures develop. These fissures serve as a portal for infection.

Vascular Disease

Coupled with the mechanical factors that contribute to diabetic foot ulceration is peripheral vascular disease. Primarily ischemic ulcers account for 15% to 20% of foot ulcers, with an additional 15% to 20% due to a mixed neuropathic-vascular etiology.[25] Involvement is most commonly localized to the tibial and peroneal arteries of the calf with sparing of the arteries of the foot.[26] Peripheral vascular disease is more prevalent, occurs at an earlier age, is more diffuse, accelerates faster, and is more extensive in patients with diabetes than in those without diabetes. Plaques develop circumferentially along the length of the vessel and calcification is seen within the tunica media. Additional factors that contribute to atherosclerosis is the dysfunction of nitric oxide. Nitric oxide is a cellular mediator that interferes with monocyte and leukocyte adhesion to the endothelium, platelet-vessel wall interaction, smooth muscle proliferation, and vascular tone. Hyperglycemia, which leads to the formation of superoxides, contributes to this dysfunction, as the reactive oxygen species bind to nitric oxide, limiting its bioavailability.[27]

The assessment of the diabetic patient should include evaluation of pedal pulses. It should be noted that the presence of pulses alone may not be predictive of clinically significant ischemia. Rivers and colleagues,[28] described a cohort of patients who required distal surgical bypass for significant ischemia in the presence of pedal pulses.

In addition to the physical examination, additional noninvasive tests have been used to quantify the severity of peripheral vascular disease. The use of the ankle-brachial index has been used to assess peripheral blood flow. Its validity in patients with diabetes may be less reliable because of the calcification present within the media layer of the distal arteries. The use of systolic toe pressure measurement by photoplethysmography or measuring transcutaneous oxygen tension may be more reliable techniques.[29,30] These measurements are performed in a vascular laboratory and provide an indication of healing potential before consideration of angiography. Arteriography would be considered a "gold standard," but must be instituted with care in this population of people in whom renal disease is often present.[31]

The ankle-brachial index is performed by dividing the segmental ankle systolic pressure by the brachial systolic pressure. Pressure changes typically correlate with flow and an index of 0.5 therefore indicates 50% of expected blood flow. A gradient of 40 mm Hg or greater between segments suggests occlusion or high level of stenosis. The thigh pressure is usually 1.3 times that of the brachial systolic pressure. As noted earlier, the value of ankle pressures may be invalid due to medial calcification. Decreased values, however, can be indicative of significant disease, as no false pressures are likely to occur. Normal indices or elevated pressures should be correlated with toe pressures.[32] The role of toe pressure measurement has been studied. It is felt that absolute toe pressures provide a highly accurate method for determining the likelihood of an ulcer or in minor amputation, thus preventing a more proximal amputation.[33] Toe pressures measuring higher than 40 mm Hg are most predictive of wound healing (**Fig. 11**).

Another method to evaluate the state of limb perfusion, and in particular the skin, is the measurement of transcutaneous partial oxygen pressure. The test is performed by placing a probe over the metatarsal region of the affected foot. After equilibrating the probe to a specific temperature, the oxygen tension of the skin is determined.[34] Although results are difficult to interpret, and may be limited by host and ambient factors, there is support for its use.[30] A transcutaneous oxygen pressure (TCpO2) reading of 40 mm Hg or higher was predictive of adequate perfusion for wound healing in patients undergoing transtibial amputation.[35] In a study by Pinzur and colleagues,[36] healing rates were correlated with TCpO2. The healing rate was 50% with a TCpO2 of 1 to

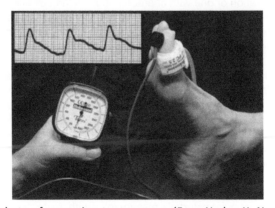

Fig. 11. Clinical photo of measuring toe-pressures. (*From* Hurley JJ. Noninvasive vascular testing in the evaluation of diabetic peripheral arterial disease. In: Bowker JH, Pfeifer MA, editors. Levin and O'Neal's the diabetic foot. 7th edition. Philadelphia: Mosby; 2008. p. 239–55; with permission.)

19 mm Hg, 75% with a TCpO2 of 20 to 29 mm Hg, and 92% at levels higher than 30 mm Hg.

Ulcer Classification

Classification of diabetic foot wounds is important to develop treatment plans, and it is important to communicate with caregivers to monitor progress and outcomes of these lesions. As has been discussed, there are several factors that need to be considered in the assessment and management of these wounds. These factors include perfusion, presence and extent of gangrenous changes, location and severity of vascular disease, location of the ulcer, shape of the ulcer, duration, the presence and depth of infection, infecting organisms, nutritional status, immunosuppression, comorbidities, bony deformity, neuropathy, previous ulcerations, gait disturbances, and abnormal foot pressures.[37] It is through recognition of these factors that we can hopefully intervene, treat, and educate patients so as to minimize risk for amputation and future ulceration.

Approximately 70% to 90% of neuropathic ulcers occur in the forefoot; the heel is the next most common area followed by the midfoot.[17]

Two common classification schemes include the Wagner-Megitt Classification and the Depth Ischemia Classification.

The Wagner-Megitt Classification is known for its simplicity and is often referred to when discussing these lesions. The original system has 6 grades of lesions. The first 4 grades (0, 1, 2 and 3) are based on the physical depth of the lesion involving the soft tissues of the foot. Grades 4 and 5 are based on the extent of lost perfusion in the foot. Most outpatient lesions are grades 0 to 1, whereas grades 2 and 3 ulcers often require hospitalization or surgical intervention. Grades 4 and 5 require amputation and control of residual infection and consideration for further limb revascularization (**Fig. 12**).

The Depth-Ischemia Classification is a modification of the Wagner-Megitt Classification. It makes it easier to distinguish between evaluation of the wound and the vascularity of the foot, which is a limitation of the Wagner-Megitt Classification. Each foot is given a number and letter grade. The number value describes the physical extent of the wound, and the letter grade describes the vascularity. Determination of grade and stage is accomplished with inspection and gentle probing with a blunt, sterile instrument. The grade 0 foot is a foot at risk and represents a foot that has had a previous ulceration or one with characteristics making ulceration likely. A grade 1 lesion is a superficial wound without exposure of deeper structures. Grade 2 lesions are deeper with exposed tendon or joint capsule, with or without infection. Grade 3 lesions are the deepest, with exposed bone and osteomyelitis or abscess (see **Fig. 12**).

Limb perfusion is next determined and assigned letters A, B, C, and D. A grade A foot will demonstrate bounding pedal pulses. These feet do not typically require vascular evaluation or intervention. A grade B foot is the most commonly encountered. It is ischemic but not gangrenous. Lesions of this nature require referral for vascular analysis. Grade C feet have partial gangrene, and grade D feet are completely gangrenous. A vascular evaluation is necessary to determine the level of adequate perfusion, level of potential healing, and the need for revascularization.

Depth-Ischemia Classification is effective at prescribing treatment (**Table 1**). Grade 0 lesions are treated with education, regular visits, and appropriate insoles and shoe wear. Grade 1 lesions require external pressure relief with a total contact cast, bracing, or shoe wear. Grade 2 lesions require surgical debridement, wound care pressure, and antibiotics. Grade 3 lesions require surgical debridement and may require partial ray amputation. Stage A lesions can be observed and followed with regular visits. Stage

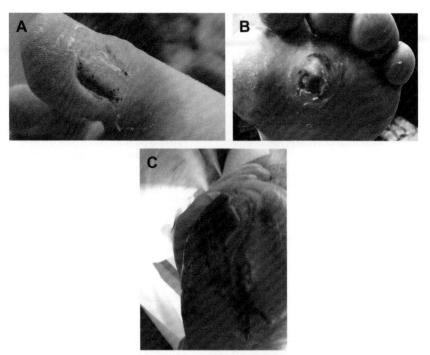

Fig. 12. (*A*) Grade 1 ulceration of hallux. (*B*) Grade 2 ulcer off plantar forefoot with exposed plantar capsule. (*C*) Grade 3 ulcer of calcaneus with necrotic wound bed and exposed calcaneus.

B requires vascular evaluation with possible vascular reconstruction. Stage C requires a proximal or distal bypass and partial amputation. Stage D lesions may require major extremity amputation (transtibial, transfemoral) with vascular reconstruction.[38]

Wound-Healing Strategies

The approach to management of foot lesions is based on the staging, grading, and etiology of the ulcer. This can be accomplished with a combination of mechanical offloading and local wound care.

Offloading can be accomplished through the use of a total contact cast. The application of the cast must be performed by experienced personnel, as serious complications may arise from its use. A patient with a nonhealing ulcer and associated deformity should be referred to a foot and ankle specialist. Other devices that have been described include removable braces and off-loading shoes. These devices, although potentially safer, require patient compliance, which historically has been poor.[39,40]

There is a wide range of wound-healing agents available. This includes, but is not limited to, saline dressings, impregnated gauze, nonadherent dressing, hydrogels, hydrocolloids, calcium alginate, silver, vacuum-assisted closure, and hyperbaric oxygen. The indications for the various agents is vast and the reader is referred to a recent review of the subject.[41]

Local wound debridement, along with application of the previously discussed modalities, are considered for chronic wounds. Office-based debridement is designed to decrease the bacterial burden of the wound. Bacterial overgrowth is a significant

Table 1
The Depth-Ischemia Classification depicting the grading and management of neuropathic foot ulcers

Grade	Definition	Treatment
Depth Classification		
0	The at-risk foot: previous ulcer or neuropathy with deformity that can cause new ulcerations	Patient education: regular examination, appropriate footwear, appropriate insoles
1	Superficial ulceration, not infected	External pressure relief; total-contact cast, walking brace, special footwear, and so forth
2	Deep ulceration exposing a tendon or joint (with or without superficial infection)	Surgical debridement, wound care, pressure relief if the lesion closes and converts to grade 1 (antibiotics as needed)
3	Extensive ulceration with exposed bone and/or deep infection (osteomyelitis) or abscess	Surgical debridement; ray or partial foot amputation; antibiotics; pressure relief if wound converts to grade 1
Ischemia Classification		
A	Not ischemic	None
B	Ischemia without gangrene	Vascular evaluation (eg, Doppler, $tcPo_2$ arteriogram); vascular reconstruction as needed
C	Partial (forefoot) gangrene of the foot	Vascular evaluation; vascular reconstruction (proximal and/or distal bypass or angioplasty); partial foot amputation
D	Complete foot gangrene	Vascular evaluation; major extremity amputation (below knee or above knee) with possible proximal vascular reconstruction

From Brodsky JW. The diabetic foot. In: Coughlin MJ, Mann RA, Saltzman CL, editors. Surgery of the foot and ankle. Philadelphia: Mosby; 2007. p. 1301; with permission.

impediment to wound healing. Enzymatic production by bacteria and the ensuing degradation of fibrin and other growth factors inhibits wound healing. Debridement of dysvascular or necrotic tissue helps decrease the bacterial count and stimulates production of local growth factors.

Finally, additional factors that predict wound healing are a total serum protein concentration of 6.2 g/dL, a serum albumin level of 3.5 g/dL, and a total lymphocyte count of 1500/mm^3.[42]

ORTHOTIC MANAGEMENT OF THE DIABETIC FOOT

All too often, institution of an orthotic or an off-loading device is undertaken after someone has healed an ulceration or has undergone a partial foot amputation from an infection created by an ulcer. The goal of a comprehensive diabetic foot program requires communication between the physician and an experienced pedorthist. The goals are to create a protective environment for the foot and to prevent recurrent ulceration.

Improper shoe wear is a common cause of ulcers.[43] There are several objectives for therapeutic shoe wear for the diabetic patient. The shoe should protect the foot from the external environment and relieve areas of pressure and distribute pressure more evenly to minimize risk of ulceration. Shoe wear should protect from shock and shear, especially in cases of significant deformity. Because many feet have significant deformities, it is important to have shoes that accommodate the neuropathic foot.[44]

The key to selecting shoe size is determined by accurately measuring the foot. This should be done both weight bearing and non–weight bearing to determine how much the foot changes. An appropriately sized shoe will have three-eighths to one-half inch between the end of the longest toe and the front of the shoe. The shoe should allow for a small amount of movement of the heel. It is important to educate the patient on proper-fitting shoes.

Foot orthoses are usually prescribed as custom-made devices. The role of the orthosis is to cushion and protect the foot. A well-made orthosis should provide shock absorption and provide shock attenuation. It should provide pressure distribution throughout in cases in which high plantar pressure exists. A total contact design should limit shear and, through the use of soft materials, it should accommodate fixed deformities. A combination of rigid and semirigid material will also limit motion and minimize ulceration.

RECOMMENDATIONS

It is critical that every health professional involved in the care of the diabetic patient take an active role in assessing an individual's risk for foot pathology. The American Diabetes Association recommends that all patients with diabetes receive a thorough foot examination on an annual basis. For patients with a previous ulcer or history of an amputation, screening should be carried out every 3 to 4 months. Patients with active wounds or Charcot arthropathy require more aggressive follow-up with weekly or biweekly visits. This assessment includes observing for protective sensation, foot structure and biomechanical imbalance and limited joint mobility, skin integrity, and vascular status.[45] An assessment of shoe wear also is essential, as improper shoe wear can lead to ulceration. One should maintain a diligent approach in looking for high-risk factors, including advancing age, a history of diabetes for more than 10 years, visual loss, inability to bend, living alone, tobacco use, and risk-taking behavior, in addition to the risk factors discussed previously.[46]

Unfortunately, there are many challenges to the treatment of these diabetic foot problems. Often patients are in denial of their disease and fail to take ownership of their illness and the necessary steps to prevent complications. A screening or prevention program may not effect change in behavior in this patient population. However, in a well-informed and motivated patient, maintaining suggested glucose control is possible through diet, exercise, and medication. It is incumbent for all practitioners to continually educate their patients about the consequences and treatment of diabetes.[47]

Screening patients for risk of ulceration is critical to prevention. Studies have demonstrated the efficacy of such screening, thereby reducing foot ulcers and their consequences.[48,49] Screening helps determine the level of risk and guide additional interventions.[50] Risk assessment is possible based on the history of ulceration, deformity, previous amputation, absence of pedal pulses, and loss of sensation.[50] A patient with risk category 0 who has a normal foot and normal neurovascular function should be educated on daily foot care and shoe wear, and have yearly examinations. A person with risk category 1 demonstrates sensory loss and is advised on daily foot inspection and to obtain soft inlays, and is advised to have the foot examined every 6 months. The patient with a risk category 2 has had a ray amputation, demonstrates sensory loss, and has deformity of the foot. These individuals require more diligent attention with more frequent visits to their physician. Custom-molded inserts are suggested and additional appliances may be necessary to further off-load the forefoot. The patient in risk category 3 has a history of ulceration, deformities, and prior multilevel amputation. These individuals also have diminished or absent pulses. These patients require extensive education and require custom-made accommodative orthoses. External modifications to shoe wear also may be required. Surveillance should be done every 2 months by a qualified health professional. These patients will typically be referred to an orthopedic foot and ankle surgeon to optimize management of the associated deformities.

The individual patient remains the most important player in prevention of foot complications. Through education of the risk factors discussed in the text and physical inspection of the foot, an individual can understand the seriousness of his or her disease. The initial responsibility for management is assigned to the primary care provider. Hopefully, with the information provided in this text, providers will have the necessary background information to understand and assess the diabetic patient at risk for ulceration and amputation and implement the necessary intervention. Any individual with loss of protective sensation, history of ulceration, or prior amputation should be referred to a foot and ankle specialist for treatment. It is important to incorporate family members, when present, into the care of these individuals. This is especially true for patients with poor vision and/or limited mobility, as they cannot adequately monitor their foot skin integrity or changes in their feet.[51] Adherence to guidelines to screening, as put forth by the American Diabetes Association, The American Board of Family Practice, and the Centers for Disease Control and Prevention, can assist the practitioner in caring for these patients with this extremely challenging disease. These recommendations include foot examination at every diabetic visit with screening for risk factors, such as age (older than 40 years), smoking, and duration of diabetes of more than 10 years. Additional recommendations include assessment of ulcer size, plain radiographs, mechanical off-loading, and metabolic control.[52]

REFERENCES

1. Atkinson AM, MacLaren NK. The pathogenesis of insulin dependent diabetes mellitus. N Engl J Med 1994;331(21):1428–36.
2. The Diabetes Control and Complications Trial Research Group. The effect of intensive treatment of diabetes on the development and progression of long term complications in insulin dependent diabetes mellitus. N Engl J Med 1993;339:977–86.
3. Geiss LS, Cowie CC. Type 2 diabetes and persons at high risk for diabetes. In: Narayan KM, Williams D, Gregg EW, et al, editors. Diabetes and public health: from data to policy. New York: Oxford University Press; 2011. p. 15–32.
4. Boyle JP, Thomson TJ, Gregg EW, et al. Projection of the year 2050 Burden of diabetes in the US adult population: dynamic modeling of incidence, mortality and prediabetes prevalence. Popul Health Metr 2010;8:29.
5. Centers for Disease Control and Prevention. National diabetes fact sheet, 2011. Atlanta (GA): Centers for Disease Control and Prevention, US Department of Health and Human Services; 2011. Available at: http://www.cdc.gov/diabetes/pubs/pdf/ndfs_2011.
6. MacLaren N, Atkinson M. Is insulin dependent diabetes mellitus environmentally induced? N Engl J Med 1992;327:348–9.

7. Foulis AK, Liddle CN, Farquharson MA, et al. The histopathology of the pancreas in type 1 (insulin dependent) diabetes mellitus: a 25 year review of deaths in patients under 20 years of age in the United Kingdom. Diabetologia 1986;29:267–74.

8. Clark CM, Lee DA. Presentation and treatment of the complications of diabetes mellitus. N Engl J Med 1995;332:1210–7.

9. Aring AM, Jones DF, Falko JM. Evaluation and prevention of diabetic neuropathy. Am Fam Physician 2005;71:2123–8.

10. Pinart J. Diabetes mellitus and its degenerative complications: a prospective study of 4400 patients observed between 1947 and 1973. Diabete Metab 1977;3:97–107.

11. Vink AI, Mehrabyan A. Understanding diabetic neuropathies. Emerg Med 2004; 5:39–44.

12. Unger J, Cole BE. Recognition and management of diabetic neuropathy. Prim Care 2007;34:887–913.

13. Edwards JL, Vincent AM, Cheng HT, et al. Diabetic neuropathy: mechanisms to management. Pharmacol Ther 2008;120:1–34.

14. Sommer TC, Lee TH. Charcot foot: the diagnostic dilemma. Am Fam Physician 2001;64:1591–8.

15. Eichenholtz SN. Charcot joints. Springfield (IL): Thomas; 1966.

16. Brodsky JW. Outpatient diagnosis and care of the diabetic foot. Instr Course Lect 1993;42:121–39.

17. Laughlin RT, Calhoun JH, Mader JT. The diabetic foot. J Am Acad Orthop Surg 1995;3:218–25.

18. Berendt AR, Lipsky B. Is this bone infected or not? Differentiating neuroarthropathy from osteomyelitis in the diabetic foot. Curr Diab Rep 2004;4(6):424–9.

19. Schauwecker DS. Osteomyelitis: diagnosis with in-111-labelled leukocytes. Radiology 1989;171(1):141–6.

20. Sanders LJ, Frykberg RG. The Charcot foot. In: Bowker JH, Pfeifer MA, editors. Levin and O'Neal's the diabetic foot. 7th edition. Philadelphia (PA): Mosby Elsevier; 2008. p. 257–83.

21. Pitocco D, Riotolo V, Caputo S, et al. Six month treatment with alendronate in acute Charcot neuroarthropathy: a randomized controlled trial. Diabetes Care 2005;28(5):1214–5.

22. Jeffcoate W. Vascular calcification and osteolysis in diabetic neuropathy: is RANKL the missing link? Diabetologia 2004;47(9):1488–92.

23. Guyton GP, Saltzman CL. The diabetic foot: basic mechanisms of disease. J Bone Joint Surg Am 2001;83(7):1084–96.

24. Katoulis EC, Ebdon-Parry M, Hollis S, et al. Postural instability in diabetic neuropathic patients at risk for foot ulceration. Diabet Med 1997;14:296–300.

25. Grunfeld C. Diabetic foot ulcers: etiology, treatment and prevention. Adv Intern Med 1991;37:103–32.

26. Logerfo W, Coffman JD. Vascular and microvascular disease of the foot in diabetes: implications for foot care. N Engl J Med 1984;311:1615–9.

27. Cosentino F, Luscher TF. Endothelial dysfunction in diabetes mellitus. J Cardiovasc Pharmacol 1998;32(Suppl 3):s54–61.

28. Rivers SD, Scher L, Veith FJ. Indications for distal arterial reconstruction in the presence of palpable pedal pulses. J Vasc Surg 1990;12(5):552–7.

29. Apelqvist J, Castenfors J, Larsson J, et al. Prognostic value of systemic ankle and toe blood pressure measurement in outcome of diabetic foot ulcer. Diabetes Care 1989;12:373–8.

30. Ballard JL, Eke CC, Bunt TJ, et al. A prospective evaluation of transcutaneous oxygen measurements in the management of diabetic foot problems. J Vasc Surg 1995;22(4):485–90.
31. Bowering CK. Diabetic foot ulcers: pathophysiology, assessment and therapy. Can Fam Physician 2001;47:1007–16.
32. Hurley JJ. Noninvasive vascular testing in the evaluation of diabetic peripheral arterial disease. In: Bowker JH, Pfeifer MA, editors. Levin and O'Neal's the diabetic foot. 7th edition. Philadelphia: Mosby; 2008. p. 239–55.
33. Holstein P, Noer I, Tonneses KH, et al. Distal blood pressure in severe arterial insufficiency. In: Bergan J, Yao J, editors. Gangrene and severe ischemia of the lower extremities. New York: Gryne and Stratton; 1978. p. 95–114.
34. Aulivola B, Craig RM. Decision making in the dysvascular lower extremity. Foot Ankle Clin 2010;15:391–409.
35. Mustapha NM, Redhead RG, Jain SK, et al. Transcutaneous partial oxygen pressure assessment of the ischemic lower limb. Surg Gynecol Obstet 1983; 156:582–4.
36. Pinzur MS, Sage R, Stuck R, et al. Transcutaneous oxygen as a predictor of wound healing in amputations of the foot and ankle. Foot Ankle 1992;13: 271–2.
37. Brodsky JW. Classification of foot lesions in diabetic patients. In: Bowker JH, Pfeiffer MA, editors. Levin and O'Neal's the diabetic foot. 7th edition. Philadelphia: Mosby; 2008. p. 221–6.
38. Brodsky JW. Outpatient diagnosis and management of the diabetic foot. Instructional course lectures, vol. 42. Rosemont (IL): American Academy of Orthopaedic Surgeons; 1993. p. 121–39.
39. Cavanagh PR, Owings TM. Nonsurgical strategies for healing and preventing recurrence of diabetic foot ulcers. Foot Ankle Clin 2006;11:735–43.
40. Armstrong D, Lavery LA, Kimbriel HR, et al. Activity patterns of patients with diabetic foot ulceration: patients with active ulceration may not adhere to a standard pressure offloading regimen. Diabetes Care 2003;26(9):2595–7.
41. Falanga V. Wound healing and its impairment in the diabetic foot. Lancet 2005; 366(9498):1736–43.
42. Wagner F Jr. A classification and treatment program for diabetic, neuropathic and dysvascular foot problems. Instr Course Lect 1979;28:143–65.
43. Reiber GE, Smith DG, Wallace C, et al. Effect of Therapeutic Footwear on Foot Reulceration in Patients with Diabetes: A Randomized Controlled Trial. JAMA 2002;287(19):2552–8.
44. Janisse DJ, Janisse EJ. Pedorthic and orthotic management of the diabetic foot. Foot Ankle Clin 2006;11:717–34.
45. Mayfield JA, Reiber G, Sanders LJ, et al. Preventive foot care in patients with diabetes. Diabetes Care 1988;21:2161–77.
46. Helfand AE. Assessing and preventing foot problems in older patients who have diabetes mellitus. Clin Podiatr Med Surg 2003;20:573–82.
47. Farber DC, Farber JS. Office based screening, prevention and management of diabetic foot disorders. Prim Care 2007;34:873–85.
48. Singh N, Armstrong DG, Lipsky BA. Preventing foot ulcers in patients with diabetes. JAMA 2005;293:217–8.
49. Willrich A, Pinzur M, McNeil M, et al. Health related quality of life, cognitive function and depression in diabetic patients with foot ulcer or amputation: a preliminary study. Foot Ankle Int 2005;26(2):128–34.

50. Berlet G, Shields N. The diabetic foot. In: Richardson EG, editor. Orthopaedic knowledge update foot and ankle 3. Rosemont (IL): American Academy of Orthopaedic Surgeons; 2004. p. 123–34.
51. Umeh L, Wallhagen M, Nicoloff N. Identifying diabetic patients at high risk for amputation. Nurse Pract 1999;24(8):56–70.
52. Zoorob RJ, Hagen MD. Guidelines on the care of diabetic nephropathy, retinopathy and foot disease. Am Fam Physician 1997;8(56):2021–8.

Offloading of the Diabetic Foot
Orthotic and Pedorthic Strategies

Brant L. McCartan, DPM, MBA, MS[a,b,*], Barry I. Rosenblum, DPM[a]

KEYWORDS

- Orthoses • Diabetes • Ulceration • Offloading • Bracing • Monitoring
- Team approach • Modifications

KEY POINTS

- Each foot must be treated independently. What works for one side may not be successful for the contralateral limb in the same patient or in other similar patients.
- The balance between what is functional and that which accommodates is a challenge for the entire team. Currently, the most appropriate materials are short lasting and must be replaced routinely.
- The diabetic foot constantly changes with time, body habitus, and systemic conditions— patients and their care takers must be educated to watch for warning signs and seek early intervention.
- Follow-up for regular monitoring, maintenance, and modifications of orthotic and pedorthic devices is crucial for successful prevention of further collapse or reulceration.
- In even the most compliant patients wearing the best devices, devices breakdown at times. The importance of always wearing a device cannot be overemphasized. Patients need to be able to apply a brace and function with the orthoses - they need to want to wear them.

INTRODUCTION: NATURE OF THE PROBLEM

The diabetic foot, at times, is an anomaly to even the most seasoned practitioners. Decreased circulation and sensation leave the limb almost destined to ulceration, collapse, or often both. Once this occurs, the susceptibility to infection and amputation is heightened. The principles of ulcer treatment have remained constant despite the technological advances of medicines, dressings, and biologic skin equivalents.

This article originally appeared in Clinics in Podiatric Medicine and Surgery, Volume 31, Issue 1, January 2014.
[a] Beth Israel Deaconess Medical Center, Harvard Medical School, 185 Pilgrim Road, Baker Span 3, Boston, MA 02215, USA; [b] Private Practice, Milwaukee Foot Specialists, 3610 Michelle Witmer Memorial Drive, Suite 110, New Berlin, WI 53151, USA
* Corresponding author. Milwaukee Foot Specialists, 3610 Michelle Witmer Memorial Drive, Suite 110, New Berlin, WI 53151, USA.
E-mail address: dr.mccartan@yahoo.com

Keys to ulcer treatment
- Infection control
- Maximizing perfusion
- Adequate nutrition
- Offloading

Offloading of the diabetic foot entails a lifetime of work and encompasses the time from initial presentation to perioperative period to postoperative management. The foot structure is in a contact flux; fluid management of patients can lead to rapid weight gains and loses. Limb swelling and neuropathy make education of patients and their caretakers paramount because regular modifications are necessary. These can be performed by a multitude of health professionals, but the best management is a team approach with regular follow-up and a watchful eye.

THERAPEUTIC OPTIONS

Orthoses and braces can be used for every type of patient. These devices are used in diabetic patients to prevent ulceration or reulceration and serve to brace or accommodate a collapsing or collapsed foot. They reduce peak plantar pressures in the foot.[1–3] There are 2 specific types of orthoses, functional and accommodative. Typically rigid orthoses are thought to best functionally correct a flexible, biomechanical abnormality. Soft orthoses accommodate a misshapen or painful rigid foot. In diabetic patients, the extremes must be avoided. There is a balance between accommodating a misshapen foot structure and helping to function as a brace to prevent further collapse. The concept of total contact, no matter if an orthotic or cast is used, helps disperse pressure evenly off of prominent areas and helps maintain current joint architecture.

Diabetic patients are at an increased risk during the intraoperative period compared with nondiabetic patients. Orthoses and bracing can help prevent surgery. Sometimes, however, surgery is unavoidable. Luckily, different devices can prolong the time to surgery. They can also serve as an intermediary in the perioperative period to help close an ulceration before an exostectomy or reconstruction. They also can be used postoperatively to bridge a patient between a cast and their normal shoe gear.

DIFFERENT INITIAL PRESENTATIONS
Ideal Foot

The diabetic foot can present in a multitude of conditions. The ideal presentation is to see a foot that has not collapsed or ulcerated in a well-educated, well-controlled patient. **Table 1** depicts a good algorithm for patients who have intact neurovascular status and are compliant with a normal-appearing foot. Certainly most standard shoes are acceptable. If a patient is neuropathic, it is beneficial to offer an extra depth shoe (**Fig. 1**) or, if hammertoes are present, a shoe with an elastic toe box (**Fig. 2**)

Table 1
Algorithm to treating an "Ideal" diabetic foot – one without collapse or calluses, in a patient with neuropathy, or increased susceptibility to deformity, collapse or ulceration

Condition of Foot	Shoes	Orthoses	Braces	Follow-up
"Ideal"	Correct fit	± for Comfort	None	Annual CDFE Education of warning signs
Ischemic/neuropathic	Extra depth	Accommodative	None	More frequent follow-up

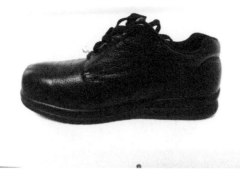

Fig. 1. Extra depth shoe – note increased height of toe box.

that stretches to accommodate the toes is helpful. An annual comprehensive diabetic foot examination (CDFE) is a good screening to help catch abnormalities before they become worse.

Diabetic Foot with Preulcerative Callus

In patients with a preulcerative callus (**Fig. 3**), the cause must be determined. Is it strictly from increased plantar pressure or too tight shoe gear? Is there increased shearing from a biomechanical abnormality? **Table 2** demonstrates a variety of scenarios. Ulcers frequently result from areas of callus.[4] The shear forces cause microseparation between skin layers and cause damage to the tissues deeper to the epidermis.[5] Routine débridements of the thickened, hypertrophic tissue help decrease pressure to the area.

Diabetic Foot with Ulceration

If a patient presents with an ulceration, it must be managed. The infection must be controlled and vascular status assessed and optimized. Depth should be analyzed, especially which tissue plane is exposed: through dermis, muscle, capsule, and

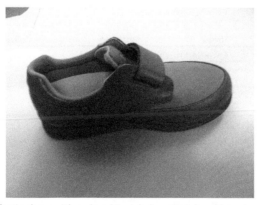

Fig. 2. Custom diabetic shoe with nylon (stretchy) material on dorsal aspect of toe box to allow room for rigid hammertoes or distal bony prominences.

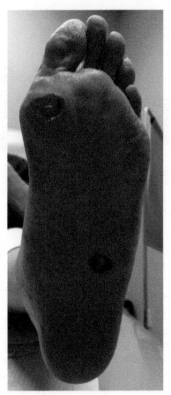

Fig. 3. Pre-ulcerative calluses on bottom of neuropathic, diabetic foot representing areas of increased pressure.

bone. Once the emergent factors are addressed, pressure reduction is the most controllable therapy for successful salvage. Again, the biomechanical cause of the ulceration must be determined. **Fig. 4** depicts a patient with a lateral foot ulceration. This ulceration results from a decreased eversion strength, leaving the foot in a varus

Table 2
Algorithm to treat diabetic patients with a pre-ulcerative callus depending on cause and location

Condition of Foot	Shoes	Orthoses	Braces	Follow-up
Dorsal calluses over IPJs	Extra depth with flexible doral toe box	± for Control	None	Regular
Medial pinch callus or styloid	Correct fit	Functional	None	Regular
Plantar forefoot or midfoot	Extra depth	Accommodative, and modified to offload prominent areas of greatest peak plantar pressure	None	Quarterly
Flexible flatfoot (*posterior tibial tendon dysfunction*)	Comfort or extra depth	Built into brace	Guantlet	Annual

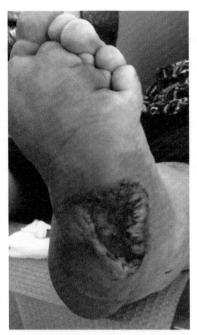

Fig. 4. Ulcer along lateral column. Note equinovarus contracture and position of foot due to lateral muscle weakness and subsequent decrease eversion strength.

attitude. Wounds like this are challenging to treat, but they are even more difficult to prevent from coming back. Bracing is a must if surgical correction is not possible. Ulceration is the precursor to amputation for most diabetic patients.[6–9] Total contact casting (TCC) remains the gold standard for ulceration offloading. TCCs are especially useful for plantar midfoot ulcerations or in patients with active Charcot joint collapse. In addition, if a patient has muscle weakness causing a deformity, such as drop foot, bracing is required. The shoes must also be able to house the brace (**Table 3**).

Table 3
Algorithm to treat diabetic patients with more severe deformities, collapse or ulcerations at specific regions of the foot

Condition of Foot	Shoes	Orthoses	Braces	Follow-up
Dorsal ulceration	Extra depth	± for Control	None	Weekly until healed
Plantar ulceration	Extra depth once healed	Accommodative and modified to offload ulcer. May need to consider regular dressing changes	TCC, felted-foam	Weekly or more frequent
Plantar cuboid, Charcot	N/A	Plastizote built into brace	CROW	
Dropfoot	Extra depth to accommodate brace	Accommodative to disperse pressure	AFO	Regular

Diabetic Foot Requiring Surgical Correction

At times, surgery is required. In the preoperative period, orthoses can be used to off-load and help reduce the ulcer size or, ideally, heal the ulceration. **Table 4** represents a variety of challenging scenarios. After this, definitive surgery can be performed. Patients with equinus as the culprit of increased forefoot pressure often require soft tissue release (tendo-Achilles lengthening, gastrocneumius recession, or targeted plantar fascia release). Boots and casts are used to maintain the correction in the perioperative period. Postoperatively, the foot adapts. Similarly to how a residual limb changes and molds for a prosthetic, the foot accommodates. Areas that were not prominent before may become the most prominent area after exostectomy.

During reconstruction and creation of an arch, there may be new areas that become more susceptible to injury and need to be addressed. During the longer-term postoperative period, adventitious bursa or bursitis can form. The bursa should diminish in size with proper offloading. If it becomes too large, it can cause reulceration and may need to be excised. The bony prominence deep to the bursa may require additional resection. During reconstructions, hardware is often placed and prevention of an ulcer (portal of entry for bacteria) is vital. As the foot changes and accommodates, so must the orthotic devices. Braces can be used to correct flexible deformities, muscle weaknesses, and wasting due to neuropathy. Many times, a normal-appearing foot is not achievable during surgery, and efforts are directed to create a foot that is functional only with a brace. **Fig. 5** is a picture of a patient's shoe and brace modification after a partial calcanectomy. Extra effort must be paid not only to supporting this patient's ankle but also directed at prevented a plantar calcaneal ulceration. Postoperatively, an amputation or fusion changes a patient's gait; bracing is required. Shoe filler helps further stabilize the foot in the shoe after single digit or multiple forefoot amputations (**Fig. 6**). Patients typically prefer wearing shoes with similar appearance. With more proximal amputations, however, this is not always possible, and a short shoe has to suffice (**Fig. 7**). Different

Table 4
Algorithm to treat or temporize diabetic patients requiring surgical intervention and methods to stabilize feet post-operatively to prevent subsequent surgeries

Condition of Foot	Shoes	Orthoses	Braces	Follow-up
Immediate postoperative	Postoperative shoe	None	Short leg cast Posterior splint Removable walking cast	Weekly or more frequent
Healed incision	Extra depth	Accommodative	Gauntlet, AFO, CROW	Very regular with multiple health professionals when applying new shoes or braces
Postamputation	Extra depth	Accommodative with shoe filler	± Based on need	Regular adjustments
Unrepairable, not a surgical candidate, failed surgery	Extra depth	Built into brace	Patellar-tendon device	Regular adjustments

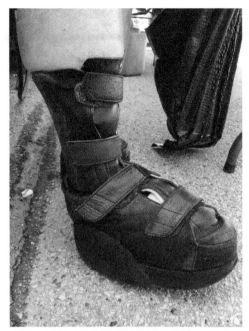

Fig. 5. Foot with calcaneal gait and subsequent partial calcanectomy. Note combination of proximal brace and rocker shoe to help off-load high pressure areas.

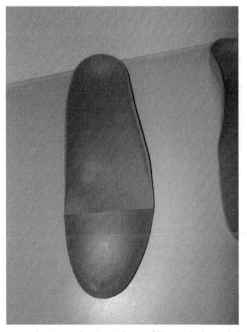

Fig. 6. Plastizote accommodative orthotic with toe filler to help stabilize foot by filling the void status post amputation.

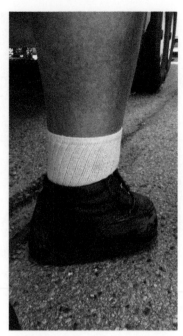

Fig. 7. Short shoe for patient status post proximal amputation.

amputation levels also result in alteration of biomechanics. Bracing can be used to restore a lever arm lost from a digital or transmetatarsal amputation.[10,11] Some patients require an ankle-foot orthosis (AFO) to compensate for the loss of lever arm or flexion strength (**Fig. 8**).

CLINICAL CORRELATION AND OUTCOMES

Improper shoe fitting can cause skin breakdown. High plantar pressure and shear force is another factor. These can be curbed by foot orthoses and bracing. If a brace does not fit properly, however, ulceration may ensue. Shoe and brace selection must be geared at making it easy for patients to maintain compliance and be easy to apply with a pleasant appearance. This becomes more difficult as the demands of and on the device increase. The devices must be modifiable as the foot changes, and they must be able to accommodate a brace.

Orthotic Materials

Orthotic materials, in general, must offload the current deformity and prevent future breakdown. This is best accomplished by dispersing plantar forces and stabilizing the foot to prevent shearing. Attention should be directed at restoring gait. If the deformities are reducible and flexible, bracing is a great conservative option. It is best to have a multilayered device. The base layer should be the most dense, and density or durometer should decrease up the device toward contact with the foot. Ethylene vinyl acetate (EVA) and 60-mm Poron are stable and easy to work with. It is the material of choice to balance out a deformity and is a good base layer. Plastizote is a great top layer or in direct contact with the foot (**Fig. 9**). It comes in varying densities and is modifiable but does break down more rapidly than cork and other materials. Some

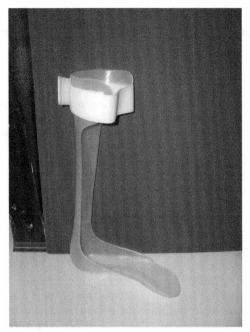

Fig. 8. Rigid ankle-foot orthoses to help keep patients ankle in a more rectus position. Used for patients with weakened extensor strength and multiplanar deformities.

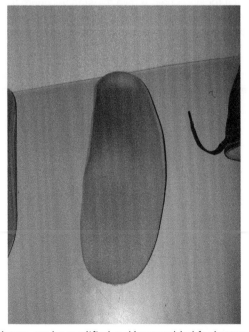

Fig. 9. Plastizote orthoses, can be modified and heat molded for better accommodation and off-loading. Typically breaks down after four months, but great at reducing pressure.

studies support a 3-layer orthotic consisting of a moldable polyethylene foam in contact with the foot, a middle urethane polymer layer for shock absorption, and a firm cork or EVA base layer for functional support and control.[12,13] Extra depth shoes are best with patients having rigid hammertoes or requiring a brace, such as an AFO.[14]

Therapeutic Shoes

Therapeutic shoes are traditionally extra depth (increased by at least one-quarter inch) and rocker soled. One study determined that "comfort shoes" are better than extra depth without an orthotic at reducing forefoot pressure.[1] Extra depth shoes with an orthotic were found, however, to greater reduce pressure, especially with a rocker bottom. If possible, the shoe should be made of breathable materials, such as leather or Gore-Tex. Slip-on shoes are easy to put on but lack stability and are often too tight once the foot slips forward. In addition, they do not hold braces or orthoses well.

Rocker Bottom

Rocker bottom shoes help offload plantar pressure in the forefoot, but are dependent on the placement of the rocker. This is particularly important because many diabetic ulcers occur in the forefoot.[15,16] Rockers help transition the foot from heel strike to toe-off. This restores normal motion as a result of collapse, stiffness, and fusion and improves the gait. Praet and Louwerens[17] discuss the rocker is the best way to offload the forefoot. The positioning of the apex of the rocker is most important. This must be custom for diabetics suffering from calluses or ulcers in specific areas or with foot collapse. Similar to a metatarsal pad, the best placement of the apex is just proximal to the area where pressure relief is desired. If there is a plantar metatarsal ulceration, the apex should be right at the neck of the metatarsals to offload the metatarsal head(s) involved. There are a handful of different rocker bottom designs.[14,18] The basic concept is just that of a rocking chair. A mild midstance (where the shoe contacts the ground) is most common and helps restore gait. Depending on severity of deformity and stiffness of joints, this can be altered and increased. It is also easy to incorporate a lift to even out a limb length discrepancy (**Fig. 10**). An example where a more severe rocker is required is a patient who has both submetatarsal head ulcerations and distal toe tip ulcerations. In patients with decreased sensation or inability to achieve toe-off, a rigid shank may be useful. This adds weight but decreases motion at the midfoot and

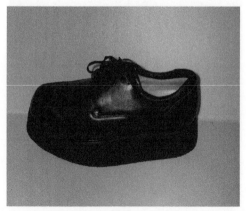

Fig. 10. Rocker bottom, extra-depth shoe. Apex of rocker is placed proximally to desired area to off-load. In this example just proximal to the metatarsal heads.

forefoot. In addition to orthoses and shoes, wearing two sets of socks can be helpful—this allows some of the shearing to take place between the two layers and decreases the movement between the skin and sock interface.

The deformity must be captured to reduce the greatest amount of plantar pressure. Scanners are easy to use; however, there is equal success with traditional casting or foam block methods. It may be easiest for patients to swing their legs over and get an impression with the foam box at a semi–weight-bearing position. As seen in (**Fig. 11**), the calluses can be marked to help the orthotic company visualize areas of pressure. Further offloading can be created when using the foam box as well (**Fig. 12**). The hips, legs, and ankle should be at right angles, and, once the subtalar joint is in neutral (assuming flexibility), even pressure must be applied to capture the contour of the foot (**Fig. 13**).[2] Again, using a modifiable material to create the orthoses is important because changes in the foot can occur even between the times of casting and application. Customization is key with multiple levels of amputation.

Braces

The proper use of a brace is important to offload the diabetic foot, whether in the acute phase, such as seen with an ulceration or Charcot deformity, or in the chronic stages, when healing is taking place and prevention is the primary goal of therapy. In this discussion, bracing techniques are any product that extends above the level of the malleoli.

For flexible deformities, a semirigid gauntlet type of device may suffice. Braces are able to restrict motion, so if there is some instability brought on my motor weakness or loss of function, this may be the ideal solution. Patients with a combination of sensory neuropathy and a collapsing medial column, whether from Charcot neuroarthropathy or posterior tibial tendon dysfunction, may benefit from a gauntlet device (**Fig. 14**).

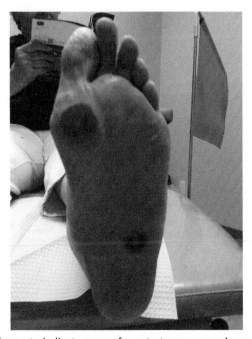

Fig. 11. Example of ways to indicate areas of greatest pressure and prominence – mark foot directly before casting.

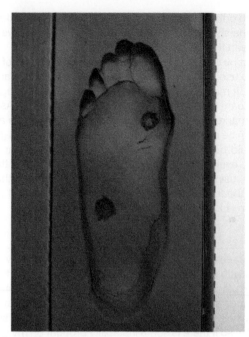

Fig. 12. Example of markings on foam-box of areas of greatest pressure to off-load in orthoses.

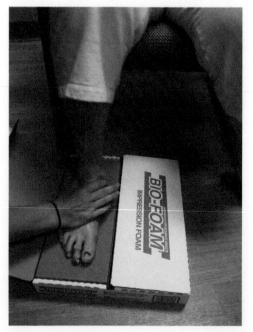

Fig. 13. Technique used to "cast" orthotic in patient that is not flexible. Notice knee is bent at 90 degrees as well as ankle. Attention directed at putting patient in subtalar joint neutral.

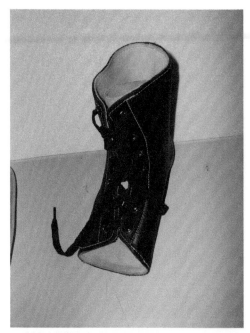

Fig. 14. Gauntlet device used for patients with ankle and or subtalar joint arthritis, Posterior Tibial Tendon dysfunction, or more severe collapse. Helps to stabilize deformity and decrease motion.

Ankle-foot Orthosis

AFO is indicated (**Fig. 15**) for more rigid deformities. Care must be taken in the neuropathic foot to avoid any areas that may be irritated or lead to additional problems. Complications may arise from any of these devices discussed, including the AFO, which, of all the braces discussed, is likely the most cost effective. For those patients with motor weakness, it helps to accommodate weakness in dorsiflexion and may also be used, along with the possibility of the gauntlet, for those who have had a partial foot amputation and have a frontal plane deformity, either in inversion or eversion.

Charcot Restraint Orthotic Walker

Charcot restraint orthotic walkers (CROWs) are often required for those patients with severe deformities or Charcot in its acute phase (**Fig. 16**). This device is custom made and is essentially a clamshell device made out of polypropylene. It is designed for the long term but is not meant to be permanent. The CROW may also be used for patients with Charcot and an active ulcer. Lastly, the CROW may be used after a Charcot reconstruction.

Total Contact Cast

Total contact cast (TCC) must be discussed, because a discussion of bracing of the foot is not complete without its mention. The standard of care is always being challenged with technology. The TCC, however, remains the gold standard for offloading.[19] An often-quoted meta analysis[20] shows the average time to heal an ulceration decreased 184 days to 44 days with the use of a TCC.[12,21,22] Possibly the greatest advantage of these is that patients cannot take them off. Some studies

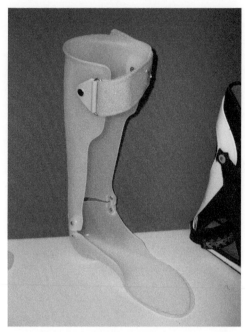

Fig. 15. Hinged ankle-foot orthotic used for patients that require some ankle motion.

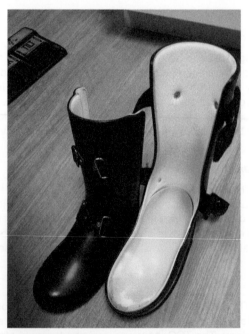

Fig. 16. Charcot restraint orthotic walker – notice plastizote interior. This clam shell appearing device is used for an unstable ankle, rearfoot and midfoot by dispersing pressures up the leg. Lower durometer plastizote is used on the plantar surface to further reduce pressure and accommodate deformity.

have shown that patients offloaded with removable cast boots walked without them 72% of the time.[12] For midfoot ulcerations where offloading is a challenge, TCCs work well. Despite all the positive evidence, a study of 895 wound care clinics in the United States showed less than 2% of clinicians use a TCC to offload a diabetic wound.[23] In the clinical setting with less challenging wounds or wounds that require daily dressing changes, felted-foam dressings can be of benefit.[24] These have less restriction, allow for dressing changes, can be applied quickly in the office, and can bridge patients while they are waiting for custom orthoses. Unfortunately, not all patients can accommodate a brace within their shoe and require an external device attached to the shoe (**Fig. 17**). This may be more cumbersome—but it allows patients to ambulate safely. A team approach using an orthotist and pedorthist is crucial because constant modifications are required—customization is the key (**Fig. 18**).

Finally, for those patients who are either not candidates for reconstruction or who have had reconstructions that have failed, it may be necessary to offload the limb more proximally. This may be accomplished with a patellar-tendon type of device (**Fig. 19**). Although essentially creating the same mechanics as a prosthetic limb, this device serves to redistribute pressure and weight-bearing forces more proximal to, as the name suggests, the prepatella area. There are many ways that this may be fabricated.

COMPLICATIONS AND CONCERNS

The clinical outcome of using orthoses or preventing reulceration status postsurgery is determined by the vigilance of patients and treating teams. As discussed in this article,

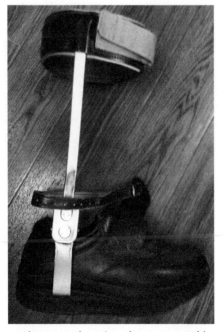

Fig. 17. External device used to control motion about an unstable ankle. Used for patients that cannot be accommodated with an internal device due to severity of deformity.

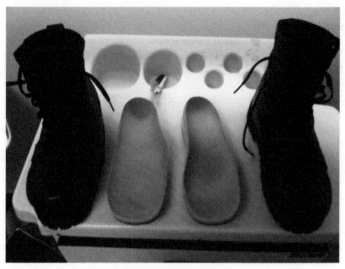

Fig. 18. Example of some of the tools required to modify devices in-office.

constant attention must be paid to hot spots and more prominent areas to prevent ulceration. Braces can cause discomfort and, if bulky in appearance, many patients refuse to wear them. They can also create new ulcerations. The highest risk factor for developing an ulceration is the history of a previous ulcer.[25,26] The highest risk times once treatment has begun are when new shoes, orthoses, or braces are used.[27,28] Time to follow-up should be short on application of new footgear. Do not

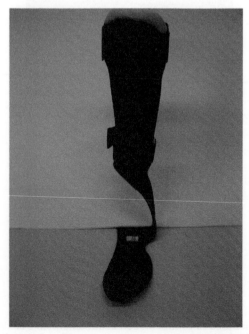

Fig. 19. Patellar-tendon device disperses pressures even more proximally up the leg.

dispense a device and discharge a patient. This is the most crucial time to prevent further breakdown.

Tips to avoid complications

- When dispensing new orthoses or braces, regular follow-up in the initial weeks to month helps quickly find and correct hot spots, or areas of unwanted pressure.
- If dispensing diabetic shoes with multiple pairs of orthoses, give patients a sticker or a reminder to put on their calendar to change orthoses every 3 to 4 months. Also, if patients are seen regularly for routine care, time their appointments around when it is right to switch out their orthoses.
- If the foot architecture is supported correctly by custom shoes, orthoses, and braces, there is less work for the lower extremity muscles and ligaments. As these structures adapt and the hypertrophied muscles return to normal size, modifications are required to maintain a good fit. Quarterly or semiannual maintenance is a good idea the first year or if patients have an increase in weight loss or weight gain.
- Do not leave patients stranded while waiting for their custom devices. Temporary support should be fabricated until the permanent shoe, orthotic, or brace is ready.
- When an ulceration is successfully closed, the new skin is not, and never will be, as strong as in its preulcerative state. Continue offloading this area until the skin strengthens and custom orthoses are ready.

SUMMARY

The diabetic foot frequently has bony prominences. These can be offloaded from the inside—surgical exostectomy or joint reconstruction—or from the outside—orthoses and bracing. Not every patient wants surgery or is even a candidate for surgery. With a well-trained team working together, orthoses can help prevent surgery as well as help avoid revisional surgery and postoperative breakdown. A recent study revealed that reulceration rate decreased from 79% to 15% 2 years after the initiation of orthotic therapy.[29] In this same study, amputation rate decreased from 54% to 6%. Education, reinforcement, and early intervention are paramount. Constant maintenance and modifications are required for lifelong success.

REFERENCES

1. Lavery LA, Vela SA, Fieischli JG, et al. Reducing plantar pressure in the neuropathic foot: a comparison of footwear. Diabetes Care 1997;20(11):1706–10.
2. Tsung BY, Zhang M, Mak AF, et al. Effectiveness of insoles on plantar pressure redistribution. J Rehabil Res Dev 2004;41(6A):767–74.
3. Viswanathan V, Madhavan S, Gopalakrishna G, et al. Effectiveness of different tyeps of footwear insoles for the diabetic neuropathic foot. Diabetes Care 2004;27(2):474–7.
4. Murray HG, Young MJ, Hollis S, et al. The association between callus formation, high pressures and neuropathy in diabetic foot population. Diabet Med 1996;13:979–82.
5. Sulzberger MB, Cortese TA, Fishman L, et al. Studies on blisters produced by friction. J Invest Dermatol 1966;47:456–65.
6. Reiber GE, Vileikyte L, Boyko EJ, et al. Causal pathways for incident lower extremity ulcers in patients with diabetes from two settings. Diabetes Care 1999;22:157–62.
7. Sedory Holzer SE, Camerota A, Martens L, et al. Costs and durations of care for lower-extremity ulcers in patients with diabetes. Clin Ther 1998;20:169–81.

8. Ollendorf DA, Kotsanos JG, Wishner WJ, et al. Potential economic benefits of lower-extremity amputation prevention strategies in diabetes. Diabetes Care 1998;21:1240–5.

9. Slater R, Ramot Y, Rapoport M. Diabetic foot ulcers: principles of assessment and treatment. Isr Med Assoc J 2001;3:59–62.

10. Philbin TM, Leyes M, Sferra JJ, et al. Orthotic and prosthetic devices in partial foot amputations. Foot Ankle Clin 2001;6(2):215–28.

11. Rheinstein J, Yanke J, Marzano R. Developing an effective prescription for a lower extremity prosthesis. Foot Ankle Clin North Am 1999;4(1):113–39.

12. Janisse DJ. A scientific approach to insole design for the diabetic foot. Foot 1993; 3:105–8.

13. Janisse DJ. Pedorthic care of the diabetic foot. In: Levin ME, O'Neal LW, Bowker JR, editors. The diabetic foot. 5th edition. St Louis (MO): Mosby-Year Book; 1993. p. 549.

14. Janisse DJ. Prescription insoles and footwear. Clin Podiatr Med Surg 1995;1: 41–61.

15. Mueller MJ, Zou D, Lott DJ. Pressure gradient as an indicator of plantar skin injury. Diabetes Care 2005;28(12):2908–12.

16. Yavuz M, Erdermir A, Botek G, et al. Peak plantar pressure and shear locations. Diabetes Care 2007;30(10):2643–5.

17. Praet SF, Louwerens JK. The influence of shoe design on plantar pressures in neuropathic feet. Diabetes Care 2003;26:441–5.

18. Marzano R. Fabricating shoe modifications and foot orthoses. In: Janisse DJ, editor. Introduction to pedorthics. Columbia (MD): Pedorthic Footwear Association; 1998. p. 221–34.

19. Pollo FE, Brodsky JW, Crenshaw SJ, et al. Plantar pressures in fiberglass total contact casts vs. a new diabetic walking boot. FAI 2003;24(1):45–9.

20. Petre M, Tokar P, Kostar D, et al. Revisiting the total contact cast: maximizing off-loading by wound isolation. Diabetes Care 2005;28(4):929–30.

21. Brodsky JW, Kourosh S, Stills M, et al. Objective evaluation of insert material for diabetic and athletic footwear. Foot Ankle 1988;9:111.

22. Armstrong DG, Laveray LA, Kimbriel HR, et al. Activity patterns of patients with diabetic foot ulceration: patients with active ulceration may not adhere to a standard pressure off-loading regimen. Diabetes Care 2003;26(9):2595–7.

23. Wu SC, Jensen JL, Weber AK, et al. Use of pressure offloading devices in diabetic foot ulcers: do we practice what we preach? Diabetes Care 2008;31:2118.

24. Zimny S, Schatz H, Pfohl U. The effects of applied felted foam on wound healing and healing times in the therapy of neuropathic diabetic foot ulcers. Diabet Med 2003;20(8):622–5.

25. Edmonds ME, Blundell MP, Morris ME, et al. Improved survival of the diabetic foot: the role of a specialized foot clnic. Q J Med 1986;60(232):763–71.

26. Apelqvist J, Larsson J, Agardh CD. Long-term prognosis for diabetic patients with foot ulcers. J Intern Med 1993;233(6):485–91.

27. Apelqvist J, Larsson J, Agardh CD. The influence of external percipitatint factors and peripheral neuropathy on the development and outcome of diabetic foot ulcers. J Diabet Complications 1990;4(1):21–5.

28. Macarlane RM, Jeffcoate WJ. Factors contributing to the presentation of diabetic foot ulcers. Diabet Med 1997;14(10):867–70.

29. Fernandez ML, Lozano RM, Diaz MI. How effective is orthotic treatment in patients with recurrent diabetic foot ulcers? J Am Podiatr Med Assoc 2013; 103(4):281–90.

Osteomyelitis in the Diabetic Foot
Diagnosis and Management

Frances L. Game, FRCP

KEYWORDS

- Diabetic foot • Osteomyelitis • Antibiotic therapy • Amputation

KEY POINTS

- Osteomyelitis of the foot in diabetes is common and frequently undiagnosed.
- Diagnosis should be clinical in the first instance and based on signs of infection, the size of the lesion, and the visibility of bone. but supported by the results of radiologic examination.
- The gold standard for diagnosis is the histologic and microbiological examination of bone, but this may not be possible or necessary in all patients. The possibility of sampling error must be taken into account.
- There is no clear consensus as to whether management should be primarily medical (antibiotics) or surgical; the pros and cons of each approach must be taken into account on an individual basis and after discussion with patients.

INTRODUCTION

Infection of the bone is a common complication of foot ulceration in diabetes and, depending on the study quoted, may complicate between 20% and 60% of the patients presenting with ulcers to a specialist clinic. Despite the existence of published guidelines,[1,2] there is little robust evidence on which much of the guidance is based and, as a result, approaches to management may vary widely. Professionals working in different countries and health care systems may hold differing views on diagnosis, the choice of antibiotics and their route and duration of administration, and the place of surgery.

PATHOLOGY

In general, the spread of infection into the bone of the foot of a patient with diabetes results from the contiguous spread of any infection of adjacent soft tissue, which may

This article originally appeared in Medical Clinics of North America, Volume 97, Issue 5, September 2013.
Conflict of Interest: Nil.
Department of Diabetes and Endocrinology, Derby Hospitals NHS Trust, Uttoxeter Road, Derby DE22 3NE, UK
E-mail address: frances.game@nhs.net

be complicating an ulcer. Bacteria enter through the cortex before spreading to the marrow. The bones affected, therefore, are those adjacent to areas where ulcers are most common—phalanges, metatarsal heads, and calcaneus. Because the spread of organisms is contiguous from the ulcers, causative organisms are similar to those isolated from complicated soft tissue infections (see the article by Peters and Lipsky elsewhere in this issue).

DIAGNOSIS
Histology and Culture of Bone

The gold standard of diagnosis of bone infection in the foot of patients with diabetes is said to be sampling of bone, which is then subjected to both histopathologic and microbiological examination.[2] This is usually done at the time of surgery or with fluoroscopic or CT guidance when surgery is not planned. In an insensate foot, a bone biopsy can be done with little or no anesthesia and the complication rate is low.[3] Histologic signs of osteomyelitis include bony necrosis and fragmentation with associated inflammatory infiltration, including leukocytes,[4] although there is currently a lack of standardized definition, which may lead to disagreement between pathologists as to the diagnosis.[5]

A condition from which it is sometimes difficult to distinguish bone infection (and may coexist) is the acute Charcot foot. Unfortunately, there are few descriptions in the literature of the histology of the acute Charcot foot to enable a histopathologist to confidently distinguish between the two. La Fontaine and colleagues[6] published the histology of a small series of 8 patients with Charcot foot in diabetes and described an inflammatory infiltrate in association with a disordered trabecular pattern. The inflammatory infiltrate was described as mainly lymphocytic in this small number of patients.

The microbiological definition of osteomyelitis relies on the culture of organisms from the bone. Care should be taken to avoid contamination, and hence, a false-positive result of the biopsy specimen, by taking a sample through skin uninvolved by ulceration. A falsely negative sample may occur from sampling error (biopsy taken from uninvolved bone) or previous treatment by antibiotics. The advantage of taking samples of bone for culture, however, is not only for diagnosis but also so that the organisms involved in the pathogenic process can be identified and targeted with appropriate and narrow-spectrum antimicrobial therapy. Unfortunately, culture of samples taken by swabbing the surface of wound has shown a less than 50% concordance with culture from bone.[7] Taking a deep tissue aspirate by needle aspiration close to bone is more accurate than surface swabs but still does not provide perfect concordance with organisms grown from bone.[8]

Although described as the gold standard, bone sampling is not performed in all patients in many specialist centers. There may be clinical reasons for this—patients are on anticoagulants, have severe ischemia, or have involvement of a very small bone, for example—but for some patients, it may be that there are doubts about whether it is a procedure that would provide an improvement in clinical outcome. A retrospective, non-randomised study from France[3] compared the outcome of patients whose management was based on biopsy-proved osteomyelitis (microbiology) versus those that were not and found an improvement in outcome in those patients who had had a biopsy (remission rates 81% vs 50%). There were other important clinical differences however, which may have affected the outcome of patients, including a higher use of Rifampicin in the centres performing bone biopsy. In addition, the outcomes of the patients who had biopsies were similar, however, to those in other reported series where no biopsies were routinely performed.[9] A further report from the same French group followed-up patients with negative biopsies for 2 years and found that 1 in 4 developed osteomyelitis after the original biopsy.[10]

Given these considerations, it is currently the recommendation of the Infectious Diseases Society of America[2] that bone biopsy be considered only in the following circumstances: (1) uncertainty regarding the diagnosis of osteomyelitis despite clinical and imaging evaluations; (2) an absence (or confusing mix) of culture data from soft tissue specimens; (3) failure of a patient to respond to empiric antibiotic therapy; and (4) a desire to use antibiotic agents that may be especially effective for osteomyelitis but have a high potential for selecting resistant organisms.

Clinical

Diagnosis is, in the first instance therefore, usually clinical and should be considered in any nonhealing wound of the foot in patients with diabetes when there is adequate perfusion and offloading has been optimized. There are various clinical features of a wound, however, that may be helpful in predicting the presence of bone infection. Of these, the depth and size of the ulcer has been considered predictive although the evidence to support this is weak. In a study where the prevalence of histology-proved osteomyelitis was 68%, the presence of exposed bone at the base of the ulcer had a sensitivity of only 32% but a specificity of 100% and an ulcer size greater than 2 cm had a sensitivity of only 52% but a specificity of 92%.[11]

Perhaps the most widely debated clinical sign is the probe-to-bone test. In one of the earliest studies,[12] a series of 76 infected ulcers were examined. Bone biopsy was not done to confirm the diagnosis in this study, but with a diagnosis on clinical criteria and in this population with a prevalence of osteomyelitis of 68%, a positive probe-to-bone test had a sensitivity of 66% and specificity of 87%, giving a positive predictive value of 89% and a negative predictive value of 56% for the diagnosis of osteomyelitis.

A subsequent UK study,[13] in a series of 81 consecutive outpatients with a total of 104 foot ulcers, both infected and noninfected, found a sensitivity of 38%, specificity of 91%, negative predictive value of 85%, and positive predictive value of only 53% for positive probe-to-bone tests to diagnose osteomyelitis (diagnosed radiologically, not by bone biopsy). The overall prevalence of osteomyelitis in this population was, however, only 23%. A further US study[14] evaluated the performance of the probe-to-bone test using the reference test of bone culture post-biopsy (not histology). In this series of 247 consecutive cases with only 12% prevalence of osteomyelitis, a positive probe-to-bone test had a sensitivity of 87%, specificity of 91%, negative predictive value of 96%, and positive predictive value of, again, only 57%. In this series, however, because only patients with a high clinical suspicion of osteomyelitis went on to have a bone biopsy and because it is uncertain whether treatment with antibiotics was started before bone culture, the prevalence of bone infection may have been higher than stated.

The only study to evaluate the probe-to-bone test in patients whose osteomyelitis was diagnosed on both bone histology and culture was performed in a series of 356 episodes of foot infections in 338 patients.[15] Almost all had surgery and biopsies were taken at the time of surgery. The prevalence of osteomyelitis was high, at 72.5%, and the sensitivity, specificity, and positive and negative predictive values for a positive probe-to-bone test for the diagnosis of osteomyelitis were 95%, 93%, 97%, and 83%, respectively.

What is clear is that the performance of the probe-to-bone test seems to vary with the prevalence of osteomyelitis in the population in which it is studied, with better positive predictive values demonstrated in populations with the highest prevalence.

What is probably more important than prevalence is the pretest probability of osteomyelitis. The 2 centers with the highest prevalence of osteomyelitis were tertiary referral centers with a population of ulcers that were infected and not responding to standard therapies. Thus, the pretest probability of osteomyelitis was high. An analysis of the available data by Wrobel and Connolly[16] suggests that at the extremes of pretest probability (ie, <20% or >80%) the probe-to-bone test makes little difference to post-test probability. When the pretest probability is approximately 50%, however, then a positive or negative probe-to-bone test could possibly improve the post-test probability to approximately 80% (positive test) or to 30% (negative test), a performance similar to plain radiographs.

The situation is complicated by none of these studies having systematically assessed all patients, whether suspected or not clinically of having bone infection, with a bone biopsy, and perhaps it is unethical to do so. It is also of concern, however, that in the only published study to investigate the interobserver variability of the probe-to-bone test between professionals there seems to be only moderate to fair concordance.[17]

Blood Tests

Unfortunately the data to support the use of blood tests to definitively diagnose osteomyelitis in the foot of patients have been disappointing. In particular, an elevated white cell count was shown in 1 retrospective study to be absent in approximately half of patients presenting with bone infection.[18] Other markers of inflammation (eg, C-reactive protein [CRP] and erythrocyte sedimentation rate [ESR]) have also been investigated. Although 2 studies have shown that an ESR greater than 70 mm/h had 100% sensitivity for the diagnosis of osteomyelitis, the specificity of this was between 28% and 50%.[11,19]

Combination Tests

A recent prospective cohort study looked at combining the ulcer depth and CRP or ESR in a cohort of 54 patients with histology-proved osteomyelitis.[20] Combing the clinical and laboratory findings (ulcer depth >3 mm or CRP >30 mmol/L, ulcer depth >3 mm or ESR >60 mm/h) improved the sensitivity of the diagnosis of osteomyelitis to 100% with a specificity of 55%.

Imaging

There have been several reviews published of the utility of imaging for the diagnosis of osteomyelitis.[21–23] A recent meta-analysis found few studies, however, that compared the use of these investigations with diagnosis by bone histology and/or microbiology.[24]

Plain Radiograph

The sensitivity of plain radiographs is poor, particularly early in the disease process, because a loss of 30% to 50% of bone mineral content is required to produce noticeable changes. The first changes in bone on radiograph may be subtle and usually indicate that the infectious process has been present for at least 2 to 3 weeks. They include periosteal thickening, lytic lesions, osteopenia, loss of trabecular architecture, and new bone apposition.[25] Observational studies have demonstrated sensitivities of between 22% and 75% and specificities of 17% and 94% for the diagnosis of osteomyelitis.[26] The lack of specificity largely results from the difficulty in differentiating infection from Charcot neuro-osteoarthropathy in patients with bony destruction.

Despite the poor predictive value of a normal radiograph, however, it is recommended[2] that a plain radiograph be taken in all patients presenting with foot ulcers, because it could also indicate the presence of foreign bodies, bony deformities, or arterial calcification.

Radionucleotide Bone Scans

There are several published studies comparing the use of technetium Tc 99m phosphate bone scans with bone pathology for the diagnosis of osteomyelitis of the foot in diabetes. A meta-analysis[24] calculated the combined sensitivity of these studies as 81%, which is better than plain radiographs in the early diagnosis of the disease, but the calculated combined specificity was only 28%. Poor specificity generally relates to the inability of technetium bone scans to distinguish osteomyelitis from any other inflammatory process in the foot, in particular, again, an acute Charcot foot or even resolving osteomyelitis.[27] In addition, it is difficult to delineate the exact anatomic location or extent of the infection.

Other radionucleotide labeling techniques, which seem more specific for infection, such as indium In 111–labeled white cell, antigranulocyte Fab' fragment antibody, or technetium Tc 99m –labeled monoclonal antigranulocyte antibody scans, should, in theory, help distinguish between an acute Charcot foot and osteomyelitis.

In 1 meta-analysis, the pooled sensitivity of indium In 111–labeled white cell scans was 74% and the pooled specificity 68%.[24] Other labeled scans have been evaluated in small studies with no real improvement in sensitivity or specificity. The downside of labeled white cell scans includes the time taken to label cells, the need to handle blood and scan at 2 time points—4 and 24 hours, and the lack of anatomic definition.[28] The sensitivity may be reduced further in an ischemic foot.[4] Combining tests, such as labeled white cell or antigranulocyte Fab' fragment antibody with technetium-labeled bone scans, should, in theory, improve specificity. Studies to prove this have been small, however, and generally of poor quality.[26] Equally, combining single-photon emission (SPECT) CT/CT with bone and leukocyte scanning should, in theory, improve the spatial location of bone infection but suffers from all the other drawbacks of labeled white cell scans. Again, early studies are small and more evidence of utility and cost-effectiveness is required.[29,30]

MRI

MRI scans have the advantage over radionucleotide bone scans of being able to accurately define the anatomic location and extent of inflammatory change in the foot as well as any soft tissue infection, including sinus tracts, deep tissue necrosis, or abscesses. In a meta-analysis of 4 studies comparing the performance of MRI scans to bone pathology for the diagnosis of osteomyelitis, the combined sensitivity was 90%[2] and the pooled specificity 79%.[24] The lower specificity in diabetes is usually attributable to the difficulty of distinguishing osteomyelitis from other causes of bone edema, in particular, Charcot neuroarthropathy.[31]

Other Types of Scan

Preliminary data suggest a possible role for combined fluorodeoxyglucose F 18–positron emission tomography/CT. The studies, however, are small, and vary not only in patient population but also in how the images are analyzed and the absence of correlation with bone pathology in the majority.[28] Standard CT scanning is more sensitive than plain radiography (and in some cases MRI) in detecting cortical disruption, periosteal reaction, and sequestrae but has low specificity.[29]

There is no single test that absolutely confirms or refutes a diagnosis of osteomyelitis in the diabetic foot. In 2008, a consensus group of the International Working Group on the Diabetic Foot described a suggested algorithm for the diagnosis of osteomyelitis based on clinical examination imaging and bone sampling methods that stratified the diagnosis into unlikely (<10% probability), possible (10%–50%), probable (51%–90%), and definite (>90%).[1] At present, however, there is no robust validation of this scheme.

MANAGEMENT CHOICES

Approaches to the management of osteomyelitis of the foot in diabetes vary widely from center to center and country to country. Clinicians differ on such fundamental management issues as the choice route and duration of antibiotics but perhaps most frequently on the place of surgery. Many specialists maintain that early surgical excision of all infected bone is essential[32,33] whereas others maintain that the majority of patients can be managed with antibiotics alone.[34] These debates will continue as long as the data to support clinical decision making are not particularly robust (as shown in the systematic reviews by the International Working Group on the Diabetic Foot[1] and the Infectious Diseases Society of America[2]).

Conservative (Primarily Nonsurgical) Treatment

In support of a conservative, that is, primarily nonsurgical, approach is the evidence from more than 500 reported cases in the literature, in which initial management was primarily with antibiotics and in which there was a mean rate of eradication of infection of greater than 60%.[4] These data are all, however, from uncontrolled observational series and may have been affected by case selection, in particular, the exclusion of those who may have required early limb salvage surgery. One series of 147 cases from a UK center did, however, study a consecutive series of patients presenting with osteomyelitis of the foot, including those who had immediate surgery.[9] In this series, 80% of those who had no initial surgery had apparent arrest of their infection with antimicrobial therapy alone, although this represented only 63% of the total series if those who had immediate limb saving surgery are counted. Overall, there was a 23% minor and 8.8% major amputation rate. These case series have been criticized by some investigators, however, as failing to specify a definition of osteomyelitis, how patients were selected, and how much nonoperative débridement of bone was performed.[2]

A further criticism of this approach is the perceived requirement for excessively prolonged antimicrobial treatment compared with those having surgical resection. In the single-center UK series above, the median length of antibiotic treatment was 61 days.[9] Other investigators have reported even more prolonged courses of antibiotic treatment, with more than 50% of patients requiring 6 months or more antibiotic treatment in a separate UK series[35] and a mean of 40 weeks' treatment in a series from Canada.[36] Using prolonged courses of broad-spectrum antibiotics in this way undoubtedly increases the risk of side-effects (including the development of Clostridium difficile diarrhea) and an increased risk of allowing the emergence of antibiotic-resistant bacteria, such as methicillin-resistant Staphylococcus aureus.

Antibiotic Choices

At present, there are few robust data to guide clinicians in the choice, duration, or route of antimicrobial therapy.[1] Because the pathogens involved are generally those involved in soft tissue infection, it makes sense that regimens should be derived from protocols for the management of this complication of foot ulceration (see the article by Peters and Lipsky elsewhere in this issue).

There has been some interest in the use of implanted antibiotic carriers (eg, polymethyl methacrylate beads or calcium sulfate pellets) in conjunction with surgery[2] but the advantages of their use have yet to be confirmed in properly designed randomized trials.[37]

Primarily Surgical Treatment

There are few published data to support the view that surgical intervention is imperative in all cases in the management of osteomyelitis of the diabetic foot. The International Working Group on the Diabetic Foot systematic review[1] found only a few small case series and no randomized studies that directly compared primarily surgical and primarily nonsurgical management. A single-center retrospective analysis[38] of 112 patients (65 with osteomyelitis) admitted for management of infection of the foot in diabetes found that those in whom surgery was delayed by 3 days or more had a worse outcome. Details on the baseline characteristics of the patients, in particular, the clinical reasons why surgery may have been delayed, are not, however, explained in the article. In a larger retrospective series of 224 patients with osteomyelitis,[33] there seemed again to be an increased risk of eventual major amputation in those who had had surgery delayed compared with those who had immediate minor amputation of the affected area. The overall major amputation rate of the cohort was, however, high, at 25%. Another study[39] looked at 32 patients with diabetic forefoot osteomyelitis who had limited débridement of the infected area (ulcerectomy plus limited débridement of the underlying phalanx or metatarsal), with an eventual healing rate of 78%. There was, however, a mean duration of antibiotic therapy of 111 days in this series.

A more recent study[40] examined 185 sequential cases of diabetic foot osteomyelitis that were treated in a single center. After initial broad-spectrum intravenous antibiotics, limited conservative surgery was performed on the majority, although 71 had initial minor and 3 major amputations. The overall major amputation rate was only 8.1%, with a minor amputation rate of 48%. This published series gives no data on antibiotic usage, but in a subsequent series from the same center,[41] the median use of antibiotics was 36 days.

One of the consistent features of the published surgical series is the number of patients reported who, despite apparent débridement of infected bone, whether conservative or minor, had recurrence of the infection, requiring further surgical intervention. In the 2 most recent series,[40,41] this is reported as 18% and 25%, respectively. A possible explanation for this observation comes from 2 small studies,[42,43] both of which examined the histology of bone specimens taken at the osteotomy site at the time of minor amputation of the diabetic foot. In both there was histologic evidence of osteomyelitis at the osteotomy site, in 60% of 54 minor amputations and 35% of 111 patients, respectively. It is possible, therefore, that the difficulty of clinically distinguishing infected from noninfected bone at the time of operation is one explanation for the finding that the surgical series with the lowest postoperative risk of amputation have included antibiotics either preoperatively or postoperatively. Although it seems from a single published surgical series[41] as if the duration of antibiotic could potentially be shorter in those having surgery compared with the published series of primarily medical management, no direct comparisons have been made.

Another identified complication of surgical solutions to osteomyelitis is that the potential alteration of foot architecture may cause transfer ulceration, that is, skin breakdown at a new high-pressure site. In a single published study, the risk of transfer ulcers postsurgery was 41% but varied depending on the site of surgery; the highest risk of ulceration followed surgery to the first metatarsal head (28%) and the lowest the 5th metatarsal head (8%).[44]

Primarily Conservative Versus Primarily Surgical Approach?

The superiority of either approach, primarily nonsurgical or early conservative surgery, is currently unclear and clinicians need to weigh the risks of prolonged antibiotics with those of repeated surgery and possible transfer ulcers. Only future well-designed controlled trials will answer this question and in which situations either approach may be clearly superior. From published series, however, those centers with the lowest major amputation rates (even allowing for the question of baseline characteristics of the patients) are those that offer a combined approach to the patient. Either initial antibiotic treatment with surgical débridement after a period of observation or conservative surgery initially with antibiotic treatment postoperatively. Thus, as in all areas of management of the diabetic foot, it is apparent that a multidisciplinary approach is imperative, with surgeons, physicians, and specialists in infectious diseases and microbiology all involved in a holistic approach to patients but with the patients' own views at the heart of the decision making.

SUMMARY

Although osteomyelitis of the foot in diabetes remains common in specialist foot clinics across the world, the quality of published work to guide clinicians in the diagnosis and management is generally poor. Diagnosis should be based primarily on clinical signs supported by results of pathologic and radiologic investigations. Although the gold standard comes from the histologic and microbiological examination of bone, clinicians should be aware of the problems of sampling error. This lack of standardization of diagnostic criteria and of consensus on the choice of outcome measures poses further difficulties when seeking evidence to support management decisions. Experts have traditionally recommended surgical removal of infected bone but available evidence suggests that in many cases (excepting those in whom immediate surgery is required to save life or limb) a nonsurgical approach to management of osteomyelitis may be effective for many, if not most, patients with osteomyelitis of the diabetic foot. The benefits and limitations of both approaches need, however, to be established in prospective trials so that appropriate therapy can be offered to appropriate patients at the appropriate time, with the patients' views taken fully into account.

REFERENCES

1. Berendt AR, Peters EJ, Bakker K, et al. Diabetic foot osteomyelitis: a progress report on diagnosis and a systematic review of treatment. Diabetes Metab Res Rev 2008;24(Suppl 1):S145–61.
2. Lipsky BA, Berendt AR, Cornia PB, et al. 2012 Infectious Diseases Society of America clinical practice guideline for the diagnosis and treatment of diabetic foot infections. Clin Infect Dis 2012;54(12):132–73.
3. Senneville E, Lombart A, Beltrand E, et al. Outcome of diabetic foot osteomyelitis treated non-surgically: a retrospective cohort study. Diabetes Care 2008;31: 637–42.
4. Jeffcoate WJ, Lipsky BA. Controversies in diagnosing and managing osteomyelitis of the foot in diabetes. Clin Infect Dis 2004;39(Suppl 2):S115–22.

5. Meyr AJ, Singh S, Zhang X, et al. Statistical reliability of bone biopsy for the diagnosis of diabetic foot osteomyelitis. J Foot Ankle Surg 2011;50(6):663–7.
6. La Fontaine J, Shibuya N, Sampson HW, et al. Trabecular quality and cellular characteristics of normal, diabetic, and charcot bone. J Foot Ankle Surg 2011; 50(6):648–53.
7. Elamurugan TP, Jagdish S, Kate V, et al. Role of bone biopsy specimen culture in the management of diabetic foot osteomyelitis. Int J Surg 2011;9:214–6.
8. Kessler L, Piemont Y, Ortega F, et al. Comparison of microbiological results of needle puncture vs. superficial swab in infected diabetic foot ulcer with osteomyelitis. Diabet Med 2006;23:99–102.
9. Game FL, Jeffcoate WJ. Primarily non-surgical management of osteomyelitis of the foot in diabetes. Diabetologia 2008;51:962–7.
10. Senneville E, Gaworowska D, Topolinski H, et al. Outcome of patients with diabetes with negative percutaneous bone biopsy performed for suspicion of osteomyelitis of the foot. Diabet Med 2012;29:56–61.
11. Newman LG, Waller J, Palestro CJ, et al. Unsuspected osteomyelitis in diabetic foot ulcers: diagnosis and monitoring by leukocyte scanning with indium in 111 oxyquinoline. JAMA 1991;266:1246–51.
12. Grayson ML, Gibbons GW, Balogh K, et al. Probing to bone in infected pedal ulcers: a clinical sign of underlying osteomyelitis in diabetic patients. JAMA 1995; 273:721–3.
13. Shone A, Burnside J, Chipchase S, et al. Probing the validity of the probe-to-bone test in the diagnosis of osteomyelitis of the foot in diabetes. Diabetes Care 2006; 29:945.
14. Lavery LA, Armstrong DG, Peters EJ, et al. Probe-to-bone test for diagnosing diabetic foot osteomyelitis: reliable or relic? Diabetes Care 2007;30:270–4.
15. Aragón-Sánchez J, Lipsky BA, Lázaro-Martínez JL. Diagnosing diabetic foot osteomyelitis: is the combination of probe-to-bone test and plain radiography sufficient for high-risk inpatients? Diabet Med 2011;28(2):191–4.
16. Wrobel JS, Connolly JE. Making the diagnosis of osteomyelitis. The role of prevalence. J Am Podiatr Med Assoc 1998;88(7):337–43.
17. Garcia Morales E, Lazaro-Martinez JL, Aragon-Sanchez FJ, et al. Inter-observer reproducibility of probing to bone in the diagnosis of diabetic foot osteomyelitis. Diabet Med 2011;28:1238–40.
18. Armstrong DG, Lavery LA, Sariaya M, et al. Leukocytosis is a poor indicator of acute osteomyelitis of the foot in diabetes mellitus. J Foot Ankle Surg 1996;35:280–3.
19. Eneroth M, Larsson J, Apelqvist J. Deep foot infections in patients with diabetes and foot ulcer: an entity with different characteristics, treatments, and prognosis. J Diabet Complications 1999;13:254–63.
20. Fleischer AE, Didyk AA, Woods JB, et al. Combined clinical and laboratory testing improves diagnostic accuracy for osteomyelitis in the diabetic foot. J Foot Ankle Surg 2009;48(1):39–46.
21. Becker W. Imaging osteomyelitis and the diabetic foot. Q J Nucl Med 1999;43: 9–20.
22. Eckman MH, Greenfield S, Mackey WC, et al. Foot infections in diabetic patients. Decision and cost-effectiveness analyses. JAMA 1995;273:712–20.
23. Tomas MB, Patel M, Marwin SE, et al. The diabetic foot. Br J Radiol 2000;73: 443–50.
24. Dinh MT, Abad CL, Safdar N. Diagnostic accuracy of the physical examination and imaging tests for osteomyelitis underlying diabetic foot ulcers: meta-analysis. Clin Infect Dis 2008;47:519–27.

25. Pineda C, Espinosa R, Pena A. Radiographic imaging in osteomyelitis: the role of plain radiography, computed tomography, ultrasonography, magnetic resonance imaging, and scintigraphy. Semin Plast Surg 2009;23(2):80–9.
26. National Institute for Health and Clinical Excellence. Diabetic foot problems Inpatient management of diabetic foot problems. 2011. Available at: http://www.nice.org.uk/nicemedia/live/13416/57943/57943.pdf. Accessed January 12, 2013.
27. Sella EJ. Current concepts review: diagnostic imaging of the diabetic foot. Foot Ankle Int 2009;30:568–76.
28. Gnanasegaran G, Vijayanathan S, Fogelman I. Diagnosis of infection in the diabetic foot using 18F-FDG PET/CT: a sweet alternative? Eur J Nucl Med Mol Imaging 2012;39:1525–7.
29. Erdman WA, Buethe J, Bhore R, et al. Indexing severity of diabetic foot infection with 99mTc-WBC SPECT/CT hybrid imaging. Diabetes Care 2012;35(9):1826–31.
30. Heiba SI, Kolker D, Mocherla B. The optimized evaluation of diabetic foot infection by dual isotope SPECT/CT imaging protocol. J Foot Ankle Surg 2010;49:529–36.
31. Craig JG, Amin MB, Wu K, et al. Osteomyelitis of the diabetic foot: MR imaging-pathologic correlation. Radiology 1997;203:849–55.
32. Lipsky BA, Berendt AR. Principles and practice of antibiotic therapy of diabetic foot infections. Diabetes Metab Res Rev 2000;16(Suppl 1):S42–6.
33. Henke PK, Blackburn SA, Wainess RW, et al. Osteomyelitis of the foot and toe in adults is a surgical disease: conservative management worsens lower extremity salvage. Ann Surg 2005;241(6):885–94.
34. Game F. Management of osteomyelitis of the foot in diabetes mellitus. Nat Rev Endocrinol 2010;6:43–7.
35. Valabhji J, Oliver N, Samarasinghe D, et al. Conservative management of diabetic forefoot ulceration complicated by underlying osteomyelitis: the benefits of magnetic resonance imaging. Diabet Med 2009;26(11):1127–34.
36. Embil JM, Rose G, Trepman E, et al. Oral antimicrobial therapy for diabetic foot osteomyelitis. Foot Ankle Int 2006;27(10):771–9.
37. Barth RE, Vogely HC, Hoepelman AI, et al. 'To bead or not to bead?' Treatment of osteomyelitis and prosthetic joint-associated infections with gentamicin bead chains. Int J Antimicrob Agents 2011;38(5):371–5.
38. Tan JS, Friedman NM, Hazelton-Miller C, et al. Can aggressive treatment of diabetic foot infections reduce the need for above-ankle amputation? Clin Infect Dis 1996;23:286–91.
39. Ha Van G, Siney H, Danan JP, et al. Treatment of osteomyelitis in the diabetic foot. Contribution of conservative surgery. Diabetes Care 1996;19:1257–60.
40. Aragón-Sánchez FJ, Cabrera-Galván JJ, Quintana-Marrero Y, et al. Outcomes of surgical treatment of diabetic foot osteomyelitis: a series of 185 patients with histopathological confirmation of bone involvement. Diabetologia 2008;51(11):1962–70.
41. Aragón-Sánchez J, Lázaro-Martínez JL, Hernández-Herrero C, et al. Does osteomyelitis in the feet of patients with diabetes really recur after surgical treatment? Natural history of a surgical series. Diabet Med 2012;29(6):813–8.
42. Hachmöller A. Outcome of minor amputations at the diabetic foot in relation to bone histopathology: a clinical audit. Zentralbl Chir 2007;132:491–6.
43. Kowalski TJ, Matsuda M, Sorenson MD, et al. The effect of residual osteomyelitis at the resection margin in patients with surgically treated diabetic foot infection. J Foot Ankle Surg 2011;50(2):171–5.
44. Molines-Barroso RJ, Lázaro-Martínez JL, Aragón-Sánchez FJ, et al. Analysis of transfer lesions in patients who underwent surgery for diabetic foot ulcers located on the plantar aspect of the metatarsal heads. Diabet Med 2013.

The Relationships Between Cardiovascular Disease and Diabetes: Focus on Pathogenesis

Jason C. Kovacic, MD, PhD[a,b], Jose M. Castellano, MD, PhD[a,b],
Michael E. Farkouh, MD[a,b,c], Valentin Fuster, MD, PhD[a,b,d],*

KEYWORDS

- Cardiovascular disease • Diabetes • Obesity • Diabetic cardiomyopathy

KEY POINTS

- Diabetes has reached an epidemic level worldwide and patients suffering from this disease are at significantly higher risk for cardiovascular disease (CVD).
- The close relationship between diabetes and CVD together with the substantial projected rise in prevalence of diabetes will likely lead to a huge increase in the future demand for health care services at a global level.
- The economic force behind the continuing rise in the cost of health care derived from caring for the 300 million projected diabetic patients in 2025 will leave policy makers no choice but to devise efficient solutions to prevent the widespread surge of this disease.
- Focus should be placed back on the mechanisms that prevent the development of diabetes and related pathologies through the promotion of cardiovascular health by smoking cessation, exercising, following a healthy diet, and weight loss strategies, all of which will improve health outcomes and reduce costs.

INTRODUCTION

Diabetes mellitus currently affects 180 million people worldwide. The epidemic of obesity and sedentary lifestyle, however, is projected to result in more than 300 million

This article originally appeared in Endocrinology and Metabolism Clinics of North America, Volume 43, Issue 1, March 2014.

No specific funding or grant was used to prepare this article. Jason Kovacic is supported by National Institutes of Health Grant K08HL111330 and has received research support from AstraZeneca.

[a] Zena and Michael A. Wiener Cardiovascular Institute, Mount Sinai School of Medicine, One Gustave L. Levy Place, Box 1030, New York, NY 10029, USA; [b] Marie-Josée and Henry R. Kravis Cardiovascular Health Center, Mount Sinai School of Medicine, One Gustave L. Levy Place, Box 1030, New York, NY 10029, USA; [c] Peter Munk Cardiac Centre and Heart and Stroke Richard Lewar Centre of Excellence, Cardiovascular Research, University of Toronto, MaRS Building 101 College Street, 3rd Floor, Toronto, ON M5G 1L7, Canada; [d] The Centro Nacional de Investigaciones Cardiovasculares (CNIC), Melchor Fernández Almagro, 3.Código Postal 28029, Madrid, Spain
* Corresponding author. Mount Sinai School of Medicine, One Gustave L. Levy Place, Box 1030, New York, NY 10029.
E-mail address: valentin.fuster@mountsinai.org

people with diabetes in 2025.[1,2] Developing countries, in particular, will be hit by this increase, with an expected 170% rise from 84 million to 228 million affected individuals. This projection is of particular importance in developing nations, where diabetes tends to arise earlier in life (at ages 40–64 years) compared with developed countries, where diabetes often occurs at age 65 years or older. The onset of diabetes at an earlier age in developing nations inevitably causes a longer duration of exposure to diabetes and, therefore, carries a potentially greater risk of diabetes-associated morbidity and mortality in later life. Although a developed nation, the projections in the United States are somber, with the number of Americans with diabetes projected to increase by 165%, from 11 million in 2000 to 29 million in 2050.[2]

Diabetes is a major risk factor for CVD and cardiovascular complications are the leading cause of mortality among diabetic patients. Recent data from the World Health Organization suggest that 50% of diabetic patients die from heart-related causes and heart disease is noted on more than two-thirds of diabetes-related death certificates among people 65 years or older.[3] Diabetes predisposes to aggressive obstructive coronary artery disease (CAD), which leads to ischemic heart disease, heart failure, and death. There is consensus in the literature about an increased prevalence of coronary plaques in diabetic hearts, with such plaques bearing a higher propensity for rupture. Furthermore, diabetes also predisposes to heart failure independent of valvular heart disease, underlying CAD, or hypertension[4]—a condition known as diabetic cardiomyopathy (DCM).[5] Nevertheless, although remaining an enormous public health burden, recent progress has been made in the ways that diabetic patients with CVD are clinically approached and treated. This article reviews some of the recent advances in the understanding of the relationships between CVD and diabetes at the vascular, cardiac, and clinical levels.

DIABETES AND THE VASCULATURE

Of the major burden of morbidity and mortality associated with diabetes, a significant proportion is attributable to vascular manifestations. In many instances these vascular manifestations are obvious, for example, when a diabetic patient presents with myocardial infarction (MI) or thromboembolic stroke, the underlying pathology is readily traceable to rampant and diffuse diabetic atherosclerosis. Beyond increased atherosclerosis, however, many of the numerous disease-related end-organ effects of diabetes include a vascular contribution. For example, although diabetic neuropathy involves direct nerve damage, microvascular changes leading to secondary neural ischemia also play a major role in the neuropathic process.[6] Similarly, alterations in the microvasculature and glomerular endothelial changes are an important aspect of diabetic nephropathy and macroalbuminuria,[7] whereas microvascular changes in the retina may lead to diabetic retinopathy and blindness. So pervasive are the effects of diabetes, that it is impossible to review in this article all of the many pathologic diabetic pathways and effects on the vascular system and, conversely, all the effects that the diabetic vasculature has on the resulting clinical end-organ phenotype. Several of the major mechanisms of interaction between diabetes and the vasculature are discussed, including oxidative stress, progenitor cell dysfunction, microvascular dysfunction, and impaired reverse cholesterol transport (**Fig. 1**).

Oxidative Stress and the Vasculature

Oxidative stress and the accumulation of reactive oxygen species (ROS) are key aspects in the development of diabetic complications and diabetic vascular disease and perhaps the most important initiating events in the cascade of diabetic vascular

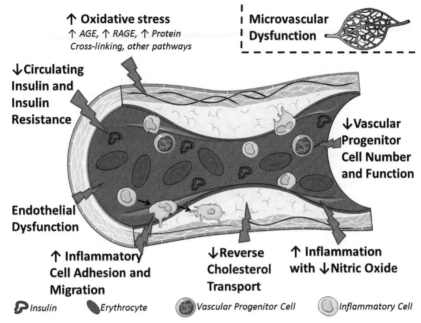

Fig. 1. Key pathologic diabetic pathways affecting the vasculature. Figure 1 produced using Servier Medical Art.

pathology. There are multiple targets of oxidative damage in the vasculature, with both endothelial and vascular smooth muscle cells (VSMCs) exposed to oxidative modifications of proteins, lipids, and nucleic acids. In turn, there are numerous consequences of this increased vascular ROS generation and oxidative damage. Impaired endothelial function is one of the key pathologic disturbances in diabetic patients, which seems due primarily to loss of nitric oxide bioactivity.[8] This is thought a seminal event in the rampant atherosclerotic process that typifies diabetes and other lipodystrophic conditions.[9]

There are multiple sources of ROS in the diabetic vasculature, including the mitochondrial electron transport chain, NADPH oxidase, xanthine oxidase, endothelial nitric oxide synthase, and cytochrome P450. The pathologic changes in these pathways that lead to increased ROS generation are diverse, but are thought to ultimately arise due to hyperglycemia or altered glucose utilization. Although debate is ongoing,[10] a popular theory to explain these vascular damage pathways was put forward in 2001 by Brownlee.[11] Referred to as the "unifying hypothesis," Brownlee argued that hyperglycemia leads to overproduction of superoxide by the mitochondrial electron transport chain, which is an upstream and central event in 4 key damage pathways: increased polyol pathway flux, increased formation of advanced glycation endproducts (AGEs), activation of protein kinase C, and increased flux through the hexosamine pathway.[10,11]

Among these damage pathways, AGE accumulation has received particular attention and is linked to multiple vascular pathologies.[12] AGE formation occurs due to several nonenzymatic reactions of glucose with lipids, proteins, and nucleic acids (glycation). This leads to the formation of a network of poorly characterized AGEs that typifies both diabetes and older age.[12] The adverse vascular effects of AGEs are multifactorial. AGEs act directly to induce cross-linking of proteins, such as vascular collagen and elastin. AGE-linked collagen and elastin are stiffer and less amenable to physiologic turnover, leading to the pathologic accumulation of structurally dysfunctional vascular proteins and a structurally rigid vascular scaffolding.[12,13] In addition to direct effects, AGE and various other ligands, such as S100B, can activate the AGE receptor, termed *RAGE*. With ligand binding to RAGE, activation of signal transduction machinery occurs, triggering further up-regulation of inflammatory and other detrimental vascular pathways, such as nuclear factor κB.[14] RAGE is expressed by endothelial cells,[15] and RAGE activation or other direct AGE effects on endothelial cells lead to multifactorial vascular dysfunction that includes increased vascular cell adhesion molecule-1 expression and inflammatory cell transmigration,[14,16,17] increased vascular permeability,[18,19] quenching of nitric oxide leading to defective endothelium-dependent vasodilatation,[20] endothelial progenitor cell (EPC) dysfunction,[21] and endothelial cell apoptosis.[22] Linking several of these aspects at the clinical level, Virmani and coworkers[23] have shown that compared with nondiabetics, plaques from diabetic subjects who died suddenly have larger mean necrotic cores and greater plaque load, increased inflammation, greater expression of RAGE, and increased VSMC apoptosis.

Diabetic Microvascular Dysfunction

Pathologic microvascular changes are a hallmark of the diabetic process and may precede the clinical diagnosis of diabetes.[24] Vascular changes seen with microvascular disease include cellular morphologic alterations, reduced cell mitochondrial content, and attenuated capillaries with thickened and fibrotic basement membranes.[12] In a meta-analysis of clinical studies, Muris and colleagues[24] identified several factors related to microvascular dysfunction that predicted a subsequent diagnosis of diabetes, including higher levels of soluble plasma E-selectin and intercellular adhesion molecule-1, a lower response to acetylcholine-mediated peripheral vascular reactivity testing, a lower retinal arteriole-to-venule ratio, and a higher albumin-to-creatinine ratio.

As an emerging but seemingly critical pathobiological disease mechanism, the authors and colleagues previously reviewed the major role played by microvascular disease in the pathology of Alzheimer disease and vascular cognitive impairment.[25] Although epidemiologic studies have documented an association between diabetes and Alzheimer disease,[26] autopsy studies have failed to find a positive relationship between diabetes and the characteristic Alzheimer pathologic changes of neurofibrillary plaques and tangles.[27] Rather, a consistent association between diabetes and ischemic cerebral vascular pathologies has been found.[27] Although other diabetes-related vascular mechanisms are also implicated, such as increased atherosclerotic burden, accumulation of ROS, and large-vessel stroke, it is now increasingly appreciated that diabetic microvascular damage is one of the fundamental pathologic pathways that culminates in degenerative brain disease.[28] Specific pathologic insults that arise due to cortical microvascular dysfunction include disruption of the blood-brain barrier and dysregulated cerebral blood flow. Given the aging of the population and concurrent obesity epidemic, the important role played by diabetic microvascular dysfunction in neurocognitive decline is certain to attract increasing research interest in the years ahead.

Vascular Progenitor Cell Dysfunction and Diabetes

Striking at the core of the vascular system, diabetes exerts a major toll on several vascular stem and vascular progenitor cell (VPC) populations. Although controversy exists regarding the precise definitions of these populations,[29] the detrimental effects of diabetes are widespread and affect both the number and functionality of VPCs.[30] This has led to the hypothesis that defective endothelial and vascular repair, arising due to these progenitor cell deficiencies, may play a role in the diabetic vascular phenotype.

The bone marrow (BM) is an important reservoir for VPCs, specifically, EPCs, in addition to its function as a reservoir for hematopoietic stem cells. Here, in this nurturing-ground for VPCs, an array of adverse changes has been described. As an example, Spinetti and colleagues[31] studied BM samples from patients with type 2 diabetes mellitus and identified a reduction of hematopoietic tissue, increased apoptosis and fat deposition, and microvascular rarefaction. Moreover, in addition to this anatomic evidence, hematopoietic and VPC numbers were reduced and molecular cell survival pathways were adversely affected in BM progenitor cells from diabetic subjects.[31]

Impaired Reverse Cholesterol Transport

Therapeutic interventions to reduce plaque burden are beginning to appear in the clinical arena. Although not all of these have lived up to expectations, therapies, such as high-dose statins and high-density lipoprotein (HDL)-raising agents, are thought to hold promise for reversing the atherosclerotic disease process. Several studies have indicated that diabetes impairs atherosclerotic regression and lipid egress from plaques. Parathath and colleagues[32] made use of a unique mouse model to show that during atherosclerotic regression there were lower reductions in plaque cholesterol (approximately 30%) and macrophages (approximately 41%) in diabetic mice compared with control mice. Diabetic (vs control) plaque macrophages also exhibited increased oxidant stress and a cellular phenotype more consistent with enhanced inflammation.[32] These findings were corroborated in humans in the prospective Reduction in Yellow Plaque by Aggressive Lipid-lowering Therapy (YELLOW) trial, in which 87 patients with multivessel CAD undergoing percutaneous coronary intervention (PCI) were randomized to intensive lipid-lowering therapy (rosuvastatin 40 mg daily) or standard-of-care lipid-lowering therapy.[33] These investigators identified that the mean reduction in plaque lipid with statin therapy was significantly greater in nondiabetic compared with diabetic subjects over an 8-week period. It was concluded that although high-dose statin therapy can reduce lipid content in obstructive coronary lesions, the magnitude of this effect is attenuated in those with diabetes versus those without diabetes, suggesting an impaired pattern for short-term regression in diabetic atherosclerosis.[33]

Summary of Relationships Between Diabetes and the Vasculature

This article reviews only a few of the many relationships between diabetes, the vasculature, and CVD. Space limitations have not permitted discussion of many other aspects, such as the role of insulin and insulin resistance,[34] altered platelet function, or the diabetes-associated circulating lipid disturbances that drive vascular disease, consisting of low HDL, increased triglycerides, and postprandial lipemia (diabetic dyslipidemia). Without question, the unifying theme of these pathways is the broad and multifaceted nature of these disease-causing insults that culminate in the diabetic vascular phenotype.

DIABETES AND THE HEART: DIABETIC CARDIOMYOPATHY

Moving from the vessels to the heart, the possibility that diabetes directly causes cardiomyopathy was first suggested more than 4 decades ago by Rubler and colleagues,[35] who reported postmortem observations from 4 patients with diabetes and congestive heart failure (CHF), where no other reason for heart failure could be determined. In the ensuing years, and not without controversy, accumulating data from experimental, pathologic, epidemiologic, and clinical studies have indicated that diabetes results in specific cardiac functional and structural changes.[36] This has led to the contemporary outlook on this disease, whereby DCM is defined as the specific cardiac dysfunction and damage present in diabetic patients, which is characterized by myocardial dilatation, hypertrophy, and decreased left ventricular (LV) systolic and diastolic functions, and which is independent of the coexistence of ischemic heart disease, MI, or hypertension.[37] Robust data now support the existence of DCM, with one of the largest epidemiologic studies, involving more than 800,000 patients, concluding that diabetes is independently associated with the occurrence of CHF after adjusting for ventricular hypertrophy, hypertension, CAD, and atrial fibrillation.[38]

Mechanisms of Disease

A clear understanding of the pathobiology of DCM is lacking at the present time. Several pathophysiologic mechanisms have been proposed, however, to explain the structural and functional changes associated with DCM that likely act in a synergistic fashion, and which include hyperglycemia, lipotoxicity, inflammation, autonomic neuropathy, and both microvascular and macrovascular changes.[39] Recent evidence has also identified mitochondrial dysfunction and epigenetic changes (alteration in gene function without changes in nucleotide sequence) as pathogenic contributors to DCM.[40] Importantly, hyperglycemia is considered a critical driver of DCM because it has the ability to trigger several adaptive and maladaptive responses that are evident during the evolution of cardiac dysfunction. In addition to the vascular effects discussed previously, hyperglycemia contributes to the generation of ROS, connective tissue damage, systemic and local cytokine elaboration, renin-angiotensin-aldosterone system activation, cardiac hypertrophy, and fibrosis. Furthermore, AGEs formed in diabetic patients not only harm the vasculature but also accumulate in cardiac tissues and are implicated in the morphologic changes that result in myocardial stiffness and impaired contractility with DCM (**Fig. 2**).[41]

Altered Substrate Metabolism

In healthy individuals, equivalent proportions of energy required for cardiac performance come from glucose metabolism and free fatty acids (FFAs). In a hyperglycemic state, increased insulin resistance leads to reductions in the glucose transporter proteins 1 and 4. Consequently, myocardial cells rely less on glucose metabolism (which accounts for only approximately 10% of myocardial energy production) and more on β-oxidation of FFAs for energy production. FFA metabolism generates several toxic intermediates that accumulate in myocardial cells, a phenomenon termed *lipotoxicity*. Lipotoxicity disrupts cellular function in several ways. First, it impairs myocyte calcium handling through reduced activity of ATPases, decreased ability of the sarcoplasmic reticulum to take up calcium, and reduced activities of other exchanges, such as sodium-calcium and the sarcolemmal calcium ATPase.[42] This impairment in calcium regulation seems to cause an overload of calcium ions in the cytosol and increased ventricular stiffness in the early stages of DCM.[43] Second, it causes increased production and release of ROS, which in turn cause oxidative stress and abnormal gene expression, resulting in cardiomyocyte death, cardiac fibrosis, and myocardial dysfunction.[44] In addition, FFAs inhibit pyruvate dehydrogenase, which leads to the accumulation of glycolytic intermediates and ceramide, which are known to enhance

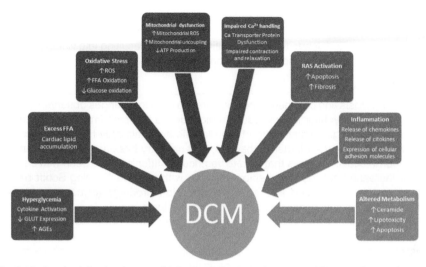

Fig. 2. Pathophysiologic triggers of DCM in diabetic patients. In addition to hyperglycemia, the combination of ROS, increased β-oxidation with elevated FFAs leading to myocardial lipotoxicity, cytokine damage, and the activation of the renin-angiotensin system (RAS) lead to the molecular and structural changes that characterize diabetic cardiomyopathy. GLUT, glucose transporter.

apoptosis.[45] FFAs have also been shown to enhance peripheral insulin resistance and trigger cell death. Abnormalities in FFA metabolism have been demonstrated in idiopathic dilated cardiomyopathy, in which the rate of FFA uptake by myocardium is inversely proportional to the severity of the myocardial dysfunction.[46] It is possible, therefore, that similar effects may be contributing to the development of DCM.

Activation of the Renin-angiotensin System

Activation of the renin-angiotensin system can exert deleterious effects on the myocardium through different mechanisms. Angiotensin II receptor density and mRNA expression are elevated in the diabetic heart.[47] Furthermore, activation of the renin-angiotensin system in the setting of diabetes is strongly associated with increased oxidative damage and cardiomyocyte and endothelial cell apoptosis and necrosis in diabetic hearts, contributing to accelerated interstitial fibrosis.[48]

Cardiac Autonomic Neuropathy

Diabetic cardiac autonomic neuropathy (CAN) occurs in 17% of patients with type 1 diabetes mellitus and 22% of patients with type 2 diabetes mellitus and is strongly associated with mortality.[39] Over time, hyperglycemia results in impaired sympathetic innervation and increases both adrenergic receptor expression and catecholamine levels.[49] One of the earliest signs of CAN is an increased resting heart rate and associated loss of heart rate variability. Resting tachycardia causes an increase in myocardial work, increased oxygen demand, reduced ventricular filling time, and reduced cardiac efficiency. These effects collectively lead to myocyte apoptosis and myocardial fibrosis, culminating in ventricular hypertrophy and dysfunction. These pathologic processes seem to increase with age, high glucose levels, and duration of disease. Not surprisingly, several studies have shown that CAN plays an important role in the deleterious effects of diabetes on the heart, causing impaired LV systolic function with reduced ejection fraction and decreased diastolic filling.[39,49] There is also evidence that autonomic neuropathy, in combination with vascular endothelial dysfunction and inflammation, leads to further insulin resistance, resulting in a vicious cycle of worsening hyperglycemia and its effects on the myocardium.[5]

Myocardial Fibrosis

Myocardial fibrosis and collagen deposition are the primary changes observed in DCM and arise in the interstitium, perivascular region, or in a combined manner. In addition to fibrosis, pathologic examination of the diabetic heart typically reveals myocardial hypertrophy, capillary endothelial changes, and capillary basal laminar thickening.[50] The pathomolecular changes that lead to ventricular stiffening have been well characterized. Increased collagen deposition interacts with glucose, forming Schiff bases, and which are reorganized into so called Amadori products (glycated collagen). Further chemical modification of the Amadori products results in the formation of AGEs, which has a profound effect on diastolic function. Furthermore, AGEs have the ability to cross-link with circulating proteins and cause impaired nitric oxide signaling and increased intracellular oxidative stress, all of which contribute to cell damage. Therefore, impaired LV function in the setting of diabetes, both diastolic and systolic, can be the result of fibrosis and altered collagen structure, specifically through the mechanisms of cross-linking and AGE formation.

Cardiovascular Findings

The complex pathogenesis of DMC ultimately leads to altered cardiac structure and function. Furthermore, frequent coexisting conditions, such as hypertension and CAD, further complicate the diabetic cardiac phenotype. Recently, in an effort to consolidate these factors into a cohesive description of the structural phenotype, a categorization of the DCM has been proposed.[39] According to this categorization, stage 1 DCM is diastolic heart failure with normal ejection fraction in the absence of other causes of heart disease. It is found in 75% of asymptomatic diabetic patients.[51] Stage 2 is defined by both diastolic and systolic dysfunction, in the absence of other contributing comorbidities for structural heart disease. Stage 3 is diastolic and/or systolic dysfunction, but in the setting of microvascular disease, uncontrolled hypertension, or other direct myopathic processes, such as infection or inflammation. Stage 4 is diastolic and/or systolic dysfunction in the setting of CAD. The advantages of the proposed scheme are 2-fold. First, it separates clinical phenotypes into those that are primarily due to DCM (stages 1 and 2) and those where other pathologies are also contributory (stages 3 and 4). Second, this classification has prognostic implications. Patients with stage 1 DCM have a 5% to 8% mortality compared with normal controls. Moreover, 37% of patients in stage 1, compared with 16.8% of normal controls, progress to symptomatic heart failure, which usually precedes the development of stage 2 DCM and systolic dysfunction.[39]

Diagnosing DCM

The diagnosis of DCM currently relies on noninvasive imaging that can demonstrate myocardial dysfunction across the continuum of ventricular dysfunction found in these patients. Although currently a consensus on the imaging definition of DCM is lacing, it is generally accepted that hypertrophy and diastolic dysfunction are responsible for (although not specific to) the clinical presentation of DCM.

Cardiac hypertrophy is a hallmark in the morphologic manifestations of DCM and can be quantified through conventional echocardiography.[52] The advent of MRI and its ability to qualitatively assess the myocardium has broadened understanding of the processes that lead to DCM and can demonstrate the presence of fatty or fibrotic infiltrates in the hypertrophied myocardium. Studies of myocardial geometry have also shown altered torsion dynamics in asymptomatic patients that could represent a subclinical phenotype with a higher propensity to develop cardiac dysfunction in the future.[53]

Changes in diastolic function have been reported in up to 75% of diabetic patients without evidence of heart disease caused by other factors, whereas it is a rare condition in healthy, nonobese individuals (where the incidence approaches 1%).[54] Consistent with this, additional studies have shown a correlation between altered transmitral Doppler inflow patterns and poor glycemic control.[54] Using tissue Doppler imaging techniques, recent studies have also shown that the prevalence of diastolic dysfunction in diabetic subjects may be as high as 50%.[55] Diastolic variables have proved especially useful in predicting the prognosis of diabetic patients without overt heart failure. A retrospective study of 486 diabetic patients demonstrated that echocardiographically derived parameter of the E/e' ratio was associated with an increase in global mortality after adjusting for age, gender, CAD, hypertension, LV ejection fraction, and left atrial volume.[56] Newer echocardiographic markers, such as total ejection isovolumic (TEI) index, are emerging as additional useful tools in the diagnosis of DCM. In a recent study of patients with type 2 diabetes mellitus without macrovascular complications, TEI index was significantly and independently associated with the presence of DCM.[37] Other modern echocardiographic techniques, such as transmitral pulsed Doppler and its applications (strain and strain rate), have recently demonstrated good sensitivity in the diagnosis of DCM.

DIABETES AND THE CARDIOVASCULAR PATIENT

Moving from the heart and DCM to the patient as a whole, the clinical implications of the association between diabetes and CVD have been well described.

Coronary Artery Disease Risk Factors

There is a strong association and overlap between diabetes and the metabolic syndrome. For patients who have developed diabetes, the strongest associations are with dyslipidemia and hypertension.

Dyslipidemia

A large number of studies both for primary and secondary prevention in diabetes have evaluated the use of statin medications. What is remarkable is that statins not only reduce coronary events by relative risk proportions equal to the nondiabetic population but also in many cases demonstrate that relative risk reduction is higher. This is one of the first demonstrations that not only is absolute risk reduction higher but also relative risk reduction.[57] This speaks to the pleotrophic effects of statins, such as reduced inflammation and thrombosis.[58] The American Diabetes Association has recommended that patients with diabetes be treated with a statin medication even if their low-density lipoprotein (LDL) cholesterol is on target. At present, for patients without coronary disease, the LDL target is less than 100 mg/dL, whereas for patients with advanced CAD and prior events, the recommended target is less than 70 mg/dL.[57] Because of the association of diabetes with hypertriglyceridemia and reduced levels of HDL, investigations are under way to find novel therapies. Fibrates have not reduced risks in diabetics in the ACCORD (Action to Control Cardiovascular Risk in Diabetes) trial,[59] however, and published data regarding the CETP inhibitors have been disappointing.[60,61] Recently, studies of niacin have also been negative for elevating HDL levels in the setting of low LDL levels.[62] As a result, statin therapy has become the gold standard therapy for hyperlipidemia in diabetic patients, with recommended LDL targets lower than those for nondiabetic patients.

Hypertension

With regards to hypertension, important recent information has shown that the goals for blood pressure control need to be carefully evaluated. In the ACCORD trial, which evaluated patients with type 2 diabetes mellitus and high cardiovascular risk, patients achieving a systolic blood pressure less than 120 mm Hg had outcomes similar to patients who achieved a systolic blood pressure less than 140 mm Hg, the traditional standard.[63] There were small reductions in stroke but for the primary cluster of death, MI, and stroke, there was no significant difference. Similar analyses from the INVEST (International Verapamil-Trandolapril Study) trial have demonstrated that the cardiovascular event rates are comparable in those patients with a systolic blood pressure less than 130 mm Hg compared with those achieving between 130 mm Hg and 140 mm Hg.[64] This speaks to the importance of less-aggressive blood pressure control than has been advocated in the past. In INVEST, it was also shown that patients with a systolic blood pressure less than 110 mm Hg experienced increased cardiovascular event rates. As a result, according to the new Eighth Report of the Joint National Committee on Prevention, Detection, Evaluation, and Treatment of High Blood Pressure guidelines and other expert opinions, it is questionable whether a blood pressure target of 130/80, as opposed to 140/90, is justified.

Glycemic control

Several pivotal trials have demonstrated that tight glycemic control (target hemoglobin A_{1c} approximately 6.0%) is not associated with improved cardiovascular outcomes.[65] This has led to a general relaxing of how aggressively physicians are treating glycemic control in their diabetic patients. Beyond this, one of the major problems with antidiabetic medications is their association with weight gain and hypoglycemia. Recently, incretin drugs in the form of glucagon-like peptide-1 agonists and dipeptidyl peptidase-4 inhibitors have entered the market. The promise of incretin therapy is the association with favorable weight changes and the relative lack of hypoglycemia.[66] Several key cardiovascular outcomes trials in type 2 diabetes mellitus are near completion and will report in the next 2 years.

Diabetes and Coronary Artery Disease

At the clinical level, the association between diabetes and CAD is well established and has been documented in several large observational cohort studies.[67,68]

Dating back to the BARI trial from the early 1990s, there has been a demonstration that patients with multivessel CAD and diabetes have improved outcomes with coronary artery bypass graft (CABG) surgery compared with PCI.[69] After BARI, researchers speculated that these findings may be related to the balloon angioplasty used in the percutaneous arm and later raised the question of whether the advent of stenting would change this outcome. Several important studies have ensued. The ARTS trial showed that there was still an increased cardiovascular event rate for diabetic patients undergoing PCI with bare metal stents compared with coronary artery bypass surgery.[70] Later, the SYNTAX trial, recruiting more than 400 diabetic patients and using drug-eluting stents (DES) (paclitaxel) with percutaneous coronary intervention (PCI) (DES-PCI), showed no difference in hard cardiovascular endpoint data at 1 year but did demonstrate and reaffirm very high repeat revascularization rates. With long-term follow-up out to 5 years, the SYNTAX study showed a clear advantage of CABG over PCI for left main and triple vessel disease.[71]

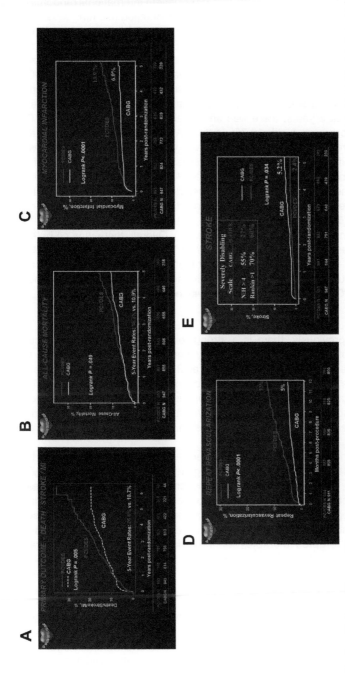

Fig. 3. Kaplan-Meier estimates from the FREEDOM study of the proportion of subjects with a clinical event by treatment assignment, as indicated: (A) primary endpoint (death/stroke/MI), (B) all-cause mortality, (C) MI, (D) repeat revascularization to 1 year, and (E) stroke. (*Reprinted with permission AHA Scientific Sessions 2012* © 2012 American Heart Association, Inc.)

The FREEDOM Trial, published in the *New England Journal of Medicine* in December 2012, provided a comprehensive insight into diabetes and multivessel CAD because it exclusively studied diabetic patients in a 1900-patient international randomized trial of DES-PCI versus CABG.[72] The majority of patients enrolled had multivessel CAD (84% had triple vessel disease). The median patient age was 63 years, with the majority having preserved LV function and an average SYNTAX score of approximately 26. FREEDOM patients were approximately 70% elective stable CAD patients, with the remainder having suffered a recent acute coronary syndrome. In the FREEDOM study, 20% of patients had off-pump CABG in the surgical arm and the mean number of treated lesions was greater than 5. For the primary endpoint, the composite of death, MI, and stroke at 5 years, there was an 8% absolute difference from 26.6% in the DES-PCI arm compared with 18.7% in the CABG arm (**Fig. 3**A). There was also an associated increase in all-cause mortality at 5 years in the DES-PCI arm, which was marginally significant ($P = .049$) (see **Fig. 3**B) as well as an increased rate of MI, which continued to accrue over the 5 years of trial ($P<.001$) (see **Fig. 3**C). Further counting against PCI, there was a significantly lower rate of repeat revascularization in the CABG arm (see **Fig. 3**D). On the other hand, there was a greater stroke rate in the bypass arm at 5 years (5.2% vs 2.4%, $P = .03$), which was most apparent in the first 30 days after the index procedure (see **Fig. 3**E). Overall, there was no heterogeneity across important subgroups, including SYNTAX score.[73] The FREEDOM trial was confirmation of the BARI findings and other meta-analysis data based on earlier trials with and without stenting,[74] and collectively these studies have clearly documented the benefits of CABG in diabetic patients with advanced CAD.

Heart Failure

As discussed previously, there is a strong relationship between diabetes and the development of CHF. In order to simplify the prescription of a clinical treatment plan, it is convenient to define heart failure as 3 distinct entities. First is systolic heart failure, which is almost always related to ischemic heart disease and is defined as an LV ejection fraction of less than 45%. Second is heart failure with preserved LV function. This is associated with diastolic abnormalities, largely related to the strong association between diabetes and hypertension. The third is DCM, as described previously.[44]

The treatment of heart failure has evolved over the past several years. In systolic heart failure, the use of β-blockers and angiotensin-converting enzyme (ACE) inhibitors has been the mainstay. Coronary revascularization for CAD with associated myocardial ischemia and CHF has also been recommended. For diastolic or preserved LV ejection fraction CHF, several therapies have been evaluated in addition to ACE inhibitors and β-blockers. This is an area of fruitful investigation at present, although targeted therapies for these forms of diabetic CHF remain to be identified.

SUMMARY

Diabetes has reached an epidemic level worldwide, and patients suffering from this disease are at significantly higher risk for CVD. Moreover, cardiovascular complications are the leading cause of diabetes-related morbidity and mortality.

The close relationship between diabetes and CVD together with the substantial rise in prevalence of diabetes will ultimately lead to a huge increase in the demand for health care services at a global level. Although FREEDOM and other studies have clarified how best to manage patients at the individual level, there are enormous challenges and opportunities in addressing the growing diabetes epidemic at the population level. Ultimately, the economic force behind the continuing rise in the cost of health care derived from caring for the 300 million projected diabetic patients in 2025 will leave policy makers no choice but to deeply revise, and come up with, efficient solutions to prevent the widespread surge of this disease. In a health care system that is continually becoming more complex, and where efficacious drugs and sophisticated devices continue to improve clinical outcomes, part of the focus should be placed back on the mechanisms that prevent the development of diabetes and related pathologies through the promotion of cardiovascular health by smoking cessation, exercising, following a healthy diet, and weight loss strategies, all of which will improve health outcomes and reduce costs.

REFERENCES

1. King H, Aubert RE, Herman WH. Global burden of diabetes, 1995-2025: prevalence, numerical estimates, and projections. Diabetes Care 1998;21:1414–31.
2. Boyle JP, Honeycutt AA, Narayan KM, et al. Projection of diabetes burden through 2050: impact of changing demography and disease prevalence in the U.S. Diabetes Care 2001;24:1936–40.
3. New WHO statistics highlight increases in blood pressure and diabetes, other noncommunicable risk factors. Cent Eur J Public Health 2012;20(134):149.
4. Chiha M, Njeim M, Chedrawy EG. Diabetes and coronary heart disease: a risk factor for the global epidemic. Int J Hypertens 2012;2012:697240.
5. Tillquist MN, Maddox TM. Update on diabetic cardiomyopathy: inches forward, miles to go. Curr Diab Rep 2012;12:305–13.
6. Johnson PC, Doll SC, Cromey DW. Pathogenesis of diabetic neuropathy. Ann Neurol 1986;19:450–7.
7. Weil EJ, Lemley KV, Mason CC, et al. Podocyte detachment and reduced glomerular capillary endothelial fenestration promote kidney disease in type 2 diabetic nephropathy. Kidney Int 2012;82:1010–7.
8. Tang Y, Li GD. Chronic exposure to high glucose impairs bradykinin-stimulated nitric oxide production by interfering with the phospholipase-C-implicated signalling pathway in endothelial cells: evidence for the involvement of protein kinase C. Diabetologia 2004;47:2093–104.
9. Kovacic JC, Martin A, Carey D, et al. Influence of rosiglitazone on flow-mediated dilation and other markers of cardiovascular risk in HIV-infected patients with lipoatrophy. Antivir Ther 2005;10:135–43.
10. Schaffer SW, Jong CJ, Mozaffari M. Role of oxidative stress in diabetes-mediated vascular dysfunction: unifying hypothesis of diabetes revisited. Vascul Pharmacol 2012;57:139–49.
11. Brownlee M. Biochemistry and molecular cell biology of diabetic complications. Nature 2001;414:813–20.
12. Kovacic JC, Moreno P, Nabel EG, et al. Cellular senescence, vascular disease, and aging: part 2 of a 2-part review: clinical vascular disease in the elderly. Circulation 2011;123:1900–10.
13. Konova E, Baydanoff S, Atanasova M, et al. Age-related changes in the glycation of human aortic elastin. Exp Gerontol 2004;39:249–54.
14. Kislinger T, Fu C, Huber B, et al. N(epsilon)-(carboxymethyl)lysine adducts of proteins are ligands for receptor for advanced glycation end products that activate cell signaling pathways and modulate gene expression. J Biol Chem 1999; 274:31740–9.

15. Brett J, Schmidt AM, Yan SD, et al. Survey of the distribution of a newly characterized receptor for advanced glycation end products in tissues. Am J Pathol 1993;143:1699–712.

16. Giri R, Shen Y, Stins M, et al. beta-amyloid-induced migration of monocytes across human brain endothelial cells involves RAGE and PECAM-1. Am J Physiol Cell Physiol 2000;279:C1772–81.

17. Kunt T, Forst T, Harzer O, et al. The influence of advanced glycation endproducts (AGE) on the expression of human endothelial adhesion molecules. Exp Clin Endocrinol Diabetes 1998;106:183–8.

18. Otero K, Martinez F, Beltran A, et al. Albumin-derived advanced glycation endproducts trigger the disruption of the vascular endothelial cadherin complex in cultured human and murine endothelial cells. Biochem J 2001;359:567–74.

19. Svensjo E, Cyrino F, Michoud E, et al. Vascular permeability increase as induced by histamine or bradykinin is enhanced by advanced glycation endproducts (AGEs). J Diabet Complications 1999;13:187–90.

20. Bucala R, Tracey KJ, Cerami A. Advanced glycosylation products quench nitric oxide and mediate defective endothelium-dependent vasodilatation in experimental diabetes. J Clin Invest 1991;87:432–8.

21. Scheubel RJ, Kahrstedt S, Weber H, et al. Depression of progenitor cell function by advanced glycation endproducts (AGEs): potential relevance for impaired angiogenesis in advanced age and diabetes. Exp Gerontol 2006;41:540–8.

22. Xiang M, Yang M, Zhou C, et al. Crocetin prevents AGEs-induced vascular endothelial cell apoptosis. Pharmacol Res 2006;54:268–74.

23. Burke AP, Kolodgie FD, Zieske A, et al. Morphologic findings of coronary atherosclerotic plaques in diabetics: a postmortem study. Arterioscler Thromb Vasc Biol 2004;24:1266–71.

24. Muris DM, Houben AJ, Schram MT, et al. Microvascular dysfunction is associated with a higher incidence of type 2 diabetes mellitus: a systematic review and meta-analysis. Arterioscler Thromb Vasc Biol 2012;32:3082–94.

25. Kovacic JC, Fuster V. Atherosclerotic risk factors, vascular cognitive impairment, and Alzheimer disease. Mt Sinai J Med 2012;79:664–73.

26. Centers for Disease Control and Prevention. Leading causes of death reports. Available at: http://webappa.cdc.gov/sasweb/ncipc/leadcaus10.html. Accessed May 19, 2011.

27. Beeri MS, Silverman JM, Davis KL, et al. Type 2 diabetes is negatively associated with Alzheimer's disease neuropathology. J Gerontol A Biol Sci Med Sci 2005;60:471–5.

28. Nelson PT, Smith CD, Abner EA, et al. Human cerebral neuropathology of Type 2 diabetes mellitus. Biochim Biophys Acta 2009;1792:454–69.

29. Kovacic JC, Moore J, Herbert A, et al. Endothelial progenitor cells, angioblasts, and angiogenesis–old terms reconsidered from a current perspective. Trends Cardiovasc Med 2008;18:45–51.

30. Tepper OM, Galiano RD, Capla JM, et al. Human endothelial progenitor cells from type II diabetics exhibit impaired proliferation, adhesion, and incorporation into vascular structures. Circulation 2002;106:2781–6.

31. Spinetti G, Cordella D, Fortunato O, et al. Global remodeling of the vascular stem cell niche in bone marrow of diabetic patients: implication of the microRNA-155/FOXO3a signaling pathway. Circ Res 2013;112:510–22.

32. Parathath S, Grauer L, Huang LS, et al. Diabetes adversely affects macrophages during atherosclerotic plaque regression in mice. Diabetes 2011;60: 1759–69.

33. Kini A, Baber U, Kovacic JC, et al. Impact of diabetes mellitus on atherosclerotic plaque lipid regression: results from the prospective. Randomized YELLOW Trial Circulation 2012;126:A17291.
34. Mather KJ, Steinberg HO, Baron AD. Insulin resistance in the vasculature. J Clin Invest 2013;123:1003–4.
35. Rubler S, Dlugash J, Yuceoglu YZ, et al. New type of cardiomyopathy associated with diabetic glomerulosclerosis. Am J Cardiol 1972;30:595–602.
36. Fang ZY, Prins JB, Marwick TH. Diabetic cardiomyopathy: evidence, mechanisms, and therapeutic implications. Endocr Rev 2004;25:543–67.
37. Voulgari C, Papadogiannis D, Tentolouris N. Diabetic cardiomyopathy: from the pathophysiology of the cardiac myocytes to current diagnosis and management strategies. Vasc Health Risk Manag 2010;6:883–903.
38. Movahed MR, Hashemzadeh M, Jamal MM. Diabetes mellitus is a strong, independent risk for atrial fibrillation and flutter in addition to other cardiovascular disease. Int J Cardiol 2005;105:315–8.
39. Maisch B, Alter P, Pankuweit S. Diabetic cardiomyopathy–fact or fiction? Herz 2011;36:102–15.
40. Singh GB, Sharma R, Khullar M. Epigenetics and diabetic cardiomyopathy. Diabetes Res Clin Pract 2011;94:14–21.
41. Avendano GF, Agarwal RK, Bashey RI, et al. Effects of glucose intolerance on myocardial function and collagen-linked glycation. Diabetes 1999;48:1443–7.
42. Cesario DA, Brar R, Shivkumar K. Alterations in ion channel physiology in diabetic cardiomyopathy. Endocrinol Metab Clin North Am 2006;35:601–10, ix–x.
43. Falcao-Pires I, Leite-Moreira AF. Diabetic cardiomyopathy: understanding the molecular and cellular basis to progress in diagnosis and treatment. Heart Fail Rev 2012;17:325–44.
44. Aneja A, Tang WH, Bansilal S, et al. Diabetic cardiomyopathy: insights into pathogenesis, diagnostic challenges, and therapeutic options. Am J Med 2008;121:748–57.
45. Park TS, Hu Y, Noh HL, et al. Ceramide is a cardiotoxin in lipotoxic cardiomyopathy. J Lipid Res 2008;49:2101–12.
46. Yazaki Y, Isobe M, Takahashi W, et al. Assessment of myocardial fatty acid metabolic abnormalities in patients with idiopathic dilated cardiomyopathy using 123I BMIPP SPECT: correlation with clinicopathological findings and clinical course. Heart 1999;81:153–9.
47. Peti-Peterdi J, Kang JJ, Toma I. Activation of the renal renin-angiotensin system in diabetes–new concepts. Nephrol Dial Transplant 2008;23:3047–9.
48. Kawasaki D, Kosugi K, Waki H, et al. Role of activated renin-angiotensin system in myocardial fibrosis and left ventricular diastolic dysfunction in diabetic patients–reversal by chronic angiotensin II type 1A receptor blockade. Circ J 2007;71:524–9.
49. Mytas DZ, Stougiannos PN, Zairis MN, et al. Diabetic myocardial disease: pathophysiology, early diagnosis and therapeutic options. J Diabet Complications 2009;23:273–82.
50. Asbun J, Villarreal FJ. The pathogenesis of myocardial fibrosis in the setting of diabetic cardiomyopathy. J Am Coll Cardiol 2006;47:693–700.
51. Boyer JK, Thanigaraj S, Schechtman KB, et al. Prevalence of ventricular diastolic dysfunction in asymptomatic, normotensive patients with diabetes mellitus. Am J Cardiol 2004;93:870–5.
52. Lang RM, Bierig M, Devereux RB, et al. Recommendations for chamber quantification: a report from the American Society of Echocardiography's Guidelines

and Standards Committee and the Chamber Quantification Writing Group, developed in conjunction with the European Association of Echocardiography, a branch of the European Society of Cardiology. J Am Soc Echocardiogr 2005;18:1440–63.

53. Chung J, Abraszewski P, Yu X, et al. Paradoxical increase in ventricular torsion and systolic torsion rate in type I diabetic patients under tight glycemic control. J Am Coll Cardiol 2006;47:384–90.

54. Galderisi M. Diastolic dysfunction and diabetic cardiomyopathy: evaluation by Doppler echocardiography. J Am Coll Cardiol 2006;48:1548–51.

55. Kiencke S, Handschin R, von Dahlen R, et al. Pre-clinical diabetic cardiomyopathy: prevalence, screening, and outcome. Eur J Heart Fail 2010;12:951–7.

56. From AM, Scott CG, Chen HH. The development of heart failure in patients with diabetes mellitus and pre-clinical diastolic dysfunction a population-based study. J Am Coll Cardiol 2010;55:300–5.

57. American Diabetes Association. Standards of medical care in diabetes–2013. Diabetes Care 2013;36(Suppl 1):S11–66.

58. Puccetti L, Santilli F, Pasqui AL, et al. Effects of atorvastatin and rosuvastatin on thromboxane-dependent platelet activation and oxidative stress in hypercholesterolemia. Atherosclerosis 2011;214:122–8.

59. Group AS, Ginsberg HN, Elam MB, et al. Effects of combination lipid therapy in type 2 diabetes mellitus. N Engl J Med 2010;362:1563–74.

60. Barter PJ, Caulfield M, Eriksson M, et al. Effects of torcetrapib in patients at high risk for coronary events. N Engl J Med 2007;357:2109–22.

61. Schwartz GG, Olsson AG, Abt M, et al. Effects of dalcetrapib in patients with a recent acute coronary syndrome. N Engl J Med 2012;367:2089–99.

62. Investigators AH, Boden WE, Probstfield JL, et al. Niacin in patients with low HDL cholesterol levels receiving intensive statin therapy. N Engl J Med 2011;365:2255–67.

63. Reboldi G, Gentile G, Angeli F, et al. Effects of intensive blood pressure reduction on myocardial infarction and stroke in diabetes: a meta-analysis in 73,913 patients. J Hypertens 2011;29:1253–69.

64. Cooper-DeHoff RM, Gong Y, Handberg EM, et al. Tight blood pressure control and cardiovascular outcomes among hypertensive patients with diabetes and coronary artery disease. JAMA 2010;304:61–8.

65. Macisaac RJ, Jerums G. Intensive glucose control and cardiovascular outcomes in type 2 diabetes. Heart Lung Circ 2011;20:647–54.

66. Ussher JR, Drucker DJ. Cardiovascular biology of the incretin system. Endocr Rev 2012;33:187–215.

67. Roger VL, Go AS, Lloyd-Jones DM, et al. Heart disease and stroke statistics–2012 update: a report from the American Heart Association. Circulation 2012;125:e2–220.

68. Smith SC Jr, Faxon D, Cascio W, et al. Prevention Conference VI: Diabetes and Cardiovascular Disease: Writing Group VI: revascularization in diabetic patients. Circulation 2002;105:e165–9.

69. Comparison of coronary bypass surgery with angioplasty in patients with multivessel disease. The Bypass Angioplasty Revascularization Investigation (BARI) Investigators. N Engl J Med 1996;335:217–25.

70. Serruys PW, Ong AT, van Herwerden LA, et al. Five-year outcomes after coronary stenting versus bypass surgery for the treatment of multivessel disease: the final analysis of the Arterial Revascularization Therapies Study (ARTS) randomized trial. J Am Coll Cardiol 2005;46:575–81.

71. Mohr FW, Morice MC, Kappetein AP, et al. Coronary artery bypass graft surgery versus percutaneous coronary intervention in patients with three-vessel disease and left main coronary disease: 5-year follow-up of the randomised, clinical SYNTAX trial. Lancet 2013;381:629–38.
72. Farkouh ME, Domanski M, Sleeper LA, et al. Strategies for multivessel revascularization in patients with diabetes. N Engl J Med 2012;367:2375–84.
73. Sianos G, Morel MA, Kappetein AP, et al. The SYNTAX Score: an angiographic tool grading the complexity of coronary artery disease. EuroIntervention 2005;1: 219–27.
74. Hlatky MA, Boothroyd DB, Bravata DM, et al. Coronary artery bypass surgery compared with percutaneous coronary interventions for multivessel disease: a collaborative analysis of individual patient data from ten randomised trials. Lancet 2009;373:1190–7.

Cardiovascular Disease in Diabetes Mellitus
Risk Factors and Medical Therapy

Magdalene M. Szuszkiewicz-Garcia, MD[a],[*],
Jaime A. Davidson, MD[b]

KEYWORDS

- Cardiovascular disease • Diabetes • Myocardial infarction • Coronary heart disease
- Hyperglycemia • Risk • Therapy

KEY POINTS

- Diabetes mellitus (DM) is a condition on the increase, carrying a high risk of cardiovascular (CV) complications.
- Diabetes carries a higher risk for cardiovascular events in women than in men.
- Clinicians still do not have the ability to precisely and reliably stratify risk among patients with diabetes.
- Treatment of known cardiovascular risks such as hypertension, hyperlipidemia, and smoking is key in decreasing the risk for cardiovascular events.
- Some glucose-lowering drugs may have a more positive impact on minimizing cardiovascular disease, but more research needs to be done to confirm this possibility.

INTRODUCTION

Diabetes mellitus (DM) is a disease on the rise. A 2011 report from the Centers for Disease Control and Prevention indicated that 25.8 million people, 8.3% of the United States population, have DM. Among adults age 65 years or older, 26.9% had diabetes in 2010.[1] Worldwide there are 240 million people with DM, and it is projected that by 2030 there will be 439 million affected by diabetes.[2] The most common cause of death among patients with diabetes is cardiovascular disease, with heart disease responsible for 70% of deaths.[3] The risk of increased cardiovascular morbidity and

This article originally appeared in Endocrinology and Metabolism Clinics of North America, Volume 43, Issue 1, March 2014.
The authors have no conflict of interest.
[a] Division of Endocrinology and Metabolism, Center for Human Nutrition, Department of Medicine, University of Texas Southwestern Medical Center, 5323 Harry Hines Boulevard, Dallas, TX 75390-8857, USA; [b] Division of Endocrinology, Diabetes and Metabolism, Touchstone Diabetes Center, University of Texas Southwestern Medical Center, 5323 Harry Hines Boulevard K5.246, Dallas, TX 75390, USA
* Corresponding author.
E-mail address: Magda.Szuszkiewicz-Garcia@UTSouthwestern.edu

Clinics Collections 1 (2014) 129–144
http://dx.doi.org/10.1016/j.ccol.2014.08.009
2352-7986/14/$ – see front matter © 2014 Elsevier Inc. All rights reserved.

mortality has been recognized for years, dubbing diabetes "cardiovascular disease equivalent."

EPIDEMIOLOGY

There is no argument that individuals with diabetes have a significantly increased risk of macrovascular complications, but how accurate is this label of "cardiovascular disease equivalent?" Fifteen years ago a landmark Finnish study attempted to answer this question. A 7-year risk of myocardial infarction in middle-aged patients with diabetes was 20%, similar to that of patients with a previous myocardial infarction.[4] Following this study there have been a flurry of epidemiologic studies arguing for or against the risk equivalence. Results are as varied as the studies themselves. The risk seems to vary by severity of diabetes as well as definition of coronary heart disease (CHD) used. For example, in patients with diet-controlled diabetes, the risk of mortality and myocardial infarction was smaller than that in patients with a previous myocardial infarction.[5,6] On the other hand, diabetic patients treated with glucose-lowering agents had a risk of mortality similar to that of patients who had a previous myocardial infarction, and a much greater risk of death than patients with angina, evidence of ischemia or infarct on electrocardiogram, but no history of an infarct. This risk was disproportionately high in women.[6,7]

In long-standing diabetes, women carried almost twice as high a hazard ratio for all-cause mortality and for death from CHD when compared with men with diabetes and patients with CHD without diabetes. The highest risk of death occurred in patients with both CHD and diabetes: hazard ratio of 4.44 for men and 5.86 for women.[8]

It is clear, therefore, that patients with diabetes are not a homogeneous group. Women are at a higher risk than men. Younger patients and those with shorter, milder disease are at a lower risk of events. Patients with type 1 diabetes may also have a lower risk when young and early in the disease course.[9]

ASSESSING THE RISK OF CARDIOVASCULAR EVENTS

There is significant amount of dispute regarding which parameters allow for most accurate assessment of risk and prediction of cardiovascular event. There is no doubt that chronic hyperglycemia imparts increased risk for mortality and events in both type 1 and type 2 diabetes; however, the association is not linear and is not consistent in all types of vascular disease. In one study, elevated fasting glucose has been found to increase the risk for all types of vascular disease, including ischemic and hemorrhagic stroke.[10] This increased risk of mortality was noted already when fasting glucose was greater than 100 mg/dL, and it was linked to a 6-year shorter life span in a 50-year-old individual with DM. Sixty percent of this risk is attributable to vascular death.[11] On the other hand, other studies show less consistent results in some groups. Postmenopausal women with established CHD and impaired fasting glucose of 100 to 125 mg/dL had no increased risk of coronary events. However, when the old definition of impaired fasting glucose was applied (glucose >110 mg/dL), women had an increased risk of myocardial infarction and cardiac death. Strokes, transient ischemic attacks (TIAs) and congestive heart failure (CHF) were not predicted by impaired fasting glucose by either definition.[12]

Postprandial glucose has been studied extensively as a predictor of cardiovascular outcomes. Hyperglycemia at 1 hour and 2 hours after a standard 75-g oral glucose tolerance test, as well as after a meal challenge, has proved to be a good predictor of cardiovascular events and mortality.[13] This relationship is linear. In some groups such as older adults and women, postprandial glucose may have a better ability to predict mortality than a fasting value, although combination of both fasting and 2-hour glucose may allow for more accurate risk estimation.[13–15] Given that acute hyperglycemia may cause vasoconstriction, there is a sound physiologic base for concern, even in patients with normal fasting glucose.

Elevation of glycosylated hemoglobin (HbA1c) appears to correlate with mortality and cardiovascular events in a linear manner as well: a 1% increase of HbA1c carries a significant increase in risk (20%–30%) for cardiovascular events or death.[16] This risk exists for coronary artery disease, fatal and nonfatal myocardial infarction and stroke, and perhaps most strongly for peripheral artery disease, in patients with both type 1 and type 2 diabetes.[17] Even in the absence of diabetes a small increase in HbA1c (>5%) is associated with an increased risk of CHD.[18]

Here again, not all data are consistent. In one study of women with no diabetes, elevation of HbA1c did not predict the risk of cardiovascular events.[19] It is controversial whether HbA1c is a better or worse prognosticator of cardiovascular events. However, attempts to lower HbA1C do not consistently lower mortality in all patients, complicating this issue further.[20]

In addition to elevated glucose, patients with diabetes have several other risk factors. Comorbidities such as renal disease, hypertension, dyslipidemia, sleep apnea, obesity, and poor physical fitness all carry a significant increase in cardiovascular risk. Some of the risks, such as macroproteinuria, may be a better predictor of mortality than glucose or HbA1c.[21] This heterogeneity of risks makes event prediction difficult. Unfortunately, treatment of cardiovascular complications is costly and, therefore, precise identification of the most vulnerable patients would be important in early prevention.

Framingham, UKPDS Risk Engine, SCORE, and DECODE are among calculators that have attempted to better estimate risk for individual patients. The results, however, are inconsistent: the accuracy varies in men and women, and none of these risk engines have been validated against a pool of American patients.[22,23]

PATHOPHYSIOLOGY

There are several potential mechanisms through which diabetes causes acceleration of atherosclerosis. Persons with type 2 diabetes have hypertension as well as abnormalities of lipid metabolism and insulin resistance, all of which are linked to increasing cardiovascular risk. Hyperglycemia likely also plays a central role in pathogenesis of vascular diseases, evidenced by the increased prevalence of atherosclerosis in people with type 1 diabetes without dyslipidemia or hypertension.

Within the blood vessels, endothelial cells come into direct contact with high glucose levels and play several key regulatory functions. These cells mediate vasodilation through production of bradykinin and nitric oxide, which acts on smooth muscle, resulting in relaxation and vasodilation. Endothelial cells also regulate vasoconstriction through local production of angiotensin-converting enzyme (ACE), prostaglandins, and endothelin. Vasoconstriction is driven by high angiotensin II levels, inducing smooth-muscle activation and bradykinin breakdown mediated by high levels of ACE. Hyperglycemia disrupts normal production of nitric oxide, leading to decreased blood flow. In addition, elevated levels of nonesterified fatty acids, often present in type 2 diabetes, further contribute by impairing vasodilation.[24]

Hyperglycemia also induces inflammation through stimulation of adipokines and upregulation of toll-like receptors (TLRs) in the endothelium. The usual function of TLRs is triggering both innate and adaptive immune response against a broad range of pathogens. When inappropriately activated, they initiate an excessive white blood cell response, resulting in ischemic reperfusion injury, restenosis, and formation of atherosclerotic plaque.[24]

Hyperglycemia may also play a role in monocytes adhering to a vessel wall and differentiating into macrophages. Glucose modulates the ability of macrophages to take up lipids and become foam cells.[24] This accumulation of lipid cells results in fatty streaks, which later become necrotic in the center and rupture.[25] Matrix metalloproteinases are also induced by hyperglycemia and may be linked to intraplaque hemorrhage, which destabilizes plaque.

There is some evidence that changes in the extracellular matrix resulting from hyperglycemia may cause collagen-matrix remodeling and smooth-muscle cell proliferation, resulting in a protective response of stabilization of a plaque. The same mechanisms may also play a deleterious role in coronary vessel restenosis after intervention.

Furthermore, hyperglycemia, hyperinsulinemia, and hypertriglyceridemia may cause excessive platelet activation and an increase in plasminogen activator inhibitor (PAI-1) levels, a major inhibitor of fibrinolysis. These changes of normal metabolism lead to a prothrombotic state.

Hyperglycemia and an increased level of fatty acids are important factors in inducing oxidative stress and inflammation in the pathogenesis of atherosclerosis, but may not be the only ones. Insulin resistance on a vascular level and a high circulating concentration of insulin may also play a role in acceleration of atherogenesis in diabetes. All of these mechanisms are still not completely understood.

MITIGATING THE RISKS
Intensive Glycemic Control

It has been well established that good glycemic control decreases the risks of microvascular complications. With regard to macrovascular complications, the answer is not as clear. It seems that treating more aggressively early in the course of DM does decrease the risk of myocardial infarction and reduces mortality. In UKPDS, a large study of patients with type 2 DM early in the disease course, there was no difference found in cardiovascular outcomes during the first 10 years between diet-controlled and intensively managed, pharmacologically treated groups. The average HbA1c difference between groups was 7.0% versus 7.9%, which was sufficient to decrease the rate of microvascular complications.[26] During the additional decade of follow-up observation with no intervention, there was a significant reduction of myocardial infarctions and death noted in the original intensive treatment group, despite the fact that the difference in HbA1c levels was lost after the first year of the follow-up study, 11 years after enrollment.[27] Similar results were found in a study of patients with type 1 DM.[28] Reduction of HbA1c from 9.1% to 7.4% early in disease course significantly reduced the risks of any cardiovascular disease by 42% and decreased the risk of strokes, myocardial infarctions, and cardiovascular death by 57% over a 17-year follow-up period.[29]

However, attempts to treat hyperglycemia aggressively in patients with long-standing diabetes did not bring similar positive results. VADT, a study of older men with long-standing diabetes, showed that reduction of HbA1c from 8.4% to 6.9% did not improve cardiovascular outcomes.[30]

Two recent large trials involving populations with previous cardiovascular events or at significant risk are the ADVANCE and ACCORD trials. The ADVANCE trial showed no beneficial effect on the rate of macrovascular events, when HbA1c was brought to 6.5% rather than the standard 7.3%.[31] On the other hand, the ACCORD trial was stopped early because of a 22% higher mortality in intensive glycemic control group.[20]

During a 5-year observational follow-up period, patients initially assigned to the intensive treatment group experience a decreased risk of myocardial infarctions, but the increased risk of mortality persisted[32]; this despite HbA1c increasing from 6.6% to 7.4% in the initial intensive control group while HbA1c remained stable in the standard group (rising from 7.7% to 7.8%). The patients in the intensive group did require a more complicated multidrug regimen. The mortality, however, did not appear to be a direct result of hypoglycemic events.[33] It is also interesting that in the intensive control group, there was a liner relationship between mortality and HbA1c: individuals with higher HbA1c had higher mortality, similarly to what was observed in the UKPDS and DCCT-EDIC trials. One possible explanation for this finding is that disproportionate mortality occurred in a group of individuals who enter the intensive arm with HbA1c higher than 8%, and whose HbA1c remains higher than 8% throughout the course of the trial despite all efforts.[34]

When these and other studies are compiled in a meta-analysis, the results are a little more reassuring. It appears that intensive glycemic control may decrease the risk of nonfatal myocardial infarction, with no positive or negative effect on mortality, strokes, and peripheral vascular disease. However, this reduction in myocardial infarcts carries a price of a 30% increased risk of hypoglycemia.[35–38]

These data indicate the need for individualization of glycemic goals. Intensive therapy may be helpful in reducing cardiovascular events and mortality when initiated in people with shorter, uncomplicated diabetes. In patients with diabetes of longer than 15 years and long-standing complications, risk of tight control may outweigh the benefit.[39] Some investigators suggest that for such patients, an HbA1c goal of 7% to 7.9% may be sufficient to optimize the risk profile for cardiovascular events (**Table 1**).[40]

There is still a significant amount of debate over what are the most appropriate goals and for whom. Part of this discussion also concerns the most beneficial manner of treating diabetes: that is, whether any particular medication or medication combination improves cardiovascular outcomes.

CHOOSING THE RIGHT AGENTS

Metformin is a first-line drug recommended by several professional associations.[41,42] Lactic acidosis is its most feared side effect, although the actual risk is likely overestimated.[43] The UKPDS trial showed that metformin was particularly efficacious, with a 33% risk reduction of myocardial infarctions and 27% reduction of death in comparison with diet therapy.[27] BARI 2D did not show a clear mortality advantage, although patients on insulin sensitizers developed less peripheral artery disease.[44,45] However, this study did not separate the effect of metformin from other sensitizers, so it is difficult to say if the beneficial effect of metformin could have been blunted by the negative effect of other drugs such as rosiglitazone. Metformin has also been associated with decreased mortality in patients with CHF, despite the fact that heart failure is listed as a relative contraindication on the insert package.[46]

Thiazolidinediones (TZDs) are another class of insulin sensitizers, but with a controversial risk profile. It is now well recognized that this class of drugs has a negative effect on heart failure, as it is associated with volume expansion through peroxisome proliferator-activated receptor (PPAR)-γ–dependent pathways. Rosiglitazone created headlines when a significantly increased risk of myocardial infarctions and cardiovascular mortality were discovered.[47] Although a follow-up study showed no mortality effect, the use of TZDs has declined.[48] Favorable data for pioglitazone with regard to decreased risk of myocardial infarctions, strokes, and death did little to restore the reputation of TZDs.[48,49]

Table 1
Major trials: effect of treatment of diabetes mellitus (DM) on cardiovascular (CV) outcomes

Study	Goal	Outcome	Notes
ACCORD[20,32]	Lowering HbA1c to <6% in intense vs standard therapy in high CV group	Increased mortality in intense therapy group	Study stopped prematurely Mortality not related to hypoglycemia
ADVANCE[31]	Lowering HbA1c to <6.5% vs standard therapy in high CV risk group	No decrease in mortality or rate of cardiovascular events	
BARI2D[44,45]	Use of insulin sensitizers vs insulin-provision therapy	No difference in CV outcomes	Analysis of events not broken down further into different class of drugs
DCCT[28]	Intense vs standard therapy (HbA1c of 7.4% vs 9.1%) in type 1 DM early in disease course	No difference in CV events during 7 y of follow-up	Low number of events in both groups (young volunteers: average age 27 y)
DCCT-EDIC[29]	17-y follow-up of patients from DCCT	Lower rates of events including death in intensive therapy group	HbA1c converged in both groups to 7.8%–7.9% at the end of study
Heart 2D 2009	Prandial vs basal insulin therapy	No difference in CV events	Stopped due to lack of efficacy. Less than expected prandial difference
LOOK AHEAD[94]	Intensive lifestyle intervention/weight loss	No effect on CV event rate at 10 y	Stopped prematurely due to futility. 6% in intervention group vs 3.5% body weight loss at the end of the study: difference may have been too small to show CV effect
UKPDS[26,27]	Diet vs medication for control of early diabetes	Lower rates of myocardial infarction and death from any cause in intense treatment group during 2nd decade of follow-up, no difference during the 1st decade	Low number of events during 1st decade of follow-up in both groups
VADT[30]	Lowering HbA1c to 1.5% below standard therapy in older men with long-standing DM and high CV risk	No difference in outcomes	

Sulfonylureas also appear to have a less favorable profile in comparison with metformin. Although they did decrease myocardial infarctions by 15% and mortality by 13% when compared with placebo in UKPDS, there are data indicating that sulfonylureas may not be optimal medications for patients with preexisting CHD and CHF.[27,50] The evidence is far from clear, and there are multiple contradictory reports.[51] Compared with other agents, including insulin, sulfonylureas carry a significant risk of hypoglycemia. It is debatable whether a specific drug has a worse profile than others, but glyburide has shown, although not consistently, to have an increased risk of acute coronary syndrome and cardiovascular death.[52,53] Some investigators suggest that if sulfonylureas must be used, glimepiride is the safest choice.[54]

Insulin is a staple of diabetes treatment. However, treatment of diabetes with insulin leads to a much higher plasma levels of insulin, potentially leading to excessive smooth-muscle activation, which may play a role in atherogenesis.[55] There are also data suggesting worse outcomes in patients with heart failure who use insulin. It is unclear whether this is a function of more severe diabetes affecting mortality or if insulin is in fact a culprit.[56] In well-controlled studies there is no conclusive evidence that insulin administration has a direct beneficial or deleterious effect on the cardiovascular system, apart from reducing hyperglycemia.[51,57]

It is possible that over the next few years clinicians may be encouraged away from insulin toward other classes of drugs. Dipeptidyl-peptidase 4 (DPP-4) inhibitors and glucagon-like peptide 1 (GLP-1) agonists are 2 classes of drugs with promising effects on cardiovascular disease. Preliminary data have suggested that there may be a lower rate of cardiovascular events and mild lipid reduction in patients on DDP-4 inhibitors. The recently published prospective trial SAVOR-TIMI53 found that saxagliptin was not cardioprotective when compared with placebo during a 2-year follow-up for patients with a high cardiovascular risk. On the other hand, there were slightly more hospitalizations for CHF in the saxagliptin group (3.5% vs 2.8% with hazard ratio of 1.27 and $P = .007$).[58] CAROLINA, a study comparing cardiovascular outcomes in patients on linagliptin versus glimepiride, is in progress and will be completed in 2018.

GLP-1 agonists induce weight loss, have a blood-pressure–lowering effect of 2 to 8 mm Hg, and improve lipids, in addition to being linked to decreased rates of cardiovascular events and hospitalizations. In experimental animals, they also improve left ventricular function and reduce infarct size caused by reperfusion.[59] Prospective studies are being conducted to confirm that this is a true effect on the cardiovascular system: the larger among these are MAGNA VICTORIA and LEADER, which will be completed in 2015 and 2016, respectively.

The newest drugs arriving on the market are sodium-glucose cotransporter-2 (SGC-2) inhibitors. Their mechanism of inducing glucosuria promises benefits of modest weight loss and possible reduction in blood pressure of 3 to 9 mm Hg, likely because of its diuretic effect. The effect on lipids is not clear as yet: it appears that treatment with SGC-2 inhibitors may slightly increase high-density lipoprotein (HDL). Data submitted to the Food and Drug Administration show a possible decreased risk of cardiovascular death and events, but long-term data is not yet available.[60] CANVAS, a canagliflozin long-term cardiovascular outcomes trial, and DECLARE-TIMI58, a 6-year cardiovascular outcomes study of dapagliflozin, are both ongoing and will be completed in 2018 and 2019, respectively.

LIPIDS

Lipid-lowering therapy is another critical intervention in improving cardiovascular outcomes. In patients with diabetes it may actually have a more profound effect than intensive glycemic control on lowering mortality and cardiovascular risk.[61] Current standard of care is to treat patients with DM to the goal of a low-density lipoprotein (LDL) level of less than 100 mg/dL, with an optional goal of less than 70 mg/dL. Patients with DM and CHD should have their LDL level lower than 70 mg/dL. Patients older than 40 years with additional risk factors should be treated with statins as well. Given the recent decline in the cost of statins and benefit of therapy, there is a debate as to whether people younger than 40 years, those with no other risk factors, and good lipid panel should also be treated with statins in the absence of CHD.[62] This proposal is prompted by data that there is a significant reduction in cardiovascular events and mortality with statin use. One study reports a 13% decline in mortality per 1 mmol/L (39 mg/dL) decrease in LDL, with a 21% reduction in major vascular events per 1 mmol/L reduction in LDL-cholesterol in people with diabetes over a period of 4 years.[63] There was no evidence of harm.[64] This treatment effect is consistent with what is observed in patients with no DM: risk reduction is effective. When results were adjusted for baseline risk, diabetic patients benefited more in both primary and secondary prevention, even though lipid reduction was similar in both groups.[65]

Fibrates have also been studied extensively, with mixed results.[66,67] In the FIELD study when fibrates were compared with placebo, there was no decrease in events, likely because of high statin use in the placebo arm, but men with low HDL and triglycerides higher than 200 mg/dL benefited from a reduction in cardiovascular events.[68] In ACCORD, fibrates as an add-on therapy to statins appeared to also have benefited men with low HDL with and without hypertriglyceridemia, whereas women might have been harmed.

Data on use of ezetimibe are still not clear. While it does lower LDL, as yet no results from prospective studies with regard to morbidity and mortality outcomes are available for ezetimibe alone or as add-on therapy. It is reassuring that at least one group found no difference in the rate of events on comparison with statins: results for patients with diabetes did not differ from the rest of the cohort.[69]

Fish oil and omega-3 fatty acid supplements enjoy popularity among physicians and lay public alike. Fish oil is an effective treatment for hypertriglyceridemia, a disorder frequently coexisting with type 2 diabetes. Earlier studies in the cardiovascular literature suggested a possible mortality decrease in patients with heart disease. However, patients with early diabetes and high cardiovascular risk did not reduce their risk of cardiovascular events or mortality by using 1 g of fish oil per day.[70]

HYPERTENSION

Hypertension is a frequent comorbidity in patients with diabetes, especially with type 2 diabetes or type 1 diabetes associated with renal disease. It significantly increases cardiovascular risks, especially strokes. Current American Diabetes Association (ADA) guidelines call for treatment of hypertension when blood pressure is higher than 140/80 mm Hg. Lowering blood pressure to less than 130/80 mm Hg is advised in younger patients if it "can be achieved without undue treatment burden."[41] This figure represents a change from previous guidelines whereby blood pressure goals were less than 130/80 mm Hg.[71] Such a change is a positive one and reflects current data, which show a clear benefit derived by lowering the blood pressure below the threshold of 140 mm Hg. ADVANCE is a clear example of this. Reduction of blood pressure from 141/77 to 135/75 mm Hg with a fixed dose of perindopril and a diuretic indapamide versus placebo resulted in an 18% reduction of cardiovascular death and a significantly lower number of coronary events.[72]

Another recent large prospective study, ACCORD, showed that lowering systolic blood pressure (SBP) to less than 120 mm Hg did not improve mortality. Risk of stroke was diminished, however, from 0.53% to 0.32% yearly, at the price of doubling the rate of serious side effects (from 1.3% to 3.3%) such as syncope and hyperkalemia.[73]

A recent meta-analysis of patients with DM and prediabetes suggested that an SBP of 130 to 135 mm Hg may be optimal. Compared with blood pressure of 140 mm Hg, SBP of less than 135 mm Hg reduced mortality by 10% and strokes by 17%. There was no further reduction in microvascualar complication, mortality or CV events, with exception of strokes when SBP was lowered to <130 mm Hg. Reducing blood pressure to less than 135 mm Hg carried a 20% increased risk of serious events, with a 40% increase with SBP lower than 130 mm Hg.[74]

Although patients with diabetes often require multiple medications to control blood pressure, blocking the renin-angiotensin system seems to decrease mortality and the risk of complications in comparison with other antihypertensive agents. Current guidelines recognize this, and recommend the use of ACE inhibitors or angiotensin receptor blockers in the treatment of hypertension in diabetes.[41] Enalapril has been shown to be superior to nisoldipine in reduction of myocardial infarctions in patients in with poorly controlled diabetes.[75]

ASPIRIN

The role of aspirin in the treatment of cardiovascular disease is well established. However, data on the use of aspirin for primary prevention is less clear. There are several prospective studies indicating to a lack of mortality benefit in the general diabetic population.[76,77] Results of subset data analysis and meta-analysis are somewhat inconsistent. Some studies find a decreased risk of fatal and nonfatal strokes and myocardial infarctions through use of low-dose aspirin only in older patients, whereas others show a similar risk reduction only in men.[75,78] One meta-analysis reported a decreased rate of major cardiovascular events and calculated that 92 patients would need to be treated to prevent 1 major cardiovascular event. There was also evidence of harm, mostly from bleeding, in 1 out of every 526 treated patients. Interestingly there was no benefit when each of the events (strokes, myocardial infarctions, mortality) was evaluated separately.[79] Decreased mortality with low-dose aspirin has been found in a study of patients with an average age of 60 years, with the most significant benefit in older and male participants.[80]

With such inconsistency in the literature, it is not surprising that various professional associations differ in their recommendations with regard to the most appropriate age at when to start aspirin in diabetes for primary prevention. Whereas the ADA recommends 75 to 162 mg aspirin for men older than 50 and women older than 60 with an additional major risk factor for cardiovascular disease, the American Heart Association advocates starting therapy for patients older than 40 with risk factors.[81] The results of ASCEND and ACCEPT-D are expected to clarify this issue.

DIAGNOSIS OF CHD IN ASYMPTOMATIC PATIENTS

There is no consensus on how to approach screening of a patient with diabetes and no symptoms of coronary artery disease, yet it is a relevant issue in practice when patients ask if they are safe to start an exercise program. Clinically significant CHD was reported in 20% to 25% of asymptomatic patients with type 2 diabetes when tested by various modalities.[82] However, whether testing is beneficial and which tests to use are unclear. Exercise stress testing with an electrocardiogram is relatively inexpensive and has a 97% negative predictive value. On the other hand, a positive predictive value is less helpful. There is also a practical limitation: some patients may not be able to complete a treadmill test because of obesity, deconditioning, or arthritis.[83]

Using coronary artery calcium scores (CACS) in patients with diabetes can have pitfalls. Asymptomatic patients with a low score of less than 100 had a 21% prevalence of CHD. When identified as low to intermediate risk by the Framingham Risk Score, a CACS score greater than 40 was an independent predictor for atherosclerotic events.[84] In the general diabetic population, an even lower CACS score of 10 or more has been shown to predict all-cause mortality and cardiovascular events with high sensitivity but low specificity. Conversely, a score of less than 10 has an excellent negative predictive value.[85]

Screening patients with adenosine-stress radionuclide myocardial perfusion imaging is widely accepted, although it does not appear to result in event reduction.[86] On the other hand, prompt revascularization in optimally medically managed patients did not result in improved outcomes or survival.[44] Of note, optimally medically managed patients with angina symptoms and those with silent ischemia did not fare any differently.[87]

REVASCULARIZATION

Although there were no differences in outcomes between patients receiving prompt revascularization and those on medical therapy in the BARI 2D trial, a group with the biggest improvement in survival was patients who had coronary artery bypass grafting (CABG).[44] The FREEDOM trial confirmed that for patients with DM and multivessel CHD, CABG was a better option than percutaneous coronary intervention (PCI) stenting. During a 5-year follow-up, the CABG group had a significantly lower mortality (10.9% vs 16.3%) and fewer myocardial infarctions (6.0% vs 13.9%). The downside was a significantly higher incidence of strokes in the postoperative period in the CABG group, 5.2% versus 2.4%.[88] Similar results were found in the past in a meta-analysis study.[89] Because the analysis incorporated studies using non–drug-eluting stents, as the technology improved the results were called to question. FREEDOM, however, compared CABG with PCI using mostly drug-eluting stents.

Men and women with diabetes treated with revascularization have similar risks of myocardial infarction, cardiovascular accidents, and death. Women, however, have more residual angina symptoms and poorer functional status even if they have less anatomic disease before revascularization.[90] After PCI stenting to a single lesion, diabetic patients have worse outcomes when compared with patients without DM. These patients are at increased risk for needing revascularization of the stented lesions during the first year after the procedure, and have an increased risk for cardiac death and myocardial infarctions during 5 years following the procedure.[91]

SUMMARY

Overall, the advanced made in care of patients with diabetes and patients with CHD are encouraging. The mean predicted risk for CHD in the entire population of 7.2% in 1999 to 2000 has dropped to 6.5% in 2009 to 2010. Risk of a cardiovascular event has also fallen from 9.2% to 8.7%, despite an increase in the prevalence of DM. Blood-pressure control, smoking cessation, and improvement in HDL-cholesterol appear to be linked to this improvement. On the other hand, minorities such as African Americans and Mexican Americans still appear to be vulnerable populations.[92]

Encouraging lifestyle modifications such as healthy diet, weight reduction, and exercise is a commonsense approach that has been a cornerstone of diabetes prevention and treatment for many years. Although as little as 5% weight loss results in

---

Box 1
Treatment strategies proved to improve cardiovascular outcomes

Lowering HbA1c to less than 8%: benefit of further lowering is controversial

Blocking angiotensin-renin system

Blood-pressure control to lower than 140/80 mm Hg

Low-dose aspirin in older individuals, especially men

Aggressive lipid-lowering therapy to low-density lipoprotein less than 100 mg/dL for primary prevention and less than 70 mg/dL for secondary prevention

Coronary artery bypass grafting is better that percutaneous coronary intervention in treatment of multivessel coronary artery disease

---

improvement of metabolic parameters, the recently completed LOOK AHEAD trial shows that it is not enough to decrease the risk for cardiovascular events in patients with diabetes.[93,94]

To date, it appears that multifactorial therapy including reduction of lipids, renin-angiotensin system suppression, personalized glycemic control, and the use of aspirin in selected patients may be the most effective way to reduce the cardiovascular complications of diabetes (**Box 1**).[61] Early diagnosis and interventions with a treat-to-target approach have been shown to be beneficial over the long term in patients with both type 1 and type 2 diabetes.

ACKNOWLEDGMENTS

Many thanks are extended to Dr Jose Enrique Garcia and Dr Zahid Ahmad for their invaluable input in editing this article.

REFERENCES

1. Centers for Disease Control and Prevention. National diabetes fact sheet: national estimates and general information on diabetes and prediabetes in the United States. 2011. Available at: http://www.cdc.gov/diabetes/pubs/factsheet11.htm. Accessed June 6, 2013.
2. Shaw JE, Sicree RA, Zimmet PZ. Global estimates of the prevalence of diabetes for 2010 and 2030. Diabetes Res Clin Pract 2010;87(1):4–14.
3. Gu K, Cowie CC, Harris MI. Mortality in adults with and without diabetes in a national cohort of the U.S. population, 1971-1993. Diabetes Care 1998;21(7):1138–45.
4. Haffner SM, Lehto S, Ronnemaa T, et al. Mortality from coronary heart disease in subjects with type 2 diabetes and in nondiabetic subjects with and without prior myocardial infarction. N Engl J Med 1998;339(4):229–34.
5. Evans JM, Wang J, Morris AD. Comparison of cardiovascular risk between patients with type 2 diabetes and those who had had a myocardial infarction: cross sectional and cohort studies. BMJ 2002;324(7343):939–42.
6. Eberly LE, Cohen JD, Prineas R, et al. Impact of incident diabetes and incident nonfatal cardiovascular disease on 18-year mortality: the multiple risk factor intervention trial experience. Diabetes Care 2003;26(3):848–54.
7. Juutilainen A, Lehto S, Rönnemaa T, et al. Type 2 diabetes as a "coronary heart disease equivalent": an 18-year prospective population-based study in Finnish subjects. Diabetes Care 2005;28(12):2901–7.

8. Whiteley L, Padmanabhan S, Hole D, et al. Should diabetes be considered a coronary heart disease risk equivalent?: results from 25 years of follow-up in the Renfrew and Paisley survey. Diabetes Care 2005;28(7):1588–93.

9. Grundy SM, Benjamin IJ, Burke GL, et al. Diabetes and cardiovascular disease: a statement for healthcare professionals from the American Heart Association. Circulation 1999;100(10):1134–46.

10. The Emerging Risk Factors Collaboration. Diabetes mellitus, fasting blood glucose concentration, and risk of vascular disease: a collaborative meta-analysis of 102 prospective studies. Lancet 2010;375(9733):2215–22.

11. Seshasai SR, Kaptoge S, Thompson A, et al. Diabetes mellitus, fasting glucose, and risk of cause-specific death. N Engl J Med 2011;364(9):829–41.

12. Kanaya AM, Herrington D, Vittinghoff E, et al. Impaired fasting glucose and cardiovascular outcomes in postmenopausal women with coronary artery disease. Ann Intern Med 2005;142(10):813–20.

13. Ceriello A, Hanefeld M, Leiter L, et al. Postprandial glucose regulation and diabetic complications. Arch Intern Med 2004;164(19):2090–5.

14. Smith NL, Barzilay JI, Shaffer D, et al. Fasting and 2-hour postchallenge serum glucose measures and risk of incident cardiovascular events in the elderly: the Cardiovascular Health Study. Arch Intern Med 2002;162(2):209–16.

15. Sorkin JD, Muller DC, Fleg JL, et al. The relation of fasting and 2-h postchallenge plasma glucose concentrations to mortality: data from the Baltimore Longitudinal Study of Aging with a critical review of the literature. Diabetes Care 2005; 28(11):2626–32.

16. Khaw KT, Wareham N, Bingham S, et al. Association of hemoglobin A1c with cardiovascular disease and mortality in adults: the European prospective investigation into cancer in Norfolk. Ann Intern Med 2004;141(6):413–20.

17. Selvin E, Marinopoulos S, Berkenblit G, et al. Meta-analysis: glycosylated hemoglobin and cardiovascular disease in diabetes mellitus. Ann Intern Med 2004; 141(6):421–31.

18. Pai JK, Cahill LE, Hu FB, et al. Hemoglobin a1c is associated with increased risk of incident coronary heart disease among apparently healthy, nondiabetic men and women. J Am Heart Assoc 2013;2(2):e000077.

19. Pradhan AD, Rifai N, Buring JE, et al. Hemoglobin A1c predicts diabetes but not cardiovascular disease in nondiabetic women. Am J Med 2007;120(8): 720–7.

20. Gerstein HC, Miller ME, Byington RP, et al. Effects of intensive glucose lowering in type 2 diabetes. N Engl J Med 2008;358(24):2545–59.

21. Cosson E, Nguyen MT, Chanu B, et al. Cardiovascular risk prediction is improved by adding asymptomatic coronary status to routine risk assessment in type 2 diabetic patients. Diabetes Care 2011;34(9):2101–7.

22. Coleman RL, Stevens RJ, Retnakaran R, et al. Framingham, SCORE, and DECODE risk equations do not provide reliable cardiovascular risk estimates in type 2 diabetes. Diabetes Care 2007;30(5):1292–3.

23. van der Heijden AA, Ortegon MM, Niessen LW, et al. Prediction of coronary heart disease risk in a general, pre-diabetic, and diabetic population during 10 years of follow-up: accuracy of the Framingham, SCORE, and UKPDS risk functions: The Hoorn Study. Diabetes Care 2009;32(11):2094–8.

24. Pasterkamp G. Methods of accelerated atherosclerosis in diabetic patients. Heart 2013;99(10):743–9.

25. Chait A, Bornfeldt KE. Diabetes and atherosclerosis: is there a role for hyperglycemia? J Lipid Res 2009;50(Suppl):S335–9.

26. UK Prospective Diabetes Study (UKPDS) Group. Intensive blood-glucose control with sulphonylureas or insulin compared with conventional treatment and risk of complications in patients with type 2 diabetes (UKPDS 33). UK Prospective Diabetes Study (UKPDS) Group. Lancet 1998;352(9131):837–53.
27. Holman RR, Paul SK, Bethel MA, et al. 10-year follow-up of intensive glucose control in type 2 diabetes. N Engl J Med 2008;359(15):1577–89.
28. The Diabetes Control and Complications Trial Research Group. The effect of intensive treatment of diabetes on the development and progression of long-term complications in insulin-dependent diabetes mellitus. The Diabetes Control and Complications Trial Research Group. N Engl J Med 1993;329(14):977–86.
29. Nathan DM, Cleary PA, Backlund JY, et al. Intensive diabetes treatment and cardiovascular disease in patients with type 1 diabetes. N Engl J Med 2005; 353(25):2643–53.
30. Duckworth W, Abraira C, Moritz T, et al. Glucose control and vascular complications in veterans with type 2 diabetes. N Engl J Med 2009;360(2):129–39.
31. Patel A, MacMahon S, Chalmers J, et al. Intensive blood glucose control and vascular outcomes in patients with type 2 diabetes. N Engl J Med 2008; 358(24):2560–72.
32. Gerstein HC, Miller ME, Genuth S, et al. Long-term effects of intensive glucose lowering on cardiovascular outcomes. N Engl J Med 2011;364(9):818–28.
33. Bonds DE, Miller ME, Bergenstal RM, et al. The association between symptomatic, severe hypoglycaemia and mortality in type 2 diabetes: retrospective epidemiological analysis of the ACCORD study. BMJ 2010;340:b4909.
34. Riddle MC. Effects of intensive glucose lowering in the management of patients with type 2 diabetes mellitus in the Action to Control Cardiovascular Risk in Diabetes (ACCORD) trial. Circulation 2010;122(8):844–6.
35. Mannucci E, Monami M, Lamanna C, et al. Prevention of cardiovascular disease through glycemic control in type 2 diabetes: a meta-analysis of randomized clinical trials. Nutr Metab Cardiovasc Dis 2009;19(9):604–12.
36. Ma J, Yang W, Fang N, et al. The association between intensive glycemic control and vascular complications in type 2 diabetes mellitus: a meta-analysis. Nutr Metab Cardiovasc Dis 2009;19(9):596–603.
37. Ray KK, Seshasai SR, Wijesuriya S, et al. Effect of intensive control of glucose on cardiovascular outcomes and death in patients with diabetes mellitus: a meta-analysis of randomised controlled trials. Lancet 2009;373(9677):1765–72.
38. Hemmingsen B, Lund SS, Gluud C, et al. Targeting intensive glycaemic control versus targeting conventional glycaemic control for type 2 diabetes mellitus. Cochrane Database Syst Rev 2011;(6):CD008143.
39. Duckworth WC, Abraira C, Moritz TE, et al. The duration of diabetes affects the response to intensive glucose control in type 2 subjects: the VA Diabetes Trial. J Diabetes Complications 2011;25(6):355–61.
40. Hoogwerf BJ. Does intensive therapy of type 2 diabetes help or harm? Seeking accord on ACCORD. Cleve Clin J Med 2008;75(10):729–37.
41. American Diabetes Association. Standards of medical care in diabetes—2013. Diabetes Care 2013;36(Suppl 1):S11–66.
42. Garber AJ, Abrahamson MJ, Barzilay JI, et al. AACE comprehensive diabetes management algorithm 2013. Endocr Pract 2013;19(2):327–36.
43. Klachko D, Whaley-Connell A. Use of metformin in patients with kidney and cardiovascular diseases. Cardiorenal Med 2011;1(2):87–95.
44. Frye RL, August P, Brooks MM, et al. A randomized trial of therapies for type 2 diabetes and coronary artery disease. N Engl J Med 2009;360(24):2503–15.

45. Althouse AD, Abbott JD, Sutton-Tyrrell K, et al. Favorable effects of insulin sensitizers pertinent to peripheral arterial disease in type 2 diabetes: results from the bypass angioplasty revascularization investigation 2 diabetes (BARI 2D) trial. Diabetes Care 2013;36(10):3269–75.

46. Eurich DT, McAlister FA, Blackburn DF, et al. Benefits and harms of antidiabetic agents in patients with diabetes and heart failure: systematic review. BMJ 2007; 335(7618):497.

47. Nissen SE, Wolski K. Effect of rosiglitazone on the risk of myocardial infarction and death from cardiovascular causes. N Engl J Med 2007;356(24):2457–71.

48. Nissen SE, Wolski K. Rosiglitazone revisited: an updated meta-analysis of risk for myocardial infarction and cardiovascular mortality. Arch Intern Med 2010; 170(14):1191–201.

49. Lincoff AM, Wolski K, Nicholls SJ, et al. Pioglitazone and risk of cardiovascular events in patients with type 2 diabetes mellitus: a meta-analysis of randomized trials. JAMA 2007;298(10):1180–8.

50. Rao AD, Kuhadiya N, Reynolds K, et al. Is the combination of sulfonylureas and metformin associated with an increased risk of cardiovascular disease or all-cause mortality?: a meta-analysis of observational studies. Diabetes Care 2008;31(8):1672–8.

51. Sillars B, Davis WA, Hirsch IB, et al. Sulphonylurea-metformin combination therapy, cardiovascular disease and all-cause mortality: the Fremantle Diabetes Study. Diabetes Obes Metab 2010;12(9):757–65.

52. Gangji AS, Cukierman T, Gerstein HC, et al. A systematic review and meta-analysis of hypoglycemia and cardiovascular events: a comparison of glyburide with other secretagogues and with insulin. Diabetes Care 2007;30(2): 389–94.

53. Abdelmoneim AS, Eurich DT, Gamble JM, et al. Risk of acute coronary events associated with glyburide compared to gliclazide use in patients with type 2 diabetes: a nested case-control study. Diabetes Obes Metab 2013. [Epub ahead of print].

54. Breen DM, Giacca A. Effects of insulin on the vasculature. Curr Vasc Pharmacol 2011;9(3):321–32.

55. Chaitman BR, Hardison RM, Adler D, et al. The bypass angioplasty revascularization investigation 2 diabetes randomized trial of different treatment strategies in type 2 diabetes mellitus with stable ischemic heart disease: impact of treatment strategy on cardiac mortality and myocardial infarction. Circulation 2009; 120(25):2529–40.

56. Smooke S, Horwich TB, Fonarow GC. Insulin-treated diabetes is associated with a marked increase in mortality in patients with advanced heart failure. Am Heart J 2005;149(1):168–74.

57. The Origin Trial Investigators. Basal insulin and cardiovascular and other outcomes in dysglycemia. N Engl J Med 2012;367(4):319–28.

58. Scirica BM, Bhatt DL, Braunwald E, et al. Saxagliptin and cardiovascular outcomes in patients with type 2 diabetes mellitus. N Engl J Med 2013;369: 1317–26.

59. Umpierrez GE, Meneghini L. Reshaping diabetes care: the fundamental role of DPP-4 inhibitors and GLP-1 receptor agonists in clinical practice. Endocr Pract 2013;19(4):1–37.

60. Basile JN. The potential of sodium glucose cotransporter 2 (SGLT2) inhibitors to reduce cardiovascular risk in patients with type 2 diabetes (T2DM). J Diabetes Complications 2013;27(3):280–6.

61. Gæde P, Lund-Andersen H, Parving HH, et al. Effect of a multifactorial intervention on mortality in type 2 diabetes. N Engl J Med 2008;358(6):580–91.
62. Steinberg D, Grundy SM. The case for treating hypercholesterolemia at an earlier age: moving toward consensus. J Am Coll Cardiol 2012;60(25):2640–2.
63. Kearney PM, Blackwell L, Collins R, et al. Efficacy of cholesterol-lowering therapy in 18,686 people with diabetes in 14 randomised trials of statins: a meta-analysis. Lancet 2008;371(9607):117–25.
64. Taylor F, Ward K, Moore TH, et al. Statins for the primary prevention of cardiovascular disease. Cochrane Database Syst Rev 2011;(1):CD004816.
65. Costa J, Borges M, David C, et al. Efficacy of lipid lowering drug treatment for diabetic and non-diabetic patients: meta-analysis of randomised controlled trials. BMJ 2006;332(7550):1115–24.
66. Ginsberg HN, Elam MB, Lovato LC, et al. Effects of combination lipid therapy in type 2 diabetes mellitus. N Engl J Med 2010;362(17):1563–74.
67. Keech A, Simes RJ, Barter P, et al. Effects of long-term fenofibrate therapy on cardiovascular events in 9795 people with type 2 diabetes mellitus (the FIELD study): randomised controlled trial. Lancet 2005;366(9500):1849–61.
68. Steiner G. How can we improve the management of vascular risk in type 2 diabetes: insights from FIELD. Cardiovasc Drugs Ther 2009;23(5):403–8.
69. Hayek S, Canepa Escaro F, Sattar A, et al. Effect of ezetimibe on major atherosclerotic disease events and all-cause mortality. Am J Cardiol 2013;111(4):532–9.
70. Bosch J, Gerstein HC, Dagenais GR, et al. n-3 fatty acids and cardiovascular outcomes in patients with dysglycemia. N Engl J Med 2012;367(4):309–18.
71. American Diabetes Association. Standards of medical care in diabetes—2012. Diabetes Care 2012;35(Suppl 1):S11–63.
72. Patel A. Effects of a fixed combination of perindopril and indapamide on macrovascular and microvascular outcomes in patients with type 2 diabetes mellitus (the ADVANCE trial): a randomised controlled trial. Lancet 2007;370(9590): 829–40.
73. Cushman WC, Evans GW, Byington RP, et al. Effects of intensive blood-pressure control in type 2 diabetes mellitus. N Engl J Med 2010;362(17):1575–85.
74. Bangalore S, Kumar S, Lobach I, et al. Blood pressure targets in subjects with type 2 diabetes mellitus/impaired fasting glucose: observations from traditional and bayesian random-effects meta-analyses of randomized trials. Circulation 2011;123(24):2799–810, 2799 p following 2810.
75. Estacio RO, Jeffers BW, Hiatt WR, et al. The effect of nisoldipine as compared with enalapril on cardiovascular outcomes in patients with non-insulin-dependent diabetes and hypertension. N Engl J Med 1998;338(10):645–52.
76. Ogawa H, Nakayama M, Morimoto T, et al. Low-dose aspirin for primary prevention of atherosclerotic events in patients with type 2 diabetes: a randomized controlled trial. JAMA 2008;300(18):2134–41.
77. Belch J, MacCuish A, Campbell I, et al. The prevention of progression of arterial disease and diabetes (POPADAD) trial: factorial randomised placebo controlled trial of aspirin and antioxidants in patients with diabetes and asymptomatic peripheral arterial disease. BMJ 2008;337:a1840.
78. De Berardis G, Sacco M, Strippoli GF, et al. Aspirin for primary prevention of cardiovascular events in people with diabetes: meta-analysis of randomised controlled trials. BMJ 2009;339:b4531.
79. Butalia S, Leung AA, Ghali WA, et al. Aspirin effect on the incidence of major adverse cardiovascular events in patients with diabetes mellitus: a systematic review and meta-analysis. Cardiovasc Diabetol 2011;10:25.

80. Ong G, Davis TM, Davis WA. Aspirin is associated with reduced cardiovascular and all-cause mortality in type 2 diabetes in a primary prevention setting: the Fremantle Diabetes study. Diabetes Care 2010;33(2):317–21.

81. Buse JB, Ginsberg HN, Bakris GL, et al. Primary prevention of cardiovascular diseases in people with diabetes mellitus: a scientific statement from the American Heart Association and the American Diabetes Association. Circulation 2007;115(1):114–26.

82. Scholte AJ, Schuijf JD, Kharagjitsingh AV, et al. Different manifestations of coronary artery disease by stress SPECT myocardial perfusion imaging, coronary calcium scoring, and multislice CT coronary angiography in asymptomatic patients with type 2 diabetes mellitus. J Nucl Cardiol 2008;15(4):503–9.

83. Upchurch CT, Barrett EJ. Clinical review: screening for coronary artery disease in type 2 diabetes. J Clin Endocrinol Metab 2012;97(5):1434–42.

84. Lau KK, Wong YK, Chan YH, et al. Prognostic implications of surrogate markers of atherosclerosis in low to intermediate risk patients with type 2 diabetes. Cardiovasc Diabetol 2012;11:101.

85. Kramer CK, Zinman B, Gross JL, et al. Coronary artery calcium score prediction of all cause mortality and cardiovascular events in people with type 2 diabetes: systematic review and meta-analysis. BMJ 2013;346:f1654.

86. Young LH, Wackers FJ, Chyun DA, et al. Cardiac outcomes after screening for asymptomatic coronary artery disease in patients with type 2 diabetes: the DIAD study: a randomized controlled trial. JAMA 2009;301(15):1547–55.

87. Dagenais GR, Lu J, Faxon DP, et al. Prognostic impact of the presence and absence of angina on mortality and cardiovascular outcomes in patients with type 2 diabetes and stable coronary artery disease: results from the BARI 2D (Bypass Angioplasty Revascularization Investigation 2 Diabetes) trial. J Am Coll Cardiol 2013;61(7):702–11.

88. Farkouh ME, Domanski M, Sleeper LA, et al. Strategies for multivessel revascularization in patients with diabetes. N Engl J Med 2012;367(25):2375–84.

89. Hlatky MA, Boothroyd DB, Bravata DM, et al. Coronary artery bypass surgery compared with percutaneous coronary interventions for multivessel disease: a collaborative analysis of individual patient data from ten randomised trials. Lancet 2009;373(9670):1190–7.

90. Tamis-Holland JE, Lu J, Korytkowski M, et al. Sex differences in presentation and outcome among patients with type 2 diabetes and coronary artery disease treated with contemporary medical therapy with or without prompt revascularization: a report from the BARI 2D Trial (Bypass Angioplasty Revascularization Investigation 2 Diabetes). J Am Coll Cardiol 2013;61(17):1767–76.

91. Lee TT, Feinberg L, Baim DS, et al. Effect of diabetes mellitus on five-year clinical outcomes after single-vessel coronary stenting (a pooled analysis of coronary stent clinical trials). Am J Cardiol 2006;98(6):718–21.

92. Ford ES. Trends in predicted 10-year risk of coronary heart disease and cardiovascular disease among U.S. Adults from 1999 to 2010. J Am Coll Cardiol 2013; 61(22):2249–52.

93. Blackburn G. Effect of degree of weight loss on health benefits. Obes Res 1995; 3(Suppl 2):211s–6s.

94. Look Ahead Research Group. Cardiovascular effects of intensive lifestyle intervention in type 2 diabetes. N Engl J Med 2013;369(2):145–54.

Type 2 Diabetes Mellitus and Hypertension: An Update

Guido Lastra, MD[a,b,c], Sofia Syed, MD[a,b], L. Romayne Kurukulasuriya, MD[a], Camila Manrique, MD[a,b,c], James R. Sowers, MD[a,b,c,d],*

KEYWORDS

- Diabetes • Hypertension • Cardiovascular disease • Chronic kidney disease
- Renin-angiotensin-aldosterone system • Sympathetic nervous system

KEY POINTS

- Patients with hypertension and type 2 diabetes are at increased risk of cardiovascular and chronic renal disease.
- Factors involved in the pathogenesis of both hypertension and type 2 diabetes include inappropriate activation of the renin-angiotensin-aldosterone system, oxidative stress, inflammation, impaired insulin-mediated vasodilatation, augmented sympathetic nervous system activation, altered innate and adaptive immunity, and abnormal sodium processing by the kidney.
- The renin-angiotensin-aldosterone system blockade is a key therapeutic strategy in the treatment of hypertension in type 2 diabetes.
- Emerging therapies include renal denervation and carotid body denervation.

INTRODUCTION

Hypertension (HTN) is present in more than 50% of patients with diabetes mellitus (DM) and contributes significantly to both microvascular and macrovascular disease in DM (**Fig. 1**).[1–4] The risk for cardiovascular disease (CVD) is 4-fold higher in patients

This article originally appeared in Endocrinology and Metabolism Clinics of North America, Volume 43, Issue 1, March 2014.

Disclosures: The authors have nothing to disclose.

Funding Sources: Dr J.R. Sowers, NIH (R01 HL73101-01A1 and R01 HL107910-01), Veterans Affairs Merit System 0018.

Conflict of Interest: Dr J.R. Sowers is on the Merck Pharmaceuticals Advisory Board.

[a] Division of Endocrinology, Diabetes & Metabolism, Department of Internal Medicine, University of Missouri Columbia School of Medicine, D109 Diabetes Center HSC, One Hospital Drive, Columbia, MO 65212, USA; [b] Diabetes and Cardiovascular Research Center, University of Missouri, One Hospital Drive, Columbia, MO 65212, USA; [c] Harry S Truman Memorial Veterans Hospital, 800 Hospital Drive, Columbia, MO 65201, USA; [d] Department of Medical Physiology and Pharmacology, University of Missouri, One Hospital Drive, Columbia, MO 65212, USA

* Corresponding author. University of Missouri, D109 Diabetes Center HSC, One Hospital Drive, Columbia, MO 65212.

E-mail address: sowersj@health.missouri.edu

http://dx.doi.org/10.1016/j.ccol.2014.08.010
2352-7986/14/$ – see front matter

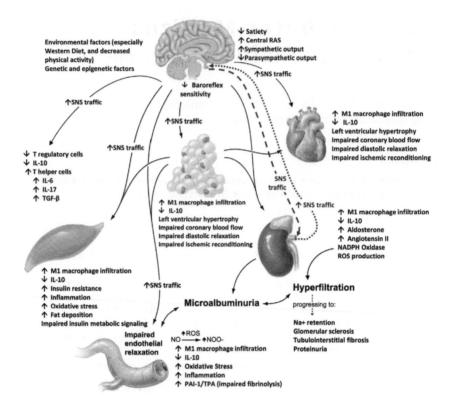

Fig. 1. Systemic and metabolic factors that promote coexistent diabetes mellitus, hypertension, cardiovascular, and chronic kidney disease. IL-10, interleukin 10; NADPH, nicotinamide adenine dinucleotide phosphate oxidase; PAI-1, plasminogen activator inhibitor 1; RAS, renin-angiotensin system; ROS, reactive oxygen species; SNS, sympathetic nervous system; TGF, tumor growth factor; TPA, tissue plasminogen activator. (*Adapted from* Sowers JR. Recent advances in hypertension. Diabetes Mellitus and Vascular Disease. Hypertension 2013;61:94; with permission.)

with both DM and HTN compared with the normotensive nondiabetic controls.[4,5] To this point, a meta-analysis of 102 prospective studies involving 698,782 individuals found that DM is responsible for approximately a 2-fold increased risk for coronary heart disease, stroke, and deaths from cardiovascular cause, including heart failure, cardiac arrhythmia, sudden death, hypertensive disease, and aortic aneurysms.[6] These data suggest that about 10% of vascular deaths in industrialized countries can be attributed to DM, and this burden will further increase as the incidence of diabetes continues to increase.[6] In the Framingham Heart Study, DM was associated with a 2-fold to 4-fold increased risk of myocardial infarction (MI), congestive heart failure, peripheral arterial disease, stroke, and death.[7] Furthermore, a more recent analysis of the Framingham data showed that the population with HTN at the time of DM diagnosis had higher rates of mortality for all causes (32 vs 20 per 1000 person-years; $P<.001$) and cardiovascular events (52 vs 31 per 1000 person-years; $P<.001$) compared with normotensive subjects with DM, thus suggesting that much of this excess risk is attributable to coexistent HTN.[8]

THE BURDEN

The National Health and Nutrition Examination Survey (NHANES) conducted from 2005 through 2008 estimated that HTN affects up to 65 million adults in the United States.[9] Only 50% of hypertensive individuals have their blood pressure (BP) under control.[10] The incidence of HTN is expected to increase further as the population ages and the frequency of obesity increases.[10,11] In a cross-sectional analysis of data from the Study to Help Improve Early Evaluation and Management of Risk Factors Leading to Diabetes (SHIELD) comparing health outcomes between patients with DM, HTN, and obesity relative to those with DM alone, obese patients with both DM and HTN had greater health care resource use, higher incidence of depression, and lower quality of life.[12] Another retrospective study assessed economic trends in patients with newly treated HTN only, DM only, and both newly treated HTN and DM for a period of time up to 24 months. Coexistent HTN and DM were associated with higher costs and resource use.[13] Furthermore, the post hoc analysis of CVD events found that the comorbid cohort had significantly more MIs and acute ischemic events, further increasing the cost of care.[13]

EPIDEMIOLOGY

In nondiabetic individuals, the prevalence of HTN is higher in men than in women until the age of 64 years when the gap closes and prevalence in women reaches that of men.[8] Women with impaired glucose tolerance (IGT) and DM have a higher incidence of HTN than men with equivalent impairment in glucose homeostasis.[14] Diabetic women also have higher relative risk for death from CVD than diabetic men.[15] The reason underlying the excess risk in diabetic women is still unclear. However, the increased risk of HTN in women with abnormal glucose tolerance may partially explain the high risk of CVD in this population.

The prevalence of HTN is different within various ethnic groups. In African Americans, the incidence of HTN is higher compared with white people between the ages of 45 and 75 years, after which it is same in both ethnicities.[16] Several mechanisms have been proposed to explain this finding, including higher rate of obesity, genetic predisposition, and environmental factors.[17] Defects in renal sodium processing have also been observed more frequently in the African American hypertensive populations, who have a greater prevalence of HTN and DM than other ethnic groups, further contributing to increased incidence of HTN.[18] In contrast, a recent analysis of the NHANES 1999 to 2008 data revealed that the Mexican-American populations, who have a high prevalence of DM, have a lower risk of coexistent uncontrolled HTN and DM compared with African Americans and white participants.[19] At present, limited data are available on the incidence of coexistent HTN and DM among Asian people in the United States.

There are several factors that contribute to increased coexistence of DM and HTN. The frequency of obesity in children and adolescents in industrialized countries has increased greatly over the last several decades, with an ominous parallel increment in the incidence of HTN and DM.[2,20] The multicenter Treatment Options for DM in Adolescents and Youth (TODAY) trial, which included 699 adolescents with DM aged 10 to 17 years, revealed that the prevalence of HTN increased from 11.6% at baseline to 33.8% by the end of study. Contrary to the adult data, the incidence of HTN was significantly increased in men versus women during the same period of time.[21]

PATHOPHYSIOLOGY: CONVERGING PATHWAYS IN COEXISTING DM AND HTN

DM and HTN share several pathophysiologic mechanisms including inappropriate activation of the renin-angiotensin-aldosterone system (RAAS), oxidative stress secondary to excessive production of reactive oxygen species (ROS), inflammation, impaired insulin-mediated vasodilatation, increased sympathetic nervous system (SNS) activation, dysfunctional innate and adaptive immune responses, and abnormal renal processing of sodium.[2,3] Obesity and increased visceral adiposity are key pathogenic factors behind the coexistence of both DM and HTN.[3] Chronic low-grade inflammation and oxidative stress in the adipose tissue lead to increased production of angiotensinogen (AGT) and angiotensin II (Ang II) with consequent tissue RAAS activation.[22,23] Further, overexpression of AGT in the white adipose tissue results in increased BP.[22] Hence, AGT and Ang II have local as well as systemic effects on BP regulation.[22,23] Ang II exerts many of its detrimental effects via activation of the Ang II type 1 receptor (AT1R).[24] The activation of AT1R in nonadrenal tissues results in multiple intracellular events, including production of ROS, reduced insulin metabolic signaling, and proliferative and inflammatory vascular responses resulting in endothelial dysfunction, insulin resistance and HTN.[24] Thus, there is often an activated RAAS in coexistent DM and HTN.

Increased aldosterone production and augmented signaling through the mineralocorticoid receptor (MR) are also key events in the pathogenesis of HTN.[25] Corticosteroids may also contribute to CVD in patients with DM via actions mediated in part through activation of the MR.[3] Adipose tissue is known to produce a lipid-soluble factor that stimulates aldosterone production from the adrenal zona glomerulosa.[26,27] Complement-C1q tumor necrosis factor (TNF)–related protein 1 (CTRP1) is a novel adipokine that promotes aldosterone production in a rodent model of obesity and insulin resistance.[28] Aldosterone activation of the MR in the renal distal tubule and collecting duct increases sodium retention leading to expansion of plasma volume and increased BP. In addition, aldosterone exerts nongenomic actions also likely through MR activation, which contribute to HTN by altering cellular redox state, signaling, and endothelial-mediated vascular relaxation.[25,27] Thus, adipose tissue contributes to systemic increases in BP, in part through local production of components of the RAAS.

ROLE OF OXIDATIVE STRESS

Increased oxidative stress is a key pathogenic factor in the development of insulin resistance, DM, and HTN.[29] ROS can be produced in different vascular cell types, including endothelial cells (ECs) and vascular smooth muscle cells (VSMCs) through activation of xanthine oxidase (XO), nitric oxide (NO) synthase, and the mitochondrial respiratory chain.[30–33] In turn, ROS can lead to impaired endothelial function by direct tissue injury, reduction of bioavailable NO, and impaired NO-mediated vasodilation.[30] One important additional source of ROS and endothelial dysfunction is endothelial NO synthase (eNOS) uncoupling. Under conditions of decreased availability of tetrahydrobiopterin (BH4, a cofactor in NO production) or the substrate L-arginine, eNOS switches from this coupled state to an uncoupled state, resulting in production of superoxide (O_2-).[31] Mitochondrial and XO-mediated oxidative stress also contribute to this excess generation of ROS in coexistent DM and HTN.[3] XO is also expressed in vascular endothelial cells and VSMC, and is another source of vascular oxidative stress, which generates O_2- by catalyzing hypoxanthine and xanthine to uric acid.[32] A major source of ROS is the membrane-bound vascular-derived nicotinamide adenine dinucleotide phosphate oxidase (NADPH), a protein enzyme composed of several subunits, including the membrane-bound subunits p22^{phox} and Nox2; the cytosolic regulatory subunits p47^{phox}, p67^{phox}, p40^{phox}; and the small GTP-binding protein Rac1/Rac2.[34] Increased ROS production in turn results in cell as well as tissue damage by activating inflammatory pathways such as nuclear factor kappa B.

Inflammation is characterized by increased activity of adhesion molecules; proinflammatory cytokines, including TNF-α, interleukin (IL)-1 and IL-6, as well as acute-phase reactants such as C-reactive protein and molecules that promote fibrosis and remodeling, such as transforming growth factor beta (TGF-β) and plasminogen activator inhibitor 1 (PAI-1).[35] Mechanical stretch (a characteristic phenomenon in HTN) can lead to membrane translocation and activation of p47[phox] and Rac1, thus leading to NADPH oxidase activation.[32] Ang II and aldosterone can also directly activate NADPH oxidase and trigger oxidative stress.[33]

INSULIN RESISTANCE AND HYPERINSULINEMIA

Insulin resistance plays an important role in the development of both DM and HTN, as shown by approximately 50% of hypertensive patients manifesting systemic insulin resistance.[3,36,37] Binding of insulin to the insulin receptor (IR) triggers 2 major pathways. A metabolic signaling pathway mediated by phosphatidylinositol 3-kinase (PI3K), downstream protein kinase B signaling, results in translocation of glucose transporter 4 (GLUT-4) to plasma membrane, thus resulting in increased insulin-mediated glucose transport in insulin-sensitive tissues such as skeletal muscle.[38] In addition, signaling through the PI3K/Akt pathway results in phosphorylation/activation of eNOS and consequent NO production promotes endothelium-mediated vasodilation.[39] Insulin also signals through the growth/proliferative signaling pathway, which is mediated by mitogen-activated protein kinase (MAPK).[38,40] By activating MAPK-dependent signaling pathways, insulin stimulates secretion of vasoconstrictor mediators, such as endothelin-1,[41,42] as well as increased expression of PAI-1, and vascular cell adhesion molecule-1.[43] In conditions of normal insulin sensitivity, the balance between these vasoconstrictor and vasodilatory actions favors vasodilation. In insulin-resistant states there is often deficient insulin metabolic signaling in concert with unchecked signaling through the growth pathway.[1–3]

Maladaptive hyperinsulinemia/insulin resistance leads to abnormalities in vascular function, vascular stiffness, hypertrophy, fibrosis, and remodeling.[44] Hyperinsulinemia also results in enhanced sympathetic output in humans through ventromedial hypothalamus mechanisms.[45,46] In addition, leptin, which is an adipokine produced in adipose tissue and is increased in obese individuals, also increases sympathetic nerve activation likely through a central nervous system effect involving leptin receptor activation.[47,48] There is increasing evidence that increased afferent traffic from, and efferent activity to, the kidney plays an important role in development of HTN associated with obesity and insulin resistance.[3]

Insulin enhances sodium reabsorption in the diluting segment of the distal nephron, in part through increased expression of sodium transporters like the epithelial sodium channel (ENaC), with consequent decreases in sodium excretion.[49] Hyperinsulinemia-mediated sodium retention could potentially contribute to the genesis of HTN via increased activation of sodium-hydrogen exchanger activity in the proximal tubule as well as through the effects on ENaC more distally. Although this is an attractive hypothesis, in an animal model of knockout of IR in the renal tubule epithelial cells, the absence of insulin action resulted in impaired natriuretic responses and HTN, likely because of reduce NO production.[50] Because of these contradictory results, further studies are needed to clarify the physiologic role of insulin on renal sodium processing.

In addition, sodium and uric acid are generally handled together; hence excess uric acid can increase along with sodium retention, thereby contributing to hyperuricemia, which is frequently seen in hypertensive patients.[51] The propensity for increased uric acid levels is increased with westernized diets that are high in fructose (see **Fig. 1**).[3]

TREATMENT OF HTN: RATIONALE, STRATEGIES, AND CHALLENGES IN HTN
Impact of BP Control

High BP is a strong independent risk factor for CVD and chronic kidney disease (CKD), and, when HTN is associated with DM, the risk is increased even further.[4,52] Although controversy exists regarding the optimal target for BP reduction,[3,52,53] consistent control of BP in patients with DM is important for preventing and delaying both microvascular and macrovascular complications.[54,55] Early data from landmark trials such as the United Kingdom Prospective Diabetes Study (UKPDS), Hypertension Optimal Treatment (HOT), Systolic Hypertension in the Elderly (SHEP), and Systolic Hypertension in Europe (Syst-Eur) showed that strict BP control was beneficial in hypertensive patients with diabetes. In a 9-year follow-up of the UKPDS cohort, patients with both HTN and DM assigned to strict BP control (mean BP, 144/82 mm Hg) achieved a significant reduction in risk for all of the end points related to DM, including death related to DM and microvascular disease, relative to patients who were treated conventionally (mean BP, 154/87 mm Hg).[55] The group allocated to tight BP control had a significant reduction in the risk of heart failure, with an additional nonsignificant reduction in the risk of MI. However, when all macrovascular diseases were combined, including MI, sudden death, stroke, and peripheral vascular disease, the group assigned to tight BP control still had a significant reduction in risk compared with the group assigned to less tight control.[55]

The HOT study revealed that, among the 1501 patients with DM at baseline, a stricter BP control (mean BP, 140/81 mm Hg) halved the risk of major cardiovascular events compared with the control group (mean BP, 144/85 mm Hg).[56] The risk for stroke decreased significantly in individuals who reached the lower target BP. In participants reaching diastolic BP less than 80 mm Hg the risk was reduced roughly 30% relative to individuals who only reached a diastolic BP less than 90 mm Hg. In addition, cardiovascular mortality was also significantly lower in this group (diastolic BP less than 80 mm Hg) than in each of the other target groups. In addition, a nonsignificant decline was seen in the risk for all (MI) in the group with stricter BP control.[56]

In the Syst-Eur trial, 492 patients (10.5%) had DM; after a 2-year follow-up, the active treatment with antihypertensive drugs reduced overall mortality by 55%, mortality from cardiovascular causes by 76%, all cardiovascular events by 69%, fatal and nonfatal stroke by 73%, as well as all cardiac events by 63%.[57] In the SHEP trial, patients with DM randomized to active treatment with antihypertensive medications had lower frequency of stroke, nonfatal MI and fatal coronary heart disease (CHD), major coronary events, and all-cause mortality relative to patients treated with placebo.[58] The Appropriate Blood Pressure Control in Diabetes (ABCD) trial showed a significant decrease in all-cause stroke with intensive (mean BP, 133/78 mm Hg) versus moderate antihypertensive therapy (mean BP, 139/86 mm Hg) in patients with DM.[59] This finding is important because of the increased risk of both fatal and nonfatal stroke in patients with coexistent DM and HTN. In summary, although specific targets are still controversial, control of HTN in the setting of DM is strongly supported by current evidence showing the critical impact that BP has on CVD in diabetic individuals.[52,55,59]

BP Targets

Clinical management guidelines derived from the widely accepted Seventh Report of the Joint National Committee on Prevention, Detection, Evaluation, and Treatment of High Blood Pressure (JNC 7) and the American Diabetes Association (ADA) have recommended strict treatment of HTN in the setting of DM, aiming at values less than 130 mm Hg for systolic BP and less than 80 mm Hg for diastolic BP.[54] Nonetheless, the additional beneficial effects of such lower BP targets remain unproved.[53,60] Hence, the recently revised ADA guidelines suggest that the BP goal for people with DM and HTN should be less than 140/80 mm Hg.[61]

Most guidelines for management of HTN are based on the landmark UKPDS and HOT trials. However, the systolic BP achieved in the tight control arm in these trials was between 140 and 150 mm Hg. Only the intensive BP control groups in the hypertensive and normotensive ABCD studies reached the consensus JNC 7 goal of less than 130/80 mm Hg. The results of the Action to Control Cardiovascular Risk in Diabetes (ACCORD) BP study,[53] recently showed that, in patients with DM, targeting systolic BP to less than 120 mm Hg did not reduce the rate of CV events (nonfatal MI and death from cardiovascular causes), compared with subjects in whom the target was less than 140 mm Hg, except for fatal and nonfatal strokes. As expected, adverse events that were attributed to BP medication were more frequent in the intensive therapy group.[53] Likewise, a post hoc analysis of the International Verapamil SR-Trandolapril (INVEST) study concluded that reducing systolic BP to less than 130 mm Hg in patients with DM and coronary artery disease was not associated with improved CVD outcomes compared with conventional BP control (systolic BP of 130–139 mm Hg).[60]

In another post hoc analysis of the Ongoing Telmisartan Alone and in Combination with Ramipril Global Endpoint Trial (ONTARGET), the relationship between BP and overall cardiovascular risk followed a similar pattern in diabetic and nondiabetic patients. With the exception of stroke, reducing systolic BP to less than 130 mm Hg did not result in improvements in either fatal or nonfatal CVD outcomes.[62] Furthermore, a recent meta-analysis of 13 major trials done in patients with DM or IGT showed that at a systolic BP of less than 130 mm Hg there was only significant reduction in the rate of stroke, with no further reduction in cardiac, renal, or retinal outcomes; however, there was an increased incidence of major adverse events such as hyperkalemia, symptomatic hypotension, bradycardia, and cardiac arrhythmias.[63] An additional concern about strict BP targets is the possible deficiency in blood perfusion to the central nervous system in diabetic patients, who already have microvascular disease and impaired cerebrovascular autoregulation.[64]

The optimal BP goal for diabetic patients should be individualized. Nevertheless, available literature suggests that a maximal benefit of BP control in patients with DM is attained with systolic BP between 130 and 135 mm Hg and diastolic BP from 80 to 85 mm Hg, except in stoke prevention, for which data suggest that further lowering BP may be beneficial.

NONPHARMACOLOGIC TREATMENT: THE ROLE OF THERAPEUTIC LIFESTYLE INTERVENTION

Despite significant advances over the last several decades, the management of HTN is still not ideal, and about 50% of hypertensive patients are still not optimally controlled. The reasons underlying these results seem to be multiple and include deficiencies in current nonpharmacologic and pharmacologic management strategies. One of these issues, access to antihypertensive medications and BP control, was studied in the cross-sectional Reasons for Geographic And Racial Differences in Stroke (REGARDS) cohort study.[65] Although access to antihypertensive medications increased significantly from 66% in 2003 to 81% in 2007, this was not independently associated with improved BP control. African American ethnicity, male sex, low income, and medication nonadherence were significant predictors of inadequate BP control, suggesting that poor BP control is multifactorial.[65]

Nonpharmacologic lifestyle interventions, which include dietary changes, low-salt diet, weight loss, increased physical activity on a regular basis, and alcohol restriction, have been shown to reduce BP in several controlled studies. Lifestyle changes including individualized counseling designed to reduce total intake of fat and intake of saturated fat, and increasing intake of fiber and physical activity, result in significant improvements in BP and reduction in the incidence of DM.[66]

The Dietary Approach to Stop Hypertension (DASH) is a nutritional strategy promoted by the United States National Heart, Lungs and Blood Institute (NHLBI) as a nonpharmacologic intervention to prevent and control HTN. The DASH diet includes foods rich in fruits, vegetables, whole grains, and low-fat dairy products, and low in total fat and saturated fat, cholesterol, refined grains, and sweets, and has been shown to provide beneficial metabolic and cardiovascular effects in DM. Adherence to the DASH diet results in lower systolic as well as diastolic BP, body weight, waist circumference, blood glucose levels, and hemoglobin A1C. It also has beneficial actions on lipid profile, and has been shown to improve high-density lipoprotein cholesterol levels and reduce low-density lipoprotein cholesterol.[67,68]

The beneficial effects of the DASH diet are probably caused by its effect on some cardiovascular risk factors. After following the DASH diet for 8 weeks, liver aminotransferase enzymes, plasma fibrinogen levels, and high-sensitivity C-reactive protein (hs-CRP) were all reduced, suggesting that this type of diet can play an important role in reducing inflammation in DM.[69] In the Lifestyle Changes Through the Use of Delivered Meals and Dietary Counseling in a Single-blind Study (STYLIST), the combination of dietary counseling by dietitians and delivery of calorie-controlled meals was effective in reducing body weight, BP, and hemoglobin A1C in patients with HTN and/or DM.[70]

In addition, sodium intake has also been associated with CVD. Results from multiple trials have shown that reduction of dietary sodium (from a daily intake of 200 mmol [4600 mg] to 100 mmol [2300 mg] of sodium per day) reduces BP and may also reduce long-term risk of cardiovascular events.[71,72] However, results from a recent meta-analysis of 7 randomized controlled trials failed to provide strong evidence that salt reduction reduced all-cause mortality or CVD morbidity in normotensive or hypertensive individuals.[73] The interventions used in this meta-analysis were capable of reducing urinary sodium excretion. Systolic and diastolic BPs were also reduced by an average of 1 mm Hg in normotensives and by an average of 2 to 4 mm Hg in persons with HTN and those with heart failure.[73] However, the methods of achieving salt reduction in the trials included in the review were modest in their impacts on sodium excretion and on BP levels, and would not be expected to have major impacts on the burden of CVD. Sodium restriction has not been tested in the diabetic population in controlled clinical trials. However, in a recent animal study, the results are in favor of oxidative stress normalization as the beneficial influence of dietary sodium deprivation on cardiovascular remodeling in the model of insulin resistance in rats. Withdrawal of sodium from the fructose diet in these rats showed prevention of CVD effects of high fructose consumption, including production of superoxide anions/oxidative stress.[74] In summary, the available literature suggests that reduction of dietary salt reduces BP and may also reduce long-term risk of CVD events in hypertensive patients; however, the data in diabetic individuals are limited. Further, more studies are need to determine whether increasing dietary potassium, calcium, and magnesium may have beneficial effects on BP, CVD, and metabolic control in patients with coexistent DM and HTN.

In addition, physical inactivity is a major underlying risk for CVD. In addition to changing the dietary patterns, increased aerobic physical activity on a regular basis (such as brisk walking) is important in this population. Between 30 and 45 minutes of brisk walking 3 to 5 days a week has been shown to improve lipid profiles, BP, and insulin resistance,[75] and is currently recommended in most management guidelines.[61] Increased physical activity may decrease the rapidity of development of both CVD and CKD events in persons with DM and HTN.

PHARMACOLOGIC THERAPY
RAAS Blockade

Use of Ang II–converting enzyme inhibitors (ACEI) reduces the activity of Ang II, which results in vasodilatation, decreased BP, and improvement in the deleterious effects of Ang II on cardiac, vascular, and renal tissues.[76,77] The Heart Outcomes Prevention Evaluation (HOPE) study compared the effects of the ACE inhibitor ramipril versus placebo on cardiovascular complications and showed 25% risk reduction in MI, stroke, or cardiovascular death after a median follow-up period of 4.5 years.[78] A subgroup of 3577 diabetic patients was analyzed in the microalbuminuria, cardiovascular, and renal outcomes (MICRO)-HOPE study, and showed similar beneficial effects of ramipril on cardiovascular and all-cause mortality in patients with DM.[79]

In contrast with ACEI, Ang II receptor blockers (ARBs) do not increase the levels of bradykinin, which can cause low patient adherence because of induction of cough. In a subset of the Losartan Intervention For Endpoint Reduction in Hypertension (LIFE) study, including 1195 type 2 diabetic patients, a significant reduction in cardiovascular morbidity and mortality was reported in patients treated with losartan compared with individuals taking a β-blocker (atenolol). A relative risk reduction of 24% for the primary composite end point of cardiovascular morbidity and mortality (cardiovascular death, stroke, or MI) was seen in patients treated with losartan compared with atenolol despite similar BP reduction.[80]

In the Antihypertensive Long-Term Use Evaluation (VALUE) and the Candesartan Antihypertensive Survival Evaluation in Japan (CASE-J) trials, cardiac morbidity and mortality were no different in patients treated with ARBs (valsartan and candesartan respectively) relative to patients treated with the long-acting calcium channel blocker (CCB) amlodipine, although they did significantly reduce the incidence of DM.[81,82] In a subgroup analysis of the ONTARGET trial in 6391 patients with DM, telmisartan (ARB) and rampril (ACEI) had similar effects on cardiovascular morbidity and mortality.[83] However, in this study the patients who received combination therapy with ACEI and ARB had an increased risk of adverse side effects including hypotension, syncope, renal dysfunction, and hyperkalemia. The combination-therapy group had a significant increase in the relative risk of impairment of renal function (1.33, $P<.001$). Also the risk of hypotension was higher in the combination group, with a relative risk of 2.75 ($P<.001$). The numbers of patients who had an increase in potassium level of more than 5.5 mmol per liter were similar in the ramipril group (283 patients) and the telmisartan group (287 patients), but the number was significantly higher in the combination-therapy group (480 patients, $P<.001$). Therefore, current literature does not recommend combined treatment with ARB and ACEI.

In addition to cardiovascular protection, available literature shows that RAAS blockade provides renal protective effects. The Bergamo Nephrologic Diabetic complications Trial (BENEDICT) and the Randomized Olmesartan and Diabetes Microalbuminuria Prevention (ROADMAP) trials found that in patients with DM, HTN, and normoalbuminuria (<30 mg/g of creatinine), RAAS blockade with an ACEI and an ARB, respectively, delayed the onset of microalbuminuria (30–300 mg/g).[84,85] Nevertheless, in the Diabetic Retinopathy Candesartan Trial (DIRECT), RAAS blockade failed to show prevention of microalbuminuria in normotensive patients with type 1 or type 2 DM.[86]

There is significant collective evidence to support RAAS blockade as the first line of therapy for HTN in DM to prevent or delay microalbuminuria; however, evidence to sustain their use in normotensive diabetic patients (type 1 or 2) to prevent or delay the development of microalbuminuria is lacking.

In addition, RAAS blockade also has potential benefits beyond BP-lowering effects, including improvements in insulin resistance, inflammation, oxidative stress, and vascular function.[87] In large clinical trials, the Randomized Aldactone Evaluation Study (RALES) and Eplerenone Post–Acute Myocardial Infarction Heart Failure Efficacy and Survival Study (EPHESUS) trials, MR blockade showed improvement in cardiovascular morbidity and mortality.

Improvement in endothelial dysfunction; decreased activation of matrix metalloproteinases; improved ventricular remodeling; along with improvements in tissue fibrosis, inflammation, oxidative stress, and insulin resistance have been postulated as the possible mechanisms responsible for these actions.[87,88]

CCBs

CCBs are an effective and well-tolerated antihypertensive therapy and have been extensively studied. In the Antihypertensive and Lipid-Lowering Treatment to Prevent Heart Attack Trial (ALLHAT), treatment with amlodipine was associated with similar rates of coronary mortality and nonfatal MI to treatment with ACEI (lisinopril) and the diuretic chlorthalidone.[77] However, the heart failure rate was higher in patients treated with CCBs compared with chlorthalidone, which could be in part caused by lower BP attained in the patients treated with the diuretic, or discontinuation of diuretic therapy in the patients in the CCB group.

In diabetic hypertensive patients, some trials have shown that ACEI significantly reduced the risk of CVD compared with CCB,[89,90] whereas another large-scale trial showed no difference.[91] As described earlier, in the VALUE and the CASE-J trials, no significant difference was seen in cardiac composite end points between ARBs and CCBs.[81,92] In the Irbesartan Diabetic Nephropathy Trial (IDNT), this ARB showed better renal protection compared with CCB, but failed to show any difference in reduction in CVD between the two.[93]

In the large diabetic subgroup (5137 patients) in the BP-lowering arm of the Anglo-Scandinavian Cardiac Outcomes Trial (ASCOT), CCB (amlodipine) showed significant reduction in total cardiovascular events compared with β-blocker.[94]

Diuretics

Thiazide-type diuretics have been the basis of antihypertensive therapy for a long time. In the ALLHAT, the diuretic chlorthalidone was e as effective as CCBs and ACEIs in reducing cardiovascular morbidity and mortality.[77] In the Hypertension in the Very Elderly Trial (HYVET), the thiazidelike diuretic indapamide reduced the rate of stroke, CHD, heart failure, and all-cause mortality in very elderly hypertensive patients.[95]

Thiazide diuretics have some significant negative metabolic effects, in particular impaired glycemic control by impairment of insulin secretion and insulin sensitivity.[96,97] They may also worsen insulin sensitivity and glucose tolerance by activation of the RAAS and the SNS, which can be attenuated by addition of MR blocker.[98]

In high doses, diuretics can result in hypokalemia, hypomagnesemia, and/or hyperuricemia, all of which have been shown to worsen glucose control.[96,97] Most of the adverse effects of thiazides are dose dependent; hence using it in low dose combined with other medications helps to avoid metabolic side effects.

Use of other agents, like β-blockers, remains controversial. There is some emerging evidence that β-blockers may be associated with weight gain, which may further worsen glucose tolerance.[96,99] However, in contrast with conventional β-blockers, nebivolol, a selective blocker of β1-adrenergic receptor with NO-potentiating vasodilatory action, has not been associated with weight gain or with worsened glucose tolerance.[99]

β-Blockers are generally not used as first-line agents for HTN in diabetic individuals; however, they are considered as add-on therapy in patients with coronary artery disease and heart failure.[61]

INCRETIN-BASED THERAPY AND HTN: BEYOND GLYCEMIC CONTROL

A better understanding of the role of gut-derived hormones and their impact on carbohydrate homeostasis has been reached over the last decade, which has led to the development of incretin-based therapy. Glucagonlike peptide 1 (GLP-1) and glucose-dependent insulinotropic peptide have been extensively studied in these regards, and are known to potentiate insulin secretion in a glucose-dependent manner in response to the presence of nutrients in the gut (ie, the incretin effect). In addition, incretin hormones slow gastric emptying, thereby slowing the absorption of nutrients in the digestive tract, and suppressing glucagon production in pancreatic alpha cells.[100]

The incretin effect is typically blunted in the setting of DM, and is restored by GLP-1 analogues such as exenatide or liraglutide, as well as inhibitors of the enzyme dipeptidyl peptidase 4 (DPP-4), which rapidly cleaves and inactivates GLP-1. In turn, reduced degradation of GLP-1 by DPP-4 inhibitors results in an enhanced incretin effect. GLP-1 action derives from activation of a highly specific G protein–coupled receptor (GLP-1R), which is expressed in several tissues, including pancreas, nervous system, kidney, cardiovascular tissue, and immune cells.[101]

In the clinical setting, GLP-1 analogues and DPP-4 inhibitors have proved to be efficacious for DM treatment because they contribute to improved beta cell function and glycemic control. In addition, there is mounting interest in the impact of incretin-based therapy on the cardiovascular and renal systems.[102–110]

Both GLP-1 agonists and DPP-4 inhibitors have been shown to modulate BP, heart rate, and contractility. Knockout of GLP-1R in mice results in impaired myocardial contractility and diastolic function.[102] GLP-1 and DPP-4 inhibitors acutely induce increases in BP and heart rate in rodents.[103,104]

In humans, the actions of GLP-1 on BP and heart rate are less clear and experimental results have been more variable. Chronic treatment with GLP-1 analogues in type 2 diabetic patients results in improvements in both systolic and diastolic BP without affecting heart rate.[103,105] In a study by Mistry and colleagues,[106] treatment with the DPP-4 inhibitor sitagliptin similarly produced a modest reduction in BP. In young Zucker obese rats, treatment with linagliptin for 8 weeks resulted in improved diastolic function, left ventricular hypertrophy, and fibrosis. These changes occurred in concert with significant improvements in BP, eNOS, and calcium processing in cardiomyocytes.[107] In the vasculature, DPP-4 inhibition also seems to affect endothelial function. Two weeks of treatment with sitagliptin improved endothelium-dependent relaxation in renal arteries, restored renal blood flow, and reduced systolic BP in spontaneously hypertensive rats (SHRs).[108] In addition, treatment with GLP-1 reduced the size of MI (23.2%–14.1% of area at risk) in rat hearts.[109]

In addition, the impact of incretin-based therapy on BP seems to be also related to activation of GLP-1R in renal tissue, which results in decreased expression of the sodium-hydrogen transporter type 3 (NH3) and leads to increased diuresis and sodium excretion in renal proximal tubules.[110] DPP-4 inhibition results in lower mean BP in young SHRs treated with sitagliptin for 8 days, in concert with increased urinary flow and decreased NH3 expression and activity.[111]

COMBINED PHARMACOLOGIC THERAPY

Although treatment of HTN is often initiated with a single agent, most diabetic patients typically require combination therapy to control their BP. In a randomized, parallel-group, double-blind international trial comparing the once-daily single-pill combination of telmisartan 80 mg and amlodipine 10 mg (telmisartan/amlodipine; T/A) with once-daily amlodipine 10 mg (A) in patients with DM and HTN, T/A provided prompt and greater BP decreases compared with A monotherapy, with most patients achieving the BP goal (<140/90 mm Hg).[112]

The Avoiding Cardiovascular Events Through Combination Therapy in Patients Living With Systolic Hypertension (ACCOMPLISH) trial, which included 6946 patients with diabetes, compared the outcome effects of the ACEI benazepril (20–40 mg/d) combined with amlodipine (5–10 mg/d) (B + A) or hydrochlorothiazide (12.5–25 mg/d; B + H). B + A was superior to the B + H combination, because there was 20% reduction in the primary end point (CV death, stroke, MI, revascularization, hospitalization for unstable angina, or resuscitated cardiac arrest) in the B + A arm compared with the B + H arm ($P = .0002$) despite a similar reduction in BP in both groups. The mean value of BP after the treatment adjustments were 131.5/72.6 mm Hg in the B + A arm and 132.7/73.7 mm Hg in the B + H arm.[113] The study was stopped early because of a difference in outcomes favoring amlodipine. The data from this study are consistent with the ASCOT study,[114] which also showed the cardiovascular benefits of the ACEI/CCB combination.

Fixed-dose combinations in a single tablet may increase compliance compared with corresponding free-drug components given separately, because they simplify treatment and thereby can improve adherence on the part of the patients.[115]

The escalation of double-drug treatment to triple-drug therapy may improve BP control in clinical practice. A subgroup analysis in African Americans and non–African Americans with HTN compared triple-combination treatment with olmesartan 40 mg, amlodipine 10 mg, and hydrochlorothiazide 25 mg with the component dual-combination treatments. Triple-combination treatment resulted in significant and similar mean reductions in diastolic and systolic BP relative to dual-combination treatment. A greater proportion of participants on triple combination reached the target BP compared with dual-combination treatments at the end of 12 weeks regardless of ethnicity.[116] Because HTN and DM generally require multiple antihypertensive agents to achieve a goal BP, triple-combination therapy may represent an important treatment option to improve BP control in this patient population.

PERSPECTIVES
Telehealth

The treatment of HTN remains challenging and demands constant reshaping. Newer strategies are currently being tried for optimal control of HTN in diabetic patients, including the use of remote services like telehealth. Telehealth encompasses the use of medical information exchange remotely via electronic communications to improve a patient's clinical health status. The use of telehealth for transmission of education and advice to the patient on an ongoing basis with close surveillance by nurses and or physicians improves clinical outcomes.[117] A randomized controlled trial conducted at the Iowa City Veterans Affairs Medical Center, evaluated the efficacy of nurse-managed home telehealth intervention to improve outcomes in veterans with comorbid DM and HTN. Intervention subjects experienced a significant decrease in systolic BP compared with the other groups at 6 months and this pattern was maintained at 12 months.[117]

Renal Denervation

Activation of renal sympathetic nerves plays an important role in the pathogenesis of HTN.[118] Renal denervation (RDN) is a percutaneous catheter-based renal sympathetic denervation procedure to disrupt renal afferent and efferent nerves using radiofrequency ablation.[119–121] In a multicenter, prospective, randomized trial (Symplicity HTN-2) evaluating the role of RDN in patients with resistant HTN, office-based BP measurements in the group assigned to the procedure (n = 52) decreased by 32/12 mm Hg (baseline of 178/96 mm Hg; $P<.0001$). This reduction persisted after 6 months.[119] However, the study did not include ambulatory BP monitoring (ABPM) in the analysis, which has been shown to be more closely related to cardiovascular morbidity and mortality than office BP.[122,123]

Another study of 50 patients investigated the effect of RDN on glucose homeostasis and BP control in patients with resistant HTN. Systolic and diastolic BP, fasting glucose, insulin, C peptide, hemoglobin A1c, and insulin sensitivity were measured before, 1 month after, and 3 months after treatment. At 1 and 3 months, office BP was reduced by 28/10 mm Hg ($P<.001$) and 32/12 mm Hg ($P<.001$) respectively in the treatment groups, without changes in concurrent antihypertensive treatment. There were also significant improvements in fasting glucose, insulin, C-peptide levels, and markers of insulin resistance.[120] In a recent multicenter study, RDN showed significant reductions in systolic and diastolic BP, taken both in the office and through 24-h ABPM.[121] In-office systolic and diastolic BP changes were significantly more pronounced than changes in 24-hour continuous measurements. Furthermore, there was no effect on ABPM in pseudoresistant patients, whereas in-office BP was reduced to a similar extent. Thus, RDN may represent an important and novel approach for selective reduction of renal sympathetic drive that results in improvement in both insulin resistance and resistant HTN. This strategy deserves additional clinical research.

ACKNOWLEDGMENTS

The authors wish to thank Brenda Hunter for editorial assistance.

REFERENCES

1. Sowers JR, Epstein M, Frohlich ED. Diabetes, hypertension, and cardiovascular disease: an update. Hypertension 2001;37:1053–9.
2. Sowers JR, Whaley-Connell A, Hayden M. The role of overweight and obesity in the cardiorenal syndrome. Cardiorenal Med 2011;1:5–12.
3. Sowers JR. Diabetes mellitus and vascular disease. Hypertension 2013;61(5): 943–7.
4. Stamler J, Vaccaro O, Neaton JD, et al. Diabetes, other risk factors, and 12-yr cardiovascular mortality for men screened in the Multiple Risk Factor Intervention Trial. Diabetes Care 1993;16:434–44.
5. Hu G, Jousilahti P, Tuomilehto J. Joint effects of history of hypertension at baseline and type 2 diabetes at baseline and during follow-up on the risk of coronary heart disease. Eur Heart J 2007;28:3059–66.

6. Sarwar N, Gao P, Seshasai SR, et al, Emerging Risk Factors Collaboration. Diabetes mellitus, fasting blood glucose concentration, and risk of vascular disease: a collaborative meta-analysis of 102 prospective studies. Lancet 2010; 375:2215–22.

7. Fox CS. Cardiovascular disease risk factors, type 2 diabetes mellitus, and the Framingham Heart Study. Trends Cardiovasc Med 2010;20:90–5.

8. Chen G, McAlister FA, Walker RL, et al. Cardiovascular outcomes in Framingham participants with diabetes: the importance of blood pressure. Hypertension 2011;57:891–7.

9. Egan BM, Zhao Y, Axon RN. US trends in prevalence, awareness, treatment, and control of hypertension, 1988-2008. JAMA 2010;303:2043.

10. Wright JD, Hughes JP, Ostchega Y, et al. Mean systolic and diastolic blood pressure in adults aged 18 and over in the United States, 2001-2008. Natl Health Stat Report 2011;35:1–22, 24.

11. Kaplan NM, Victor RG. Hypertension in the population at large. In: Kaplan NM, Victor RG, editors. Kaplan's clinical hypertension. 10th edition. Philadelphia: Wolter's Kluwer; 2010. p. 1.

12. Green AJ, Bazata DD, Fox KM, et al. Quality of life, depression, and healthcare resource utilization among adults with type 2 diabetes mellitus and concomitant hypertension and obesity: a prospective survey. Cardiol Res Pract 2012. http://dx.doi.org/10.1155/2012/404107.

13. Eaddy MT, Shah M, Lunacsek O, et al. The burden of illness of hypertension and comorbid diabetes. Curr Med Res Opin 2008;24:2501–7.

14. Haffner SM, Valdez R, Morales PA, et al. Greater effect of glycemia on incidence of hypertension in women than in men. Diabetes Care 1992;15:1277–84.

15. Hu G, DECODE Study Group. Gender difference in all-cause and cardiovascular mortality related to hyperglycaemia and newly-diagnosed diabetes. Diabetologia 2003;46:608–17.

16. Carson AP, Howard G, Burke GL, et al. Ethnic differences in hypertension incidence among middle-aged and older adults: the multi-ethnic study of atherosclerosis. Hypertension 2011;57:1101–7.

17. Dyer AR, Liu K, Walsh M, et al. Ten-year incidence of elevated blood pressure and its predictors: the CARDIA Study, Coronary Artery Risk Development in (Young) Adults. J Hum Hypertens 1999;13:13–21.

18. Etkin N, Mahoney J, Forsthoefel M, et al. Racial differences in hypertension-associated red cell sodium permeability. Nature 1982;297:588–9.

19. Liu X, Song P. Is the association of diabetes with uncontrolled blood pressure stronger in Mexican Americans and Blacks than in Whites among diagnosed hypertensive patients? Am J Hypertens 2013. [Epub ahead of print].

20. Ogden CL, Carroll MD, Kit BK, et al. Prevalence of obesity and trends in body mass index among US children and adolescents, 1999-2010. JAMA 2012;307:483–90.

21. TODAY Study Group. Rapid rise in hypertension and nephropathy in youth with type 2 diabetes: the TODAY clinical trial. Diabetes Care 2013;36:1735–41.

22. Massiera F, Bloch-Faure M, Ceiler D, et al. Adipose angiotensinogen is involved in adipose tissue growth and blood pressure regulation. FASEB J 2001;15:2727–9.

23. Boustany CM, Bharadwaj K, Daugherty A, et al. Activation of the systemic and adipose renin-angiotensin system in rats with diet-induced obesity and hypertension. Am J Physiol Regul Integr Comp Physiol 2004;287:R943–9.

24. Mehta PK, Griendling KK. Angiotensin II cell signaling: physiological and pathological effects in the cardiovascular system. Am J Physiol Cell Physiol 2007; 292:C82–97.

25. Williams JS, Williams GH. 50th anniversary of aldosterone. J Clin Endocrinol Metab 2003;88:2364–72.
26. Whaley-Connell A, Johnson MS, Sowers JR. Aldosterone: role in the cardiometabolic syndrome and resistant hypertension. Prog Cardiovasc Dis 2010;52: 401–9.
27. Caprio M, Feve B, Claes A, et al. Pivotal role of the mineralocorticoid receptor in corticosteroid-induced adipogenesis. FASEB J 2007;21:2185–94.
28. Jeon JH, Kim KY, Kim JH, et al. A novel adipokine CTRP1 stimulates aldosterone production. FASEB J 2008;22:1502–11.
29. Cooper SA, Whaley-Connell A, Habibi J, et al. Renin-angiotensin-aldosterone system and oxidative stress in cardiovascular insulin resistance. Am J Physiol Heart Circ Physiol 2007;293:H2009–23.
30. Taniyama Y, Griendling KK. Reactive oxygen species in the vasculature: molecular and cellular mechanisms. Hypertension 2003;42:1075–81.
31. Madamanchi NR, Vendrov A, Runge MS. Oxidative stress and vascular disease. Arterioscler Thromb Vasc Biol 2005;25:29–38.
32. Dröge W. Free radicals in the physiological control of cell function. Physiol Rev 2002;82:47–95.
33. Johar S, Cave AC, Narayanapanicker A, et al. Aldosterone mediates angiotensin II-induced interstitial cardiac fibrosis via a Nox2-containing NADPH oxidase. FASEB J 2006;20:1546–8.
34. Barhoumi T, Kasal DA, Li MW, et al. T regulatory lymphocytes prevent angiotensin II-induced hypertension and vascular injury. Hypertension 2011;57: 469–76.
35. Brown NJ. Aldosterone and vascular inflammation. Hypertension 2008;51: 161–7.
36. Ferrannini E, Buzzigoli G, Bonadonna R, et al. Insulin resistance in essential hypertension. N Engl J Med 1987;317:350–7.
37. Bonora E, Capaldo B, Perin PC, et al. Hyperinsulinemia and insulin resistance are independently associated with plasma lipids, uric acid and blood pressure in non-diabetic subjects. The GISIR database. Nutr Metab Cardiovasc Dis 2008; 18:624–31.
38. Muniyappa R, Quon MJ. Insulin action and insulin resistance in vascular endothelium. Curr Opin Clin Nutr Metab Care 2007;10:523–30.
39. Vincent MA, Montagnani M, Quon MJ. Molecular and physiologic actions of insulin related to production of nitric oxide in vascular endothelium. Curr Diab Rep 2003;3:279–88.
40. Taniguchi CM, Emanuelli B, Kahn CR. Critical nodes in signalling pathways: insights into insulin action. Nat Rev Mol Cell Biol 2006;7:85–96.
41. Potenza MA, Marasciulo FL, Chieppa DM, et al. Insulin resistance in spontaneously hypertensive rats is associated with endothelial dysfunction characterized by imbalance between NO and ET-1 production. Am J Physiol Heart Circ Physiol 2005;289:H813–22.
42. Formoso G, Chen H, Kim JA, et al. Dehydroepiandrosterone mimics acute actions of insulin to stimulate production of both nitric oxide and endothelin 1 via distinct phosphatidylinositol 3-kinase- and mitogen-activated protein kinase-dependent pathways in vascular endothelium. Mol Endocrinol 2006;20: 1153–63.
43. Mukai Y, Wang CY, Rikitake Y, et al. Phosphatidylinositol 3-kinase/protein kinase Akt negatively regulates plasminogen activator inhibitor type-1 expression in vascular endothelial cells. Am J Physiol Heart Circ Physiol 2006;292:H1937–42.

44. Kim J, Montagnani M, Kwaug KK, et al. Reciprocal relationship between insulin resistance and endothelial dysfunction. Circulation 2006;113:1888–904.
45. Heagerty AM, Heerkens EH, Izzard AS. Small artery structure and function in hypertension. J Cell Mol Med 2010;14:1037–43.
46. Anderson EA, Hoffman RP, Balon TW, et al. Hyperinsulinemia produces both sympathetic neural activation and vasodilation in normal humans. J Clin Invest 1991;87:2246–52.
47. Landsberg L. Insulin-mediated sympathetic stimulation: role in the pathogenesis of obesity-related hypertension (or, how insulin affects blood pressure, and why). J Hypertens 2001;19:523–8.
48. Haynes WG, Morgan DA, Walsh SA, et al. Receptor-mediated regional sympathetic nerve activation by leptin. J Clin Invest 1997;100:270–8.
49. Song J, Hu X, Riazi S, et al. Regulation of blood pressure, the epithelial sodium channel (ENaC), and other key renal sodium transporters by chronic insulin infusion in rats. Am J Physiol Renal Physiol 2006;290:F1055–64.
50. Tiwari S, Sharma N, Gill PS, et al. Impaired sodium excretion and increased blood pressure in mice with targeted deletion of renal epithelial insulin receptor. Proc Natl Acad Sci U S A 2008;105:6469–774.
51. Muscelli E, Natali A, Bianchi S, et al. Effect of insulin on renal sodium and uric acid handling in essential hypertension. Am J Hypertens 1996;9:746–52.
52. Garcia-Touza M, Sowers JR. Evidence-based hypertension treatment in patients with diabetes. J Clin Hypertens (Greenwich) 2012;14:97–102.
53. Cushman WC, Evans GW, Byington RP, et al, ACCORD Study Group. Effects of intensive blood-pressure control in type 2 diabetes mellitus. N Engl J Med 2010; 362:1575–85.
54. American Diabetes Association. Standards of medical care in diabetes–2011. Diabetes Care 2011;34:S11–61.
55. UK Prospective Diabetes Study Group. Tight blood pressure control and risk of macrovascular and microvascular complications in type 2 diabetes: UKPDS 38. BMJ 1998;317:703–13.
56. Hansson L, Zanchetti A, Carruthers SG, et al. Effects of intensive blood pressure lowering and low-dose aspirin in patients with hypertension: principal results of the Hypertension Optimal Treatment (HOT) randomised trial. HOT Study Group. Lancet 1998;351:1755–62.
57. Tuomilehto J, Rastenyte D, Birkenhäger WH, et al. Effects of calcium-channel blockade in older patients with diabetes and systolic hypertension. Systolic Hypertension in Europe Trial Investigators. N Engl J Med 1999;340:677–84.
58. Curb JD, Pressel SL, Cutler JA, et al. Effect of diuretic-based antihypertensive treatment on cardiovascular disease risk in older diabetic patients with isolated systolic hypertension. JAMA 1996;276:1886–92.
59. Schrier RW, Estacio RO, Jeffers B. Appropriate blood pressure control in NIDDM (ABCD) trial. Diabetologia 1996;39:1646–54.
60. Cooper-DeHoff RM, Gong Y, Handberg EM, et al. Tight blood pressure control and cardiovascular outcomes among hypertensive patients with diabetes and coronary artery disease. JAMA 2010;304:61–8.
61. American Diabetes Association. Standards of medical care in diabetes-2013. Diabetes Care 2013;36:S11–66.
62. Redon J, Mancia G, Sleight P, et al, ONTARGET Investigators. Safety and efficacy of low blood pressures among patients with diabetes: subgroup analyses from the ONTARGET (Ongoing Telmisartan Alone and in combination with Ramipril Global Endpoint Trial). J Am Coll Cardiol 2012;59:74–83.

63. Bangalore S, Kumar S, Lobach I, et al. Blood pressure targets in subjects with type 2 diabetes mellitus/impaired fasting glucose: observations from traditional and bayesian random-effects meta-analyses of randomized trials. Circulation 2011;123:2799–810.
64. Kim YS, Davis SC, Truijen J, et al. Intensive blood pressure control affects cerebral blood flow in type 2 diabetes mellitus patients. Hypertension 2011;57: 738–45.
65. Cummings DM, Letter AJ, Howard G, et al. Generic medications and blood pressure control in diabetic hypertensive subjects: results from the REasons for Geographic And Racial Differences in Stroke (REGARDS) study. Diabetes Care 2013;36:591–7.
66. Tuomilehto J, Lindström J, Eriksson JG, et al, Finnish Diabetes Prevention Study Group. Prevention of type 2 diabetes mellitus by changes in lifestyle among subjects with impaired glucose tolerance. N Engl J Med 2001;344: 1343–50.
67. Sacks FM, Svetky LP, Vollmer WM, et al. Effects on blood pressure of reduced dietary sodium and the Dietary Approaches to Stop Hypertension (DASH) diet. DASH-Sodium Collaborative Research Group. N Engl J Med 2001;344:3–10.
68. Azadbakht L, Fard NR, Karimi M, et al. Effects of the dietary approaches to stop hypertension (DASH) eating plan on cardiovascular risks among type 2 diabetic patients. Diabetes Care 2011;34:55–7.
69. Azadbakht L, Surkan PJ, Esmaillzadeh A, et al. The dietary approaches to stop hypertension eating plan affects C-reactive protein, coagulation abnormalities, and hepatic function tests among type 2 diabetic patients. J Nutr 2011;141: 1083–8.
70. Noda K, Zhang B, Iwata A, et al, STYLIST Study Investigators. Lifestyle changes through the use of delivered meals and dietary counseling in a single-blind study. The STYLIST study. Circ J 2012;76:1335–44.
71. Cook NR, Cutler JA, Obarzanek E, et al. Long term effects of dietary sodium reduction on cardiovascular disease outcomes: observational follow-up of the trials of hypertension prevention (TOHP). BMJ 2007;334:885–8.
72. Cook NR, Kumanyika SK, Cutler JA. Effect of change in sodium excretion on change in blood pressure corrected for measurement error. The Trials of Hypertension Prevention, Phase I. Am J Epidemiol 1998;148:431–44.
73. Taylor RS, Ashton KE, Moxham T, et al. Reduced dietary salt for the prevention of cardiovascular disease: a meta-analysis of randomized controlled trials (Cochrane Review). Am J Hypertens 2011;24:843–53.
74. Rugale C, Oudot C, Desmetz C, et al. Sodium restriction prevents cardiovascular remodeling associated with insulin-resistance in the rat. Ann Cardiol Angeiol (Paris) 2013;62:139–43.
75. Whelton SP, Chin A, Xin X, et al. Effect of aerobic exercise on blood pressure: a metaanalysis of randomized, controlled trials. Ann Intern Med 2002;136: 493–503.
76. Hansson L, Lindholm LH, Niskanen L, et al. Effect of angiotensin-converting-enzyme inhibition compared with conventional therapy on cardiovascular morbidity and mortality in hypertension: the Captopril Prevention Project (CAPPP) randomized trial. Lancet 1999;353:611–6.
77. ALLHAT Collaborative Research Group. Major outcomes in high-risk hypertensive patients randomized to angiotensin-converting enzyme inhibitor or calcium channel blocker vs diuretic: the Antihypertensive and Lipid-Lowering Treatment to Prevent Heart Attack Trial (ALLHAT). JAMA 2002;288:2981–97.

78. The Heart Outcomes Prevention Evaluation Study Investigators. Effects of an angiotensin-converting-enzyme inhibitor, ramipril, on cardiovascular events in high risk patients. N Engl J Med 2000;342:145–53.

79. Heart Outcomes Prevention Evaluation (HOPE) Study Investigators. Effects of ramipril on cardiovascular and microvascular outcomes in people with diabetes mellitus: results of the HOPE study and MICRO-HOPE substudy. Lancet 2000; 355:253–9.

80. Lindholm LH, Ibsen H, Dahlöf B, et al, LIFE Study Group. Cardiovascular morbidity and mortality in patients with diabetes in the Losartan Intervention For Endpoint reduction in hypertension study (LIFE): a randomised trial against atenolol. Lancet 2002;359:1004–10.

81. Ogihara T, Nakao K, Fukui T, et al, Candesartan Antihypertensive Survival Evaluation in Japan Trial Group. Effects of candesartan compared with amlodipine in hypertensive patients with high cardiovascular risks: Candesartan Antihypertensive Survival Evaluation in Japan Trial. Hypertension 2008;51:393–8.

82. Fretheim A. VALUE: analysis of results. Lancet 2004;364:934–5.

83. Yusuf S, Teo KK, Pogue J, et al, ONTARGET Investigators. Telmisartan, ramipril, or both in patients at high risk for vascular events. N Engl J Med 2008;358: 1547–59.

84. Ruggenenti P, Perna A, Ganeva M, et al. Impact of blood pressure control and angiotensin-converting enzyme inhibitor therapy on new-onset microalbuminuria in type 2 diabetes: a post hoc analysis of the BENEDICT trial. J Am Soc Nephrol 2006;17:3472–81.

85. Haller H, Ito S, Izzo J, et al. Olmesartan for delay or prevention of microalbuminuria in type 2 diabetes. N Engl J Med 2011;364:907–17.

86. Bilous R, Chatuverdi N, Sjolie AK, et al. Effect of candesartan on microalbuminuria and albumin excretion rate in diabetes: three randomized trials. Ann Intern Med 2009;5:11–20.

87. Lastra G, Whaley-Connell A, Manrique C, et al. Low-dose spironolactone reduces reactive oxygen species generation and improves insulin-stimulated glucose transport in skeletal muscle in the TG(mRen2)27 rat. Am J Physiol Endocrinol Metab 2008;295:E110–6.

88. Lastra-Lastra G, Sowers JR, Restrepo-Erazo K, et al. Role of aldosterone and angiotensin II in insulin resistance: an update. Clin Endocrinol 2009;71:1–6.

89. Estacio RO, Jeffers BW, Hiatt WR, et al. The effect of nisoldipine as compared with enalapril on cardiovascular outcomes in patients with non-insulin-dependent diabetes and hypertension. N Engl J Med 1998;338:645–52.

90. Tatti P, Pahor M, Byington RP, et al. Outcome results of the Fosinopril Versus Amlodipine Cardiovascular Events Randomized Trial (FACET) in patients with hypertension and NIDDM. Diabetes Care 1998;21:597–603.

91. Leenen FH, Nwachuku CE, Black HR, et al, Antihypertensive and Lipid-Lowering Treatment to Prevent Heart Attack Trial Collaborative Research Group. Clinical events in high-risk hypertensive patients randomly assigned to calcium channel blocker versus angiotensin-converting enzyme inhibitor in the Antihypertensive and Lipid-lowering Treatment to Prevent Heart Attack trial. Hypertension 2006;48:374–84.

92. Julius S, Kjeldsen SE, Weber M, et al, VALUE Trial Group. Outcomes in hypertensive patients at high cardiovascular risk treated with regimens based on valsartan or amlodipine: the VALUE randomised trial. Lancet 2004;363:2022–31.

93. Berl T, Hunsicker LG, Lewis JB, et al, Irbesartan Diabetic Nephropathy Trial, Collaborative Study Group. Cardiovascular outcomes in the Irbesartan Diabetic

Nephropathy Trial of patients with type 2 diabetes and overt nephropathy. Ann Intern Med 2003;138:542–9.

94. Ostergren J, Poulter NR, Sever PS, et al, ASCOT Investigators. The Anglo-Scandinavian Cardiac Outcomes Trial: blood pressure-lowering limb: effects in patients with type II diabetes. J Hypertens 2008;26:2103–11.

95. Beckett NS, Peters R, Fletcher AE, et al, HYVET Study Group. Treatment of hypertension in patients 80 years of age or older. N Engl J Med 2008;358: 1887–98.

96. Manrique C, Johnson M, Sowers JR. Thiazide diuretics alone or with beta-blockers impair glucose metabolism in hypertensive patients with abdominal obesity. Hypertension 2010;55:15–7.

97. Cooper-DeHoff RM, Wen S, Beitelshees AL, et al. Impact of abdominal obesity on incidence of adverse metabolic effects associated with antihypertensive medications. Hypertension 2010;55:61–8.

98. Raheja P, Price A, Wang Z, et al. Spironolactone prevents chlorthalidone-induced sympathetic activation and insulin resistance in hypertensive patients. Hypertension 2012;60:319–25.

99. Zhou X, Ma L, Habibi J, et al. Nebivolol improves diastolic dysfunction and myocardial remodeling through reductions in oxidative stress in the Zucker obese rat. Hypertension 2010;55:880–8.

100. Campbell JE, Drucker DJ. Pharmacology, physiology, and mechanisms of incretin hormone action. Cell Metab 2013;17:819–37.

101. Thorens B, Porret A, Buhler L, et al. Cloning and functional expression of the human islet GLP-1 receptor: demonstration that exendin-4 is an agonist and exendin-(9–39) an antagonist of the receptor. Diabetes 1993;42:1678–82.

102. Gros R, You X, Baggio LL, et al. Cardiac function in mice lacking the glucagon-like peptide-1 receptor. Endocrinology 2003;144:2242–52.

103. Grieve DJ, Cassidy RS, Green BD. Emerging cardiovascular actions of the incretin hormone glucagon-like peptide-1: potential therapeutic benefits beyond glycaemic control? Br J Pharmacol 2009;157:1340–51.

104. Ussher JR, Drucker DJ. Cardiovascular biology of the incretin system. Endocr Rev 2012;33:187–215.

105. Horton ES, Silberman C, Davis KL, et al. Weight loss, glycemic control, and changes in cardiovascular biomarkers in patients with type 2 diabetes receiving incretin therapies or insulin in a large cohort database. Diabetes Care 2010;33: 1759–65.

106. Mistry GC, Maes AL, Lasseter KC. Effect of sitagliptin, a dipeptidyl peptidase-4 inhibitor, on blood pressure in nondiabetic patients with mild to moderate hypertension. J Clin Pharmacol 2008;48:592–8.

107. Aroor AR, Sowers JR, Bender SB, et al. Dipeptidylpeptidase inhibition is associated with improvement in blood pressure and diastolic function in insulin-resistant male Zucker obese rats. Endocrinology 2013;154:2501–13.

108. Liu L, Liu J, Wong WT, et al. Dipeptidyl peptidase 4 inhibitor sitagliptin protects endothelial function in hypertension through a glucagon-like peptide 1-dependent mechanism. Hypertension 2012;60:833–41.

109. Ossum A, van Deurs U, Engstrøm T, et al. The cardioprotective and inotropic components of the postconditioning effects of GLP-1 and GLP-1(9-36)a in an isolated rat heart. Pharmacol Res 2009;60:411–7.

110. Girardi AC, Fukuda LE, Rossoni LV, et al. Dipeptidyl peptidase IV inhibition downregulates Na+ - H+ exchanger NHE3 in rat renal proximal tubule. Am J Physiol Renal Physiol 2008;294:F414–22.

111. Pacheco BP, Crajoinas RO, Couto GK, et al. Dipeptidyl peptidase IV inhibition attenuates blood pressure rising in young spontaneously hypertensive rats. J Hypertens 2011;29:520–8.
112. Sharma AM, Bakris G, Neutel JM, et al. Single-pill combination of telmisartan/amlodipine versus amlodipine monotherapy in diabetic hypertensive patients: an 8-week randomized, parallel-group, double-blind trial. Clin Ther 2012;34: 537–51.
113. Weber MA, Bakris GL, Jamerson K, et al, ACCOMPLISH Investigators. Cardiovascular events during differing hypertension therapies in patients with diabetes. J Am Coll Cardiol 2010;56:77–85.
114. Dahlof B, Swever PS, Poulter NR, et al, ASCOT Investigators. Prevention of cardiovascular events with an antihypertensive regimen of amlodipine adding perindopril as required versus atenolol adding bendroflumethiazide as required, in the Anglo-Scandinavian Cardiac Outcomes Trial-Blood Pressure Lowering Arm (ASCOT-BPLA); a multicenter randomised controlled trial. Lancet 2005;366: 895–906.
115. Gupta AK, Arshad S, Poulter NR. Compliance, safety, and effectiveness of fixed-dose combinations of antihypertensive agents: a meta-analysis. Hypertension 2010;55:399–407.
116. Chrysant SG, Littlejohn T 3rd, Izzo JL Jr, et al. Triple-combination therapy with olmesartan, amlodipine, and hydrochlorothiazide in black and non-black study participants with hypertension: the TRINITY randomized, double-blind, 12-week, parallel-group study. Am J Cardiovasc Drugs 2012;12:233–43.
117. Wakefield BJ, Holman JE, Ray A, et al. Effectiveness of home telehealth in comorbid diabetes and hypertension: a randomized, controlled trial. Telemed J E Health 2011;17:254–61.
118. Johns EJ, Abdulla MH. Renal nerves in blood pressure regulation. Curr Opin Nephrol Hypertens 2013;22:504–10.
119. Symplicity HTN-2 Investigators, Esler MD, Krum H, et al. Renal sympathetic denervation in patients with treatment-resistant hypertension (The Symplicity HTN-2 Trial): a randomised controlled trial. Lancet 2010;376:1903–9.
120. Mahfoud F, Schlaich M, Kindermann I, et al. Effect of renal sympathetic denervation on glucose metabolism in patients with resistant hypertension: a pilot study. Circulation 2011;123:1940–6.
121. Mahfoud F, Ukena C, Schmieder RE, et al. Ambulatory blood pressure changes after renal sympathetic denervation in patients with resistant hypertension. Circulation 2013;128:132–40.
122. Fagard RH, Celis H, Thijs L, et al. Daytime and nighttime blood pressure as predictors of death and cause-specific cardiovascular events in hypertension. Hypertension 2008;51:55.
123. Pickering TG, Shimbo D, Haas D. Ambulatory blood-pressure monitoring. N Engl J Med 2006;354:2368–74.

Comanagement of Diabetic Kidney Disease by the Primary Care Provider and Nephrologist

Brendan T. Bowman, MD[a], Amanda Kleiner, MD[b],
W. Kline Bolton, MD[a],*

KEYWORDS

- Comanagement • Internist • Collaborative care • Diabetic kidney disease

KEY POINTS

- Diabetic kidney disease (DKD) is a common but complex and multifaceted disorder, and few patients achieve current therapeutic targets described in clinical guidelines.
- A coordinated approach to the care of these patients offers the opportunity to improve patient outcomes.
- Guidelines outlining the specifics of coordinating care for patients with DKD do not currently exist.
- Careful collaboration between all health care providers, particularly primary care physicians, nephrologists, and endocrinologists, and the creation of disorder-specific health care systems, offer the best opportunity for improving the management and clinical outcomes of these patients.

INTRODUCTION

Estimates of chronic kidney disease (CKD) prevalence in the United States vary but suggest upwards of 26 million affected individuals, inclusive of all stages of CKD.[1] Within this population, diabetes mellitus (DM) is both a comorbid condition and a cause of kidney disease.[2–4] True prevalence remains difficult to estimate because a definitive diagnosis of diabetic kidney disease (DKD) requires biopsy[5]; however, of the 26 million Americans diagnosed with some form of DM, 20% to 40% will develop renal involvement according to the American Diabetes Association (ADA).[6] Diabetes

This article originally appeared in Medical Clinics of North America, Volume 97, Issue 1, January 2013.

[a] Division of Nephrology, Department of Medicine, University of Virginia "Health System", Box 800133, Charlottesville, VA 22908, USA; [b] Division of Endocrinology, Department of Medicine, University of Virginia "Health System", Box 801406, Charlottesville, VA 22908, USA
* Corresponding author.
E-mail address: wkb5s@virginia.edu

Clinics Collections 1 (2014) 165–181
http://dx.doi.org/10.1016/j.ccol.2014.08.011

remains the most common cause of incident end stage renal disease (ESRD) according to the United States Renal Data System's (USRDS) Annual Report.[3] For most clinicians, DKD is generally encountered as proteinuria with or without impaired glomerular filtration rate (GFR) in the appropriate clinical setting,[2] although pathologic changes of DM may be present years before clinical signs.[7] Large randomized controlled trials have shown that glycemic control reduces microvascular complications and delays progression of proteinuria[8,9] - important as the risk of ESRD and cardiovascular disease (CVD) increase with progression of proteinuria.[10,11]

Given the significant morbidity and mortality associated with DM, CKD, and ESRD,[3,11] guidelines to assist in diagnosing, stabilizing, and managing DKD have been proposed by various government agencies and professional societies.[2,6,12] CKD alone has been shown to increase mortality but the presence of DM more than doubles mortality, primarily because of CVD.[3]

Although the risks of DKD are better appreciated, evidence suggests that care for CKD and DKD has significant room for improvement.[3,6,13,14] Unfortunately, primary care physicians (PCPs) and nephrologists face increased patient loads and projected workforce shortages, making dedicated time for DKD care difficult to provide.[15,16] These increased demands require PCPs and nephrologists to find more efficient and effective ways to work together.

Proposed primary care delivery models such as accountable care organizations (ACO) and the patient-centered medical home (PCMH) have sought to improve outcomes and reduce costs by integrating the major health care entities (PCPs, hospitals, and specialists) into a single functional entity emphasizing primary care and care coordination.[17–19] Within these models, clear roles and responsibilities of the PCP and specialist have not been assigned. Current practice patterns in DKD management vary widely from the PCP who performs comprehensive care to the physician who refers to the nephrologist for preventive care in any diabetic patient. Regardless of practice styles, evidence exists for the benefits of nephrology involvement in the management of DKD and CKD that persists even after initiation of dialysis.[20–22]

However, barriers to effective collaboration between health care providers exist both in DKD and CKD management. These barriers include low rates of screening, poor recognition of renal disease, late referral for nephrology care, and perceptions of poor communication following referral.[3,23,24] Interventions to address these barriers have been evaluated, but few of these studies take the form of large-scale randomized controlled trials, which is a common problem in renal literature.[25] Most interventions related to collaborative care take the form of improved referral communication, educational interventions, and quality improvement (QI) projects.[26–28] There is no large body of data regarding DKD-specific interventions to improve outcomes, but evaluating the larger body of CKD literature can help inform the topic.

This article discusses areas of weakness in the PCP-nephrology interface, attitudes and perceptions of comanagement, options for attaining euglycemia in DKD, and lastly, proposes a model for DKD care delivery.

SCREENING AND DIAGNOSIS IN DKD

Benefits of early screening and detection in diabetic renal disease derive primarily from early interventions to retard progression of proteinuria and preserve GFR.[8,9,29] In the United States, patients with CKD and diabetes are most often seen by the PCP,[3] making the primary care clinic the logical target of screening and early detection.

Several organizations provide resources for PCPs regarding screening and interpretation of test results. The National Kidney Foundation (NKF) publishes the Kidney

Disease Outcomes Quality Initiative (KDOQI) set of clinical practice guidelines, whereas the ADA separately publishes guidelines for diabetes, including renal disease.[2,6] The NKF also operates the Kidney Early Evaluation Program, which promotes screening for at-risk groups, algorithms for confirmatory testing, and results interpretation.[12] The National Institute of Diabetes and Digestive and Kidney Disease promotes screening and management via the National Kidney Disease Education Program. In addition, annual screening targets have been set for DKD as a Healthy People 2020 goal at a modest 37% of the diabetic Medicare population.[3]

The NKF and ADA both recommend annual screening for GFR and proteinuria with follow-up confirmatory testing.[2,6] Recently, the US Preventive Services Task Force concluded there were insufficient data to support routine screening for CKD but, that recommendation did not address DKD.[30] A 2010 Canadian study by Manns and colleagues[31] evaluated cost-effectiveness of screening for CKD and found benefit specifically in diabetic patients, with an acceptable cost per quality-adjusted life year (QALY) of $C22,600. For reference, an intervention less than $50,000 per QALY is considered reasonable from a public health perspective. A summary of screening recommendations for DKD is presented in **Table 1**.

Despite these recommendations, USRDS data show low rates of annual testing for proteinuria, with creatinine testing performed 3 times more frequently.[3] Given the specificity of urine microalbumin testing to the investigation of renal disease, this may be a better indicator of low DKD screening rates. The USRDS Medicare data set also shows low rates of annual microalbuminuria screening at 37.3%.[3] The likelihood of diabetics receiving the recommended combination of urine protein, creatinine, lipid, and eye screening in a given year is a low 25%.[3]

Although screening rates for DKD remain too low, other studies suggest that, even in the presence of diagnostic laboratory values, DKD may simply be underdiagnosed. In a study by Meyers and colleagues,[23] the investigators reviewed a large electronic medical record (EMR) clinical data base, and approximately 35% of diabetic patients showed renal impairment by estimated GFR (eGFR) criteria (eGFR<60 mL/min/1.73 m^2). Despite this, only 20% of the DKD group was documented as having any stage of CKD. Ryan and colleagues[32] found similar results for patients with CKD in reviewing standardized laboratory data and EMRs from 13 primary care clinics. In the study by Ryan and colleagues,[32] these low rates of diagnosis were reported despite the addition of automated eGFR reporting.

Both studies are limited by their retrospective nature and reliance on diagnosis codes or characteristic actions (ie, nephrology referral) to interpret PCP awareness of renal impairment. A more direct method of assessing PCP recognition of DKD was used by Boulware and colleagues[24] using a national survey of family physicians, internists, and nephrologists. In their study, 304 physicians were presented with a clinical vignette and laboratory data including a progressively worsening creatinine (2.1 mg/dL to 2.3 mg/dL) at the time of initial office visit. The investigators purposely did not provide eGFR but did provide all variables necessary to calculate it. Participants were asked to identify the presence and stage of CKD and to assess the need for referral. Responses showed that 59% of family physicians and 78% of internists were able to accurately categorize the patient as having CKD and to stage appropriately (stage 4) versus 97% of nephrologists. KDOQI guidelines recommend referral to a nephrologist at Stage 4; however, fewer PCPs recommended referral (76% family medicine and 81% internal medicine) compared with 99% of nephrologists. These studies suggest an element of decreased awareness of renal disease in primary care.

Recognizing this problem, others have successfully improved renal disease awareness through a variety of interventions. In the CKD literature, Humphreys and

Table 1
Screening guidelines for DKD from major professional societies

Organization	Year Reviewed	Target Populations	Acceptable Tests	Frequency of Screening
NKF/KDOQI	2007	All patients with type 1 diabetes of at least 5 y duration. All type 2 diabetics at diagnosis	Serum creatinine with eGFR by MDRD, Cockroft-Gault methods. Measurement of albumin/creatinine ratio in a spot urine sample	Annually. Increased albumin/creatinine ratio confirmed twice within following 3–6 mo
ADA	2012	All patients with type 1 diabetes of at least 5 y duration. All type 2 diabetics at diagnosis	Serum creatinine. Test of urine albumin excretion	Annually. Increased albumin/creatinine ratio confirmed twice within following 3–6 mo

Abbreviations: eGFR, estimated GFR; MDRD, modification of diet in renal disease.
Data from Klahr S, Levey AS, Beck GJ, et al. The effects of dietary protein restriction and blood-pressure control on the progression of chronic renal disease. N Engl J Med 1994;330:877–84.

colleagues[33] reported a 31% improvement in CKD identification and 40% improvement in blood pressure target achievement with implementation of a QI project using the Plan-Do-Study-Act methodology. Similar findings were reported by Fox and colleagues[34] implementing a QI and education plan in 2 family practice clinics. In the latter study, a mixed intervention of education and process improvements facilitated by specially trained CKD nurses led to improvements in both diagnosis and medication adjustments. Neither study specifically required a nephrologist.

Kaiser Permanente of Southern California published results from a CKD identification initiative that resulted in a 79% usage rate of CKD diagnosis codes in their prevalent CKD population.[35] This contrasts with the low CKD diagnosis code rate ($\sim$20%) noted in the retrospective chart reviews discussed earlier.[23,32] Here again, most of these patients were never seen by nephrologists, with PCPs performing CKD diagnosis and early stage care.

In the aggregate, these studies suggest that current screening methods may suffer from lack of implementation and, when blood tests alone are used, under-recognition of DKD. Although nephrologists may diagnose DKD more reliably, screening remains most opportunistic in the PCP's office. The United Kingdom and Southern California Kaiser Permanente experiences suggest that dedicated renal disease identification interventions in the primary care office can markedly improve diagnosis.

REFERRAL: OPENING THE DOOR TO COLLABORATION

The benefits of nephrology referral as well as the harms of late referral have previously been described in CKD and DKD literature. A brief list of reported benefits includes reduction in rate of GFR decline, increased use of renin-angiotensin-aldosterone system (RAAS) blockers, and improved mortality.[20–22,36,37] Potential harms of late referral include suboptimal management of mineral bone disorders and anemia, higher rates of dialysis catheter use versus fistulas when initiating renal replacement therapy (RRT), and increased mortality both overall and in the first year of dialysis.[21,38] The KDOQI and ADA recommendations for referral[2,6] are listed in **Table 2**.

Definitions of late referral vary among studies but generally imply a rapid initiation of RRT following referral (<1–4 months) without adequate time to counsel patients on options for ESRD care (including transplantation) or to obtain a fistula if possible, or

Table 2 Summary of indications for nephrology referral related to DKD from KDOQI and ADA guidelines		
Organization	**Year Published**	**Excerpts of Referral Guidelines/Recommendations in DKD/CKD**
NKF/KDOQI	2007	Patients with CKD should be referred to a specialist for consultation and comanagement if the clinical action plan cannot be prepared, the prescribed evaluation of the patient cannot be carried out, or the recommended treatment cannot be carried out. In general, patients with GFR <30 mL/min/1.73 m^2 should be referred to a nephrologist
ADA	2012	GFR 45–60 mL/min/1.73 m^2: referral to nephrology if possibility for non-DKD exists (duration type 1 diabetes <10 y, heavy proteinuria, abnormal findings on renal ultrasound, resistant hypertension, rapid decrease in GFR, or active urinary sediment on ultrasound) GFR <30 mL/min/1.73 m^2: referral to nephrologist

otherwise a graft. The prevalence of late referrals varies by study and definition, but is commonly reported to be between 20% and 40% in the CKD population.[38,39]

Perhaps the largest study of referral patterns and outcomes of patients with diabetes and CKD was performed by Tseng and colleagues,[22] and involved a retrospective review of more than 39,000 Veterans Administration (VA) patients. In that study, the investigators found a mortality benefit proportional to the frequency of nephrology follow-up in patients with stage 3 and 4 kidney disease. In another study, Martinez-Ramirez and colleagues[20] performed one of the few prospective evaluations of referral benefit in patients with CKD and DM. The investigators assigned patients with DM and proteinuria to early nephrology referral, and compared outcomes with a cohort of patients remaining under their family physician's care. Within cohorts, patients were categorized by degree of proteinuria and followed for 1 year. At the conclusion, nephrology care was associated with stable GFR in the study group versus loss in controls, better blood pressure control, increased use of RAAS blocking agents, and decreased nonsteroidal antiinflammatory medication use.

In addition to GFR preservation, the study group also saw decreased progression of proteinuria, with the microalbuminuric group showing the greatest benefit.

Causes of late referral vary, from the patient with rapid decline in GFR making timely referral impossible, to those with insidious disease recognized late in their course. Fischer and colleagues[40] proposed 3 broad causative categories for late referral: patient factors, PCP factors, and health care system factors. PCP-related factors include poor renal disease recognition and lack of screening. Health care system–related factors include fragmented care organizations (part VA, part Medicare, for example) and lack of access to nephrology care. Patient-related factors include older age (>75 years), lack of health insurance, undiagnosed rapid progression of CKD, and poor compliance. A systematic review of late referral causes by Naveneethan and colleagues[41] used a similar system and added poor communication between PCPs and nephrologists to this list.

Boulware and colleagues[24] further explored PCP-nephrologist referral perceptions, surveying both groups regarding comfort with general KDOQI guidelines, ideal referral timing, and desired information from referral. Forty-seven percent of family practitioners and 31% of internists reported difficulty in referring patients at least "a little of the time", and 52% and 29%, respectively, of family practice and internal medicine physicians cited difficulty referring because of lack of local nephrologists. Only a small percentage (<10% in both groups) noted concern that a nephrologist may want to completely take over the patient's care. The investigators found that PCPs electing to refer were more likely to be recent graduates (in practice <10 years) and to self-identify as being familiar with CKD guidelines.

Age may also play a factor as referral rates in CKD are generally lower in the elderly, although not all studies have found this.[39,41,42] Campbell and colleagues[42] reviewed referral decision making by PCPs in the elderly using a clinical vignette and survey. PCP referral decisions were influenced not only by CKD stage but also comorbidities and cognitive abilities, suggesting nuanced referral decisions. This finding suggests the lower rates of elderly CKD referral may be appropriate.

Few studies have evaluated interventions to improve referral in DKD specifically. One study by Stoves and colleagues[26] in the United Kingdom used an e-consult to increase access to and facilitate communication with nephrologists. This study involved electronic review of referrals and patient records by nephrologists followed by electronically communicated recommendations to general practitioners (GPs) through an automated e-consult. This e-consult allowed GPs and nephrologists to determine the necessity of a full clinic visit referral versus providing focused guidance to the GP.

Although this intervention reduced total referrals, the appropriateness of referrals was improved in a collaborative manner.

Despite evidence of improved outcomes in DKD with early referral, 20% to 40% of patients initiating dialysis are referred late, with subsequently increased mortality that persists into the period of RRT. Factors specific to patients, health care systems, and providers contribute to this problem. Difficulties in providing access to nephrology care, both real and perceived, are a barrier to referral. Interventions allowing virtual access to nephrology care and educating PCPs on recognition may improve the quality and timeliness of DKD referrals. Allowing PCPs and nephrologists to communicate before referral to determine appropriate referrals may be helpful in reducing rates of unnecessary referrals.

ATTITUDES TOWARD COLLABORATIVE CARE

To our knowledge, the attitudes and expectations of PCPs and nephrologists regarding comanagement of DKD have not been studied. There is no body of literature describing how PCPs and nephrologists divide clinical responsibilities (dietary counseling, prescriptions, lipid management, glycemic control) in day-to-day practice. These matters remain at the discretion of individual providers and are functions of practice patterns and interrelationships. Although there are few DKD-specific data, there are survey data regarding referral in general and CKD comanagement between PCPs and specialists.

In 2000, Gandhi and colleagues[43] performed an electronic survey of PCPs and specialists to determine satisfaction with their current referral and information sharing. Large percentages of both groups were dissatisfied with the information received from the other (28% of PCPs and 43% of specialists). Nearly half of both groups were dissatisfied with the timeliness of communication, suggesting a need for improvement in communication between colleagues.

Specific to CKD, Boulware and colleagues[24] and Diamantidis and colleagues[44] both reported attitudes toward collaboration between PCPs and nephrologists using a stage 4 CKD vignette. The investigators surveyed both groups' preferences in referral communication, frequency of specialist input, transition of primary care activities, and types of information sought. PCPs most often preferred periodic input (every 4–6 months). Most clinicians in both the PCP and nephrology groups agreed on communication regarding confirmation of diagnosis and evaluation, performance of additional testing and evaluation, nutritional advice, and medication regimen advice. Nephrologists were more likely than PCPs to prioritize information related to preparation for RRT and electrolyte disorders.

Regarding longitudinal care, PCPs and nephrologists overwhelmingly preferred the PCP to remain the primary caregiver, which suggests that neither group desires nephrology to "take over" the CKD patients primary care.

In summary, it seems that PCPs and specialists both note problematic communication, with lack of timely reporting and necessary content missing. When PCPs and nephrologists are surveyed, both groups prefer collaboration in which the PCP remains the main caregiver. However, the groups diverge on the timing and importance of CKD complications such as mineral bone disorders, anemia, and preparation for RRT.

DKD CARE DELIVERY MODEL

DKD is a multifaceted entity affecting many organ systems with increased risk for CVD and subsequent mortality, particularly in patients with advanced GFR loss and macroalbuminuria.[10,11] Because of the number of health care professionals involved, and also because the multiple areas of management overlap, there is no definitive model of comanagement in general use. The ADA officially endorses use of the 6-component Chronic Disease Model (CDM) for DM care; however, the data for use of this model are unproven in kidney disease care.[45] Although further studies of structured interventions are needed, based on current published literature, surveys, and data from CKD and DM, a model of DKD care should consist of at least the following elements:

- Clearly delineated areas of clinical practice agreed on between all providers in advance
- An effective outcomes measurement system and QI strategy
- Integration of multidisciplinary teams with multifactorial interventions
- Effective communication strategy using a shared EMR with access to a fully functional patient chart

In primary care, 2 recent models of care have been promoted heavily: the ACO and PCMH. Both seek to improve patient outcome through emphasizing primary care, improved coordination, and quality metric tracking.[17,18] Both also provide an emphasis on integrated care to maximize the benefits of the PCP-specialist management of comorbidities. The elements of a DKD care model listed earlier can be integrated into these frameworks and differ from the traditional model of 2 to 3 providers that is common at present. **Fig. 1** depicts a traditional 3-provider model with PCP, nephrologist, and endocrinologist. **Fig. 2** depicts the elements of an idealized DKD care delivery model. As shown in the figure, providers, patient, and multidisciplinary team are able to interact through an EMR, and the primacy of the patient-PCP relationship remains intact through an entity such as the PCMH. An integrated QI methodology such as the Plan-Do-Study-Act cycle is embraced by all providers.

ELEMENTS OF THE DKD CARE DELIVERY MODEL

Clear definitions of clinical areas and responsibilities are essential to eliminate overlap and avoid duplicate effort in DKD care. Although all providers have different practice patterns and preferences, the previously discussed survey data suggest that most PCPs and nephrologists have broadly similar views on frequency of referral, information of value expected from referral, and the patient's appropriate medical home.[24,44] Reviewing these surveys suggests that most PCPs prefer nephrology input periodically and would prefer that most health care remain with the PCP. These preferences

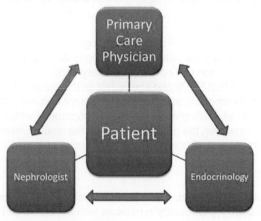

Fig. 1. Traditional model of care for DKD.

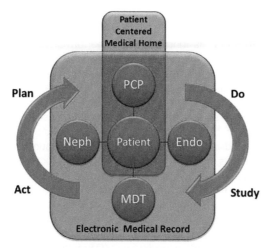

Fig. 2. Proposed model using the PCMH as the primary care entity, with the Plan-Do-Study-Act (PDSA) cycle for QI overlying the EMR as a communication vehicle between providers. The multidisciplinary team (MDT) may be a stand-alone entity, part of a PCMH/ACO or a component of the PCP/specialist practice. The PCMH model is chosen here for example only. ACO structure could be substituted depending on the clinical needs. Many iterative QI programs are acceptable, and the PDSA cycle is selected for example purposes only. Endo, endocrinologist; Neph, nephrologist; PCP, primary care physician.

exclude management of those conditions unique to kidney disease, such as mineral bone disorders (secondary hyperparathyroidism, hyperphosphatemia, and so forth), anemia of CKD, and preparation for RRT. Using survey data regarding preferred roles by the clinicians, a responsibility matrix can be built to assign areas of management to providers. **Fig. 3** suggests how those roles may transition based on progression of

Clinical Focus Areas	Stage 3			Stage 4			Stage 5		
	PCP	Nephro	Endo	PCP	Nephro	Endo	PCP	Nephro	Endo
Health Maint	+			+			+		
DM Mgt	+		+	+		+	+		+
HTN Mgt.	+				+			+	
Lipid Mgt	+			+			+		
Diet & Lifestyle	+	+	+	+	+	+	+	+	+
MBD	+	+			+			+	
Anemia of CKD	+	+			+			+	

Fig. 3. Areas of focus for PCP, nephrologist, and endocrinologist with progression of DKD following development of stage 3 CKD. HTN, hypertension; MBD, mineral bone disorders; Mgt, management; Nephro, nephrologist.

underlying renal disease. These are only suggested role assignments and providers should customize these roles to the individual provider's strengths, weaknesses, and preferences.[46] In short, as long as clinical performance measures (CPMs) are monitored and achieved, it is unimportant which provider assumes a specific role.

Given the overall need for improvement in achieving clinical targets in the care of DKD,[6,13,14] a continuous QI process should be an integral part of a DKD care delivery model. Evaluation and review cycles such as the Plan-Do-Study-Act cycle have been proposed by entities such as the Agency for Healthcare Research and Quality in the care of chronic disease.[47,48] These methods have been used successfully to improve performance in areas as diverse as attainment of blood pressure targets and improvement in quality of referrals.[26,33] The Renal Physicians Association (RPA) provides a CKD toolkit with suggested CPMs that can be applied to DKD to ensure high-quality care delivery.[49] Given the number of health care professionals engaged in DKD management, more potential process flow bottlenecks and breakdowns are possible, necessitating that a QI methodology be integrated into the care model. These concepts are also embraced in the ACO and PCMH models.

A third component of an effective model for DKD would be integration of a multidisciplinary team (MDT). MDTs are groups of care providers, usually physician led, tasked with improving outcomes through multifactorial interventions (diet, lifestyle, social services). Teams typically include a dietician/nutritionist, clinical pharmacist, social worker, nurse practitioners, physician assistant, and specially trained nursing staff.[50–53] MDTs have been studied in diabetes care and are now included specifically in ADA guidelines.[6,54,55] Team-based care was recently the subject of an Institute of Medicine work group, suggesting the high value of team-based care as a permanent change to the way health care is delivered in the United States.[56]

The effect of MDTs on patients has been best evaluated in CKD, but some studies address DKD specifically. One prospective multicenter 2-year study of a structured care intervention using nurse educators, endocrinologists, and pharmacists in Hong Kong showed improved attainment of glycosylated hemoglobin and blood pressure targets. Patients in the structured care group were also more likely to meet treatment targets, which conveyed a 60% relative risk reduction in reaching ESRD compared with the usual care group.[57] Studies in CKD, on balance, favor the MDT approach.[58–60] For example, a study by Thanamayooran and colleagues[61] showed improved adherence to clinical targets such as blood pressure goals and glycosylated hemoglobin. Wu and colleagues[60] in Taiwan prospectively studied 2 cohorts, 1 assigned to usual care, the other to a structured MDT intervention, and were able to show decreased progression to dialysis and decreased mortality in the intervention group. Hemmelgarn and colleagues[58] retrospectively evaluated elderly patients exposed to MDT and also showed mortality benefit compared with matched controls.

The driver for the effect of MDTs on CKD outcomes is difficult to assess. By nature, these are multifactorial interventions and controlling for each individual intervention is difficult. Nonetheless, the existing data from CKD and DM studies generally show improved achievement of clinical targets, decreased incidence of ESRD, and improved mortality.

The final component of a DKD care delivery model is effective communication between PCPs and specialists. However, both groups perceive important shortfalls in timely, complete, and accurate communication, as shown in provider surveys.[43] Many studies have used EMR systems to improve communication between specialists and PCPs. Stoves and colleagues[26] showed the value of the e-consultation in improving appropriate referrals and reducing total volume of referrals overall using an EMR. Kim-Hwang and colleagues[62] similarly described implementation of an e-referral system resulting in improved clarity of referral reason, reduction of inappropriate referrals, and reduced unnecessary follow-up visits.

Other elements of EMRs suggest promise for improved outcomes but study data are limited or mixed. Chang and colleagues[63] recently reviewed available literature on the use of computerized provider order entry (CPOE) and clinical decision support systems (CDSS) in acute kidney injury and CKD care but this mostly excluded office-based chronic care. A small randomized trial of CDSS for CKD care in a primary clinic noted no clear benefit but was limited in size and duration.[64] A larger 2008 study using a multifactorial intervention of education, practice enhancement assistants, and CDSS to manage CKD in a primary care setting showed improved diagnosis of CKD, but the driver of the improvements was unclear.[34] To our knowledge, data specific to DKD outcomes related to use of CPOE or CDSS have not been separately studied. Supporting data for diabetes care alone using EMRs and CDSSs is more robust but also mixed.[65] We think that, although CPOE and CDSS hold promise, more studies are needed to support the inclusion of these technologies in routine DKD care.

SPECIAL CONSIDERATIONS IN DKD: THE ROLE OF GLYCEMIC CONTROL

Hyperglycemia is the principal metabolic defect occurring in both type 1 and type 2 DM, and euglycemia remains the central management goal.[6] Multiple large, multi-center, randomized controlled trials consistently show the role of glycemic control in reducing the risk of DKD.[8,66,67] It remains controversial whether tight glycemic control prevents the progression of existing microalbuminuria to macroalbuminuria in diabetic patients, with the Kumamoto Study[68] showing a protective effect of tight glycemic control in type 2 DM, whereas the Diabetes Control and Complication Trial (DCCT) was underpowered to show a similar effect in type 1 DM.[8] However, prolonged euglycemia can slow the rate of progression in renal injury, even in the presence of known DKD,[69] and guidelines support tight glycemic targets in this group.[6,70,71]

Glycemic control should be a focus in the prevention and management of DKD,[71] but achieving this remains an elusive goal.[72] Most glycemic management for diabetic patients is provided by PCPs working independently, yet few have the resources and support necessary to achieve the glycemic control required to prevent complications of diabetes.[73]

There are several challenges to achieving glycemic control and only a minority of patients achieve these targets.[74] The reasons for this are multifactorial and include patient factors, such as medication nonadherence, health care costs, poor attention to diet, and difficulty with blood glucose self-monitoring,[75,76] and physician factors, such as lack of time for counseling, inadequate education and experience, and clinical inertia.[77,78] Compounding these challenges is the complexity of modifying medication regimens in the presence of underlying renal disease.

Given the complexity of glycemic management in patients with DKD, the ADA recommends all such patients be referred to an endocrinologist.[6] There is evidence showing the benefits of the role of the endocrinologist on glycemic control, either directly, through a traditional referral program, or indirectly, though creation of treatment protocols, supervision and education of other providers, or the creation of specialist diabetes clinics[79–82] Hardy and colleagues[83] showed improvement in DKD-specific end points, such as decline in the rate of decrease in GFR, in an endocrinologist-supervised diabetes nephropathy clinic. The investigators used protocols for the monitoring and management of DKD care, including glycosylated hemoglobin, lipid, and blood pressure targets, patient education, and dietary counseling. All protocols were created in conjunction with an affiliated nephrologist, with whom the care of all patients with advanced DKD was collaboratively managed. Fundamental to the success of this model was the delineation of clinical responsibility, as well as the communication of clear guidelines for the ongoing management of patients by PCPs.

SPECIAL CONSIDERATIONS IN DKD: RENAL DISEASE AND EUGLYCEMIA

The achievement of glycemic control in patients with CKD in general, and DKD in particular, is made more challenging by the pathologic impairments in the production and handling of carbohydrates and insulin that accompany these diseases.

The kidney is a major site of intrinsic glucose production in the fasting state, accounting for approximately 25% of gluconeogenesis.[84] This capacity of the kidney to accomplish gluconeogenesis is impaired with progression of CKD, at a rate that varies between individuals. In addition, the kidneys are the major site of removal and inactivation of circulating insulin, via glomerular filtration, and the intracellular degradation of insulin through a variety of intracellular processes and the action of insulinase.[85,86] The ability of the kidney to remove and inactivate insulin is impaired in CKD, and the resulting reduction in insulin metabolism and clearance induces a prolonged duration of insulin action.

Countering this process is evidence that tissue resistance to insulin is present at all stages of renal impairment, even before a measurable decrease in GFR.[87] This increase in insulin resistance is further compounded by the effect of hyperparathyroidism, low levels of calcitriol, and anemia on pancreatic islet cells and glucose tolerance in CKD.[88,89]

It has long been reported that severe DKD can result in cures of diabetes, or even episodes of spontaneous hypoglycemia.[90] These findings reflect the complex interaction of reduced caloric intake, progressive weight loss, intermittent acidosis, impaired gluconeogenesis, and reduced drug and insulin metabolism that can occur in ESRD. The balance between these processes is variable among individuals, and can translate into a challenging clinical scenario for any single provider. The complexity of disease in DKD alone suggests a need for close collaboration between the PCP, endocrinologist, and nephrologist.

SUMMARY

DKD is a complex and multifaceted disease. A substantial portion of patients remain unable to attain clinical targets for glycosylated hemoglobin, lipids, and blood pressure.[3,14] Improving outcomes requires multifactorial interventions that are best delivered through collaborative care.

Targets for improvement should include screening, diagnosis, and early referral. Following referral, the patient should be cared for in an integrated framework using the 4 elements of an effective DKD care delivery model: clear roles and responsibilities, integrated QI programs, MDT approach, and effective communication facilitated through access to a shared EMR.

Given the differences in the pathophysiology of DM in the renal population, a nephrologist and endocrinologist can be invaluable in improving care for this population. Large-scale trials are needed to validate the cost and usefulness of collaborative care as current data are insufficient. Based on available data, models such as the one proposed here should serve to maximize the strengths of individual providers and provide improved quality of care to patients.

REFERENCES

1. Castro AF, Coresh J. CKD surveillance using laboratory data from the population-based National Health and Nutrition Examination Survey (NHANES). Am J Kidney Dis 2009;53(3 Suppl 3):S46–55.
2. KDOQI clinical practice guidelines and clinical practice recommendations for diabetes and chronic kidney disease. Am J Kidney Dis 2007;49(2 Suppl 2): S12–154.
3. Collins AJ, Foley RN, Chavers B, et al. United States Renal Data System 2011 Annual Data Report: atlas of chronic kidney disease & end-stage renal disease in the United States. Am J Kidney Dis 2012;59(1 Suppl 1):A7 e1–420.
4. Lou Arnal LM, Campos GB, Cuberes IM, et al. Prevalence of chronic kidney disease in patients with type 2 diabetes mellitus treated in primary care. Nefrologia 2010;30(5):552–6 [in Spanish].
5. Olsen S, Mogensen CE. How often is NIDDM complicated with non-diabetic renal disease? An analysis of renal biopsies and the literature. Diabetologia 1996;39(12):1638–45.
6. American Diabetes Association. Standards of medical care in diabetes - 2012. Diabetes Care 2012;35(Suppl 1):S11–63.
7. Najafian B, Mauer M. Progression of diabetic nephropathy in type 1 diabetic patients. Diabetes Res Clin Pract 2009;83:1–8.
8. The Diabetes Control and Complications Trial Research Group. The effect of intensive treatment of diabetes on the development and progression of long-term complications in insulin-dependent diabetes mellitus. N Engl J Med 1993;329:977–86.
9. Effect of intensive blood-glucose control with metformin on complications in overweight patients with type 2 diabetes (UKPDS 34). UK Prospective Diabetes Study (UKPDS) Group. Lancet 1998;352(9131):854–65.
10. Yokoyama H, Araki S, Haneda M, et al. Chronic kidney disease categories and renal-cardiovascular outcomes in type 2 diabetes without prevalent cardiovascular disease: a prospective cohort study (JDDM25). Diabetologia 2012;55(7):1911–8.
11. Go A, Chertow GM, Fan D, et al. Chronic kidney disease and the risks of death, cardiovascular events, and hospitalization. N Engl J Med 2004;351:1296–305.
12. Evaluate Patients with CKD. National Institutes of Health 2012. Available at: http://nkdep.nih.gov/identify-manage/evaluate-patients.shtml. Accessed on September 13th, 2012.
13. Owen WF Jr. Patterns of care for patients with chronic kidney disease in the United States: dying for improvement. J Am Soc Nephrol 2003;14(7 Suppl 2): S76–80.
14. Snyder JJ, Collins AJ. KDOQI hypertension, dyslipidemia, and diabetes care guidelines and current care patterns in the United States CKD population: National Health and Nutrition Examination Survey 1999-2004. Am J Nephrol 2009; 30(1):44–54.
15. Kohan DE, Rosenberg ME. The chronic kidney disease epidemic: a challenge for nephrology training programs. Semin Nephrol 2009;29(5):539–47.
16. The impact of health care reform on the future supply and demand for physicians updated projections through 2025. 2012. Ref Type: Online Source.
17. Accountable Care Organizations (ACO). 4-5-0012. Centers for Medicare & Medicaid Services. Ref Type: Online Source.
18. Understanding the patient-centered medical home. 2012. American College of Physicians. Ref Type: Online Source.

19. DuBose TD Jr, Behrens MT, Berns A, et al. The patient-centered medical home and nephrology. J Am Soc Nephrol 2009;20(4):681–2.
20. Martinez-Ramirez HR, Jalomo-Martinez B, Cortes-Sanabria L, et al. Renal function preservation in type 2 diabetes mellitus patients with early nephropathy: a comparative prospective cohort study between primary health care doctors and a nephrologist. Am J Kidney Dis 2006;47(1):78–87.
21. Khan SS, Xue JL, Kazmi WH, et al. Does predialysis nephrology care influence patient survival after the initiation of dialysis? Kidney Int 2005;67(3):1038–46.
22. Tseng CL, Kern EF, Miller DR, et al. Survival benefit of nephrologic care in patients with diabetes mellitus and chronic kidney disease. Arch Intern Med 2008;168(1):55–62.
23. Meyers JL, Candrilli SD, Kovacs B. Type 2 diabetes mellitus and renal impairment in a large outpatient electronic medical records database: rates of diagnosis and antihyperglycemic medication dose adjustment. Postgrad Med 2011;123(3):133–43.
24. Boulware L, Troll M, Jaar B, et al. Identification and referral of patients with progressive CKD: a national study. Am J Kidney Dis 2006;48(2):192–204.
25. Strippoli GF, Craig JC, Schena FP. The number, quality, and coverage of randomized controlled trials in nephrology. J Am Soc Nephrol 2004;15(2):411–9.
26. Stoves J, Connolly J, Cheung CK, et al. Electronic consultation as an alternative to hospital referral for patients with chronic kidney disease: a novel application for networked electronic health records to improve the accessibility and efficiency of healthcare. Qual Saf Health Care 2010;19(5):e54.
27. Cortes-Sanabria L, Cabrera-Pivaral CE, Cueto-Manzano AM, et al. Improving care of patients with diabetes and CKD: a pilot study for a cluster-randomized trial. Am J Kidney Dis 2008;51(5):777–88.
28. Rayner HC, Hollingworth L, Higgins R, et al. Systematic kidney disease management in a population with diabetes mellitus: turning the tide of kidney failure. BMJ Qual Saf 2011;20(10):903–10.
29. de Boer IH, Sun W, Cleary PA, et al. Intensive diabetes therapy and glomerular filtration rate in type 1 diabetes. N Engl J Med 2011;365(25):2366–76.
30. Moyer VA. Screening for chronic kidney disease: U.S. Preventive Services Task Force Recommendation Statement. Ann Intern Med 2012;157(8):567–70.
31. Manns B, Hemmelgarn B, Tonelli M, et al. Population based screening for chronic kidney disease: cost effectiveness study. BMJ 2010;341:c5869.
32. Ryan TP, Sloand JA, Winters PC, et al. Chronic kidney disease prevalence and rate of diagnosis. Am J Med 2007;120(11):981–6.
33. Humphreys J, Harvey G, Coleiro M, et al. A collaborative project to improve identification and management of patients with chronic kidney disease in a primary care setting in Greater Manchester. BMJ Qual Saf 2012;21(8):700–8.
34. Fox CH, Swanson A, Kahn LS, et al. Improving chronic kidney disease care in primary care practices: an Upstate New York Practice-based Research Network (UNYNET) study. J Am Board Fam Med 2008;21(6):522–30.
35. Rutkowski M, Mann W, Derose S, et al. Implementing KDOQI CKD definition and staging guidelines in Southern California Kaiser Permanente. Am J Kidney Dis 2009;53(3 Suppl 3):S86–99.
36. Campbell GA, Bolton WK. Referral and comanagement of the patient with CKD. Adv Chronic Kidney Dis 2011;18(6):420–7.
37. Herget-Rosenthal S, Quellmann T, Linden C, et al. How does late nephrological co-management impact chronic kidney disease? - an observational study. Int J Clin Pract 2010;64(13):1784–92.

38. Ritz E. Consequences of late referral in diabetic renal disease. Acta Diabetol 2002;39(Suppl 1):S3–8.

39. Arora P, Obrador GT, Ruthazer R, et al. Prevalence, predictors, and consequences of late nephrology referral at a tertiary care center. J Am Soc Nephrol 1999;10:1281–6.

40. Fisher M, Ahya S, Gordon E. Interventions to reduce late referrals to nephrologists. Am J Nephrol 2011;33:60–9.

41. Navaneethan SD, Aloudate S, Singh S. A systematic review of patient and health system characteristics associated with late referral in CKD. BMC Nephrol 2009;9:3.

42. Campbell KH, Smith SG, Hemmerich J, et al. Patient and provider determinants of nephrology referral in older adults with severe chronic kidney disease: a survey of provider decision making. BMC Nephrol 2011;12:47.

43. Gandhi TK, Sittig DF, Franklin M, et al. Communication breakdown in the outpatient referral process. J Gen Intern Med 2000;15(9):626–31.

44. Diamantidis CJ, Powe NR, Jaar BG, et al. Primary care-specialist collaboration in the care of patients with chronic kidney disease. Clin J Am Soc Nephrol 2011; 6(2):334–43.

45. Ronksley PE, Hemmelgarn BR. Optimizing care for patients with CKD. Am J Kidney Dis 2012;60(1):133–8.

46. Bolton WK, Owen WF Jr. Preparing the kidney failure patient for renal replacement therapy. Teamwork optimizes outcomes. Postgrad Med 2002;111(6): 97–108.

47. Clancy CM. Kidney-related diseases and quality improvement: AHRQ's role. Clin J Am Soc Nephrol 2011;6(10):2531–3.

48. Diabetes care quality improvement: resource guide. 9-14-2012. Ref Type: Online Source. Available at: http://www.ahrq.gov/qual/diabqual/diabqguidemod5.htm.

49. Bolton WK. Renal Physicians Association. Clinical practice guideline: appropriate patient preparation for renal replacement therapy. Guideline Number 3. Renal Physicians Association Guideline. J Am Soc Nephrol 2003;14(5):1406–10.

50. Bolton WK. The role of the nephrologist in ESRD/pre-ESRD care: a collaborative approach. J Am Soc Nephrol 1998;9:S90–5.

51. Bolton WK. Nephrology nurse practitioners in a collaborative care model. Am J Kidney Dis 1998;31:786–93.

52. Holley JL, McGuirl K. Advanced practice nurses in ESRD: varied roles and a cost analysis. Nephrol News Issues 2000;14(3):18–20.

53. Bolton WK, Kliger AS. Chronic renal insufficiency: current understandings and their implications. Am J Kidney Dis 2000;36(6):S4–12.

54. Renders CM, Valk GD, Griffin S, et al. Interventions to improve the management of diabetes mellitus in primary care, outpatient and community settings. Cochrane Database Syst Rev 2001;(1):CD001481.

55. Pimouguet C, Le GM, Thiebaut R, et al. Effectiveness of disease-management programs for improving diabetes care: a meta-analysis. CMAJ 2011;183(2): E115–27.

56. Wynia MK, Von KI, Mitchell PH. Challenges at the intersection of team-based and patient-centered health care: insights from an IOM working group. JAMA 2012;308(13):1327–8.

57. Saxena R, Bygren P, Butkowski RJ, et al. Specificity of kidney-bound antibodies in Goodpasture's syndrome. Clin Exp Immunol 1989;78:31–6.

58. Hemmelgarn BR, Manns BJ, Zhang J, et al. Association between multidisciplinary care and survival for elderly patients with chronic kidney disease. J Am Soc Nephrol 2007;18:993–9.

59. Richards N, Whitfield M, O'Donoghue D, et al. Primary care-based disease management of chronic kidney disease (CKD), based on estimated glomerular filtration rate (eGFR) reporting, improves patient outcomes. Nephrol Dial Transplant 2008;23(2):549–55.

60. Wu IW, Wang SY, Hsu KH, et al. Multidisciplinary predialysis education decreased the incidence of dialysis and reduces mortality-a controlled cohort study based on the NKF/DOQI guidelines. Nephrol Dial Transplant 2009;24: 3426–33.

61. Thanamayooran S, Rose C, Hirsch DJ. Effectiveness of a multidisciplinary kidney disease clinic in achieving treatment guideline targets. Nephrol Dial Transplant 2005;20:2385–93.

62. Kim-Hwang JE, Chen AH, Bell DS, et al. Evaluating electronic referrals for specialty care at a public hospital. J Gen Intern Med 2010;25(10):1123–8.

63. Chang J, Ronco C, Rosner MH. Computerized decision support systems: improving patient safety in nephrology. Nat Rev Nephrol 2011;7(6):348–55.

64. Abdel-Kader K, Fischer GS, Li J, et al. Automated clinical reminders for primary care providers in the care of CKD: a small cluster-randomized controlled trial. Am J Kidney Dis 2011;58(6):894–902.

65. O'Reilly D, Holbrook A, Blackhouse G, et al. Cost-effectiveness of a shared computerized decision support system for diabetes linked to electronic medical records. J Am Med Inform Assoc 2012;19(3):341–5.

66. UKPDS 3. Intensive blood-glucose control with sulphonylureas or insulin compared with conventional treatment and risk of complications in patients with type 2 diabetes. Lancet 1998;352(9131):837–53.

67. Ohkubo Y, Kishikawa H, Araki E, et al. Intensive insulin therapy prevents the progression of diabetic microvascular complications in Japanese patients with non-insulin-dependent diabetes mellitus: a randomized prospective 6-year study [see comments]. Diabetes Res Clin Pract 1901;28(2):103–17.

68. Shichiri M, Kishikawa H, Ohkubo Y, et al. Long-term results of the Kumamoto Study on optimal diabetes control in type 2 diabetic patients. Diabetes Care 2000;23(Suppl 2):B21–9.

69. Coppelli A, Giannarelli R, Vistoli F, et al. The beneficial effects of pancreas transplant alone on diabetic nephropathy. Diabetes Care 2005;28(6):1366–70.

70. Gross JL, de Azevedo MJ, Silveiro SP, et al. Diabetic nephropathy: diagnosis, prevention, and treatment. Diabetes Care 2005;28(1):164–76.

71. American Diabetes Association. Nephropathy in Diabetes. Position Statement. Diab Care 2004;27:S79–83.

72. Grant RW, Buse JB, Meigs JB. Quality of diabetes care in U.S. academic medical centers: low rates of medical regimen change. Diabetes Care 2005;28(2): 337–442.

73. Quinn DC, Graber AL, Elasy TA, et al. Overcoming turf battles: developing a pragmatic, collaborative model to improve glycemic control in patients with diabetes. Jt Comm J Qual Improv 2001;27(5):255–64.

74. Del PS, Felton AM, Munro N, et al. Improving glucose management: ten steps to get more patients with type 2 diabetes to glycaemic goal. Recommendations from the Global Partnership for Effective Diabetes Management. Int J Clin Pract Suppl 2007;157:47–57.

75. Cramer JA. A systematic review of adherence with medications for diabetes. Diabetes Care 2004;27(5):1218–24.

76. Odegard PS, Gray SL. Barriers to medication adherence in poorly controlled diabetes mellitus. Diabetes Educ 2008;34(4):692–7.

77. Phillips LS, Branch WT, Cook CB, et al. Clinical inertia. Ann Intern Med 2001; 135(9):825–34.
78. Shah BR, Hux JE, Laupacis A, et al. Clinical inertia in response to inadequate glycemic control: do specialists differ from primary care physicians? Diabetes Care 2005;28(3):600–6.
79. Phillips LS, Ziemer DC, Doyle JP, et al. An endocrinologist-supported intervention aimed at providers improves diabetes management in a primary care site: improving primary care of African Americans with diabetes (IPCAAD) 7. Diabetes Care 2005;28(10):2352–60.
80. de Sonnaville JJ, Bouma M, Colly LP, et al. Sustained good glycaemic control in NIDDM patients by implementation of structured care in general practice: 2-year follow-up study. Diabetologia 1997;40(11):1334–40.
81. Verlato G, Muggeo M, Bonora E, et al. Attending the diabetes center is associated with increased 5-year survival probability of diabetic patients: the Verona Diabetes Study. Diabetes Care 1996;19(3):211–3.
82. Graber AL, Elasy TA, Quinn D, et al. Improving glycemic control in adults with diabetes mellitus: shared responsibility in primary care practices. South Med J 2002;95(7):684–90.
83. Hardy K, Furlong N, Hulme S, et al. Delivering improved management and outcomes in diabetic kidney disease in routine clinical care. Br J Diabetes Vasc Dis 2007;7:172–82.
84. Gerich JE, Meyer C, Woerle HJ, et al. Renal gluconeogenesis: its importance in human glucose homeostasis. Diabetes Care 2001;24(2):382–91.
85. Valera Mora ME, Scarfone A, Calvani M, et al. Insulin clearance in obesity. J Am Coll Nutr 2003;22(6):487–93.
86. Mak RH, DeFronzo RA. Glucose and insulin metabolism in uremia. Nephron 1992;61(4):377–82.
87. Becker B, Kronenberg F, Kielstein JT, et al. Renal insulin resistance syndrome, adiponectin and cardiovascular events in patients with kidney disease: the mild and moderate kidney disease study. J Am Soc Nephrol 2005;16(4):1091–8.
88. Hajjar SM, Fadda GZ, Thanakitcharu P, et al. Reduced activity of Na(+)-K+ ATPase of pancreatic islets in chronic renal failure: role of secondary hyperparathyroidism. J Am Soc Nephrol 1992;2(8):1355–9.
89. Chagnac A, Weinstein T, Zevin D, et al. Effects of erythropoietin on glucose tolerance in hemodialysis patients. Clin Nephrol 1994;42(6):398–400.
90. Runyan JW Jr, Hurwitz D, Robbins SL. Effect of Kimmelstiel-Wilson syndrome on insulin requirements in diabetes. N Engl J Med 1955;252(10):388–91.

Diabetic Kidney Disease and the Cardiorenal Syndrome: Old Disease, New Perspectives

Ankur Jindal, MD[a,b], Mariana Garcia-Touza, MD[b,c],
Nidhi Jindal, MD[d], Adam Whaley-Connell, DO, MSPH[b,c,d,e],
James R. Sowers, MD[b,c,e,f],*

KEYWORDS

- Diabetes • Cardiorenal syndrome • Diabetic nephropathy • Chronic kidney disease
- Blood pressure variability • Albuminuria • Proteinuria

KEY POINTS

- Diabetic nephropathy should be studied and treated in the context of cardiorenal syndrome, with a focus on the complex intertwined metabolic changes, which increase risk for chronic kidney disease and cardiovascular disease.
- Blood pressure and glycemic control are crucial for prevention and treatment of diabetic kidney disease.
- Newer drugs for achieving glycemic control have an important role in the treatment of type 2 diabetes mellitus in patients with cardiorenal syndrome.

This article originally appeared in Endocrinology and Metabolism Clinics of North America, Volume 42, Issue 4, December 2013.

Funding Sources: NIH (R01 HL73101-01A1 & R01 HL107910-01), Veterans Affairs Merit System 0019 (J.R. Sowers); NIH (R-03 AG040638), Veterans Affairs System (CDA-2), ASN-ASP Junior Development Grant in Geriatric Nephrology, supported by a T. Franklin Williams Scholarship Award (A. Whaley-Connell).

Conflict of Interest: Merck Pharmaceuticals Advisory Board (J.R. Sowers).

[a] Hospital Medicine, Department of Internal Medicine, University of Missouri, One Hospital Drive, Columbia, MO 65212, USA; [b] Diabetes and Cardiovascular Research Center, University of Missouri, One Hospital Drive, Columbia, MO 65212, USA; [c] Division of Endocrinology, Diabetes & Metabolism, Department of Internal Medicine, University of Missouri Columbia School of Medicine, One Hospital Drive, Columbia, MO 65212, USA; [d] Division of Nephrology and Hypertension, Department of Internal Medicine, University of Missouri Columbia School of Medicine, One Hospital Drive, Columbia, MO 65212, USA; [e] Department of Internal Medicine, Harry S Truman Memorial Veterans Hospital, Five Hospital Drive, Columbia, MO 65201, USA; [f] Department of Medical Physiology and Pharmacology, University of Missouri, One Hospital Drive, Columbia, MO 65212, USA

* Corresponding author. University of Missouri, D109 Diabetes Center HSC, One Hospital Drive, Columbia, MO 65212.

E-mail address: sowersj@health.missouri.edu

Clinics Collections 1 (2014) 183–202
http://dx.doi.org/10.1016/j.ccol.2014.08.012

INTRODUCTION

Prevalent chronic kidney disease (CKD) in the United States has increased over last few decades and comprises an alarming 13% of the US general population.[1] Diabetes is recognized as the leading cause of CKD and end-stage renal disease (ESRD), and accounts for about 40% of ESRD cases in the United States.[2–4] It is estimated that CKD affects more than 35% of adults with diabetes and nearly 20% of adults with hypertension.[5] The expansion of CKD can be explained, in part, by the increased prevalence of obesity and diabetes, thus raising concerns for even more pronounced trends in the future.[1] Regardless of cause, CKD is prevalent enough to be considered a critical public health concern, especially with the associated increased morbidity and mortality from cardiovascular disease (CVD).[1,6] In this context, diabetic kidney disease (DKD) is a clinical syndrome characterized by early glomerular hyperfiltration and albuminuria, followed by increasing proteinuria and a decline in glomerular filtration rate (GFR), blood pressure increase, and high risk of CVD morbidity and mortality.[7] The cause of this disease, although it is increasingly common because of the global expansion of diabetes and obesity, is poorly understood.

PATHOLOGY OF DKD

DKD has been studied extensively over the years, but our understanding of this complex disease process is far from complete. It is generally accepted that diabetes is associated with diverse structural changes in the kidney; all structural compartments are affected, leading to functional impairments at all levels of the nephron. Three basic steps have been described in progression of DKD[8]: (1) glomerular hypertrophy and hyperfiltration, (2) inflammation of the glomeruli and tubulointerstitial area, and (3) apoptosis of cells and accumulation of extracellular matrix.

The hyperglycemia observed in diabetes contributes to a microinflammatory, oxidative stress milieu and extracellular matrix expansion within the kidney.[8] There are 3 critical abnormalities including intracellular metabolism, formation of advanced glycation end products, and intraglomerular hypertension implicated in development of glomerular endothelial and mesangial cell injury. These pathologic changes are associated with cellular injury, expression of adhesion molecules, and macrophage infiltration in kidney tissue.[8]

Expansion of the mesangium, thickening of the glomerular basement membrane (GBM), and hyalinosis of afferent and efferent arterioles are the characteristic lesions of DKD.[9] It is generally believed that thickening of GBM and expansion of mesangium occur early in the course of diabetes. Diffuse global mesangial expansion is seen in diabetes, and it is primarily caused by an increase in extracellular matrix, with limited contribution from increase in mesangial cell volume.[9] Kimmelstiel-Wilson nodules (acellular to paucicellular nodular accumulations of mesangial matrix) have been described in DKD. These nodular sclerotic lesions occur in patients with advanced DKD, and their presence is considered to mark the transition from early to more advanced stages of DKD.[10] Kimmelstiel-Wilson nodules are not pathognomonic of DKD, because these lesions can be seen in other conditions like monoclonal immunoglobulin deposition disorders, membranoproliferative glomerulonephritis, postinfectious glomerulonephritis, and amyloidosis.[9,10] In parallel, hyaline deposition in the glomerular arterioles is another typical histologic feature of DKD. Hyalinosis and the resultant hyaline appearance (homogeneous and glassy) is caused by insinuation of plasma proteins into the vascular wall.

Alternatively, loss of integrity of the filtration barrier and podocyte injury with effacement of foot processes and loss of podocytes are other microscopic changes evident in DKD that play important roles in the development of progressive sclerosis and proteinuria.[9]

Recently, DKD in type 1 diabetes mellitus and type 2 diabetes mellitus (T2DM) has been classified based on severity of glomerular lesions. Classification based on glomerular lesions has been chosen over interstitial or vascular lesions, because of ease of recognition and good interobserver reproducibility. In addition, it has been suggested that severity of chronic interstitial and glomerular lesions corelate closely. The pathologic classification of DKD as proposed by the Renal Pathology Society[10] is: class 1, diabetic injury with GBM thickening (>2 standard deviations from normal); class 2, mesangial expansion; 2a, mild mesangial expansion; 2b, severe mesangial expansion; class 3, nodular sclerosis (Kimmelstiel-Wilson lesion); class 4, advanced diabetic glomerulosclerosis: global sclerosis involving more than 50% of glomeruli in addition to the changes described earlier. Ongoing basic science and clinical research is helping shape our understanding of DKD pathogenesis and correlation between histologic lesions of DKD and progression of clinical DKD.

THE CARDIORENAL SYNDROME AND DKD

Involvement of both kidneys and the cardiovascular system is common in conjunction with overweight/obesity, metabolic abnormalities, hypertension and early T2DM. Thus, it is important to understand how involvement of 1 organ system contributes to the dysfunction of the other, and these complex interactions have been captured with the emergence of the concept of cardiorenal syndrome (CRS).[7,11–13] Risk factors that influence heart and kidney disease like overweight or obesity, hypertension, insulin resistance, and metabolic dyslipidemic function are the defining components of CRS (**Fig. 1**).[11] The presence of hypertension, obesity, and hyperinsulinemia are independently associated with reductions in kidney function.[12] The interaction of these factors and their metabolic and immunologic effect should be referred to as the CRS. Obesity is associated with altered intrarenal physical forces, inappropriate activation of the renin-angiotensin system (RAS) and sympathetic nervous system, and decreased activity of endogenous natriuretic peptides, which contribute to increases in blood pressure and altered responses to handling of glucose in individuals with insulin resistance.[14] Thus, the various components of CRS interact via complex intertwined pathways and result in the loss of renal structure and function.

IMPACT OF HYPERTENSION ON DKD

There have been several seminal studies describing the importance of hypertension to cardiovascular mortality in individuals with DKD. In this context, approximately 66% of individuals with an estimated GFR (eGFR) less than 60 mL/min/1.73 m^2 have hypertension and as eGFR diminishes over time, the prevalence rates increase from 36% in stage 1 to 84% in stages 4 to 5 CKD.[15] Because increases in blood pressure dictate cardiovascular mortality to some extent, it has been noted that mortality caused by CVD is 10 to 30 times higher in individuals with kidney disease compared with the general population: a relationship that extends into earlier stages of DKD.[16] This relationship has been described as a continuous relationship: with reductions in GFR and increases in proteinuria comes a graded increase in CVD.[17] Moreover, recent studies support the notion that even early stages of CKD pose a significant risk of CVD.[18]

Control of blood pressure in diabetes has been studied extensively, and stricter blood pressure targets have been tested overtime. Many studies have shown the beneficial effects of blood pressure control on various outcomes in patients with diabetes; however, blood pressure targets have been a source of debate for several

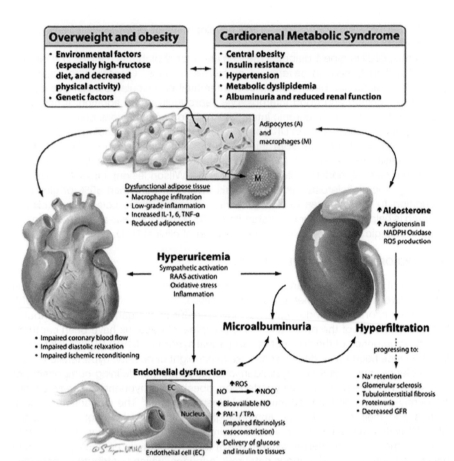

Fig. 1. The interrelationship between adiposity and maladaptive changes in the heart and kidney in CRS. IL, interleukin; PAI, plasminogen activator inhibitor; RAAS, renin-angiotensin-aldosterone system; ROS, reactive oxygen species; TNF, tumor necrosis factor; TPA, tissue plasminogen activator. (*From* Sowers JR, Whaley-Connell A, Hayden MR. The role of overweight and obesity in the cardiorenal syndrome. Cardiorenal Med 2011;1:5–12; with permission.)

years.[19] There are sufficient data to support blood pressure control in T2DM, because this control reduces proteinuria and progression of DKD.[20] The United Kingdom Prospective Diabetes Study (UKPDS) suggests the potential microvascular benefits of blood pressure control in patients with diabetes, wherein 758 patients with T2DM were randomized to tight blood pressure control (<150/85 mm Hg) and 390 to less tight control (<180/105 mm Hg). Mean blood pressures of 144/82 mm Hg and 154/87 mm Hg were achieved in the 2 groups, respectively. Fewer patients in the tight control group had urine albumin concentration greater than 50 mg/L than in the less tight control group at 6 years, although these differences were not significant at 9 years of follow-up.[21] Data from the ADVANCE (Action in Diabetes and Vascular Disease: Preterax and Diamicron Modified Release Controlled Evaluation) trial along with the AASK (African American Study of Kidney Disease and Hypertension) trial suggest that tight blood pressure control (<120/70 mm Hg) in the context of diabetes and proteinuria improves kidney-specific outcomes. In the ADVANCE trial, there were

11,140 enrolled patients with T2DM, who were randomly assigned to blood pressure treatment with fixed combination perindopril-indapamide or placebo. During the follow-up, mean systolic blood pressure (SBP) 134.7 and 140.3, and mean diastolic blood pressure (DBP) 74.8 and 77.0 mm Hg was attained in the active treatment and placebo groups, respectively. Active treatment not only decreased the risk for onset and progression of microalbuminuria, it also increased the chance of regression of microalbuminuria.[20]

Over time, evidence has accumulated to suggest renal benefits of tight blood pressure control in hypertensive patients with diabetes, and has raised questions about treatment threshold. This question was addressed in the Appropriate Blood Pressure Control in Diabetics (Normotensive ABCD) study. Normotensive ABCD is a prospective randomized trial designed to study the effects of decreasing blood pressure in normotensive (blood pressure <140/90 mm Hg) patients with diabetes. A total of 480 patients were randomly assigned to intensive DBP control (target DBP of 10 mm Hg < baseline) and moderate DBP control (target DBP 80–89 mm Hg). The intensive treatment group was treated with nisoldipine or enalapril, and the moderate-treatment group with placebo. Over a 5-year follow-up period, intensive blood pressure control (mean blood pressure 128/75 mm Hg) was associated with decreased risk for progression to incipient nephropathy and diabetic nephropathy in patients who were normotensive at baseline.[22]

The importance of blood pressure control in patients with diabetes cannot be over-emphasized. Blood pressure control is paramount for preservation of kidney function in patients with diabetes, especially because risk for progression to ESRD is increased up to 7-fold in patients with concomitant T2DM and hypertension.[23]

NONDIPPING BLOOD PRESSURE/PULSE PATTERN IN DIABETES

A characteristic of diabetes includes a disproportionate increase in SBP, with a loss of nocturnal dipping of blood pressure and heart rate, commonly referred to as nondipping.[24] In normotensive patients, there is a circadian regulation of blood pressure wherein there are nocturnal drops in blood pressure of approximately 10% to 15%, commonly referred to as dipping. Alternatively, nondippers have less than the usual 10% decline at night. Nondipping is frequent among diabetic patients, as shown on ambulatory blood pressure monitoring. This nondipping pattern is caused, in part, by dysfunction of the autonomic nervous system, which is often present in individuals with T2DM and is characterized by a reduction in relative parasympathetic activity; it is believed to contribute to the 5-fold to 7-fold increase in sudden death in diabetic patients.[24,25] Studies have shown that the nondipping pattern of blood pressure is associated with microalbuminuria, overt proteinuria, and higher morbidity and mortality in patients with diabetes.[26] In this context, use of ambulatory blood pressure for measurement of dipping status is superior to office blood pressure in predicting target organ involvement, such as proteinuria and left ventricular hypertrophy.[24]

BLOOD PRESSURE VARIABILITY AS A RISK FACTOR FOR DKD

There are several modifiable risk factors that predict development of incipient and overt kidney disease in people with obesity and diabetes.[27,28] Traditional risk factors for DKD include long-term poor glycemic control, systemic and glomerular hypertension, hypercholesterolemia, urine albumin excretion (UAE) rate, intrauterine growth retardation, and smoking.[27-29] With regard to hypertension, attention has traditionally been focused on systolic, diastolic, and mean blood pressure with the assumption that conventional clinic readings depict a patient's true blood pressure and predict adverse outcomes.[30] Blood pressure variability has been considered a random phenomenon of little clinical significance, although accumulating data suggest that visit-to-visit variability in blood pressure and episodic hypertension might affect cardiovascular and other target organ outcomes.[30,31] Emerging data also suggest that different drug classes affect blood pressure variability differently. Calcium channel blockers and nonloop diuretics decrease blood pressure variability, whereas β-blockers, angiotensin-converting enzyme (ACE) inhibitors, and angiotensin receptor blockers (ARB) increase the blood pressure variability.[32]

A post hoc analysis of data from DCCT (Diabetes Control and Complications Trial) shows that a patient with SBP variability of 13.3 mm Hg has a risk 2.34 times higher for kidney disease compared with a patient with variability of 3.7 mm Hg.[33] Observational data from a retrospective cohort study involving 354 patients with T2DM suggest that individuals who have greater visit-to-visit SBP variability might be at risk for development and progression of proteinuria.[34] Recent data from multiple cohorts involving patients with previous transient ischemic attacks and treated hypertension show a strong predictive value of visit-to-visit variability in SBP and maximum SBP for stroke and coronary events, independent of mean systolic pressures. Data from this study emphasize the risks of episodic hypertension, but do not prove a causal link between stroke and blood pressure variability or maximum SBP.[35] Data from a relatively small longitudinal retrospective observational study involving 374 elderly patients with CKD showed association between visit-to-visit blood pressure variability and all-cause mortality. This study failed to show association between blood pressure variability and progression of CKD.[36] Data accumulating from other studies points that visit-to-visit SBP variability might be associated with all-cause mortality and progression of vascular disease independent of mean arterial pressures in patients with or without diabetes.[34–39]

Results of a meta-analysis[40] suggest that variability of SBP between arms could be helpful for identification of people at increased risk for vascular disease. These findings have prompted investigators to study the role of blood pressure difference between arms further and to explore its predictive value for other outcomes. Recently, investigators have studied the role of difference in SBP between arms and between lower limbs, in predicting risk for DKD. Initial data suggest that such blood pressure differences could be novel risk markers for DKD.[41]

Accumulating data challenges the notion that mean arterial pressure or usual blood pressure is a sufficient predictor of vascular events and stresses the need to analyze the available data and to explore the roles of other factors like blood pressure variability. Blood pressure variability is difficult to quantify and it is unclear how to incorporate it in to clinical practice. Further research is needed to better quantify associated risks and treatment parameters.

USE OF ACE INHIBITORS OR ARBS IN DKD

The treatment of hypertension in those with DKD includes both nonpharmacologic and pharmacologic approaches. However, in the presence of reduced blood pressure in DKD, use of pharmacologic strategies with interruption of the RAS with ACE inhibitors or ARBs is a primary risk-reduction strategy.[23,42–45] Available data suggest that ARBs might have renal benefits independent of the SBP decreasing effect in patients with T2DM.[43,44,46] Data from a study that compared the renoprotective effects of telmisartan and enalapril suggest that ARBs and ACE inhibitors are equally effective in preventing loss of kidney function in patients with T2DM and early DKD.[47] Data from another large study show that losartan has significant beneficial effects on kidney function in patients with T2DM. Small differences in blood pressure were noted between the losartan and placebo-treated groups, and it remains unclear to what extent the renal benefits in the group treated with losartan could be attributed to the lower blood pressure.[46] Data from the ROADMAP (Randomized Olmesartan and Diabetes Microalbuminuria Prevention) trial also showed that the use of olmesartan was associated with delay in onset of microalbuminuria, but again there were subtle differences in blood pressure between the 2 treatment groups.[45]

However, the benefit of dual RAS blockade has been in question. Data from ONTARGET (Ongoing Telmisartan Alone and in Combination with Ramipril Global Endpoint Trial) suggest that combined treatment with an ACE inhibitor and ARB was more effective than ACE inhibitor alone in reducing proteinuria, but the combination was associated with less desirable renal outcomes and faster decline in GFR.[48] Available data suggest that individual components of RAS blockade help preserve kidney function better than other antihypertensives, at least in people with proteinuria.[48]

EFFECTS OF CKD ON GLUCOSE HOMEOSTASIS AND ASSESSMENT OF GLYCEMIC CONTROL

Diabetes has been implicated in the development and progression of CKD, but progressive renal dysfunction also induces complex changes in insulin metabolism and clearance and affects glucose homeostasis in patients with diabetes. CKD is associated with increased insulin resistance on one hand and decreased insulin clearance on other. A decrease in GFR is associated with decrease in metabolic clearance of insulin, which becomes apparent as GFR decreases lower than 15 to 20 mL/min/1.73 m^2. Usually, as renal function declines, peritubular insulin uptake increases and maintains insulin clearance, but as GFR declines to levels lower than 15 to 20 mL/min/1.73 m^2, peritubular insulin uptake is unable to compensate for decreased renal function.[49] With progression of CKD, the degradation of insulin in the liver and muscle is also impaired because of accumulation of the uremic by-products. This decreased insulin clearance can decrease the insulin requirements in diabetes and can lead to hypoglycemic episodes. The decreased insulin clearance in CKD is counterbalanced by increased insulin resistance and decreased insulin production in patients with CKD.[50] Many other factors like loss of appetite, malnutrition and deficient renal gluconeogenesis and catecholamine release affect glucose homeostasis in renal disease.[50] Complex interactions of multiple divergent pathways make the determination of insulin requirement challenging in patients with DKD.

Lack of a standardized clinical test for monitoring glycemic control in DKD complicates management of diabetes in this patient subgroup. Glycated hemoglobin (HbA1c), which is widely used to evaluate glycemic control in diabetes, provides a retrospective assessment of glycemic control. HbA1c has been found to reliably access glycemic control in patients with diabetes, but its accuracy in patients with DKD is questionable. HbA1c levels are affected by high urea levels, uremic acidosis, reduced red blood cell survival, and frequent blood transfusions, and hence there is a potential for erroneous glycemic control estimates in patients with DKD.[51]

Other markers of glycemic control such as glycated albumin and serum fructosamine assess glycemic control over 2 weeks, but these are unreliable in conditions affecting albumin metabolism.[52] These tests have not been standardized and are not used frequently in clinical practice.[53] Further studies are required to assess their use for diagnosis of diabetes and evaluation of glycemic control.

MARKERS OF DKD AND PROGNOSTIC VALUE OF EGFR AND MICROALBUMINURIA

Traditionally, eGFR and UAE have been used to define and to follow progression of DKD. In clinical practice, eGFR is estimated using clearance of endogenous creatinine. Release of creatinine into circulation is variable and depends on factors like age, gender, muscle mass, diet, volume status, medications, and so forth. Creatinine clearance further tends to overestimate GFR, because of tubular secretion of creatinine. Several equations like Cockcroft-Gault and Modification of Diet in Renal Disease 4-variable (MDRD) have been used to improve the accuracy of GFR estimation, but these equations are less than perfect.[2] Recently, the Chronic Kidney Disease Epidemiologic Collaboration) (CKD-EPI) equation was developed in an attempt to overcome the limitations of the MDRD equation. The CKD-EPI equation estimates GFR more accurately, especially at eGFR greater than 60 mL/min/1.73 m².[54]

Other markers of GFR such as cystatin C have been studied, but have not received widespread acceptance in clinical practice because of associated costs. Limitations of biomarkers for acute kidney injury and CKD have prompted active interest in study of biomarkers. Many biomarkers are under investigation, including urinary podocytes, neutrophil gelatinase-associated lipocalin, kidney injury molecule 1, Smad-1, connective tissue growth factor, and transforming growth factor β.[2]

Along with eGFR, UAE is used to monitor progression and for staging of DKD. Although debatable, microalbuminuria is considered a risk predictor for progression to overt DKD and for CVD. Screening for microalbuminuria is widely recommended for risk stratification. Numerous population-based and intervention studies support microalbuminuria as a risk factor for CVD and as a strong predictor of cardiovascular morbidity and mortality in patients with diabetes.[55,56] Data from a study of 3431 diabetic patients in the United Kingdom[57] show that eGFR declined rapidly in people with macroalbuminuria and microalbuminuria, at rates of 5.7% and 1.5% per annum, respectively. The progression of DKD was slower in patients with normoalbuminuria: an eGFR decline of only 0.3% per year. Recently, a post hoc analysis of the HUNT-2 (Nord-Trøndelag Health) study[58] showed that CKD progression risk increases substantially, in presence of microalbuminuria or macroalbuminuria. Data from this analysis suggest a strong synergistic interaction between albuminuria and reduced eGFR, which together confer higher risk of progression to ESRD than is attributable to either risk factor individually.[58] This study highlights the importance of using UAE in combination with eGFR for better classification and risk stratification of patients with CKD.[58]

The risk for all-cause and cardiovascular mortality increases with increase in UAE and decrease in eGFR. Data from a large retrospective study involving 1,120,295 adult patients showed that low eGFR (≤60 mL/min/1.73 m²) was independently associated with increased risk of death, cardiovascular events, and hospitalization. The risks were substantially increased when eGFR decreased further to levels lower than 45 mL/min/1.73 m². The adjusted hazard ratios for death were 1.2 (95% confidence interval [CI], 1.1–1.2), 1.8 (95% CI, 1.7–1.9), 3.2 (95% CI, 3.1–3.4), and 5.9 (95% CI, 5.4–6.5) for eGFR 45 to 59, 30 to 44, 15 to 29, and less than 15, respectively.[17] Data from RIACE (Renal Insufficiency And Cardiovascular Events), a cross-sectional study involving 15,773 patients with T2DM,[59] led to similar conclusions. The data further showed that low eGFR and albuminuria ≥10.5 mg/24 h are associated with coronary artery disease in patients with T2DM. A meta-analysis of albumin-to-creatinine ratio (ACR) data from more than 1 million participants and urine protein dipstick data from 112,310 participants showed a significant increase in mortality risk at low eGFR (≤60 mL/min/1.73 m²) compared with optimum eGFR (90–104 mL/min/1.73 m²).[6] Albuminuria was measured by ACR or urine dipstick in the included studies. The analyses showed that even trace protein on urine dipstick is associated with increased mortality in the general population, independent of eGFR and traditional cardiovascular risk factors.[6] The hazard ratios for all-cause mortality were 1.20 (95% CI, 1.15–1.26), 1.63 (95% CI, 1.50–1.77) and 2.22 (95% CI, 1.97–2.51) for ACR 1.1 mg/mmol, 3.4 mg/mmol, and

33.9 mg/mmol, respectively, compared with ACR of 0.6 mg/mmol.[6] These findings highlight the importance of urine dipstick, an imprecise but inexpensive measure of albuminuria, in detection of DKD.[6]

Although some data suggest that CKD is not an independent risk factor for cardiovascular mortality,[60,61] many believe that CKD is independently associated with cardiovascular mortality and all-cause mortality.[62–67] Confounding by previous CVD and by traditional and nontraditional CVD risk in patients with established CKD makes data interpretation challenging.[17] It is unclear if the increased cardiovascular mortality in CKD is an independent effect or if it can be attributed to confounding factors. The role of other pathologic changes like hypercoagulability, endothelial dysfunction, arterial stiffness, and increased inflammatory response as cardiovascular outcome modulators in people with CKD is an area of active interest.[17]

The literature supports the simultaneous use of eGFR and UAE for better risk stratification of patients with DKD. When used simultaneously, these markers help predict CKD progression and cardiovascular risk in patients with DKD.

DKD WITHOUT ALBUMINURIA

Proteinuria has traditionally been considered a diagnostic and prognostic marker of DKD, and its presence prompts interventions such as initiation of ACE inhibitors or ARBs. Absence of proteinuria can render a false sense of reassurance for clinicians and often delays diagnosis and treatment of DKD. Development and progression of microalbuminuria in patients with DKD are not rules, and there is a distinct population who do not develop any level of proteinuria until late in disease. There is a possibility of stabilization and even regression of microalbuminuria in patients with diabetes.[68] DKD is believed to arise from microvascular damage, which leads to increased UAE.[69] Over time, data have accumulated to suggest a high prevalence of kidney disease in patients with diabetes and normal UAE, suggesting the presence of renal lesions other than classic diabetic glomerulosclerosis in this population subgroup. This finding has prompted investigators to consider other explanations like interstitial fibrosis, ischemic vascular disease, cholesterol microemboli, atherosclerotic involvement of the renal vasculature, and so forth.[69,70]

Recently, researchers studied the development of nephropathy in the Cohen diabetic rat (an experimental model of human T2DM). The Cohen diabetic sensitive rats develop CKD with reduced eGFR and histologic changes consistent with DKD, as shown by light and electron microscopy, in absence of proteinuria, when fed a diabetogenic diet. These rats develop changes suggestive of nonproliferative retinopathy as well, although these changes appeared later than development of DKD.[71]

The characteristic histologic lesions seen in classic diabetic glomerulosclerosis are often seen with other systemic manifestations of microvascular disease. These lesions include increased basement membrane thickness, diffuse mesangial sclerosis with nodular formation, hyalinosis, microaneurysm, and hyaline arteriosclerosis.[70,71]

Data from DEMAND (Developing Education on Microalbuminuria for Awareness of Renal and Cardiovascular Risk in Diabetes), a global cross-sectional study,[72] showed that kidney dysfunction is not uncommon in T2DM with normal UAE. Kramer and colleagues[70] performed a cross-sectional analysis of a nationally representative sample of adults with T2DM and found that about 30% individuals with eGFR less than 60 did not have retinopathy or microalbuminuria. Data from other cross-sectional studies like RIACE, and longitudinal studies like ARIC (Atherosclerosis Risk in Communities) and UKPDS suggest that normoalbuminuric renal impairment occurs frequently in patients with T2DM.[68,73–75] Macroangiopathy could be the underlying renal disease as opposed to microangiopathy, in diabetic patients with normoalbuminuric CKD.[73] This change in phenotype of DKD could be related to better control of risk factors like hyperglycemia, hyperlipidemia, hypertension, and early use of ACE inhibitors and ARBs.[73]

Recent findings have encouraged investigators to think of microalbuminuria and reduced eGFR as markers of different pathologic processes. Microalbuminuria could be a phenotypic expression of endothelial dysfunction, whereas reduced eGFR could be a renal manifestation of systemic atherosclerosis.[67]

DOES BETTER GLYCEMIC CONTROL REDUCE DKD?

Data from DCCT and UKPDS have shaped the understanding and management of diabetes over the years for risk reduction of cardiovascular and kidney disease. In UKPDS, patients with T2DM were randomly assigned to intensive or conventional glycemic control using insulin or oral hypoglycemic agents. Over 10 years, HbA1c levels of 7% and 7.9% were achieved in the intensive and conventional groups, respectively. The patients assigned to intensive treatment protocols had decreased risk of microvascular complications, but the intensive treatment was associated with more hypoglycemic episodes and weight gain. The data also suggested that intensive control was associated with decreased progression of albuminuria.[76] Posttrial monitoring of patients enrolled in UKPDS, without any attempt to maintain previous diabetes therapies, showed an early loss (at 1 year) of glycemic differences between the 2 cohorts. Over a 10-year follow-up, sustained benefit and continued risk reduction for microvascular complications were observed in the cohort previously subject to intensive diabetes therapy.[77]

ADVANCE is a multicenter randomized controlled trial designed to study the effects of intensive glucose control (target HbA1c <6.5%) on vascular outcomes in T2DM. Mean HbA1c levels of 6.5% and 7.3% were achieved in the intensive and standard therapy groups, respectively. Data from this trial showed significant reduction in the incidence of nephropathy with intensive glycemic control. Intensive treatment was also associated with decreased need for renal replacement therapy and death from complications related to kidney disease.[78]

Previously, data from DCCT showed beneficial effects of intensive versus conventional glycemic control on kidney function in patients with type 1 diabetes. Conventional therapy aimed at prevention of symptoms attributable to glycosuria or hyperglycemia and maintenance of normal growth and development, whereas intensive therapy aimed at achieving preprandial blood glucose levels of 70 to 120 mg/dL and postprandial blood glucose concentration less than 180 mg/dL. Over a mean follow-up period of 6.5 years, microalbuminuria and albuminuria developed in fewer patients on intensive treatment, compared with patients on conventional treatment, leading to conclusions that intensive management of blood glucose in patients with insulin-dependent diabetes can delay the onset and slow the progression of diabetic nephropathy.[79] The DCCT participants were followed in the EDIC (Epidemiology of Diabetes Interventions and Complications) study, an observational study after the DCCT closeout. The DCCT intensive treatment cohort were encouraged to continue the intensive treatment, and the conventional treatment cohort were encouraged to switch to intensive treatment. Over 8 years of further follow-up, the HbA1c difference between the 2 groups narrowed, with mean values of 8.0% and 8.2% in the 2 cohorts, respectively. The incidence of microalbuminuria and clinical albuminuria was significantly lower in the group subject to intensive treatment during the DCCT trial.[80] Further follow-up data have shown the extension of benefits of early intensive diabetes treatment in patients with insulin-dependent diabetes for up to 22 years. The patients in the intensive treatment arm of DCCT had a 50% lower risk of impaired GFR at 22 years of follow-up, compared with patients in the conventional treatment arm, suggesting a metabolic memory effect.[81] These data further suggest that intensive therapy for insulin-dependent diabetes in 29 patients for 6.5 years can prevent impaired GFR in 1 patient over 20 years.[82]

Data from these well-designed prospective trials indicate that better glycemic control has an important role in delaying the onset and slowing the progression of nephropathy in patients with diabetes.

Although good glycemic and blood pressure control remain the cornerstones of treatment strategy, to prevent or to slow progression of DKD, other treatment approaches are being explored. Recently, effects of treatment with linagliptin, either alone or in combination with telmisartan, were studied in a mouse model of diabetic nephropathy. The combination seemed to have beneficial effects on albuminuria in mice, but its role in treatment or prevention of DKD in humans needs to be explored.[83]

PHARMACOLOGIC TREATMENT OF HYPERGLYCEMIA IN DKD/USE OF OLD AND NEW DRUGS OTHER THAN INSULIN

CKD affects metabolism of oral hypoglycemic agents and leads to accumulation of their metabolites, thus limiting the therapeutic options for patients with DKD. As discussed previously, renal dysfunction alters glucose homeostasis in unpredictable ways via multiple mechanisms in patients with DKD. This finding makes management of diabetes, especially glycemic control, challenging in DKD. The alterations in glucose and insulin handling by kidneys and other body tissues in DKD lead to a state of glycemic dysregulation, which is associated with increased risk of hypoglycemia as well as hyperglycemia.[53]

Selection of an appropriate therapeutic modality is complicated by pharmacokinetic alterations caused by reduced kidney function (**Table 1**).

Sulfonylureas

Sulfonylureas are insulin secretagogues and they increase endogenous insulin secretion. There is a high risk of hypoglycemia, especially with the use of longer-acting sulfonylureas like glyburide.[84]

Second-generation sulfonylureas like glipizide and glimepiride can be used in patients with diabetes and CKD. Glyburide should be avoided because of its long half-life. Glimepiride should be initiated at a low dose in patients with CKD and should be avoided in patients on dialysis.

Glipizide is the preferred second-generation sulfonylurea for patients with diabetes and CKD, and no dosage adjustment is required for patients with CKD or for those on dialysis.[84]

Meglitinides

These are insulin secretagogues with rapid onset of action and short half-life. Repaglinide and nateglinide are the 2 meglitinides available in the United States.[85]

No dose adjustment is required while using repaglinide in patients with CKD or for those on dialysis, but it is recommended that repaglinide be initiated at a lower dose (0.5 mg before each meal) in patients with GFR less than 40.[84] Use in people with GFR less than 20 or those on dialysis has not been studied. Nateglinide should be initiated at a lower dose (60 mg before each meal) in patients with CKD and should be avoided in patients on dialysis.[84]

Table 1
Dosage of drugs used to manage hyperglycemia in patients with diabetes and CKD/DKD

Drug Class	Drug	Major Action	Dosing Recommendation in CKD	Dosing Recommendation in Dialysis
Sulfonylureas	Glipizide	Insulin secretagogue	No dose adjustment required	No dose adjustment required
	Glimepiride	Insulin secretagogue	Initiate at 1 mg/d and titrate slowly	Avoid
	Glyburide	Insulin secretagogue	Not recommended	Not recommended
α-Glucosidase inhibitors	Acarbose	Slow carbohydrate absorption	Not recommended in sCr >2 mg/dL	Not recommended
	Miglitol	Slow carbohydrate absorption	Not recommended if sCr >2 mg/dL	Not recommended
Meglitinides	Repaglinide	Insulin secretagogue	Initiate at a lower dose 0.5 mg before each meal if GFR <40	Use not studied
	Nateglinide	Insulin secretagogue	Initiate at a low dose 60 mg before each meal	Avoid
Biguanides	Metformin	Liver insulin sensitizer	Contraindicated if sCr ≥1.5 mg/dL in men, and ≥1.4 mg/dL in women	Not recommended
Thiazolidinediones	Rosiglitazone	Peripheral insulin sensitizer	No dose adjustment	No dose adjustment
	Pioglitazone	Peripheral insulin sensitizer	No dose adjustment	No dose adjustment

Class	Drug	Mechanism	Dosing	Simplified recommendation
Incretin mimetics	Exenatide	Improved insulin secretion	GFR >50 no dose adjustment GFR 30–50 cautious use, but no dose adjustment suggested GFR <30 use not recommended	Use not recommended
	Liraglutide	Improved insulin secretion	No dose adjustment	No dose adjustment
Dipeptidylpeptidase-4 inhibitors	Sitagliptin	Improved insulin secretion	GFR >50 no dose adjustment, use 100 mg/d GFR 30–50 use 50 mg/d GFR <30 use 25 mg/d	Use 25 mg/d
	Alogliptin	Improved insulin secretion	GFR >50 no dose adjustment GFR 50–30 use 12.5 mg/d GFR <30 use 6.25 mg/d	Use 6.25 mg/d
	Linagliptin	Improved insulin secretion	No dose adjustment	No dose adjustment
	Saxagliptin	Improved insulin secretion	GFR >50 no dose adjustment GFR <50 use 2.5 mg/d	Use 2.5 mg/d
Amylin analogue	Pramlintide	Increased satiety and decreased glucagon	GFR >20 no dose adjustment	Lacks clinical data
Sodium glucose cotransporter 2 inhibitors	Canagliflozin	Glucuresis	GFR ≥60 no dose adjustment (use 100–300 mg daily) GFR 45–60 (maximum dose 100 mg/d) GFR 30–45 use not recommended GFR <30 contraindicated	Contraindicated

Abbreviation: sCr, serum creatinine level.
Adapted from Refs.[84,86–90]

α-Glucosidase Inhibitors

α-Glucosidase inhibitors prevent or decrease postprandial hyperglycemia. They work by decreasing the rate of breakdown of complex carbohydrates in the intestine, and thus decrease the amount of glucose available for absorption.[86] Acarbose has minimal systemic absorption, but the drug and its metabolite tend to accumulate in patients with severe renal dysfunction. Similarly, higher plasma levels of miglitol are present in patients with severe renal failure compared with patients with normal renal function, when on equal doses of miglitol. Acarbose and miglitol are available in the United States, but are not recommended for patients with serum creatinine greater than 2 mg/dL or on dialysis, because long-term safety of these drugs in patients with CKD has not been studied.[84]

Biguanides

Metformin suppresses gluconeogenesis by decreasing hepatic insulin resistance. It effectively decreases glucose concentration in fasting as well as postprandial states.[85]

Metformin should be avoided in patients with moderate and severe renal failure, because renal clearance of metformin is decreased in patients with renal impairment, leading to accumulation of the drug and increased risk of lactic acidosis. Its use in contraindicated in men with serum creatinine level 1.5 mg/dL or greater and women with serum creatinine level 1.4 mg/dL or greater.[84]

Thiazolidinedione

Thiazolidinediones are agonists of peroxisome proliferator-activated receptor γ. The stimulation of this receptor increases insulin-stimulated glucose uptake in muscles and adipose tissue and decreases hepatic glucose production and insulin resistance.[85]

Rosiglitazone and pioglitazone are available in the United States, and these can be used in patients with CKD without dose adjustment. However, these drugs should be used with caution in those with advanced CKD, because of concerns of volume retention. Careful attention should be given to volume status of patients, because thiazolidinediones can cause fluid retention, hemodilution, and exacerbation of heart failure.[84]

Incretin Mimetics

Glucagonlike peptide 1 (GLP-1) is an incretin that increases glucose-dependent insulin secretion. It also slows gastric emptying and increases satiety, and thus decreases food intake.[85] Exenatide and liraglutide are the GLP-1 analogues available in the United States. Use of an exenatide is not recommended in patients with creatinine clearance less than 30 mL/min, or in those on dialysis.[84] Close monitoring is required while initiating or up-titrating the dose of exenatide, especially in patients with mild to moderate renal dysfunction, because use of exenatide is associated with nausea and vomiting, and potential for volume depletion and worsening of renal function. No renal dose adjustment is required for liraglutide, and it can be used safely in patients with CKD or ESRD, although attention to volume status is warranted because of associated nausea and vomiting.[84]

Dipeptidylpeptidase-4 Inhibitors

Dipeptidylpeptidase-4 (DPP-4) inhibitors inhibit DPP-4 and thus prevent degradation of GLP-1. Sitagliptin, linagliptin, saxagliptin, and alogliptin are the DPP-4 inhibitors available in the United States. The dose of sitagliptin and alogliptin needs to be decreased by 50% and 75% for GFR 50 to 30 mL/min/1.73 m^2 and less than 30 mL/min/1.73 m^2, respectively.[84] Saxagliptin can be dosed at 2.5 to 5 mg daily if the GFR is greater than 50, but for patients with lower GFR or ESRD, a dose of 2.5 mg/d should be used.[87] No dosage adjustment is required in patients with CKD for linagliptin.[88]

Amylin Analogue

Amylin is secreted along with insulin by pancreatic β cells. Pramlintide is a synthetic analogue of amylin, and preprandial administration of pramlintide is associated with decreased plasma glucagon, slower gastric emptying, and increased satiety.[85] This medication is metabolized primarily in the kidney, but no change in dose is required if the creatinine clearance is more than 20 mL/min/1.73 m^2. Data are lacking to recommend use of pramlintide in patients on dialysis.[84]

Sodium Glucose Cotransporter 2 Inhibitors

Sodium glucose cotransporter 2 (SGLT2) inhibitors decrease renal threshold for glucose and induce glucuresis independent of insulin action. These agents induce renal excretion of glucose and have the potential to cause weight loss, by disposing excess calories/glucose.[89] Canagliflozin is an SGLT2 inhibitor that has been recently approved in the United States. Its efficacy in patients with diabetes and stage 3 CKD (eGFR ≥30 and <50 mL/min/1.73 m^2) has been shown in a placebo-controlled randomized, controlled trial.[90] Efficacy of canagliflozin depends on renal function and this drug is not expected to be effective in patients with eGFR less than 30 mL/min/1.73 m^2 or in those on dialysis.[90] SGLT2 inhibitors have an osmotic diuretic effect and can lead to plasma volume depletion, so kidney function should be monitored while initiating this drug in patients with DKD.

Many new therapeutic agents have been introduced for treatment of diabetes in patients with or without CKD, but special attention to renal function is warranted when choosing the appropriate agent, and dose adjustments should be made to prevent any deleterious effects.

SUMMARY

Diabetes is increasingly prevalent and is an important cause of CKD and ESRD. Recently, attention has been focused on DKD without albuminuria, and its pathogenesis is being studied. There are some indications that pathogenesis of diabetic nephropathy, in the absence of albuminuria, might differ from that of traditional diabetic nephropathy with microalbuminuria. Review of recent trial data indicates that better glycemic and blood pressure control can delay the onset and slow the progression of kidney disease in patients with diabetes. Use of several older oral hypoglycemic agents is either contraindicated or requires dosage adjustment in CKD. New medications for diabetes have been approved recently and many can be used safely in patients with CKD, thus providing treatment alternatives for better glycemic control in patients who are reluctant to use insulin. We further suggest that DKD should be considered in a broader context of cardiorenal metabolic syndrome rather than just diabetes, and close attention should be paid to other modifiable cardiorenal risk factors.

REFERENCES

1. Coresh J, Selvin E, Stevens LA, et al. Prevalence of chronic kidney disease in the United States. JAMA 2007;298:2038–47.

2. Reeves WB, Rawal BB, Abdel-Rahman EM, et al. Therapeutic modalities in diabetic nephropathy: future approaches. Open J Nephrol 2012;2:5–18.

3. Molitch ME, DeFronzo RA, Franz MJ, et al. Nephropathy in diabetes. Diabetes Care 2004;27:S79–83.

4. Whaley-Connell A, Chaudhary K, Misra M, et al. A case for early screening for diabetic kidney disease. Cardiorenal Med 2011;1:235–42.

5. Centers for Disease Control and Prevention. National chronic kidney disease fact sheet 2010. Available at: http://www.cdc.gov/diabetes/pubs/factsheets/kidney.htm. Accessed April 5, 2013.

6. Matsushita K, van der Velde M, Astor BC, et al. Association of estimated glomerular filtration rate and albuminuria with all-cause and cardiovascular mortality in general population cohorts: a collaborative meta-analysis. Lancet 2010;375:2073–81.

7. Sowers JR. Metabolic risk factors and renal disease. Kidney Int 2007;71:719–20.

8. Wada J, Makino H. Inflammation and the pathogenesis of diabetic nephropathy. Clin Sci 2013;124:139–52.

9. Najafian B, Alpers CE, Fogo AB. Pathology of human diabetic nephropathy. Contrib Nephrol 2011;170:36–47.

10. Tervaert TW, Mooyaart AL, Amann K, et al. Pathologic classification of diabetic nephropathy. J Am Soc Nephrol 2010;21:556–63.

11. Sowers JR, Whaley-Connell A, Hayden MR. The role of overweight and obesity in the cardiorenal syndrome. Cardiorenal Med 2011;1:5–12.

12. Jindal A, Brietzke S, Sowers JR. Obesity and the cardiorenal metabolic syndrome: therapeutic modalities and their efficacy in improving cardiovascular and renal risk factors. Cardiorenal Med 2012;2:314–27.

13. Bakris G, Vassalotti J, Ritz E, et al. National Kidney Foundation consensus conference on cardiovascular and kidney diseases and diabetes risk: an integrated therapeutic approach to reduce events. Kidney Int 2010;78:726–36.

14. Whaley-Connell A, Pavey BS, Afroze A, et al. Obesity and insulin resistance as risk factors for chronic kidney disease. J Cardiometab Syndr 2006;1:209–14.

15. US Renal Data System. USRDS 2010 annual data report: atlas of chronic kidney disease and end-stage renal disease in the United States. Bethesda (MD): National Institutes of Health, National Institute of Diabetes and Digestive and Kidney Diseases; 2010.

16. Sarnak MJ, Levey AS, Schoolwerth AC, et al. Kidney disease as a risk factor for development of cardiovascular disease: a statement from the American Heart Association Councils on Kidney in Cardiovascular Disease, High Blood Pressure Research, Clinical Cardiology, and Epidemiology and Prevention. Circulation 2003;108:2154–69.

17. Go AS, Chertow GM, Fan D, et al. Chronic kidney disease and the risks of death, cardiovascular events, and hospitalization. N Engl J Med 2004;351:1296–305.

18. Anavekar NS, McMurray JJ, Velazquez EJ, et al. Relation between renal dysfunction and cardiovascular outcomes after myocardial infarction. N Engl J Med 2004;351:1285–95.

19. Jindal A, Connell AW, Sowers JR. Type 2 diabetes in older people: the importance of blood pressure control. Curr Cardiovasc Risk Rep 2013;7(3):233–7.

20. de Galan BE, Perkovic V, Ninomiya T, et al. Lowering blood pressure reduces renal events in type 2 diabetes. J Am Soc Nephrol 2009;20:883–92.

21. Tight blood pressure control and risk of macrovascular and microvascular complications in type 2 diabetes: UKPDS 38. UK Prospective Diabetes Study Group. BMJ 1998;317:703–13.

22. Schrier RW, Estacio RO, Esler A, et al. Effects of aggressive blood pressure control in normotensive type 2 diabetic patients on albuminuria, retinopathy and strokes. Kidney Int 2002;61:1086–97.
23. Ruggenenti P, Perna A, Ganeva M, et al. Impact of blood pressure control and angiotensin-converting enzyme inhibitor therapy on new-onset microalbuminuria in type 2 diabetes: a post hoc analysis of the BENEDICT trial. J Am Soc Nephrol 2006;17:3472–81.
24. Pickering TG, Kario K. Nocturnal non-dipping: what does it augur? Curr Opin Nephrol Hypertens 2001;10:611–6.
25. Nielsen FS, Hansen HP, Jacobsen P, et al. Increased sympathetic activity during sleep and nocturnal hypertension in type 2 diabetic patients with diabetic nephropathy. Diabet Med 1999;16:555–62.
26. Ohkubo T, Hozawa A, Yamaguchi J, et al. Prognostic significance of the nocturnal decline in blood pressure in individuals with and without high 24-h blood pressure: the Ohasama study. J Hypertens 2002;20:2183–9.
27. Rossing P, Hougaard P, Parving HH. Risk factors for development of incipient and overt diabetic nephropathy in type 1 diabetic patients: a 10-year prospective observational study. Diabetes Care 2002;25:859–64.
28. Gall MA, Hougaard P, Borch-Johnsen K, et al. Risk factors for development of incipient and overt diabetic nephropathy in patients with non-insulin dependent diabetes mellitus: prospective, observational study. BMJ 1997;314:783–8.
29. Parving HH. Renoprotection in diabetes: genetic and non-genetic risk factors and treatment. Diabetologia 1998;41:745–59.
30. Rothwell PM. Limitations of the usual blood-pressure hypothesis and importance of variability, instability, and episodic hypertension. Lancet 2010;375:938–48.
31. Rossignol P, Kessler M, Zannad F. Visit-to-visit blood pressure variability and risk for progression of cardiovascular and renal diseases. Curr Opin Nephrol Hypertens 2013;22:59–64.
32. Webb AJ, Fischer U, Mehta Z, et al. Effects of antihypertensive-drug class on interindividual variation in blood pressure and risk of stroke: a systematic review and meta-analysis. Lancet 2010;375:906–15.
33. Kilpatrick ES, Rigby AS, Atkin SL. The role of blood pressure variability in the development of nephropathy in type 1 diabetes. Diabetes Care 2010;33:2442–7.
34. Okada H, Fukui M, Tanaka M, et al. Visit-to-visit blood pressure variability is a novel risk factor for the development and progression of diabetic nephropathy in patients with type 2 diabetes. Diabetes Care 2013;36(7):1908–22.
35. Rothwell PM, Howard SC, Dolan E, et al. Prognostic significance of visit-to-visit variability, maximum systolic blood pressure, and episodic hypertension. Lancet 2010;375:895–905.
36. Di Iorio B, Pota A, Sirico ML, et al. Blood pressure variability and outcomes in chronic kidney disease. Nephrol Dial Transplant 2012;27:4404–10.
37. Hsieh YT, Tu ST, Cho TJ, et al. Visit-to-visit variability in blood pressure strongly predicts all-cause mortality in patients with type 2 diabetes: a 5.5-year prospective analysis. Eur J Clin Invest 2012;42:245–53.
38. Okada H, Fukui M, Tanaka M, et al. Visit-to-visit variability in systolic blood pressure is correlated with diabetic nephropathy and atherosclerosis in patients with type 2 diabetes. Atherosclerosis 2012;220:155–9.
39. Muntner P, Shimbo D, Tonelli M, et al. The relationship between visit-to-visit variability in systolic blood pressure and all-cause mortality in the general population: findings from NHANES III, 1988 to 1994. Hypertension 2011;57:160–6.

40. Clark CE, Taylor RS, Shore AC, et al. Association of a difference in systolic blood pressure between arms with vascular disease and mortality: a systematic review and meta-analysis. Lancet 2012;379:905–14.

41. Okada H, Fukui M, Tanaka M, et al. A difference in systolic blood pressure between arms and between lower limbs is a novel risk marker for diabetic nephropathy in patients with type 2 diabetes. Hypertens Res 2013;17:207.

42. Ravid M, Brosh D, Levi Z, et al. Use of enalapril to attenuate decline in renal function in normotensive, normoalbuminuric patients with type 2 diabetes mellitus. A randomized, controlled trial. Ann Intern Med 1998;128:982–8.

43. Parving HH, Lehnert H, Brochner-Mortensen J, et al. The effect of irbesartan on the development of diabetic nephropathy in patients with type 2 diabetes. N Engl J Med 2001;345:870–8.

44. Lewis EJ, Hunsicker LG, Clarke WR, et al. Renoprotective effect of the angiotensin-receptor antagonist irbesartan in patients with nephropathy due to type 2 diabetes. N Engl J Med 2001;345:851–60.

45. Haller H, Ito S, Izzo JL Jr, et al. Olmesartan for the delay or prevention of microalbuminuria in type 2 diabetes. N Engl J Med 2011;364:907–17.

46. Brenner BM, Cooper ME, de Zeeuw D, et al. Effects of losartan on renal and cardiovascular outcomes in patients with type 2 diabetes and nephropathy. N Engl J Med 2001;345:861–9.

47. Barnett AH, Bain SC, Bouter P, et al. Angiotensin-receptor blockade versus converting-enzyme inhibition in type 2 diabetes and nephropathy. N Engl J Med 2004;351:1952–61.

48. Mann JF, Schmieder RE, McQueen M, et al. Renal outcomes with telmisartan, ramipril, or both, in people at high vascular risk (the ONTARGET study): a multicentre, randomised, double-blind, controlled trial. Lancet 2008;372:547–53.

49. Mak RH. Impact of end-stage renal disease and dialysis on glycemic control. Semin Dial 2000;13(1):4–8.

50. Kovesdy CP, Park JC, Kalantar-Zadeh K. Glycemic control and burnt-out diabetes in ESRD. Semin Dial 2010;23:148–56.

51. Ansari A, Thomas S, Goldsmith D. Assessing glycemic control in patients with diabetes and end-stage renal failure. Am J Kidney Dis 2003;41:523–31.

52. Koga M, Murai J, Saito H, et al. Glycated albumin and glycated hemoglobin are influenced differently by endogenous insulin secretion in patients with type 2 diabetes. Diabetes Care 2010;33:270–2.

53. Kovesdy CP, Sharma K, Kalantar-Zadeh K. Glycemic control in diabetic CKD patients: where do we stand? Am J Kidney Dis 2008;52:766–77.

54. Levey AS, Stevens LA, Schmid CH, et al. A new equation to estimate glomerular filtration rate. Ann Intern Med 2009;150:604–12.

55. Dinneen SF, Gerstein HC. The association of microalbuminuria and mortality in non-insulin-dependent diabetes mellitus. A systematic overview of the literature. Arch Intern Med 1997;157:1413–8.

56. Jensen T, Borch-Johnsen K, Kofoed-Enevoldsen A, et al. Coronary heart disease in young type 1 (insulin-dependent) diabetic patients with and without diabetic nephropathy: incidence and risk factors. Diabetologia 1987;30:144–8.

57. Hoefield RA, Kalra PA, Baker PG, et al. The use of eGFR and ACR to predict decline in renal function in people with diabetes. Nephrol Dial Transplant 2011;26:887–92.

58. Hallan SI, Ritz E, Lydersen S, et al. Combining GFR and albuminuria to classify CKD improves prediction of ESRD. J Am Soc Nephrol 2009;20:1069–77.

59. Solini A, Penno G, Bonora E, et al. Diverging association of reduced glomerular filtration rate and albuminuria with coronary and noncoronary events in patients with type 2 diabetes: the renal insufficiency and cardiovascular events (RIACE) Italian multicenter study. Diabetes Care 2012;35:143–9.
60. Garg AX, Clark WF, Haynes RB, et al. Moderate renal insufficiency and the risk of cardiovascular mortality: results from the NHANES I. Kidney Int 2002;61: 1486–94.
61. Culleton BF, Larson MG, Wilson PW, et al. Cardiovascular disease and mortality in a community-based cohort with mild renal insufficiency. Kidney Int 1999;56: 2214–9.
62. Drey N, Roderick P, Mullee M, et al. A population-based study of the incidence and outcomes of diagnosed chronic kidney disease. Am J Kidney Dis 2003;42: 677–84.
63. Muntner P, He J, Hamm L, et al. Renal insufficiency and subsequent death resulting from cardiovascular disease in the United States. J Am Soc Nephrol 2002;13:745–53.
64. Nakamura K, Okamura T, Hayakawa T, et al. Chronic kidney disease is a risk factor for cardiovascular death in a community-based population in Japan: NIPPON DATA90. Circ J 2006;70:954–9.
65. Manjunath G, Tighiouart H, Coresh J, et al. Level of kidney function as a risk factor for cardiovascular outcomes in the elderly. Kidney Int 2003;63:1121–9.
66. Manjunath G, Tighiouart H, Ibrahim H, et al. Level of kidney function as a risk factor for atherosclerotic cardiovascular outcomes in the community. J Am Coll Cardiol 2003;41:47–55.
67. Ninomiya T, Perkovic V, de Galan BE, et al. Albuminuria and kidney function independently predict cardiovascular and renal outcomes in diabetes. J Am Soc Nephrol 2009;20:1813–21.
68. Retnakaran R, Cull CA, Thorne KI, et al. Risk factors for renal dysfunction in type 2 diabetes: U.K. Prospective Diabetes Study 74. Diabetes 2006;55:1832–9.
69. MacIsaac RJ, Panagiotopoulos S, McNeil KJ, et al. Is nonalbuminuric renal insufficiency in type 2 diabetes related to an increase in intrarenal vascular disease? Diabetes care 2006;29:1560–6.
70. Kramer HJ, Nguyen QD, Curhan G, et al. Renal insufficiency in the absence of albuminuria and retinopathy among adults with type 2 diabetes mellitus. JAMA 2003;289:3273–7.
71. Yagil C, Barak A, Ben-Dor D, et al. Nonproteinuric diabetes-associated nephropathy in the Cohen rat model of type 2 diabetes. Diabetes 2005;54: 1487–96.
72. Dwyer JP, Parving HH, Hunsicker LG, et al. Renal dysfunction in the presence of normoalbuminuria in type 2 diabetes: results from the DEMAND study. Cardiorenal Med 2012;2:1–10.
73. Penno G, Solini A, Bonora E, et al. Clinical significance of nonalbuminuric renal impairment in type 2 diabetes. J Hypertens 2011;29:1802–9.
74. Bash LD, Selvin E, Steffes M, et al. Poor glycemic control in diabetes and the risk of incident chronic kidney disease even in the absence of albuminuria and retinopathy: Atherosclerosis Risk in Communities (ARIC) Study. Arch Intern Med 2008;168:2440–7.
75. MacIsaac RJ, Tsalamandris C, Panagiotopoulos S, et al. Nonalbuminuric renal insufficiency in type 2 diabetes. Diabetes Care 2004;27:195–200.
76. Intensive blood-glucose control with sulphonylureas or insulin compared with conventional treatment and risk of complications in patients with type 2 diabetes

(UKPDS 33). UK Prospective Diabetes Study (UKPDS) Group. Lancet 1998;352: 837–53.

77. Holman RR, Paul SK, Bethel MA, et al. 10-year follow-up of intensive glucose control in type 2 diabetes. N Engl J Med 2008;359:1577–89.

78. Patel A, MacMahon S, Chalmers J, et al. Intensive blood glucose control and vascular outcomes in patients with type 2 diabetes. N Engl J Med 2008;358: 2560–72.

79. The effect of intensive treatment of diabetes on the development and progression of long-term complications in insulin-dependent diabetes mellitus. The Diabetes Control and Complications Trial Research Group. N Engl J Med 1993;329: 977–86.

80. Writing Team for the Diabetes Control and Complications Trial/Epidemiology of Diabetes Interventions and Complications Research Group. Sustained effect of intensive treatment of type 1 diabetes mellitus on development and progression of diabetic nephropathy: the Epidemiology of Diabetes Interventions and Complications (EDIC) study. JAMA 2003;290:2159–67.

81. de Boer IH, Sun W, Cleary PA, et al. Intensive diabetes therapy and glomerular filtration rate in type 1 diabetes. N Engl J Med 2011;365:2366–76.

82. de Boer IH, Rue TC, Cleary PA, et al. Long-term renal outcomes of patients with type 1 diabetes mellitus and microalbuminuria: an analysis of the Diabetes Control and Complications Trial/Epidemiology of Diabetes Interventions and Complications cohort. Arch Intern Med 2011;171:412–20.

83. Alter ML, Ott IM, von Websky K, et al. DPP-4 inhibition on top of angiotensin receptor blockade offers a new therapeutic approach for diabetic nephropathy. Kidney Blood Press Res 2012;36:119–30.

84. Abe M, Okada K, Soma M. Antidiabetic agents in patients with chronic kidney disease and end-stage renal disease on dialysis: metabolism and clinical practice. Curr Drug Metab 2011;12:57–69.

85. Rodbard HW, Jellinger PS, Davidson JA, et al. Statement by an American Association of Clinical Endocrinologists/American College of Endocrinology consensus panel on type 2 diabetes mellitus: an algorithm for glycemic control. Endocr Pract 2009;15:540–59.

86. Hanefeld M, Schaper F. Acarbose: oral anti-diabetes drug with additional cardiovascular benefits. Expert Rev Cardiovasc Ther 2008;6:153–63.

87. Boulton DW, Li L, Frevert EU, et al. Influence of renal or hepatic impairment on the pharmacokinetics of saxagliptin. Clin Pharmacokinet 2011;50:253–65.

88. Friedrich C, Emser A, Woerle HJ, et al. Renal impairment has no clinically relevant effect on the long-term exposure of linagliptin in patients with type 2 diabetes. Am J Ther 2013;13:13.

89. Whaley JM, Tirmenstein M, Reilly TP, et al. Targeting the kidney and glucose excretion with dapagliflozin: preclinical and clinical evidence for SGLT2 inhibition as a new option for treatment of type 2 diabetes mellitus. Diabetes Metab Syndr Obes 2012;5:135–48.

90. Yale JF, Bakris G, Cariou B, et al. Efficacy and safety of canagliflozin in subjects with type 2 diabetes and chronic kidney disease. Diabetes Obes Metab 2013; 15:463–73.

Obesity and Diabetic Kidney Disease

Christine Maric-Bilkan, PhD

KEYWORDS

- Kidney • Obesity • Diabetes • Proteinuria • Hyperfiltration • Hypertension
- Glomerulopathy • Diabetic nephropathy

KEY POINTS

- The prevalence of obesity has risen to epidemic proportions and continues to be a major health problem worldwide.
- The high prevalence of obesity is closely linked to the increased incidence of several chronic diseases, including type 2 diabetes, hypertension, and cardiovascular disease.
- Obesity, type 2 diabetes, hypertension, and cardiovascular disease are all risk factors for chronic kidney disease (CKD) and end-stage renal disease (ESRD).
- The mechanisms by which obesity independently, or in concert with type 2 diabetes and hypertension, contributes to the development and/or progression of ESRD are not completely understood.

INTRODUCTION

The prevalence of obesity (body mass index [BMI] ≥ 30 kg/m^2) has risen to epidemic proportions and continues to be a major health problem worldwide.[1-3] The high prevalence of obesity is closely linked to the increased incidence of several chronic diseases, including type 2 diabetes, hypertension, and cardiovascular disease.[2,4-8] Obesity, type 2 diabetes, hypertension, and cardiovascular disease are all risk factors for chronic kidney disease (CKD) and end-stage renal disease (ESRD),[9-13] inasmuch as the presence of 1 or more of these risk factors multiplies the overall risk for disease development and progression (**Fig. 1**). In addition, evidence suggests that obesity may also increase the risk of ESRD independently of type 2 diabetes and hypertension.[14-16] However, the precise mechanisms by which obesity independently, or in concert with type 2 diabetes and hypertension, contributes to the development and/or progression of CKD and ESRD are not completely understood.

This article originally appeared in Medical Clinics of North America, Volume 97, Issue 1, January 2013.
The authors acknowledge the financial support of NIH/NIDDK (RO1DK075832 to C. Maric-Bilkan).
Department of Physiology and Biophysics, University of Mississippi Medical Center, 2500 North State Street, Jackson, MS 39216-4505, USA
E-mail address: cmaric@umc.edu

Clinics Collections 1 (2014) 203–218
http://dx.doi.org/10.1016/j.ccol.2014.08.013

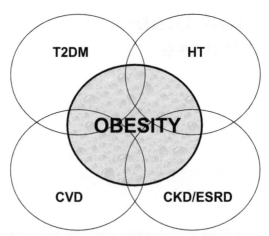

Fig. 1. Clustering of risk factors for obesity-related renal disease. Obesity, type 2 diabetes (T2DM), hypertension (HT), and cardiovascular disease (CVD) are all risk factors for chronic kidney disease (CKD) and end-stage renal disease (ESRD). The presence of 1 or more of these risk factors multiplies the overall risk for disease development and progression.

The two leading causes of ESRD are type 2 diabetes and hypertension, which together account for more than 70% of patients with ESRD.[17,18] Because the growing prevalence of obesity is a major driving force for the continued increase in the prevalence of type 2 diabetes,[7,19] it is often difficult to separate out the individual contribution of either obesity, type 2 diabetes, or hypertension to the development of ESRD. The pathophysiology of type 2 diabetes–related renal disease (ie, diabetic nephropathy) and obesity-related renal disease is almost identical. They both evolve in a sequence of stages beginning with initial increases in glomerular filtration rate (GFR) and intraglomerular capillary pressure (P_{Gc}), glomerular hypertrophy, and microalbuminuria.[20,21] Increased systolic blood pressure further exacerbates the disease progression to proteinuria, nodular glomerulosclerosis, and tubulointerstitial injury and a decrease in GFR leading to ESRD.[22,23] Diabetes-related and obesity-related renal disease also have common initiating events, which include interactions among multiple metabolic and hemodynamic factors that activate common intracellular signaling pathways that in turn trigger the production of cytokines and growth factors, leading to renal disease. The purpose of this review is to provide perspectives regarding the mechanisms by which obesity may lead to ESRD and to discuss prevention strategies and the treatment of obesity-related renal disease.

EPIDEMIOLOGY OF OBESITY AND DIABETES-RELATED KIDNEY DISEASE
Prevalence of Obesity and Type 2 Diabetes

Based on the most recent report from the National Health and Nutrition Examination Survey (NHANES) examining obesity prevalence among US adults, adolescents, and children, more than one-third of adults and almost 17% of children and adolescents were obese in 2009/2010.[24,25] Although there has been a significant increase in obesity prevalence among men and boys over the last decade, no changes were seen among women and girls. The prevalence of obesity is 35.5% among adult men, 35.8% among adult women, and 16.9% amongst children and adolescents of both sexes. Thus, the Healthy People 2010 goals of 15% obesity among adults and 5% obesity among children are far from being met.

Similar to obesity, the global prevalence of type 2 diabetes has more than doubled in the last 30 years and is predicted to continue to increase at an alarming rate. According to the World Health Organization, in 2008, almost 350 million people worldwide have diabetes, 90% of whom have type 2 diabetes.[26] Although the major driving force for the increase in the prevalence of type 2 diabetes is obesity, other factors, including genetic and environmental factors, are also important contributors to the development of type 2 diabetes. Accumulating evidence suggests that this markedly high prevalence of both obesity and type 2 diabetes contributes to the increased incidence of chronic diseases, including CKD and ESRD.[9-13]

Obesity, Diabetes, and CKD

Obesity is a well-recognized risk factor for both type 2 diabetes and hypertension, which are leading causes of CKD and ESRD.[27] Analysis of data from the Framingham Heart Study, which included more than 2600 patients with no CKD at baseline, showed an increased risk of developing stage 3 CKD in obese (BMI $\geq$30 kg/m^2) but not overweight (BMI 25–30 kg/m^2) patients after 18.5 years of follow-up.[9] However, this relationship was no longer significant after adjustment for known cardiovascular disease risk factors, including diabetes and hypertension. Numerous other studies have also demonstrated that the association between obesity and CKD is mediated through risk factors including diabetes, hypertension, and other elements of the metabolic syndrome.[10,16,28-30]

Although studies clearly indicate that the high risk of obesity-related CKD is driven by diabetes and hypertension, there are several other studies that suggest that obesity can lead to the development of CKD independently of either diabetes or hypertension. Specifically, the data from the Hypertension Detection and Follow-Up Program show that, in a cohort of 5897 patients with hypertension and no CKD at baseline, the incidence of CKD after a 5-year follow-up was 28% in patients with normal BMI, 31% in overweight patients, and 34% in obese patients.[16] This risk for CKD persisted in the overweight and obese patients even after adjustment for covariates, including type 2 diabetes, suggesting that obesity increases the risk of CKD independently of type 2 diabetes. Also supporting the notion that obesity increases the risk of CKD independently of diabetes and hypertension is the Physician's Health Study, a large cohort of initially healthy men, in which BMI was associated with increased risk for CKD over 14 years.[31] Furthermore, in 74,986 prehypertensive individuals participating in the first Health Study in Nord-Trøndelag in Norway, the risk of CKD over 21 years was shown to increase dramatically with obesity.[32] In addition to increasing the risk of CKD, obesity has also been suggested to have a higher rate of decline of GFR and progress faster to ESRD.[33]

Obesity, Diabetes, and ESRD

Several studies have shown that increased BMI is an independent risk factor for ESRD. In a cohort of 320,252 adult patients of Kaiser Permanente who were followed for 15 to 35 years, BMI was found to be a strong and common risk factor for ESRD.[10] This relationship between BMI and ESRD persisted even after controlling for baseline blood pressure and diabetes. Similarly, in a population-based, case-control study in Sweden, obesity was shown to be an important and potentially preventable risk factor for ESRD.[11] This study also showed that the coexistence of obesity and diabetes doubled the risk of new onset kidney disease. One study compared the temporal trends in mean BMI and obesity prevalence among incident ESRD by year of dialysis initiated between 1995 and 2002, and these trends were compared with those in the US population during this same period.[34] This study found that among incident patients with ESRD, mean BMI at the start of dialysis increased from 25.7 to 27.5 kg/m^2, and total obesity and stage 2 obesity increased by 33 and 63%, respectively. The slope of mean BMI at initiation of dialysis over the 8 years of follow-up was ~2-fold higher in the incident ESRD population compared with the US population for all age groups.[34]

In contrast to most of the studies suggesting that obesity is a risk factor for CKD and ESRD, some studies have reported that high BMI is associated with greater survival in patients on maintenance hemodialysis.[35,36] This phenomenon, commonly referred to as the obesity paradox, reasons that in patients receiving long-term hemodialysis, larger body size (ie, larger BMI) with more muscle mass (ie, higher serum creatinine concentration) is associated with greater survival. These observations indicate that it is the increase in muscle mass rather than increase in total body weight that confers protection, suggesting that BMI may not always be the most reliable index of CKD risk, at least in certain patient populations. Other studies indicate that visceral or central obesity, but not BMI, is associated with incident CKD[37] and increased cardiovascular disease in patients with CKD.[38] Thus, it is conceivable that overall weight loss with a concomitant increase in muscle mass may be an effective treatment strategy in preventing obesity-associated CKD and ESRD.

PATHOPHYSIOLOGY OF OBESITY AND DIABETES-RELATED KIDNEY DISEASE

Obesity-related renal disease, similar to diabetes-related renal disease, is associated with physiologic, anatomic, and pathologic changes in the kidney (**Fig. 2**). Both obesity and diabetes renal disease evolve in a sequence of stages beginning with initial increases in GFR and P_{Gc}, glomerular hypertrophy, and microalbuminuria.[20,21] Increased systolic blood pressure further exacerbates the disease progression to proteinuria, nodular glomerulosclerosis and tubulointerstitial injury, and a decline in GFR leading to ESRD.[22,23] Obesity-related and diabetes-related renal disease also share common initiating events, which include interactions among multiple metabolic

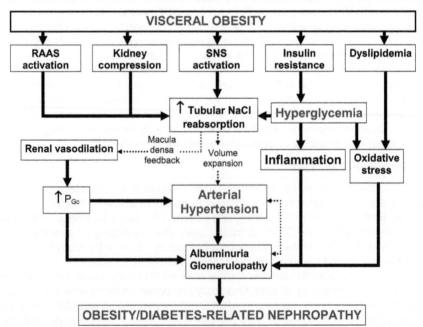

Fig. 2. Interaction between metabolic and hemodynamic pathways in the pathophysiology of obesity-related and diabetes-related renal disease. P_{Gc}, intraglomerular capillary pressure; RAAS, renin angiotensin aldosterone system; SNS, sympathetic nervous system.

and hemodynamic factors that activate common intracellular signaling pathways that in turn trigger the production of cytokines and growth factors, leading to renal disease (**Fig. 3**).

Obesity, Diabetes, and Glomerular Hemodynamics

Experimental studies in diet-induced obese dogs and genetically induced obese rats show that one of the earliest changes in renal hemodynamics in response to the obese state is glomerular hyperfiltration. Specifically, dogs fed a high-fat diet for only 5 to 6 weeks and obese Zucker rats show an increase in GFR.[39,40] These changes in GFR are reversible, at least in the obese Zucker rats, in which food restriction was associated with attenuation of glomerular hyperfiltration, possibly due to decreased protein intake or overall weight loss.[40] These observations in experimental models have also been confirmed in obese humans. Studies have shown that obese individuals have around 50% higher GFR compared with lean individuals.[41] Although there is still some debate about the mechanisms underlying obesity-related glomerular hyperfiltration, the most likely explanation is increased sodium reabsorption by the proximal tubule or loop of Henle, leading to tubuloglomerular feedback (TGF)–mediated reduction in afferent arteriolar resistance, increased P_{Gc}, and thus increased GFR.[42] This TGF-driven dilation of afferent arterioles and resultant impairment of renal autoregulation, in turn, allows increases in blood pressure to be transmitted to the glomerulus causing further increases in P_{Gc} and subsequent glomerular injury.[43] This may be especially important in individuals with a reduced number of nephrons in whom there is a greater risk of enhanced glomerular blood pressure transmission due to the substantially greater preglomerular vasodilation.[43] There is also evidence for increased activation of the renin-angiotensin-aldosterone system (RAAS) and increased renal sympathetic tone as important stimuli for increased sodium reabsorption exacerbating the renal hemodynamic changes associated with obesity.[44–46]

It is generally believed that the initial increase in GFR associated with obesity likely serves as an early compensatory response that allows for restoration of salt balance despite continued increases in tubular reabsorption. However, in the long term, glomerular hyperfiltration may contribute to the development of renal injury, especially

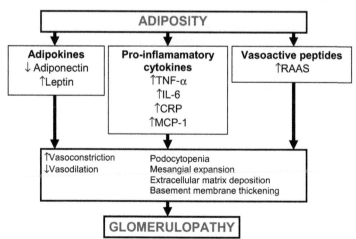

Fig. 3. Mechanisms of obesity-related glomerulopathy. CRP, C-reactive protein; IL-6, interleukin-6; MCP-1, monocyte chemoattractant protein-1; RAAS, renin angiotensin aldosterone system; TNF-α, tumor necrosis factor α.

if combined with hypertension. Studies supporting this notion show that weight loss reduces glomerular hyperfiltration and subsequent renal injury.[41,47]

Similar to obesity-associated glomerular hyperfiltration, renal vasodilation and increases in GFR and P_{Gc} also characterize the early stages of diabetes-associated renal disease.[48] Although the precise mechanisms underlying diabetes-associated glomerular hyperfiltration remain inconclusive, it is believed that mechanisms similar to those occurring in obesity drive the initial increase in GFR. Specifically, reduced delivery of salt to the macula densa, as a consequence of increased proximal reabsorption of glucose and sodium, reduces afferent arteriolar resistance leading to increased P_{Gc} and GFR via attenuated TGF.[49–51] In addition, afferent vasodilation and efferent vasoconstriction in response to circulating or locally formed vasoactive factors (eg, angiotensin II (Ang II) and endothelin) produced in response to hyperglycemia or shear stress are also believed to contribute to the development of diabetes-associated glomerular hyperfiltration.[52,53]

Although most studies suggest that the mechanisms underlying glomerular hyperfiltration due to obesity and diabetes are similar, there is some evidence to suggest that hyperglycemia and obesity may have at least partially additive effects on glomerular hemodynamics. Because obesity and diabetes coexist with elements of the metabolic syndrome, including hypertension, it is often difficult to separate the effects of each element on glomerular hemodynamics and progression of renal injury, at least in humans. However, experimental studies provide some mechanistic insights. Specifically, mice lacking the gene for the melanocortin-4 receptor are obese, hyperinsulinemic, and hyperleptinemic but normotensive at 55 weeks of age and exhibit moderately increased GFR compared with their wild-type counterparts.[54] However, when rendered hypertensive via treatment with N(G)-nitro-L-arginine methyl ester (L-NAME), they develop prominent glomerular hyperfiltration, suggesting that increases in blood pressure may exacerbate obesity-related increases in GFR. These data support the concept of a synergistic effect of various components of obesity, metabolic syndrome, diabetes, and hypertension on glomerular hemodynamics.

Although the early stages of obesity-related and diabetes-related renal disease are characterized by glomerular hyperfiltration, one of the hallmarks of the advanced stages of the disease is the decline in GFR. Unlike studies examining the mechanisms underlying glomerular hyperfiltration, much less is known about the mechanisms underlying the decline in GFR characteristic of advanced diabetic and obesity-related nephropathy. The main reason for this lack of knowledge is the lack of appropriate experimental models that mimic the advanced stages of the disease; most experimental models of obesity-related or diabetes-related renal injury never really develop overt nephropathy and are in a permanent state of glomerular hyperfiltration. However, the existing evidence suggests that obesity and diabetes are states of low-grade inflammation and oxidative stress, both of which may lead to kidney damage, progressive loss of nephrons, and decrease in GFR over time. In addition, hyperlipidemia has been linked to reduced GFR associated with advanced diabetic nephropathy. Several clinical studies have demonstrated the importance of lipid control in preserving GFR in patients with diabetes.[55] However, additional studies are warranted to examine whether the beneficial effects of lipid lowering in diabetes-related and obesity-related nephropathy are caused by improvement in the lipid profile or more direct renoprotection.

Hypertension as a Driving Force for Obesity-Related and Diabetes-Related Kidney Disease

The nearly linear relationship between BMI and blood pressure in diverse populations throughout the world[35,56–58] has led to the notion that obesity contributes to the development of hypertension. Numerous clinical, population, and basic research studies have shown that visceral obesity, the main driver of type 2 diabetes, increases blood pressure.[59,60] Data from the Framingham Heart Study and other population-based studies indicate that excess weight gain may account for as much as 78% of primary (essential) hypertension in men and 65% in women.[61,62] In addition, obese individuals have a 3.5-fold increase in the risk for developing hypertension.[56,63] Clinical studies also indicate that weight loss reduces blood pressure in most patients with hypertension and is effective in the primary prevention of hypertension.[60] Discussing the mechanisms underlying obesity-driven hypertension is beyond the scope of this review, but accumulating evidence suggests that physiologic, environmental, and genetic factors all contribute to obesity-related hypertension.[64] Given that the focus of this review is the contribution of obesity to the development of renal disease, the question to be asked is how does obesity-related hypertension lead to the development of renal disease?

Several studies have suggested that visceral (but not subcutaneous) obesity induces hypertension, initially by increasing renal tubular sodium reabsorption and causing a hypertensive shift of renal-pressure natriuresis via activation of multiple pathways including the sympathetic nervous system and the RAAS.[39,64,65] In addition, physical compression of the kidneys caused by visceral obesity has also been suggested to contribute to the increase in blood pressure, at least in some experimental models.[39] This increase in blood pressure, alongside increases in P_{Gc} and GFR (discussed later), and other metabolic abnormalities (eg, dyslipidemia, hyperglycemia) all likely interact to contribute to the initial renal insult. A similar sequence of events has been proposed to contribute to renal injury in the setting of type 2 diabetes, independent of obesity, suggesting that hypertension plays a major role in obesity as well as diabetes-associated renal disease. Hypertension, in addition to contributing to the initial development of renal injury is also an important factor in the disease progression. Progressive renal injury only occurs when hypertension is superimposed on obesity or diabetes.[54] The importance of tight blood pressure control for treating diabetic nephropathy is recognized in current guidelines, with a recommended target blood pressure of less than 130/80 mm Hg.[66] Several studies have shown clear renoprotection with respect to slowing progression of nephropathy in patients with type 2 diabetes by lowering blood pressure.[67–71]

Obesity, Diabetes, and Albuminuria

The earliest clinical manifestation of obesity-related and diabetes-related renal injury is microalbuminuria (30–300 mg/d) which, over time, can progresses to overt proteinuria (300–3000 mg/d).[72–74] Microalbuminuria, in turn, signifies increased risk of progression to ESRD and cardiovascular disease.[74] Studies in nondiabetic and diabetic overweight individuals have shown that increases in urine albumin excretion strongly correlate with increases in body weight and other markers of obesity, including BMI, waist circumference, and waist-to-hip ratio.[75–78] In the Prevention of Renal and Vascular End stage Disease (PREVEND) study, the prevalence of microalbuminuria in lean and obese individuals correlated with central obesity even after correction for confounding variables.[79] Retrospective analysis of the database of a population study showing that the prevalence of microalbuminuria increased from 9.5% in men with normal BMI to 18.3% in overweight men, and 29.3% in obese men further supports the notion of a direct correlation between BMI and microalbuminuria.[77] In a cross-sectional study of a cohort of African Americans, microalbuminuria was most prevalent in patients with newly diagnosed type 2 diabetes and was independently associated with BMI.[78] Others have shown that even moderate weight reduction in patients with type 2 diabetes with proteinuria reduces urine protein excretion by approximately 30%.[80] Furthermore, weight reduction achieved by either dietary caloric restriction or bariatric surgery has been shown to attenuate progression of proteinuria in obese nondiabetic individuals.[81,82]

The development of microalbuminuria in either nondiabetic or diabetic individuals was traditionally believed to result from damage to the glomerular filtration barrier as a consequence of an increase in blood pressure which is transmitted to the glomeruli, increasing P_{Gc} and GFR. In addition, in the setting of diabetes, hyperglycemia-associated inflammation and oxidative stress have been shown to contribute to the damage to the glomerular filtration barrier, contributing to increased leakage of protein across the ie membrane leading to the development of albuminuria.[72] In the setting of obesity, cytokines including adiponectin have been suggested to play a role in the development of albuminuria. Specifically, the adiponectin knockout mouse exhibits increased baseline albuminuria and podocyte foot process effacement, suggesting that adiponectin regulates podocyte function and thus contributes to the initial development of albuminuria.[83] Apart from the glomerulocentric view of the origin of albuminuria, a more recent theory on the mechanisms of albuminuria, especially in the setting of diabetes, is that the diabetic milieu also impairs proximal tubular reabsorption of albumin leading to increased urine albumin excretion.[84]

Obesity, Diabetes, and Glomerulopathy

Accompanying the hemodynamic changes, the early stage of obesity is associated with up to a 40% increase in kidney weight.[39,85] Histologically, the obese kidney is characterized by glomerulomegaly, mesangial expansion, and podocytopenia, leading to focal segmental glomerulosclerosis.[43,86,87] These features, which precede overt renal insufficiency, have been observed in biopsies from obese humans[88] and experimental models of obesity-related kidney disease, namely the obese Zucker rat[89,90] and dogs fed a high-fat diet.[39] However, the degree of glomerulosclerosis seems to be highly variable amongst different experimental models and obese individuals,[91] and some studies indicate that some obese individuals do not even develop glomerulosclerosis, despite the glomerulomegaly.[87] A review of native 6818 renal biopsies indicated that obesity-related glomerulopathy is characterized by lesser segmental sclerosis, less podocyte effacement, but more glomerulomegaly compared with idiopathic glomerulosclerosis.[91] However, despite the less pronounced glomerular lesions in obesity-related glomerulopathy, the long-term prognosis of the disease is just as poor. It has been reported that the probabilities of renal survival are 77% and 51% at 5 and 10 years, respectively,[92] and that nephron number may play a significant role in the renal prognosis.[93] Specifically, in patients with unilateral renal agenesis, the decline in renal function is most pronounced in obese patients, suggesting that obesity accelerates renal dysfunction in patients with severe reductions in renal mass.[93]

Similar to obesity-related glomerulopathy, early diabetic nephropathy is accompanied by hyperfiltration and microalbuminuria. Histologically, the diabetic kidney exhibits glomerular hypertrophy, widening of the glomerular basement membrane, mesangial expansion, podocytopenia leading to nodular (Kimmelstiel-Wilson) glomerulosclerosis, and tubulointerstitial fibrosis.[22] Thus, given the similarities in the histologic appearance of the renal lesions from diabetic and obese individuals, it is not surprising that the mechanisms underlying these changes have many similarities.

Mechanisms of Obesity-Related and Diabetes-Related Glomerulopathy

Obesity (ie, visceral adiposity) and diabetes (hyperglycemia) both promote a low-grade inflammatory state and are associated with infiltration of macrophages into the kidney.

The infiltrated macrophages, in turn, become a source of a whole host of proinflammatory mediators such as tumor necrosis factor-α (TNF-α), interleukin-6 (IL-6), C-reactive protein, monocyte chemoattractant protein-1, and macrophage migration inhibitory factor.[94,95] In addition, visceral fat releases adipokines such as adiponectin and leptin into the circulation which also play a role in the pathophysiology of renal injury.[95] Apart from adipokines and inflammatory mediators, vasoactive peptides such as Ang II also contribute to obesity-associated and diabetes-associated glomerulopathy.

Adiponectin
Obese humans are characterized by consistently low levels of circulating adiponectin. However, in patients with CKD and ESRD due to obesity or diabetes, adiponectin levels are increased, possibly because of impaired renal function.[96,97] Experimental studies have shown that genetic deletion of adiponectin is associated with albuminuria and podocyte effacement, which are further exacerbated by diabetes.[98] Treatment of these mice with exogenous adiponectin results in normalization of albuminuria, improvement of podocyte foot process effacement, increased activation of glomerular AMP-activated kinase, and reduced urinary and glomerular markers of oxidative stress.[83] These observations suggest that adiponectin may have a renoprotective effect.

Leptin
Although the primary action of leptin is to act on the satiety center to limit food intake, leptin has also been linked to renal disease. Circulating leptin levels are increased in CKD and in patients on hemodialysis.[99,100] Leptin levels are also typically increased in obese individuals. Mice overexpressing leptin have more renal disease than leptin-deficient mice.[101] Long-term infusion of recombinant leptin in rats is associated with proteinuria, increased expression of extracellular matrix proteins (collagen type IV), transforming growth factor-beta (TGF-β) and other proinflammatory cytokines, macrophage infiltration, and glomerulosclerosis.[102] These observations suggest that, unlike adiponectin, leptin promotes the development of renal injury in both obese and lean individuals.

Inflammatory markers
Both obesity and diabetes are characterized by increased levels of circulating cytokines, including TNF-α and IL-6,[103,104] and markers of inflammation are inversely associated with measures of kidney function and positively with albuminuria. It is believed that the major source of proinflammatory cytokines in obese and diabetic individuals that directly contribute to renal injury are infiltrated macrophages.[101] In addition, renal parenchyma has also been shown to release proinflammatory cytokines in response to hyperglycemia or locally active vasoactive peptides, such as Ang II.[105] Once released, these proinflammatory mediators contribute to a low-grade chronic inflammatory state that contributes to obesity-associated and diabetes-associated glomerulopathy. In particular, TNF-α has been shown to reduce the expression of key components of the slit diaphragm, nephrin and podocin, thus contributing to podocytopathy.[106] Similarly, IL-6 promotes the expression of adhesion molecules and subsequent oxidative stress,[107] whereas blocking the IL-6 receptor prevents progression of proteinuria, renal lipid deposition, and mesangial cell proliferation associated with severe hyperlipoproteinemia.[108] Thus, there is strong evidence for the contribution of inflammation in obesity-associated and diabetes-associated renal disease.

Other factors
Although several vasoactive peptides have been implicated in the pathogenesis of obesity-associated and diabetes-associated glomerulopathy, the most prominent,

and certainly the best described vasoactive hormonal pathway is the RAAS; Ang II is the most biologically active component. Both obesity and persistent hyperglycemia are associated with upregulation of the intrarenal RAAS.[109,110] Activation of the RAAS leads to both hemodynamic and cellular effects. Ang II leads to increases in efferent arteriolar vasoconstriction and glomerular pressure, sodium retention, and cell proliferation.[111–113] On a cellular level, Ang II activates protein kinase C and mitogen-activated protein kinase, and transcription factors such as nuclear factor-κB that lead to alteration in the gene expression of several growth factors and cytokines including TGF-β. TGF-β, in turn, promotes podocyte apoptosis, mesangial cell proliferation, and extracellular matrix synthesis, cellular events that are important in the development of obesity-associated and diabetes-associated glomerulopathy.[114]

Although there are many similarities between the obese and diabetic kidney, there are some features unique to obesity in the absence of diabetes. Glomerular/mesangial lipid deposits (foam cells) are frequently seen in the kidneys of obese individuals, supporting the concept of lipotoxicity (ie, lipid-induced renal injury). This lipid accumulation in the glomerulus then leads to upregulation of the sterol-regulatory element-binding proteins (SREBP-1 and -2), which, in turn, promote podocyte apoptosis and mesangial cell proliferation and cytokine synthesis.[115]

SUMMARY

Obesity and diabetes are major causes of CKD and ESRD, and are thus enormous health concerns worldwide. Both obesity and diabetes, along with other elements of the metabolic syndrome including hypertension, are highly interrelated and contribute to the development and progression of renal disease. Studies show that multiple factors act in concert to initially cause renal vasodilation, glomerular hyperfiltration, and albuminuria, leading to the development of glomerulopathy. The coexistence of hypertension contributes to the disease progression, which, if not treated, may lead to ESRD. Although early intervention and management of body weight, hyperglycemia, and hypertension are imperative, novel therapeutic approaches are also necessary to reduce the high morbidity and mortality associated with both obesity-related and diabetes-related renal disease.

REFERENCES

1. Yanovski SZ, Yanovski JA. Obesity prevalence in the United States–up, down, or sideways? N Engl J Med 2011;364(11):987–9.
2. Flegal KM, Carroll MD, Ogden CL, et al. Prevalence and trends in obesity among US adults, 1999-2008. JAMA 2010;303(3):235–41.
3. World Health Organization. Obesity and overweight fact sheet. 2012. Available at: http://www.who.int/mediacentre/factsheets/fs311/en/index.html. Accessed on October 2nd, 2012.
4. Kopelman P. Health risks associated with overweight and obesity. Obes Rev 2007;8(Suppl 1):13–7.
5. Eknoyan G. Obesity, diabetes, and chronic kidney disease. Curr Diab Rep 2007;7(6):449–53.
6. Hall JE, Crook ED, Jones DW, et al. Mechanisms of obesity-associated cardiovascular and renal disease. Am J Med Sci 2002;324(3):127–37.
7. Ogden CL, Carroll MD, Curtin LR, et al. Prevalence of overweight and obesity in the United States, 1999-2004. JAMA 2006;295(13):1549–55.
8. Neeland IJ, Turer AT, Ayers CR, et al. Dysfunctional adiposity and the risk of prediabetes and type 2 diabetes in obese adults. JAMA 2012;308(11):1150–9.

9. Foster MC, Hwang SJ, Larson MG, et al. Overweight, obesity, and the development of stage 3 CKD: the Framingham Heart Study. Am J Kidney Dis 2008; 52(1):39–48.
10. Hsu CY, McCulloch CE, Iribarren C, et al. Body mass index and risk for end-stage renal disease. Ann Intern Med 2006;144(1):21–8.
11. Ejerblad E, Fored CM, Lindblad P, et al. Obesity and risk for chronic renal failure. J Am Soc Nephrol 2006;17(6):1695–702.
12. Praga M, Morales E. Obesity, proteinuria and progression of renal failure. Curr Opin Nephrol Hypertens 2006;15(5):481–6.
13. Wang Y, Chen X, Song Y, et al. Association between obesity and kidney disease: a systematic review and meta-analysis. Kidney Int 2008;73(1):19–33.
14. Ogden CL, Yanovski SZ, Carroll MD, et al. The epidemiology of obesity. Gastroenterology 2007;132(6):2087–102.
15. Coresh J, Selvin E, Stevens LA, et al. Prevalence of chronic kidney disease in the United States. JAMA 2007;298(17):2038–47.
16. Kramer H, Luke A, Bidani A, et al. Obesity and prevalent and incident CKD: the hypertension detection and follow-up program. Am J Kidney Dis 2005;46(4): 587–94.
17. de Zeeuw D, Ramjit D, Zhang Z, et al. Renal risk and renoprotection among ethnic groups with type 2 diabetic nephropathy: a post hoc analysis of RENAAL. Kidney Int 2006;69(9):1675–82.
18. Remuzzi G, Macia M, Ruggenenti P. Prevention and treatment of diabetic renal disease in type 2 diabetes: the BENEDICT study. J Am Soc Nephrol 2006; 17(4 Suppl 2):S90–7.
19. US Renal Data System. USRDS 2009 annual data report: atlas of chronic kidney disease and end-stage renal disease in the United States. Bethesda (MD): National Institutes of Health, National Institute of Diabetes and Digestive and Kidney Diseases; 2009.
20. Thomson SC, Vallon V, Blantz RC. Kidney function in early diabetes: the tubular hypothesis of glomerular filtration. Am J Physiol Renal Physiol 2004;286(1):F8–15.
21. Hostetter TH. Hyperfiltration and glomerulosclerosis. Semin Nephrol 2003;23(2): 194–9.
22. Caramori ML, Mauer M. Diabetes and nephropathy. Curr Opin Nephrol Hypertens 2003;12(3):273–82.
23. Leon CA, Raij L. Interaction of haemodynamic and metabolic pathways in the genesis of diabetic nephropathy. J Hypertens 2005;23(11):1931–7.
24. Ogden CL, Carroll MD, Kit BK, et al. Prevalence of obesity and trends in body mass index among US children and adolescents, 1999-2010. JAMA 2012; 307(5):483–90.
25. Flegal KM, Carroll MD, Kit BK, et al. Prevalence of obesity and trends in the distribution of body mass index among US adults, 1999-2010. JAMA 2012;307(5): 491–7.
26. Danaei G, Finucane MM, Lin JK, et al. National, regional, and global trends in systolic blood pressure since 1980: systematic analysis of health examination surveys and epidemiological studies with 786 country-years and 5.4 million participants. Lancet 2011;377(9765):568–77.
27. US Renal Data System. USRDS 2006 annual data report: atlas of end-stage renal disease in the United States. Bethesda (MD): National Institutes of Health, National Institute of Diabetes and Digestive and Kidney Diseases; 2006.
28. Kurella M, Lo JC, Chertow GM. Metabolic syndrome and the risk for chronic kidney disease among nondiabetic adults. J Am Soc Nephrol 2005;16(7):2134–40.

29. Chen J, Muntner P, Hamm LL, et al. The metabolic syndrome and chronic kidney disease in U.S. adults. Ann Intern Med 2004;140(3):167–74.
30. Stengel B, Tarver-Carr ME, Powe NR, et al. Lifestyle factors, obesity and the risk of chronic kidney disease. Epidemiology 2003;14(4):479–87.
31. Gelber RP, Kurth T, Kausz AT, et al. Association between body mass index and CKD in apparently healthy men. Am J Kidney Dis 2005;46(5):871–80.
32. Munkhaugen J, Lydersen S, Wideroe TE, et al. Prehypertension, obesity, and risk of kidney disease: 20-year follow-up of the HUNT I study in Norway. Am J Kidney Dis 2009;54(4):638–46.
33. Iseki K, Ikemiya Y, Kinjo K, et al. Body mass index and the risk of development of end-stage renal disease in a screened cohort. Kidney Int 2004;65(5):1870–6.
34. Kramer HJ, Saranathan A, Luke A, et al. Increasing body mass index and obesity in the incident ESRD population. J Am Soc Nephrol 2006;17(5):1453–9.
35. Kalantar-Zadeh K, Kopple JD. Obesity paradox in patients on maintenance dialysis. Contrib Nephrol 2006;151:57–69.
36. Kalantar-Zadeh K, Streja E, Kovesdy CP, et al. The obesity paradox and mortality associated with surrogates of body size and muscle mass in patients receiving hemodialysis. Mayo Clin Proc 2010;85(11):991–1001.
37. Elsayed EF, Sarnak MJ, Tighiouart H, et al. Waist-to-hip ratio, body mass index, and subsequent kidney disease and death. Am J Kidney Dis 2008;52(1):29–38.
38. Elsayed EF, Tighiouart H, Weiner DE, et al. Waist-to-hip ratio and body mass index as risk factors for cardiovascular events in CKD. Am J Kidney Dis 2008; 52(1):49–57.
39. Henegar JR, Bigler SA, Henegar LK, et al. Functional and structural changes in the kidney in the early stages of obesity. J Am Soc Nephrol 2001;12(6):1211–7.
40. Maddox DA, Alavi FK, Santella RN, et al. Prevention of obesity-linked renal disease: age-dependent effects of dietary food restriction. Kidney Int 2002;62(1): 208–19.
41. Chagnac A, Weinstein T, Herman M, et al. The effects of weight loss on renal function in patients with severe obesity. J Am Soc Nephrol 2003;14(6):1480–6.
42. Hall JE. The kidney, hypertension, and obesity. Hypertension 2003;41(3 Pt 2): 625–33.
43. Griffin KA, Kramer H, Bidani AK. Adverse renal consequences of obesity. Am J Physiol Renal Physiol 2008;294(4):F685–96.
44. Hall JE, Kuo JJ, da Silva AA, et al. Obesity-associated hypertension and kidney disease. Curr Opin Nephrol Hypertens 2003;12(2):195–200.
45. Esler M, Rumantir M, Wiesner G, et al. Sympathetic nervous system and insulin resistance: from obesity to diabetes. Am J Hypertens 2001;14(11 Pt 2):304S–9S.
46. Blanco S, Bonet J, Lopez D, et al. ACE inhibitors improve nephrin expression in Zucker rats with glomerulosclerosis. Kidney Int Suppl 2005;(93):S10–4.
47. Chagnac A, Herman M, Zingerman B, et al. Obesity-induced glomerular hyperfiltration: its involvement in the pathogenesis of tubular sodium reabsorption. Nephrol Dial Transplant 2008;23(12):3946–52.
48. Yip JW, Jones SL, Wiseman MJ, et al. Glomerular hyperfiltration in the prediction of nephropathy in IDDM: a 10-year follow-up study. Diabetes 1996;45(12): 1729–33.
49. Vallon V, Schroth J, Satriano J, et al. Adenosine A(1) receptors determine glomerular hyperfiltration and the salt paradox in early streptozotocin diabetes mellitus. Nephron Physiol 2009;111(3):p30–8.
50. Woods LL, Mizelle HL, Hall JE. Control of renal hemodynamics in hyperglycemia: possible role of tubuloglomerular feedback. Am J Physiol 1987;252(1 Pt 2):F65–73.

51. Persson P, Hansell P, Palm F. Tubular reabsorption and diabetes-induced glomerular hyperfiltration. Acta Physiol (Oxf) 2010;200(1):3–10.
52. Cherney DZ, Scholey JW, Miller JA. Insights into the regulation of renal hemodynamic function in diabetic mellitus. Curr Diabetes Rev 2008;4(4):280–90.
53. Carmines PK. The renal vascular response to diabetes. Curr Opin Nephrol Hypertens 2010;19(1):85–90.
54. do Carmo JM, Tallam LS, Roberts JV, et al. Impact of obesity on renal structure and function in the presence and absence of hypertension: evidence from melanocortin-4 receptor-deficient mice. Am J Physiol Regul Integr Comp Physiol 2009;297(3):R803–12.
55. Fried LF, Orchard TJ, Kasiske BL. Effect of lipid reduction on the progression of renal disease: a meta-analysis. Kidney Int 2001;59(1):260–9.
56. Must A, Spadano J, Coakley EH, et al. The disease burden associated with overweight and obesity. JAMA 1999;282(16):1523–9.
57. Wilson PW, D'Agostino RB, Sullivan L, et al. Overweight and obesity as determinants of cardiovascular risk: the Framingham experience. Arch Intern Med 2002;162(16):1867–72.
58. Doll S, Paccaud F, Bovet P, et al. Body mass index, abdominal adiposity and blood pressure: consistency of their association across developing and developed countries. Int J Obes Relat Metab Disord 2002;26(1):48–57.
59. Hall JE, Jones DW, Kuo JJ, et al. Impact of the obesity epidemic on hypertension and renal disease. Curr Hypertens Rep 2003;5(5):386–92.
60. Neter JE, Stam BE, Kok FJ, et al. Influence of weight reduction on blood pressure: a meta-analysis of randomized controlled trials. Hypertension 2003;42(5):878–84.
61. Garrison RJ, Kannel WB, Stokes J 3rd, et al. Incidence and precursors of hypertension in young adults: the Framingham Offspring Study. Prev Med 1987;16(2):235–51.
62. Kannel WB, Zhang T, Garrison RJ. Is obesity-related hypertension less of a cardiovascular risk? The Framingham Study. Am Heart J 1990;120(5):1195–201.
63. Mokdad AH, Ford ES, Bowman BA, et al. Prevalence of obesity, diabetes, and obesity-related health risk factors, 2001. JAMA 2003;289(1):76–9.
64. Kotchen TA. Obesity-related hypertension: epidemiology, pathophysiology, and clinical management. Am J Hypertens 2010;23(11):1170–8.
65. Hall JE, Henegar JR, Dwyer TM, et al. Is obesity a major cause of chronic kidney disease? Adv Ren Replace Ther 2004;11(1):41–54.
66. Van Buren PN, Toto R. Hypertension in diabetic nephropathy: epidemiology, mechanisms, and management. Adv Chronic Kidney Dis 2011;18(1):28–41.
67. Mancia G. Effects of intensive blood pressure control in the management of patients with type 2 diabetes mellitus in the Action to Control Cardiovascular Risk in Diabetes (ACCORD) trial. Circulation 2010;122(8):847–9.
68. Heerspink HJ, de Zeeuw D. The kidney in type 2 diabetes therapy. Rev Diabet Stud 2011;8(3):392–402.
69. Rayner HC, Hollingworth L, Higgins R, et al. Systematic kidney disease management in a population with diabetes mellitus: turning the tide of kidney failure. BMJ Qual Saf 2011;20(10):903–10.
70. Williams ME. The goal of blood pressure control for prevention of early diabetic microvascular complications. Curr Diab Rep 2011;11(4):323–9.
71. Grossman E, Messerli FH. Management of blood pressure in patients with diabetes. Am J Hypertens 2011;24(8):863–75.

72. Jauregui A, Mintz DH, Mundel P, et al. Role of altered insulin signaling pathways in the pathogenesis of podocyte malfunction and microalbuminuria. Curr Opin Nephrol Hypertens 2009;18(6):539–45.

73. de Boer IH, Sibley SD, Kestenbaum B, et al. Central obesity, incident microalbuminuria, and change in creatinine clearance in the epidemiology of diabetes interventions and complications study. J Am Soc Nephrol 2007;18(1):235–43.

74. Eijkelkamp WB, Zhang Z, Remuzzi G, et al. Albuminuria is a target for renoprotective therapy independent from blood pressure in patients with type 2 diabetic nephropathy: post hoc analysis from the Reduction of Endpoints in NIDDM with the Angiotensin II Antagonist Losartan (RENAAL) trial. J Am Soc Nephrol 2007; 18(5):1540–6.

75. Klausen KP, Parving HH, Scharling H, et al. Microalbuminuria and obesity: impact on cardiovascular disease and mortality. Clin Endocrinol (Oxf) 2009; 71(1):40–5.

76. Savage S, Nagel NJ, Estacio RO, et al. Clinical factors associated with urinary albumin excretion in type II diabetes. Am J Kidney Dis 1995;25(6):836–44.

77. de Jong PE, Verhave JC, Pinto-Sietsma SJ, et al. Obesity and target organ damage: the kidney. Int J Obes Relat Metab Disord 2002;26(Suppl 4):S21–4.

78. Kohler KA, McClellan WM, Ziemer DC, et al. Risk factors for microalbuminuria in black Americans with newly diagnosed type 2 diabetes. Am J Kidney Dis 2000; 36(5):903–13.

79. Pinto-Sietsma SJ, Navis G, Janssen WM, et al. A central body fat distribution is related to renal function impairment, even in lean subjects. Am J Kidney Dis 2003;41(4):733–41.

80. Morales E, Valero MA, Leon M, et al. Beneficial effects of weight loss in overweight patients with chronic proteinuric nephropathies. Am J Kidney Dis 2003;41(2):319–27.

81. Praga M, Morales E. Obesity-related renal damage: changing diet to avoid progression. Kidney Int 2010;78(7):633–5.

82. Mohan S, Tan J, Gorantla S, et al. Early improvement in albuminuria in non-diabetic patients after Roux-en-Y bariatric surgery. Obes Surg 2012; 22(3):375–80.

83. Sharma K, Ramachandrarao S, Qiu G, et al. Adiponectin regulates albuminuria and podocyte function in mice. J Clin Invest 2008;118(5):1645–56.

84. Comper WD, Russo LM. The glomerular filter: an imperfect barrier is required for perfect renal function. Curr Opin Nephrol Hypertens 2009;18(4):336–42.

85. Kasiske BL, Cleary MP, O'Donnell MP, et al. Effects of genetic obesity on renal structure and function in the Zucker rat. J Lab Clin Med 1985;106(5):598–604.

86. Tran HA. Obesity-related glomerulopathy. J Clin Endocrinol Metab 2004;89(12): 6358.

87. Ritz E, Koleganova N, Piecha G. Is there an obesity-metabolic syndrome related glomerulopathy? Curr Opin Nephrol Hypertens 2011;20(1):44–9.

88. Kasiske BL, Napier J. Glomerular sclerosis in patients with massive obesity. Am J Nephrol 1985;5(1):45–50.

89. Coimbra TM, Janssen U, Grone HJ, et al. Early events leading to renal injury in obese Zucker (fatty) rats with type II diabetes. Kidney Int 2000;57(1):167–82.

90. O'Donnell MP, Kasiske BL, Cleary MP, et al. Effects of genetic obesity on renal structure and function in the Zucker rat. II. Micropuncture studies. J Lab Clin Med 1985;106(5):605–10.

91. Kambham N, Markowitz GS, Valeri AM, et al. Obesity-related glomerulopathy: an emerging epidemic. Kidney Int 2001;59(4):1498–509.

92. Praga M, Hernandez E, Morales E, et al. Clinical features and long-term outcome of obesity-associated focal segmental glomerulosclerosis. Nephrol Dial Transplant 2001;16(9):1790–8.
93. Praga M. Synergy of low nephron number and obesity: a new focus on hyperfiltration nephropathy. Nephrol Dial Transplant 2005;20(12):2594–7.
94. King GL. The role of inflammatory cytokines in diabetes and its complications. J Periodontol 2008;79(Suppl 8):1527–34.
95. Tang J, Yan H, Zhuang S. Inflammation and oxidative stress in obesity-related glomerulopathy. Int J Nephrol 2012;2012:608397.
96. Guebre-Egziabher F, Bernhard J, Funahashi T, et al. Adiponectin in chronic kidney disease is related more to metabolic disturbances than to decline in renal function. Nephrol Dial Transplant 2005;20(1):129–34.
97. Saraheimo M, Forsblom C, Thorn L, et al. Serum adiponectin and progression of diabetic nephropathy in patients with type 1 diabetes. Diabetes Care 2008; 31(6):1165–9.
98. Ma K, Cabrero A, Saha PK, et al. Increased beta-oxidation but no insulin resistance or glucose intolerance in mice lacking adiponectin. J Biol Chem 2002; 277(38):34658–61.
99. Kastarinen H, Kesaniemi YA, Ukkola O. Leptin and lipid metabolism in chronic kidney failure. Scand J Clin Lab Invest 2009;69(3):401–8.
100. Sharma K, Considine RV, Michael B, et al. Plasma leptin is partly cleared by the kidney and is elevated in hemodialysis patients. Kidney Int 1997;51(6):1980–5.
101. Mathew AV, Okada S, Sharma K. Obesity related kidney disease. Curr Diabetes Rev 2011;7(1):41–9.
102. Wolf G, Ziyadeh FN. Leptin and renal fibrosis. Contrib Nephrol 2006;151: 175–83.
103. Park HS, Park JY, Yu R. Relationship of obesity and visceral adiposity with serum concentrations of CRP, TNF-alpha and IL-6. Diabetes Res Clin Pract 2005;69(1): 29–35.
104. Gupta J, Mitra N, Kanetsky PA, et al. Association between albuminuria, kidney function, and inflammatory biomarker profile. Clin J Am Soc Nephrol 2012. http://dx.doi.org/10.2215/CJN.03500412.
105. Ruiz-Ortega M, Ruperez M, Lorenzo O, et al. Angiotensin II regulates the synthesis of proinflammatory cytokines and chemokines in the kidney. Kidney Int Suppl 2002;(82):S12–22.
106. Ikezumi Y, Suzuki T, Karasawa T, et al. Activated macrophages down-regulate podocyte nephrin and podocin expression via stress-activated protein kinases. Biochem Biophys Res Commun 2008;376(4):706–11.
107. Patel NS, Chatterjee PK, Di Paola R, et al. Endogenous interleukin-6 enhances the renal injury, dysfunction, and inflammation caused by ischemia/reperfusion. J Pharmacol Exp Ther 2005;312(3):1170–8.
108. Tomiyama-Hanayama M, Rakugi H, Kohara M, et al. Effect of interleukin-6 receptor blockage on renal injury in apolipoprotein E-deficient mice. Am J Physiol Renal Physiol 2009;297(3):F679–84.
109. Ahmed SB, Fisher ND, Stevanovic R, et al. Body mass index and angiotensin-dependent control of the renal circulation in healthy humans. Hypertension 2005;46(6):1316–20.
110. Kennefick TM, Anderson S. Role of angiotensin II in diabetic nephropathy. Semin Nephrol 1997;17(5):441–7.
111. Zhuo JL, Li XC. Novel roles of intracrine angiotensin II and signalling mechanisms in kidney cells. J Renin Angiotensin Aldosterone Syst 2007;8(1):23–33.

112. Griffin KA, Bidani AK. Progression of renal disease: renoprotective specificity of renin-angiotensin system blockade. Clin J Am Soc Nephrol 2006;1(5):1054–65.
113. Crowley SD, Gurley SB, Coffman TM. AT(1) receptors and control of blood pressure: the kidney and more. Trends Cardiovasc Med 2007;17(1):30–4.
114. Ziyadeh FN. Mediators of diabetic renal disease: the case for tgf-Beta as the major mediator. J Am Soc Nephrol 2004;15(Suppl 1):S55–7.
115. Jiang G, Li Z, Liu F, et al. Prevention of obesity in mice by antisense oligonucleotide inhibitors of stearoyl-CoA desaturase-1. J Clin Invest 2005;115(4):1030–8.

Gastrointestinal Complications of Diabetes

Brigid S. Boland, MD[a],*, Steven V. Edelman, MD[b,c], James D. Wolosin, MD[d]

KEYWORDS

- Gastrointestinal symptoms • Glycemic control • Gastroparesis • Celiac
- Nonalcoholic fatty liver disease

KEY POINTS

- Gastrointestinal symptoms are common in the general population and frequently are related to irritable bowel syndrome.
- The incidence of multiple gastrointestinal diseases is more common in diabetic patients for a variety of reasons.
- Diabetic neuropathy may lead to abnormal gastrointestinal motility that causes gastroparesis, small bacterial intestinal overgrowth, diabetic diarrhea, and fecal incontinence.

INTRODUCTION

When practitioners think about complications of diabetes, they may focus on the microvascular, macrovascular, and peripheral neuropathic complications that are known to be associated with the disease. Although gastrointestinal problems are extremely common, with upper gastrointestinal symptoms alone affecting more than 40% of the general population,[1] the incidence of certain gastrointestinal symptoms is more common in diabetes, and health care professionals should be aware of these associations. Gastrointestinal symptoms have not only a detrimental effect on quality of life but also significant medical consequences. Poor control of diabetes can affect any segment of the gut from the mouth to the rectum. However, unfamiliarity

This article originally appeared in Endocrinology and Metabolism Clinics of North America, Volume 42, Issue 4, December 2013.

Funding Sources: None.

Conflict of Interest: None.

[a] Division of Gastroenterology, Department of Medicine, University of California, San Diego, 9500 Gilman Drive, La Jolla, CA 92093, USA; [b] Division of Endocrinology and Metabolism, University of California, San Diego, 9350 Campus Point Drive, Suite 2G, La Jolla, CA 92093-9111, USA; [c] Division of Endocrinology and Metabolism, Diabetes Care Clinic, Veterans Affairs Medical Center, 3350 La Jolla Village Drive (111G), San Diego, CA 92161, USA; [d] Division of Gastroenterology, Sharp Rees-Stealy Medical Group, 2929 Health Center Drive, San Diego, CA 92123, USA

* Corresponding author.

E-mail address: bboland@ucsd.edu

http://dx.doi.org/10.1016/j.ccol.2014.08.014
2352-7986/14/$ – see front matter

with these symptoms can delay treatment or referrals to appropriate specialists. The purpose of this review is to highlight the incidence, diagnosis, and treatment of some of the more common gastrointestinal complications of diabetes.

ESOPHAGEAL DISORDERS
Esophageal Motility Dysfunction in Diabetes

The term esophageal motility dysfunction is a phrase used to describe a multitude of esophageal complications that can occur in diabetic patients. Abnormalities seen include reduced lower esophageal sphincter tone, diminished amplitude of esophageal contractions, reduced coordination of esophageal contractions, prolonged esophageal transit, and increased acid reflux.[2] Esophageal motility disorders appear to be driven by neuropathy, a known complication of diabetes. Specifically, vagal nerve dysfunction is thought to drive the underlying pathophysiology. However, recent studies have also implicated motor nerve dysfunction as playing a role.[3]

Symptoms of Esophageal Motility Disorders

Symptoms of esophageal motility disorders may include heartburn after eating and/or drinking, chest pain, odynophagia, and dysphagia. More commonly, these abnormalities are asymptomatic but have been incidentally observed in clinical studies. Treatment options for esophageal hypomotility are limited but may entail lifestyle modification.

Gastroesophageal Reflux Disease in Patients with Diabetes

Just as many motility abnormalities are clinically silent in diabetic patients, the prevalence of asymptomatic gastroesophageal reflux confirmed by pH study is significantly higher in diabetic patients than in healthy controls.[4] Furthermore, the prevalence of gastroesophageal reflux disease (GERD) is higher in patients with diabetes with neuropathy as compared with the general population (41% as compared to 14%).[5] Practitioners should be mindful of this association and be aware of the incidence of GERD when a diagnosis of neuropathy is established. As GERD is a common clinical entity, it is worth familiarizing one's self with the common presentation and treatment modalities.

Risk Factors for Gastroesophageal Reflux in Diabetes

- Cardiovascular autonomic dysfunction
- Elevated body mass index
- Longer duration of disease
- Poor glycemic control

Management of GERD

In patients with reflux, initial recommendations should include lifestyle modifications, such as avoidance of trigger foods (coffee, tomato sauce, spicy foods, and alcohol being common offenders), reduction in meal size, avoidance of eating before sleeping, smoking cessation, elevation of head at night, and weight loss. Frequently, patients will require medical therapy. Management may entail antacids as needed or H2 blockers, such as rantidine, for mild disease. For more significant or persistent symptoms, proton pump inhibitors (PPIs), such as omeprazole or pantoprazole, are extremely effective in the treatment of reflux. Interestingly, a recent randomized clinical trial showed that PPIs improve glycemic control, suggesting additional benefits of

PPIs in diabetic patients with GERD.[6] In patients with classic symptoms of postprandial reflux that responds to antacids, further diagnostic testing is not necessary.

Diagnostic Testing for GERD

When the symptoms of GERD do not respond to a PPI, the underlying diagnosis should be questioned. A referral to a gastroenterologist is appropriate to guide further diagnostic evaluation, such as upper endoscopy, 24-hour esophageal pH monitoring, or manometry. Esophageal pH monitoring directly measures acid in the esophagus and quantifies acid reflux, providing a definitive diagnosis. Technological advances have significantly enhanced diagnostic capabilities with the development of a wireless pH-detection capsule that is placed during endoscopy. Manometry, a study that measures esophageal pressure and muscular contractions, may be used to evaluate for a motility disorder causing GERD-like symptoms. In patients with a long-standing history of GERD, especially middle-aged, overweight Caucasian men, upper endoscopy should be considered to evaluate for Barrett esophagus and assess for esophageal cancer risks.

Esophageal Candidiasis

Individuals with diabetes are at higher risk for oral or esophageal candidiasis that is typically caused by *Candida albicans*. Poor glycemic control allows for favorable conditions for the yeast to grow, increasing the risk of fungal infection. The incidence of esophageal candidiasis in patients with diabetes is not well defined.

Signs and Symptoms of Candidiasis
• Odynophagia
• Dysphagia with solids
• Avoidance of oral intake
• Erythematous friable lesions in oropharynx
• White patches in oropharynx

Management of Oropharyngeal and Esophageal Candidiasis

Candidiasis limited to the oropharyngeal cavity may be treated with nystatin. A typical dosage is 4 to 6 mL (400,000 to 600,000 units) 4 times per day in a swish-and-swallow fashion. Patients continue this therapy until 48 hours after symptoms have resolved. However, if the symptoms are not responding, oral fluconazole should be the treatment of choice. Similarly, the presence of odynophagia in combination with oral thrush is highly predictive of esophageal involvement and is an indication for fluconazole therapy. Therefore, the presence of thrush should always key a practitioner to inquire about pain with swallowing. A loading dose of fluconazole 200 mg is given, followed by 100 to 200 mg daily for 7 to 14 days. Symptoms should resolve in 1 week with treatment, and lack of response should prompt further evaluation with upper endoscopy.[7]

GASTRIC DISORDERS
Gastroparesis

Gastroparesis is defined as delayed gastric emptying in the absence of mechanical obstruction. The condition can result in a wide array of symptoms, ranging from none to a complete inability to tolerate oral nutrients with chronic nausea and vomiting.

Delayed gastric emptying may be seen in up to 40% of patients with diabetes but only 10% or fewer of these patients will have any symptoms. Severe symptoms can result in a significant decrease in quality of life and can further potentiate poor glycemic control, as matching mealtime insulin with slow emptying can be extremely difficult. Patients will often complain of early satiety that may be accompanied by postprandial nausea, vomiting, belching, reflux, palpitations, and/or abdominal pain. The tremendous overlap with symptoms of functional dyspepsia may obscure the diagnosis of gastroparesis.

Although gastroparesis does not independently increase mortality, it is associated with a worse prognosis as compared with age-matched and gender-matched individuals with normal gastric emptying. The 5-year survival of individuals with gastroparesis is 67% as compared with the expected 81% survival.[8]

Epidemiology

The overall incidence of gastroparesis is 4.8% in type 1 diabetes mellitus (DM1), 1% in type 2 diabetes mellitus (DM2), and 0.1% in the general population.[9] Although the incidence of gastroparesis is higher in patients with DM1 as compared with DM2, the overall higher prevalence of DM2 makes gastroparesis more commonly seen by health care providers in this patient population. The incidence and prevalence in women is nearly 4 times that in men.[8] Although onset of gastroparesis appears to occur after 10 years of disease duration, a recent population-based study found no association between diabetes duration and gastroparesis.[9–11]

Pathophysiology of Gastroparesis

Normal gastric emptying is a complex process involving synchronization of smooth muscle and autonomic nerves. This process is coordinated in the interstitial cells of Cajal (ICC), or the pacemakers of the stomach. The ICCs integrate fundic tone, antral contractions, and relaxation of the pylorus to facilitate postprandial emptying. Consequences of diabetes may lead to disruptions in different components of this process, interfering with the normal function of the stomach. Hyperglycemia, even at modest levels, disrupts gastric coordination and emptying in healthy volunteers as well as diabetic patients.[12] Reductions in ICC quantity are seen in biopsies from individuals with gastroparesis.[13]

Autonomic neuropathy, inflammation, and oxidative stress appear to be critical components driving patients with diabetic gastroparesis.[11] The effects of autonomic neuropathy have been demonstrated by gastric biopsies from diabetic patients with gastroparesis showing reduced number of nerve fibers.[14] Vagal nerve functional studies are abnormal in diabetic patients with gastroparesis, showing reduction in postprandial gastric acid section.[15] Oxidative stress has been implicated, given that loss of nitric oxide from enteric cells has been documented in mouse and human

Symptoms of Gastroparesis
• Nausea
• Vomiting
• Early satiety
• Bloating
• Upper abdominal discomfort

models of patients with diabetic gastroparesis and appears to occur early after diabetes onset.[16,17] Similarly, loss of a cytoprotective enzyme, heme oxidase-1, has been linked to the pathogenesis of gastroparesis in mouse models.[18] Further, oxidative stress and loss of survival signals from insulin and insulinlike growth factor (IGF)-1 contribute to ICC death.[11,18]

Diagnosis of Gastroparesis

- Symptoms of gastroparesis
- Absence of gastric outlet obstruction based on imaging or endoscopy
- Presence of retained food in the stomach on endoscopy after a fast of more than 12 hours
- Slowed gastric emptying based on scintigraphy

Overall, the symptoms lack sensitivity and specificity, but nausea, vomiting, and early satiety are the best predictors of gastroparesis.[19] The presence of food in the stomach on endoscopy after a 12-hour fast suggests delayed gastric emptying and should raise suspicion for gastroparesis. Consensus guidelines recommend diagnostic testing to confirm the diagnosis of gastroparesis, and scintigraphy is typically the test of choice.[20] For this examination, patients ingest radioisotope technetium-99m–labeled test meals of defined caloric amount. After ingestion of the solid-phase meal, images will be obtained at 60 minutes, 120 minutes, 180 minutes, and 240 minutes. The most reliable predictor of gastroparesis is percentage of retained food at 4 hours. If possible, medications that delay or accelerate gastric emptying, should be discontinued approximately 48 to 72 hours before the study. Acute hyperglycemia may delay gastric emptying, so practitioners may want to delay scintigraphy until blood sugar has been stabilized.[21] Many patients with diabetes may have abnormal emptying studies in the absence of symptoms, and others may have mildly abnormal gastric emptying along with functional dyspepsia that is not directly related to diabetes. It is important to take a good history and be certain that symptoms are suggestive of delayed gastric emptying before making a diagnosis of gastroparesis.

Management of Gastroparesis

- Evaluation and correction of nutritional status
- Improvement of gastric emptying
- Symptomatic treatment

Nutritional Optimization

Gastroparesis may interfere with oral intake and nutritional status; therefore, the first goals of management are to restore hydration, replete electrolytes, and ensure sufficient long-term oral intake. Alcohol and cigarette smoking should be avoided, as they slow gastric emptying. Dietary modifications for gastroparesis aim to optimize emptying of the stomach, while avoiding foods that may delay motility, such as those with high fat and fiber content. A gastroparesis diet entails small, frequent, low-fat, and low-residue meals. If individuals are unable to tolerate modified diets, liquid meals may be trialed, as gastric emptying of liquids is frequently maintained in gastroparesis.

Consultation with a nutritionist may be quite useful in helping patients deal with multiple dietary restrictions. In severe cases, unintentional weight loss greater than 10% of body weight over 3 to 6 months suggests refractory gastroparesis and should prompt consideration for feeding tube placement. To bypass abnormal gastric motility, feeding tubes should be placed beyond the pylorus to bypass the abnormal motility in the stomach.[20]

Management of Glycemic Control in Gastroparesis

Based on experimental models, hyperglycemia delays gastric emptying in patients with diabetes as well as healthy patients.[12,22] Management of gastroparesis should include optimization of glycemic control that may improve short-term symptoms. For patients on mealtime insulin, the timing of their mealtime bolus may have to be adjusted. Rapid-acting insulin can be dosed at the start of the meal or 15 minutes *after* starting a meal in an attempt to match peak insulin levels with glucose appearance. Similarly, switching from rapid-acting analogues to regular insulin may be appropriate for the same reason. Using the square and dual-wave bolus function that is a feature with insulin pumps can be helpful. In addition, current medical treatments, including pramlintide and GLP-1 analogs, cause delayed gastric emptying and may exacerbate symptoms of gastroparesis.[23,24] The drugs may still be used in mild cases, but their use should be discouraged in any case where prokinetic agents must be initiated.

Management of Gastroparesis in Diabetes

Metoclopramide is the first-line prokinetic drug for treatment of gastroparesis. Metoclopramide is a D2 dopamine receptor antagonist (with less potent stimulation of 5-HT4) that increases lower esophageal sphincter tone, gastric pressure, and antral contractions that aids in emptying of the stomach. Metoclopramide also provides anti-emetic action by acting centrally and inhibiting the D2 dopamine and 5-HT3 receptors in the chemoreceptor trigger zone, a center in the medulla that integrates sensory input and stimulates vomiting.[25] Although this is the only prokinetic medication for gastroparesis that is approved by the Food and Drug Administration (FDA), its use is approved for only 3 months. The strongest evidence supporting use of metoclopramide comes from 4 placebo-controlled studies that showed improvement in symptoms ranging from 25% to 50%. However, these studies were of shorter duration, on the order of 3 weeks.[26–29] Prolonged use of the medication necessitates an evaluation of the benefits versus potential risks of ongoing therapy.

Metoclopramide carries a black box warning for an increased risk of tardive dyskinesia; a disorder characterized by involuntary movements of the face or extremities induced by dopamine inhibition.[25] Although the incidence of tardive dyskinesia is estimated at approximately 0.2%, the potential irreversible nature of the condition makes even a low incidence concerning. Groups at higher risk for developing tardive dyskinesia include patients on higher doses, those of younger age, and women.[30] Other side effects include QT prolongation, parkinsonian movements, akathisia, and hyperprolactinemia. Guidelines on use of metoclopramide recommend use of a minimal effective dose beginning with 5 mg before meals, monitoring for early signs of tardive dyskinesia, and drug holidays.[31]

Domperidone, a type II dopamine antagonist, has a similar mechanism of action as metoclopramide but with reduced central nervous system effects, and, thus, tardive dyskinesia. Three large randomized controlled trials with domperidone in patients with diabetic gastroparesis have been published and showed symptomatic improvement as compared with baseline or placebo.[32–34] Dosing typically starts at 10 mg with meals. Baseline electrocardiogram is recommended before initiation of therapy based on potential QT prolongation. Less common side effects also include prolactinemia, and potential drug interactions. Although the makers of domperidone have never applied for FDA approval, there are programs for obtaining this medication in the United States.[20]

Intravenous erythromycin lactobionate, a motilin agonist, has been shown to be effective in short-term treatment of hospitalized patients with diabetic gastroparesis. However, ongoing administration of intravenous or oral erythromycin over longer periods of time leads to tachyphylaxis by downregulation of receptors for motilin.[35] In addition, erythromycin itself may induce abnormal gastric motility with resultant nausea and vomiting.

Another technique that has been used in clinical practice is endoscopic intrapyloric injection of botulinum toxin. Manometry studies show that the pylorus has increased tone in patients with gastroparesis. Injection of botulinum toxin to block neurotransmission showed promise in open-label trials, but a randomized clinical trial including diabetic patients showed improvement in gastric emptying without symptomatic improvement.[36] Thus, routine use of botulinum toxin for the treatment of gastroparesis is not advised (**Table 1**).[20]

Management of the nausea and vomiting associated with gastroparesis typically relies on off-label use of medications. Therapies that are used include prochlorperazine, promethazine, ondansetron, scopolamine, and dronabinol; however, there are no evidence-based guidelines for management.

Pain remains extremely challenging, as opiates further slow gastric emptying and exacerbate symptoms. Clinical trials are lacking. Practitioners should discontinue opiates and recommend nonopiate alternatives, including tricyclic antidepressants (TCAs), tramadol, selective serotonin receptor inhibitors, or gabapentin. Low-dose tricyclic antidepressants and selective serotonin receptor inhibitors may modulate pain and improve glycemic control. TCAs have the added benefit of treating pain from coexisting peripheral neuropathy; however, this class of medications has varying anticholinergic effects that may worsen gastroparesis.[20]

Gastric Electric Stimulation for Refractory Gastroparesis

The gastric electrical stimulator (GES) is a neurostimulator that is implanted surgically into the abdomen and provides high-frequency stimulation to the stomach. GES was approved by the FDA under the humanitarian device exemption. A randomized

Table 1 Summary of prokinetic medications for gastroparesis			
Drug	**Starting Dose**	**Side Effects**	**Considerations**
Metoclopramide	5 mg with meals	Tardive dyskinesia, QT prolongation, akathisia, parkinsonian movements, hyperprolactinemia	Use minimum effective dose >4 wk of use needs to be re-evaluated
Domperidone	10 mg with meals	QT prolongation, hyperprolactinemia	Baseline electrocardiogram Not readily available in the United States Better side-effect profile
Erythromycin	3 mg/kg intravenous	Tachyphylaxis	Evidence supports short-term use in hospital

crossover trial showed a reduction in weekly vomiting frequency from 13 to 7, but in the subgroup of patients with diabetes there were no significant differences in symptoms and vomiting frequency.[37] A recent meta-analysis included 10 studies and concluded that GES improved symptoms with small mean differences in symptom scores, and diabetic gastroparesis was the most responsive to GES.[38] Although randomized trials and availability are lacking, GES may be an option for refractory cases.

Salvage and Alternative Therapies for Gastroparesis

There is little evidence to guide management of refractory cases of gastroparesis; however, salvage therapies for symptom management may include venting gastrostomy with or without jejunostomy feeding tube or gastectomy. Alternative treatments remain under investigation with acupuncture showing promise based on symptom improvement in a randomized study.[39]

Accelerated Gastric Emptying

Accelerated gastric emptying has emerged as a new entity, but few studies have been done to further understand this condition. Vagal dysfunction impairs gastric accommodation, leading to elevated pressures and rapid emptying. Symptoms are typically consistent with dumping syndrome, with the developmental of abdominal discomfort, nausea, vomiting, and diarrhea within an hour of eating. Although patients may have disproportionately more difficulty with postprandial glucose control and weight loss, the symptoms may be difficult to distinguish from gastroparesis. Gastric transit measured by scintigraphy typically establishes the diagnosis. Treatments are not well defined at this time, but amylin analogs and glucagonlike peptide-1 (GLP-1) agonists that can slow gastric emptying may improve symptoms.[11]

SMALL INTESTINAL DISORDERS
Celiac Disease Overview

Celiac disease is an immune-mediated enteropathy in which ingestion of gluten leads to atrophy of the small intestinal villi and malabsorption. Celiac disease affects approximately 1% of the US population; however, this risk is much higher in patients with DM1. Approximately 3% to 8% of patients with DM1 have celiac disease.[40–42] From 1951 to 2001, the incidence of celiac disease has increased incrementally; an increase that mirrors the increased incidence of DM1.[43,44] In the vast majority of cases, the diagnosis of DM1 precedes that of celiac disease.[45]

Pathogenesis of Celiac Disease

Gluten is a storage protein derived from wheat, rye, or barley. Gluten has high proline and glutamine content, which makes digestion difficult; α-gliadin is among the polypeptides that remain undigested in the small intestine. If there is a defect in the intestinal epithelium, then α-gliadin crosses into the lamina propria. In patients with celiac disease, α-gliadin initiates an innate and adaptive immune response that leads to an inflammatory infiltrate of the small bowel with villous destruction. The mechanism responsible for the epithelium defect is not well understood, but an infectious etiology has been proposed.[46,47] In the lamina propria, tissue transglutaminase, a celiac autoantigen, binds to gliadin and enhances its affinity for HLA DQ2 and DQ8 molecules on antigen-presenting cells that initiates humoral and cell-mediated immune responses. The immune response leads to significant inflammation in the small intestine as well as distant organs. Simultaneously, activation of intraepithelial lymphocytes initiates an innate immune response contributing to the pathology. Ultimately, destruction of small intestinal enterocytes leads to villous atrophy and impaired nutritional absorption, causing the classic symptoms associated with celiac disease.[46,47]

Genetic Predisposition to Celiac Disease

Celiac disease essentially develops only in genetically predisposed individuals who possess certain HLA genes that encode for antigen-presenting cell surface markers. HLA DQ2 and DQ8 are the susceptibility serotypes that are present in 25% to 40% of the general population. Only a small subset of individuals with DQ2 or DQ8 will develop celiac disease. If an individual carries multiple susceptibility alleles, there is an additive risk of celiac disease.[48]

Association of Celiac Disease and DM1

The mechanism underlying the increased incidence of celiac disease in patients with DM1 is not completely understood. Celiac disease and DM1 are autoimmune phenomena that share HLA and non-HLA susceptibility genes. A common environmental, microbial, or immunologic entity has been postulated, but has not been fully elucidated. Given this known association, diarrhea, weight loss, or new-onset hypoglycemic episodes in a patient with DM1 should prompt evaluation for celiac disease. The topic of whether to screen asymptomatic patients with DM1 for celiac disease remains somewhat controversial, although routinely occurs in the pediatric population. Furthermore, if an individual with DM1 undergoes upper endoscopy, obtaining duodenal biopsies is recommended to screen for celiac disease (**Table 2**).[49]

Childhood Presentation of Celiac Disease

Celiac disease may present with a wide variety of symptoms and historically was thought to be a disease of childhood. In infancy, typical presentations include development of abdominal pain and/or distension, steatorrhea, and vomiting after introduction of cereal into the diet. Falling off of the growth curve or failure to thrive should elicit concern for celiac disease. Older children may present with anemia or nutritional deficiencies, or in patients with diabetes, sudden improvement in hemoglobin A1c should prompt evaluation for celiac disease.

Table 2 Celiac disease	
Type of Celiac Disease	**Definition**
Classic	Patients with abnormal duodenal histology with typical gastrointestinal symptoms
Atypical	Lack of gastrointestinal symptoms but may present with extraintestinal findings related to celiac disease (eg, iron deficiency anemia, dermatitis herpetiformis)
Silent	Diagnosed based on serologies or during endoscopy for another indication. Lack of gastrointestinal symptoms
Latent	Individual with celiac disease on gluten-free diet with resolution of symptoms and duodenal changes based on histology or patients with normal duodenal histology with gluten-containing diet who will later develop celiac disease
Potential	Individuals with positive serologies but negative duodenal biopsies without symptoms who are at high risk for development of classic celiac disease

Adult Presentation of Celiac Disease
• Diarrhea
• Steatorrhea
• Abdominal pain
• Weight loss

Celiac symptoms are predominantly related to malabsorption. The severity of diarrhea and weight loss correlates with the degree of the intestinal inflammation. However, symptoms of celiac disease may be nonspecific and frequently overlap with symptoms of irritable bowel syndrome. It is important to consider the diagnosis of celiac disease in any patient undergoing evaluation for irritable bowel syndrome.

Extraintestinal Manifestations of Celiac Disease

Adults with celiac disease may present with extraintestinal manifestations of the systemic disease, rather than classic gastrointestinal symptoms. Iron deficiency anemia can result from decreased iron absorption in the proximal small intestine. Less frequently, celiac disease will affect the terminal ileum and interfere with vitamin B12 absorption. Nutritional deficiencies may lead to other extraintestinal signs or symptoms, such as peripheral neuropathy, ataxia, and osteoporosis. The most common dermatologic manifestation of celiac disease is dermatitis herpetiformis, a pruritic, erythematous blistering lesion located on extensor surfaces. Gluten mediates the pathogenesis of dermatitis herpetiformis, and recent studies suggest that immunoglobulin A (IgA) antiepidermal tissue transglutaminase antibody deposition in the dermis may cause the rash.[50]

Diagnosis of Celiac Disease: Utility of Serologic Testing

The first step in evaluating for celiac disease should be serologic testing; however, definitive diagnosis of celiac disease is made by duodenal biopsies in the setting of gluten exposure. Current guidelines recommend testing for tissue transglutaminase IgA (TTG IGA) as the preferred serologic test for celiac disease. Based on multiple studies, the overall specificity is greater than 95%, with sensitivity ranging from 89% to 96%.[51,52] The antiendomysial antibody (EMA) test has a similar profile but is more expensive. Antigliadin antibodies are of limited value because of decreased sensitivity and specificity. Patients with IgA deficiency will not, however, have detectable serum TTG IGA antibodies. It may be reasonable to routinely check IgA levels when evaluating individuals at high risk for celiac with the TTG IGA antibody. In individuals with low or absent IgA levels, deamidated gliadin peptide IgG antibody may be a useful screening tool. In the setting of DM1, the overlapping susceptibility genes render HLA-DQ2 and DQ8 testing less useful.

Duodenal Biopsies: Gold Standard for Diagnosis

If serologies are positive, upper endoscopy with duodenal bulb and distal duodenal biopsies should be obtained to confirm the diagnosis. Upper endoscopy should also be performed in the setting of negative serologies if there is high clinical suspicion. Endoscopic appearance of the duodenum may be abnormal with scalloping or flattening of folds. Duodenal biopsies may reveal a spectrum of changes including crypt hypertrophy, villous atrophy, and a lymphocytic inflammatory infiltrate. Dietary intake at time of endoscopy must be assessed and taken into account when interpreting the results of the endoscopy, as reductions in gluten consumption may lessen the intestinal inflammation and damage. Initiation of a 4-week gluten challenge may enable diagnosis of celiac disease in patients adhering to a gluten-free diet.[52,53]

Treatment of Celiac Disease: Gluten-Free Diet

Elimination of dietary wheat, rye, and barley is the current therapy for celiac disease. A gluten-free diet has been shown to improve symptoms, improve mortality, and possibly reduce the risk of cancer.[54,55] Nutritional consultation and support groups may offer assistance in helping patients adhere to a gluten-free diet. In a patient with concomitant diabetes, competing dietary restrictions may further complicate management of both diseases, and adequate nutrition remains a significant concern in the patients. Patients should be assessed for nutritional deficiencies in folic acid, vitamin B12, iron, calcium, and fat-soluble vitamins, as well as osteoporosis.[46]

Failure of a Gluten-Free Diet

Inadvertent exposure to gluten is the most common reason for failure to respond to a gluten-free diet. Failure should prompt reevaluation of the diagnosis of celiac disease and assessment of adherence to diet. If this evaluation is unrevealing, practitioners should consider alternative etiologies for the symptoms. Diseases that are associated with celiac disease and may cause similar symptoms include pancreatic insufficiency, small intestinal bacterial overgrowth, microscopic colitis, lactose intolerance, and irritable bowel syndrome.[56] In addition, celiac disease is associated with increased risk of small bowel adenocarcinoma and enteropathy-associated T-cell lymphoma.[46]

Small Bowel Bacterial Overgrowth Overview

Small bowel bacterial overgrowth (SIBO) is characterized by alterations in the type and quantity of bacteria within the small intestine. Significant changes in the microbiota of the small intestine may cause gastrointestinal symptoms, such as bloating, abdominal pain, diarrhea, and gas, and may lead to nutritional deficiencies.

Epidemiology

The prevalence of SIBO in the general population is difficult to estimate, although studies of healthy controls suggest a prevalence of 6% that increases with aging.[57] In one recent study, 43% of patients with diabetes with diarrhea had SIBO and improved with antibiotic therapy.[58]

Pathogenesis

The physiologic mechanisms for controlling intestinal bacterial growth include secretion of acid in the stomach and normal gastrointestinal motility. Specifically, in the small bowel, the migrating motor complex (MMC) clears any residual intestinal contents every 90 to 120 minutes. However, gastroparesis or abnormal motility of the small intestine enables bacterial stasis and subsequent overgrowth. Furthermore, any structural abnormalities from surgeries, particularly blind loops, may also create reservoirs that enable overgrowth of bacteria. The excessive growth of organisms leads to generation of ammonia, inflammatory cytokines, short-chain fatty acids, bile acid deconjugation, and toxins. Ultimately, the bacterial by-products interfere with normal absorption of fat and carbohydrates.[59]

Nutritional Complications of Untreated SIBO

If the bacterial overgrowth is severe and goes untreated, individuals may eventually develop nutritional deficiencies. Bacterial deconjugation of bile salts creates bile acids that may cause direct toxic damage to villi. This process impairs absorption and disrupts micelle formation. Disruption of fat absorption leads to deficiencies in vitamins A, D, E, and K. In addition, anaerobic intestinal bacteria metabolize vitamin B12 before absorption can occur.[60]

Symptoms of Bacterial Overgrowth

The typical symptoms associated with SIBO are abdominal pain with bloating, gas, and diarrhea. Other frequently reported symptoms include flatulence, abdominal distension, and weakness. The symptoms are frequently vague and overlap significantly with those of irritable bowel syndrome. Practitioners should consider this diagnosis when diabetic patients develop diarrhea and abdominal bloating.

Jejunal Aspirate: Gold Standard for Diagnosis of SIBO

SIBO is generally defined as greater than 100,000 colony-forming units(CFU)/mL in the small bowel as compared with the normal value of less than 10,000 CFU/mL. Historically, the gold standard for diagnosis is quantification of bacteria obtained from proximal jejunal aspirate during upper endoscopy; however, costs associated with endoscopy, rigorous specimen handling procedures, and difficulty culturing bacteria limit the widespread use of the test.[61]

Use of Breath Tests in Diagnosis of SIBO

Breath tests for diagnosis of SIBO are used to evaluate the ability of intestinal bacteria to produce analytes, such as hydrogen or radiolabeled carbon dioxide. In healthy individuals, glucose is absorbed in the small intestines; however, the excess bacteria in SIBO metabolize glucose into carbon dioxide and hydrogen that can be detected by breath test. The specificity and sensitivity of each specific test varies and fails in the setting of abnormal motility. In comparison with small bowel aspirate, the glucose hydrogen test has a sensitivity and specificity of 62% and 83%, respectively.[62] Given the low sensitivity, there is some debate over the utility of testing as compared with empiric treatment.

Treatment of Underlying Etiology

Treatment and reversal of the underlying etiology of SIBO may be difficult in certain circumstances. In the setting of gastroparesis or slow small intestinal transit as a predisposing factor, one should aim to optimize treatment of the motility disorder. Goals should include improvement of glycemic control and potential use of a prokinetic agent, such as metoclopramide or domperidone, as mentioned previously.

Nutritional Assessment

Individuals should be assessed for weight loss, malnutrition, or electrolyte imbalances. Significant weight loss should prompt discussion about nutritional supplementation. One may consider evaluating for deficiencies in fat-soluble vitamins and vitamin B12.

Antibiotic Treatment in SIBO

Antibiotic treatment for SIBO typically provides significant symptomatic relief. Although many different antibiotics are used, few randomized clinical trials have rigorously compared different regimens and durations. The most extensively studied medication in treatment of SIBO is rifaximin, a minimally absorbed antibiotic with activity against gram-negative and gram-positive bacteria. Based on a review of existing trials, rifaximin improved symptoms in 33% to 92% with eradication of SIBO in more than 80%.[63] Rifaximin, 1200 to 1600 mg daily for 7 to 10 days, is the first-line treatment; however, other antibiotics, such as doxycycline, augmentin, and flagyl, are less expensive and frequently used in clinical practice with success. Recurrence of SIBO is common and may respond to repeated courses of antibiotics. In refractory cases, patients may require continuous cycling of antibiotics to control symptoms.

Diabetic Diarrhea

Diarrhea is a frequent gastrointestinal symptom encountered in diabetic patients with a wide variety of potential etiologies. Diarrhea may be related to ingestion of artificial sweeteners, concomitant celiac disease, bacterial overgrowth, irritable bowel syndrome, or medication side effects. The biguanide derivative, metformin, frequently causes diarrhea. This effect may occur either early or late in use. The α-glucosidase inhibitors, such as acarbose, may also cause diarrhea in a significant proportion of patients. Diabetic diarrhea typically occurs in insulin-dependent patients who have had diabetes for at least 8 years. Many of these patients suffer from peripheral and autonomic neuropathy.[64,65]

Epidemiology of Diabetic Diarrhea

Significant variation in estimates of the prevalence of diabetic diarrhea may be related to referral basis in tertiary care settings. The prevalence of diabetic diarrhea is higher in patients with DM1 when compared with DM2, with rates of 5.0% and 0.4% respectively. Factors associated with diabetic diarrhea are disease duration, A1c levels, male sex, and autonomic neuropathy.[64] The lack of specific diagnostic markers for diabetic diarrhea makes differentiation from irritable bowel syndrome very difficult and undoubtedly there is some degree of overlap.

Pathogenesis of Diabetic Diarrhea

The pathogenesis of diabetic diarrhea is not well understood but appears to be closely related to autonomic neuropathy. The MMC, organized small bowel contractions while fasting, may be abnormal in patients with diabetes, slowing motility. Sympathetic denervation is found frequently in patients with autonomic neuropathy. Interruption of sympathetic nerves and adrenergic stimulation of electrolyte and fluid absorption may be the etiology of diarrhea.[66]

Symptoms of Diabetic Diarrhea
• Watery, voluminous diarrhea
• Nocturnal symptoms
• Steatorrhea
• Fecal incontinence
• Episodic symptoms with intervening normal bowel habits or constipation
• Absence of abdominal pain

Diabetic diarrhea is typically watery, voluminous, and explosive, with or without steatorrhea. Although the symptoms of diabetic diarrhea may relatively straightforward, patients may accept these symptoms and fail to disclose these symptoms.

Diagnosis

Diabetic diarrhea is a diagnosis of exclusion, and diagnostic evaluation includes obtaining a detailed history about diet and medication use for alternative etiologies. Specifically, diarrhea is a frequent side effect of metformin. Diagnostic evaluation may include stool studies for parasitic infection, serology for celiac disease, and consideration of flexible sigmoidoscopy or colonoscopy to evaluate for inflammatory bowel disease or microscopic colitis. If there is a significant history of incontinence, one may consider anorectal manometry to evaluate defecation.[64]

Treatment

Treatment may begin with optimization of glycemic control and removal of medications that may be exacerbating symptoms. Medications are almost uniformly needed to control symptoms. Initial treatment should be empiric with use of standard antidiarrheal agents, such as loperamide, diphenoxylate with atropine, and codeine sulfate, as well as fiber supplementation. Cholestyramine may be of benefit, especially if there is a component of bile salt malabsorption. A trial of fiber supplementation or probiotics may also be helpful. The α2-adrenergic agonist, clonidine, may provide adrenergic stimuli to facilitate fluid and electrolyte absorption in the intestines that appears to be disrupted in diabetic diarrhea. Small studies demonstrated that clonidine reduced stool volume in diabetic patients with profuse diarrhea.[67] Clonidine should be started at 0.1 mg twice daily but may be increased to 0.6 mg twice daily. If the medication is discontinued, a slow taper is recommended to prevent rebound hypertension. Octreotide, a long-acting somatostatin, has also been used to treat diabetic diarrhea with symptomatic improvement in small case series; however, it may slow small bowel motility and increase risk of bacterial overgrowth.[68] Additionally, octreotide is an inhibitor of glucagon and insulin, which places patients with diabetes at risk for both hyperglycemia and hypoglycemia.

LARGE INTESTINE DISORDERS
Fecal Incontinence

Fecal incontinence, the involuntary passage of fecal matter, appears to be a consequence of autonomic neuropathy. Incidence in the general population is estimated at 1%, although increases with age.[69] Symptoms of fecal incontinence frequently start with concomitant low-volume diarrhea. Nocturnal symptoms are frequent, and a subset of patients may have steatorrhea. Fecal incontinence typically occurs in patients with long disease duration and management is frequently challenging. Most of these patients are older and may have alternative etiologies for fecal incontinence, such as prior anal sphincter injuries from childbirth or surgery.

Pathophysiology of Fecal Incontinence

Autonomic neuropathy in diabetes appears to be responsible for nerve damage that leads to fecal incontinence. Multiple mechanisms help maintain fecal continence, and numerous insults are required to disrupt the process. Diabetic patients with incontinence have abnormal resting tone of the internal anal sphincter that is responsible for maintaining continence. Sensation of rectal distension also appears to be diminished in patients with diabetes, impairing the recto-anal reflex that leads to relaxation of the internal sphincter.[70] Furthermore, studies show that hyperglycemia independently impairs internal anal sphincter tone and rectal compliance, potentiating underlying deficits.[71]

Evaluation of Fecal Incontinence

Evaluation for fecal incontinence should include an evaluation for alternative etiologies for incontinence, including fecal impaction, infection, colonic mucosal disease, or primary diarrhea. A rectal examination will indicate whether fecal impaction with overflow incontinence is responsible for the symptoms and will allow for assessment of the anal sphincter. Evaluation of diarrhea should include stool cultures and flexible sigmoidoscopy or colonoscopy to evaluate for mucosal inflammation or structural etiology for the incontinence.[72]

Diagnosis of Fecal Incontinence

Anorectal manometry is the primary method used to define the deficits in fecal incontinence and typically quantifies sphincter pressure, rectal sensation, rectal compliance, and rectal reflexes. Recent technical advances in high-resolution manometry have greatly enhanced the ability to define underlying mechanisms causing fecal incontinence and may guide potential biofeedback therapy.[72]

Treatment of Fecal Incontinence

- Optimization of glycemic control
- Supportive lifestyle modification
- Antidiarrheal medications
- Biofeedback therapy
- Sacral stimulator or surgery

Management of fecal incontinence primarily begins with optimization of glycemic control and initiation of antidiarrheal medications. Loperamide and diphenoxylate with atropine reduce incontinence episodes and may suffice in managing modest symptoms. Cholestyramine may decrease diarrhea and improve continence. Biofeedback therapy aims to train individuals to become more aware of, and increase control of, anorectal muscles. It may improve anal sphincter strength, coordination of muscles, and sensory perception. Clinical improvement appears to be variable, as a result of differing symptom severity and lack of uniformity in biofeedback therapy. Small non-randomized studies of biofeedback have shown clinical efficacy in diabetic patients with fecal incontinence.[73] In refractory fecal incontinence, sacral nerve stimulation device implantation and surgery may improve symptoms; however, studies of fecal incontinence in diabetic patients have not been performed.

HEPATOBILIARY DISORDERS
Nonalcoholic Fatty Liver Disease Overview

Nonalcoholic fatty liver disease (NAFLD) is defined by fat deposition in the liver in the absence of alcohol abuse or other known hepatotoxins. It is a spectrum that includes nonalcoholic fatty liver (NAFL; fat deposition in the liver without inflammation) and nonalcoholic steatohepatitis (NASH; fat deposition with associated inflammation or hepatitis). Fatty liver is typically defined by the accumulation of fat in the liver without associated inflammation or elevated liver enzymes. In contrast, NASH is defined by the presence of fatty infiltrate in the liver with associated inflammation. Distinguishing between these 2 entities remains a significant clinical challenge (**Table 3**).

Table 3
Spectrum of nonalcoholic fatty liver disease

Term	Definition
Nonalcoholic fatty liver disease (NAFLD)	Encompasses spectrum of liver disease from fatty infiltrate without inflammation to cirrhosis
Nonalcoholic fatty liver (NAFL)	Liver fat accumulation in the liver without inflammation
Nonalcoholic steatohepatitis (NASH)	Liver fat accumulation *with* inflammation
NASH cirrhosis	End stage of NASH

Epidemiology

Incidence of NAFLD in the general population is not well defined. The incidence reported by different studies varies dramatically depending on the population, definition of NAFLD, and diagnostic modalities. Based on 2 histology-based studies of potential living liver donors, the prevalence of NAFLD is estimated to be between 20% and 51%.[74,75] The prevalence of NAFLD in DM2 may be as high as 69%, with diabetes as an independent predictor for progression of liver disease.[76] Risk factors include obesity, diabetes, hyperlipidemia, and age. The highest incidence appears to be in Hispanic individuals, and the lowest incidence occurs in African American individuals.[76]

Natural History of NAFLD

Based on limited studies, individuals with NAFLD have increased mortality as compared with matched control populations. Although liver-associated mortality is higher in NAFLD, the most common cause of death in this population is cardiovascular disease.[77] The survival of patients with NASH with associated inflammation as compared with those with benign hepatic fat is significantly worse.[78] Individuals with NASH, but probably not NAFL, have a significant risk of progression to cirrhosis, which will occur in up to 30%.[23]

Pathogenesis of NAFLD

The pathogenesis of NAFLD is poorly understood, and the lack of adequate animal models has limited research. The accumulation of fat in the liver appears to be related to an imbalance where lipogenesis exceeds lipolysis, and the amount of hepatic free-fatty acids exceeds requirements for mitochondrial oxidation, cholesterol synthesis, and phospholipid synthesis. This process appears to be driven by insulin levels and insulin resistance that drives free-fatty acid synthesis, inhibits synthesis of very low-density lipoproteins (VLDL), and enhances susceptibility to hepatic injury.[79] Free-fatty acids are toxic to hepatocytes through multiple mechanisms and play a role in induction of inflammation, but the precise mechanism underlying the progression from fatty liver to steatohepatitis is not completely understood, although it may be related to oxidative stress and mitochondrial dysfunction.[66,80]

Signs and Symptoms of NAFLD

NAFLD is typically asymptomatic and is frequently incidentally detected during an evaluation for an unrelated condition. Some individuals may report right upper quadrant abdominal pain, fatigue, or malaise. Although patients may have an enlarged liver on physical examination, concomitant obesity makes this physical finding difficult to appreciate. Serum alanine aminotransferase (ALT) and aspartate aminotransferase (AST) are frequently elevated, with ALT usually higher than AST. In the absence of advanced liver disease, total bilirubin, prothrombin time, and albumin levels remain normal. Imaging studies may show fat infiltrating the liver with the appearance varying by imaging modality.

Definition of NAFLD

- Presence of hepatic steatosis based on imaging or histology
- Absence of significant alcohol use
- Absence of secondary etiologies for liver disease
- Absence of coexisting chronic liver disease

Diagnosis of NAFLD or NASH is a clinical and pathologic diagnosis. Clinically, practitioners must exclude other etiologies for liver disease, including significant alcohol use, medications causing hepatic injury, viral hepatitis, Wilson's disease, autoimmune hepatitis, hemochromatosis, or alternative etiologies. The definition of significant alcohol use varies by gender and ultimately becomes a clinical assessment. Without histology, one cannot distinguish between benign fatty liver deposition and NASH, the latter being associated with a worse prognosis.

New Diagnostic Tools for NAFLD

Although practitioners typically begin with abdominal ultrasound when evaluating those suspected for NAFLD, this modality is not sensitive, nor specific. Computed tomography and magnetic resonance imaging (MRI) are more sensitive and specific in detecting steatosis. Newer forms of MRI are being developed to detect individuals with NASH or advanced fibrosis. Specifically, MR transient elastography measures liver stiffness noninvasively and successfully detects the presence of fibrosis in NAFLD, although is less accurate in the setting of obesity.[24] Other composite scores of simple laboratory parameters are being validated for detecting advanced fibrosis.[69]

The Role of Liver Biopsy

The role of liver biopsy in diagnosis remains somewhat debated. In some cases, biopsy is clearly needed to rule out concomitant liver disease. Although liver biopsy is an expensive and morbid procedure, it remains the gold standard for diagnosis and staging of disease. Fat deposition in the form of steatosis may be present on histology in fatty liver and NASH, but cellular damage with hepatocyte ballooning and/or fibrosis occurs only in NASH and distinguishes the progressive disease from benign fat infiltration. An active area of investigation is the development of noninvasive testing to identify NASH or advanced fibrosis.[81]

Management of NAFLD

Current management involves addressing any modifiable risk factors for NAFLD, including insulin resistance, diabetes, obesity, and hyperlipidemia, as well as the liver disease. Medications aimed at reversing the liver disease are reserved for individuals with NASH.

Lifestyle Modification

First-line treatment for NAFLD is initiation of diet and exercise. Based on current studies, weight loss of 3% to 5% of body weight may improve steatosis, but greater weight loss may be required to improve fibrosis. Exercise even without weight loss improves steatosis but may not reverse fibrosis.[77]

Medical Therapies for NASH and Diabetes

The medical therapies for NASH evaluated to date focus on enhancing insulin sensitivity but have had limited success. Metformin initially showed promise; however, a meta-analysis shows that metformin does not decrease liver enzymes or improve histology.[76] Conversely, a meta-analysis of 4 randomized clinical trials concluded that pioglitazone, a thiazolidinedione (TZD), significantly reduced steatosis and inflammation in NASH. However, the trials enrolled patients without diabetes, limiting the generalizability to diabetic patients, and long-term cardiovascular safety data are lacking.[77] Furthermore, recent associations of TZDs with bladder cancer have limited their overall use.[82] Similarly, vitamin E (800 IU per day) may improve histology in NASH; however, few data support use of vitamin E in diabetic patients with NASH, particularly given the potential association with prostate cancer.[83] Bariatric surgery appears to improve liver histology and will likely be a future treatment; however, randomized clinical trials are needed to support its use and determine which surgeries are most efficacious.[84] Overall, studies of NASH in diabetic patients are lacking and will be essential going forward to guide management; however, there are no approved treatments currently for liver disease associated with NASH.

Statin Use in NAFLD

Central to management of NAFLD is risk factor modification. Statins are extremely effective for dyslipidemia but may cause elevations in AST and ALT. As a result of this potential side effect, practitioners may be reluctant to use statins in the setting of NAFLD. The use of statins in the setting of NAFLD appears safe without increased risk of hepatotoxicity, and post hoc analyses suggest that statins improve cardiovascular outcomes and liver enzymes in NAFLD.[77] Although there are no guidelines to guide practitioners, a twofold increase in liver enzymes should be tolerated without cessation of therapy.

Cholelithiasis and Association with Diabetes

Gallstone disease and its complications, such as cholangitis, cholecystitis, and gallstone pancreatitis, occur more frequently in diabetic patients based on epidemiologic studies. However, these 2 diseases are both quite common and share risk factors, making it difficult to tease out the relationship between these entities. Mouse and human studies have shown relative bile stasis within the gallbladder and reduced cholecystokinin levels that may drive gallbladder stone formation.[85] Prophylactic cholecystectomy should not be performed for asymptomatic gallstones in diabetic patients.

PANCREATIC DISEASE
Pancreatic Insufficiency

Pancreatic exocrine insufficiency occurs in patients with DM1 and DM2. Historical studies demonstrated biochemical insufficiency in nearly 50% and 30% to 50% of patients with insulin-dependent diabetes and noninsulin-dependent diabetes, respectively.[86] Most of these patients have minor pancreatic exocrine insufficiency that is not clinically significant. If exocrine insufficiency is clinically significant and leads to fat malabsorption, individuals may benefit from mealtime pancreatic enzyme supplementation containing amylase, lipase, and protease. Clinically, pancreatic insufficiency may be a difficult entity to diagnose, and at times a clinical trial of pancreatic enzyme supplementation may be appropriate.

Acute Pancreatitis in Diabetes

Diabetic patients have an elevated risk of pancreatitis that appears to be intrinsic to the diseases as well as related to medications. Patients with DM1 have a twofold increased risk of pancreatitis, and patients with DM2 have a nearly threefold increased risk of pancreatitis as compared with the general population. The highest risk was in patients with DM2 who were younger than 30 years old.[66,87] The precise mechanism is not completely understood but may be related to ongoing inflammation. DM2 and pancreatitis share obesity and hypertriglyceridemia as common risk factors. Based on a review of the FDA adverse event reporting, GLP-1 agonists and dipeptidyl peptidase 4 inhibitors are associated with a sixfold increased risk of pancreatitis with a possible increased risk of pancreatic cancer.[88]

Pancreatic Cancer

Diabetes is a risk factor for pancreatic cancer but may also be a presenting sign. The etiologic role of diabetes in development of pancreatic cancer is poorly understood, although may be related to low-grade chronic inflammation of the pancreas. The relative risk of pancreatic cancer appears to be nearly 2 in patients with diabetes. The highest risk was in newly diagnosed diabetic patients, underscoring that new-onset diabetes may be an early sign of pancreatic malignancy.[89]

SUMMARY

The gastrointestinal complications of diabetes can affect essentially any organ in the gastrointestinal tract, are associated with significant morbidity and mortality, and can directly impair quality of life. With this in mind, the health care professional should be aware of these associated conditions, as well as the high prevalence of overlapping gastrointestinal symptoms unrelated to diabetes. Although screening for heart disease, retinopathy, neuropathy, and nephropathy typically make their way into preformed electronic records for a clinic visit, gastrointestinal symptoms are frequently not screened for and may be underreported. Abnormalities uncovered should be investigated with consideration of referral to a gastroenterology specialist when appropriate. In this way, screening and treating gastrointestinal-related complications may enhance comprehensive care of diabetic patients.

REFERENCES

1. Camilleri M, Dubois D, Coulie B, et al. Prevalence and socioeconomic impact of upper gastrointestinal disorders in the United States: results of the US Upper Gastrointestinal Study. Clin Gastroenterol Hepatol 2005;3:543–52.
2. Gatopoulou A, Papanas N, Maltezos E. Diabetic gastrointestinal autonomic neuropathy: current status and new achievements for everyday clinical practice. Eur J Intern Med 2012;23:499–505.
3. Kinekawa F, Kubo F, Matsuda K, et al. Relationship between esophageal dysfunction and neuropathy in diabetic patients. Am J Gastroenterol 2001;96: 2026–32.
4. Lluch I, Ascaso JF, Mora F, et al. Gastroesophageal reflux in diabetes mellitus. Am J Gastroenterol 1999;94:919–24.

5. Wang X, Pitchumoni CS, Chandrarana K, et al. Increased prevalence of symptoms of gastroesophageal reflux diseases in type 2 diabetics with neuropathy. World J Gastroenterol 2008;14:709–12.

6. Singh PK, Hota D, Dutta P, et al. Pantoprazole improves glycemic control in type 2 diabetes: a randomized, double-blind, placebo-controlled trial. J Clin Endocrinol Metab 2012;97:E2105–8.

7. Wilcox CM, Karowe MW. Esophageal infections: etiology, diagnosis, and management. Gastroenterologist 1994;2:188–206.

8. Jung HK, Choung RS, Locke GR 3rd, et al. The incidence, prevalence, and outcomes of patients with gastroparesis in Olmsted County, Minnesota, from 1996 to 2006. Gastroenterology 2009;136:1225–33.

9. Choung RS, Locke GR 3rd, Schleck CD, et al. Risk of gastroparesis in subjects with type 1 and 2 diabetes in the general population. Am J Gastroenterol 2012; 107:82–8.

10. Keshavarzian A, Iber FL, Vaeth J. Gastric emptying in patients with insulin-requiring diabetes mellitus. Am J Gastroenterol 1987;82:29–35.

11. Camilleri M, Bharucha AE, Farrugia G. Epidemiology, mechanisms, and management of diabetic gastroparesis. Clin Gastroenterol Hepatol 2011;9:5–12 [quiz: e17].

12. Schvarcz E, Palmer M, Aman J, et al. Physiological hyperglycemia slows gastric emptying in normal subjects and patients with insulin-dependent diabetes mellitus. Gastroenterology 1997;113:60–6.

13. Farrugia G. Interstitial cells of Cajal in health and disease. Neurogastroenterol Motil 2008;20(Suppl 1):54–63.

14. Harberson J, Thomas RM, Harbison SP, et al. Gastric neuromuscular pathology in gastroparesis: analysis of full-thickness antral biopsies. Dig Dis Sci 2010;55: 359–70.

15. Schwartz TW. Pancreatic polypeptide: a hormone under vagal control. Gastroenterology 1983;85:1411–25.

16. Tomita R, Tanjoh K, Fujisaki S, et al. The role of nitric oxide (NO) in the human pyloric sphincter. Hepatogastroenterology 1999;46:2999–3003.

17. Watkins CC, Sawa A, Jaffrey S, et al. Insulin restores neuronal nitric oxide synthase expression and function that is lost in diabetic gastropathy. J Clin Invest 2000;106:803.

18. Choi KM, Gibbons SJ, Nguyen TV, et al. Heme oxygenase-1 protects interstitial cells of Cajal from oxidative stress and reverses diabetic gastroparesis. Gastroenterology 2008;135:2055–64, 2064.e1–2.

19. Sarnelli G, Caenepeel P, Geypens B, et al. Symptoms associated with impaired gastric emptying of solids and liquids in functional dyspepsia. Am J Gastroenterol 2003;98:783–8.

20. Camilleri M, Parkman HP, Shafi MA, et al, American College of Gastroenterology. Clinical guideline: management of gastroparesis. Am J Gastroenterol 2013;108: 18–37 [quiz: 38].

21. Abell TL, Camilleri M, Donohoe K, et al, American Neurogastroenterology and Motility Society and the Society of Nuclear Medicine. Consensus recommendations for gastric emptying scintigraphy: a joint report of the American Neurogastroenterology and Motility Society and the Society of Nuclear Medicine. J Nucl Med Technol 2008;36:44–54.

22. Fraser RJ, Horowitz M, Maddox AF, et al. Hyperglycaemia slows gastric emptying in type 1 (insulin-dependent) diabetes mellitus. Diabetologia 1990; 33:675–80.

23. Fassio E, Alvarez E, Dominguez N, et al. Natural history of nonalcoholic steato-hepatitis: a longitudinal study of repeat liver biopsies. Hepatology 2004;40:820–6.
24. Musso G, Gambino R, Cassader M, et al. Meta-analysis: natural history of non-alcoholic fatty liver disease (NAFLD) and diagnostic accuracy of non-invasive tests for liver disease severity. Ann Med 2011;43:617–49.
25. Lee A, Kuo B. Metoclopramide in the treatment of diabetic gastroparesis. Expert Rev Endocrinol Metab 2010;5:653–62.
26. McCallum RW, Ricci DA, Rakatansky H, et al. A multicenter placebo-controlled clinical trial of oral metoclopramide in diabetic gastroparesis. Diabetes Care 1983;6:463–7.
27. Perkel MS, Moore C, Hersh T, et al. Metoclopramide therapy in patients with de-layed gastric emptying: a randomized, double-blind study. Dig Dis Sci 1979;24:662–6.
28. Snape WJ Jr, Battle WM, Schwartz SS, et al. Metoclopramide to treat gastropa-resis due to diabetes mellitus: a double-blind, controlled trial. Ann Intern Med 1982;96:444–6.
29. Miller LG, Jankovic J. Metoclopramide-induced movement disorders. Clinical findings with a review of the literature. Arch Intern Med 1989;149:2486–92.
30. Bateman DN, Rawlins MD, Simpson JM. Extrapyramidal reactions with metoclo-pramide. Br Med J (Clin Res Ed) 1985;291:930–2.
31. Parkman HP, Mishra A, Jacobs M, et al. Clinical response and side effects of metoclopramide: associations with clinical, demographic, and pharmacoge-netic parameters. J Clin Gastroenterol 2012;46:494–503.
32. Silvers D, Kipnes M, Broadstone V, et al. Domperidone in the management of symptoms of diabetic gastroparesis: efficacy, tolerability, and quality-of-life out-comes in a multicenter controlled trial. DOM-USA-5 Study Group. Clin Ther 1998;20:438–53.
33. Patterson D, Abell T, Rothstein R, et al. A double-blind multicenter comparison of domperidone and metoclopramide in the treatment of diabetic patients with symptoms of gastroparesis. Am J Gastroenterol 1999;94:1230–4.
34. Franzese A, Borrelli O, Corrado G, et al. Domperidone is more effective than cis-apride in children with diabetic gastroparesis. Aliment Pharmacol Ther 2002;16:951–7.
35. Janssens J, Peeters TL, Vantrappen G, et al. Improvement of gastric emptying in diabetic gastroparesis by erythromycin. Preliminary studies. N Engl J Med 1990;322:1028–31.
36. Adams LA, Angulo P. Role of liver biopsy and serum markers of liver fibrosis in non-alcoholic fatty liver disease. Clin Liver Dis 2007;11:25–35, viii.
37. Abell T, McCallum R, Hocking M, et al. Gastric electrical stimulation for medi-cally refractory gastroparesis. Gastroenterology 2003;125:421–8.
38. Chu H, Lin Z, Zhong L, et al. Treatment of high-frequency gastric electrical stim-ulation for gastroparesis. J Gastroenterol Hepatol 2012;27:1017–26.
39. Wang CP, Kao CH, Chen WK, et al. A single-blinded, randomized pilot study evaluating effects of electroacupuncture in diabetic patients with symptoms suggestive of gastroparesis. J Altern Complement Med 2008;14:833–9.
40. Sjoberg K, Eriksson KF, Bredberg A, et al. Screening for coeliac disease in adult insulin-dependent diabetes mellitus. J Intern Med 1998;243:133–40.
41. Talal AH, Murray JA, Goeken JA, et al. Celiac disease in an adult population with insulin-dependent diabetes mellitus: use of endomysial antibody testing. Am J Gastroenterol 1997;92:1280–4.

42. Cronin CC, Feighery A, Ferriss JB, et al. High prevalence of celiac disease among patients with insulin-dependent (type I) diabetes mellitus. Am J Gastroenterol 1997;92:2210–2.
43. Fasano A, Berti I, Gerarduzzi T, et al. Prevalence of celiac disease in at-risk and not-at-risk groups in the United States: a large multicenter study. Arch Intern Med 2003;163:286–92.
44. Ludvigsson JF, Rubio-Tapia A, van Dyke CT, et al. Increasing incidence of celiac disease in a North American population. Am J Gastroenterol 2013;108(5):818–24.
45. Cronin CC, Shanahan F. Insulin-dependent diabetes mellitus and coeliac disease. Lancet 1997;349:1096–7.
46. Green PH, Cellier C. Celiac disease. N Engl J Med 2007;357:1731–43.
47. Kagnoff MF. Celiac disease: pathogenesis of a model immunogenetic disease. J Clin Invest 2007;117:41–9.
48. Rostom A, Dube C, Cranney A, et al. Celiac disease. Evid Rep Technol Assess (Summ) 2004;(104):1–6.
49. Sud S, Marcon M, Assor E, et al. 2010 Celiac disease and pediatric type 1 diabetes: diagnostic and treatment dilemmas. Int J Pediatr Endocrinol 2010;2010: 161285.
50. Nakajima K. 2012 Recent advances in dermatitis herpetiformis. Clin Dev Immunol 2012;2012:914162.
51. van der Windt DA, Jellema P, Mulder CJ, et al. Diagnostic testing for celiac disease among patients with abdominal symptoms: a systematic review. JAMA 2010;303:1738–46.
52. Rostom A, Murray JA, Kagnoff MF. American Gastroenterological Association (AGA) Institute technical review on the diagnosis and management of celiac disease. Gastroenterology 2006;131:1981–2002.
53. Rostom A, Dube C, Cranney A, et al. The diagnostic accuracy of serologic tests for celiac disease: a systematic review. Gastroenterology 2005;128:S38–46.
54. Corrao G, Corazza GR, Bagnardi V, et al. Mortality in patients with coeliac disease and their relatives: a cohort study. Lancet 2001;358:356–61.
55. Loftus CG, Loftus EV Jr. Cancer risk in celiac disease. Gastroenterology 2002; 123:1726–9.
56. Leffler DA, Dennis M, Hyett B, et al. Etiologies and predictors of diagnosis in nonresponsive celiac disease. Clin Gastroenterol Hepatol 2007;5:445–50.
57. Parlesak A, Klein B, Schecher K, et al. Prevalence of small bowel bacterial overgrowth and its association with nutrition intake in nonhospitalized older adults. J Am Geriatr Soc 2003;51:768–73.
58. Virally-Monod M, Tielmans D, Kevorkian JP, et al. Chronic diarrhoea and diabetes mellitus: prevalence of small intestinal bacterial overgrowth. Diabete Metab 1998;24:530–6.
59. Dukowicz AC, Lacy BE, Levine GM. Small intestinal bacterial overgrowth: a comprehensive review. Gastroenterol Hepatol 2007;3:112–22.
60. Saltzman JR, Russell RM. Nutritional consequences of intestinal bacterial overgrowth. Compr Ther 1994;20:523–30.
61. Bures J, Cyrany J, Kohoutova D, et al. Small intestinal bacterial overgrowth syndrome. World J Gastroenterol 2010;16:2978–90.
62. Corazza GR, Menozzi MG, Strocchi A, et al. The diagnosis of small bowel bacterial overgrowth. Reliability of jejunal culture and inadequacy of breath hydrogen testing. Gastroenterology 1990;98:302–9.
63. Pimentel M. Review of rifaximin as treatment for SIBO and IBS. Expert Opin Investig Drugs 2009;18:349–58.

64. Lysy J, Israeli E, Goldin E. The prevalence of chronic diarrhea among diabetic patients. Am J Gastroenterol 1999;94:2165–70.
65. Miller LJ. Small intestinal manifestations of diabetes mellitus. Yale J Biol Med 1983;56:189–93.
66. Feldman M, Friedman LS, Brandt LJ, editors. Sleisenger and Fordtran's gastro-intesitnal and liver disease: pathophysiology/diagnosis/management. 9th edition. Philadelphia: Elsevier; 2010.
67. Fedorak RN, Field M, Chang EB. Treatment of diabetic diarrhea with clonidine. Ann Intern Med 1985;102:197–9.
68. Meyer C, O'Neal DN, Connell W, et al. Octreotide treatment of severe diabetic diarrhoea. Intern Med J 2003;33:617–8.
69. Angulo P, Hui JM, Marchesini G, et al. The NAFLD fibrosis score: a noninvasive system that identifies liver fibrosis in patients with NAFLD. Hepatology 2007;45:846–54.
70. Schiller LR, Santa Ana CA, Schmulen AC, et al. Pathogenesis of fecal incontinence in diabetes mellitus: evidence for internal-anal-sphincter dysfunction. N Engl J Med 1982;307:1666–71.
71. Russo A, Botten R, Kong MF, et al. Effects of acute hyperglycaemia on anorectal motor and sensory function in diabetes mellitus. Diabet Med 2004;21:176–82.
72. Rao SS. Diagnosis and management of fecal incontinence. American College of Gastroenterology Practice Parameters Committee. Am J Gastroenterol 2004;99:1585–604.
73. Wald A, Tunuguntla AK. Anorectal sensorimotor dysfunction in fecal incontinence and diabetes mellitus. Modification with biofeedback therapy. N Engl J Med 1984;310:1282–7.
74. Lee JY, Kim KM, Lee SG, et al. Prevalence and risk factors of non-alcoholic fatty liver disease in potential living liver donors in Korea: a review of 589 consecutive liver biopsies in a single center. J Hepatol 2007;47:239–44.
75. Marcos A, Fisher RA, Ham JM, et al. Selection and outcome of living donors for adult to adult right lobe transplantation. Transplantation 2000;69:2410–5.
76. Vernon G, Baranova A, Younossi ZM. Systematic review: the epidemiology and natural history of non-alcoholic fatty liver disease and non-alcoholic steatohepatitis in adults. Aliment Pharmacol Ther 2011;34:274–85.
77. Chalasani N, Younossi Z, Lavine JE, et al, American Gastroenterological Association, American Association for the Study of Liver Diseases, American College of Gastroenterologyh. The diagnosis and management of non-alcoholic fatty liver disease: practice guideline by the American Gastroenterological Association, American Association for the Study of Liver Diseases, and American College of Gastroenterology. Gastroenterology 2012;142:1592–609.
78. Soderberg C, Stal P, Askling J. Decreased survival of subjects with elevated liver function tests during a 28-year follow-up. Hepatology 2010;51:595–602.
79. Chitturi S, Abeygunasekera S, Farrell GC, et al. NASH and insulin resistance: insulin hypersecretion and specific association with the insulin resistance syndrome. Hepatology 2002;35:373–9.
80. Browning JD, Horton JD. Molecular mediators of hepatic steatosis and liver injury. J Clin Invest 2004;114:147–52.
81. Farrell GC, Larter CZ. Nonalcoholic fatty liver disease: from steatosis to cirrhosis. Hepatology 2006;43:S99–112.
82. Lewis JD, Ferrara A, Peng T, et al. Risk of bladder cancer among diabetic patients treated with pioglitazone: interim report of a longitudinal cohort study. Diabetes Care 2011;34:916–22.

83. Sanyal AJ, Chalasani N, Kowdley KV, et al. Pioglitazone, vitamin E, or placebo for nonalcoholic steatohepatitis. N Engl J Med 2010;362:1675–85.
84. Chavez-Tapia NC, Tellez-Avila FI, Barrientos-Gutierrez T, et al. Bariatric surgery for non-alcoholic steatohepatitis in obese patients. Cochrane Database Syst Rev 2010;(1):CD007340.
85. Pazzi P, Scagliarini R, Gamberini S, et al. Review article: gall-bladder motor function in diabetes mellitus. Aliment Pharmacol Ther 2000;14(Suppl 2):62–5.
86. Hardt PD, Ewald N. 2011 Exocrine pancreatic insufficiency in diabetes mellitus: a complication of diabetic neuropathy or a different type of diabetes? Exp Diabetes Res 2011;2011:761950.
87. Shen HN, Chang YH, Chen HF, et al. Increased risk of severe acute pancreatitis in patients with diabetes. Diabet Med 2012;29:1419–24.
88. Elashoff M, Matveyenko AV, Gier B, et al. Pancreatitis, pancreatic, and thyroid cancer with glucagon-like peptide-1-based therapies. Gastroenterology 2011; 141:150–6.
89. Ben Q, Xu M, Ning X, et al. Diabetes mellitus and risk of pancreatic cancer: a meta-analysis of cohort studies. Eur J Cancer 2011;47:1928–37.

Diabetic Retinopathy
Current Concepts and Emerging Therapy

Daniel F. Rosberger, MD, PhD, MPH[a,b]

KEYWORDS

- Diabetic retinopathy • Anti-VEGF therapy • Intravitreal medications
- Microvascular complications of diabetes • Laser photocoagulation

KEY POINTS

- The epidemiology of diabetic retinopathy indicates that although diabetes remains the leading cause of blindness among Americans, tight glucose control and lifestyle modification can reduce its prevalence.
- Although laser photocoagulation remains the mainstay of treatment of both proliferative diabetic retinopathy and clinically significant macular edema, the paradigm is shifting toward treatment with intravitreal medications.
- Emerging therapy with anti–vascular endothelial growth factor agents, long-acting corticosteroids, protein kinase C inhibitors, tumor necrosis factor modulators, and other medications may dramatically improve the treatment of diabetic retinopathy in the coming years.
- The Diabetes Retinopathy Clinical Research Network is a National Institutes of Health–funded collaborative network of more than 300 physicians dedicated to multicenter clinical research of diabetic retinopathy, diabetic macular edema, and associated conditions.

INTRODUCTION

Diabetic retinopathy is a disease that eventually affects nearly all patients with long-standing diabetes mellitus. The earliest visualized lesions are generally intraretinal hemorrhages and microaneurysms. With progression, fibrovascular proliferation and neovascularization can occur. Visual loss eventually results from macular edema, macular ischemia from capillary nonperfusion, vitreous hemorrhage, fibrous distortion of the macula, neovascular glaucoma, and tractional or rhegmatogenous retinal detachments (RD). The Diabetes Control and Complications Trial (DCCT) and the United Kingdom Prospective Diabetes Study (UKPDS) have clearly demonstrated that tight glucose control in both type 1 and type 2 diabetes can significantly delay the onset and progression of retinopathy. (**Table 1** lists the commonly used abbreviations in diabetic retinopathy.) For both diabetic macular edema (DME) and proliferative diabetic

This article originally appeared in Endocrinology and Metabolism Clinics of North America, Volume 42, Issue 4, December 2013.
[a] Weill-Cornell Medical College of Cornell University, 1300 York Avenue, New York, NY 10021, USA; [b] MaculaCare, PLLC, 52 East 72nd Street, New York, NY 10021, USA
E-mail address: drosberger@gmail.com

Table 1
Commonly used abbreviations in diabetic retinopathy

CSME	Clinically significant diabetic retinopathy
CWS	Cotton wool spot
DCCT	Diabetes Control and Complications Trial
DME	Diabetic macular edema
DRCR net	Diabetic Retinopathy Clinical Research network
DRS	Diabetic Retinopathy Study
ETDRS	Early Treatment Diabetic Retinopathy Study
FA	Fluorescein angiography
FVP	Fibrovascular proliferation
HR	High risk
IRH	Intraretinal hemorrhage
IVTA	Intravitreal triamcinolone acetonide
ma	Microaneurysm
NHR	Non–high risk
NPDR	Nonproliferative diabetic retinopathy
NVA	Neovascularization of the trabecular angle
NVD	Neovascularization of the optic disk
NVE	Neovascularization elsewhere (other than the optic disk)
NVG	Neovascular glaucoma
NVI	Neovascularization of the iris
OCT	Optical coherence tomography
POAG	Primary open angle glaucoma
PDR	Proliferative diabetic retinopathy
RD	Retinal detachment
SLE	Slit lamp examination
UKPDS	United Kingdom Prospective Diabetes Study
VH	Vitreous hemorrhage
WESDR	Wisconsin Epidemiologic Study of Diabetic Retinopathy

retinopathy (PDR), the mainstay of treatment has been laser photocoagulation. However, in the past few years, new agents and new delivery systems have been developed that are fundamentally changing the treatment paradigm.

EPIDEMIOLOGY

Diabetic retinopathy remains one of the most common complications of chronic diabetes mellitus and the leading cause of new cases of blindness (defined by central visual acuity worse than 20/200) in the United States in people aged 20 to 74 years. An estimated 50 000 new cases of retinal neovascularization and macular edema occur yearly.[1–3] Despite this, as many as half of the patients who would benefit from treatment remain untreated.[4] The DCCT demonstrated a marked reduction in the development and progression of diabetic retinopathy in intensively treated type 1 diabetes compared with those treated conventionally.[5–7] The UKPDS showed similar results in patients with type 2 diabeties.[8]

Much of what we know about the epidemiology of diabetic retinopathy in the United States comes from the Wisconsin Epidemiologic Study of Diabetic Retinopathy

(WESDR), which received its initial funding from the National Institutes of Health (NIH) in 1979. The primary aims of this study were to (1) describe the prevalence and severity of retinopathy and visual loss in people with diabetes and their relationship to other systemic complications and mortality, (2) quantitate the association of risk factors with retinopathy, and (3) provide information on health care delivery and quality of life in people with diabetes.

Table 2 summarizes the baseline prevalence and disease severity in WESDR. In an 11-county region of southwestern Wisconsin, 452 of the 457 physicians who provided primary medical care to patients with diabetes participated by collecting lists of all the patients with diabetes they saw during the 1-year period from July 1, 1979 through June 30, 1980.[9,10] A total of 10 135 patients were identified, and an initial sample of 2990 patients was selected for a baseline examination. The sample was divided into 2 groups. The first, type 1 diabetes, was referred to as *younger onset* and consisted of 1210 patients diagnosed with diabetes before 30 years of age who were taking insulin. The second group, referred to as *older onset*, consisted of a probability sample of 1780 patients taken from all eligible patients who were diagnosed with diabetes at 30 years of age or older with a postprandial serum glucose measurement of 11.1 mmol/L or more or a fasting serum glucose measurement of 7.8 mmol/L or more on at least 2 separate occasions. The older-onset group was further stratified by (1) the duration of diabetes (less than 5 years [576 patients], 5 to 14 years [579 patients], and greater than 15 years [625 patients]) and (2) insulin usage (824 patients were taking insulin and 956 were not).

At the study initiation visit, approximately 70% of the younger-onset patients had some degree of diabetic retinopathy and 23% had PDR.[11] In the older-onset arm, 70% of the patients taking insulin had some degree of retinopathy, whereas only 39% of the patients not taking insulin did. Moreover, 14% of the older-onset patients taking insulin and 3% of the patients who were not on insulin had PDR.[12] Clinically significant macular edema (CSME) was present in approximately 6% of the younger-onset patients, 12% of the older-onset patients taking insulin, and 4% of the older-onset patients not taking insulin.[13]

A recent study analyzed a cross-sectional, nationally representative sample of the National Health and Nutrition Examination Survey 2005–2008 (n = 1006).[14] Among US adults with diabetes, the estimated prevalence of diabetic retinopathy and vision-threatening diabetic retinopathy was 28.5%. Retinopathy was slightly more

Table 2
Baseline prevalence and disease severity in the WESDR

Retinopathy Status	Younger Onset, (N = 996)	Older Onset, Taking Insulin (N = 673)	Older Onset, Not Taking Insulin (N = 673)
None (%)	29.3	29.9	61.3
Mild NPDR (%)	30.4	30.6	27.3
Moderate and severe NPDR (%)	17.6	25.7	8.5
PDR without HR characteristics (%)	13.2	9.1	1.4
Proliferative with HR characteristics or worse (%)	9.5	4.8	1.4
CSME (%)	5.9	11.6	3.7

Abbreviations: CSME, clinically significant diabetic retinopathy; HR, high risk; NPDR, nonproliferative diabetic retinopathy.

prevalent among men than women. Non-Hispanic blacks with diabetes had a higher crude prevalence than non-Hispanic whites of diabetic retinopathy (38.8% vs 26.4%) and vision-threatening diabetic retinopathy (9.3% vs 3.2%). Independent risk factors for the presence of diabetic retinopathy included male sex, higher hemoglobin A1c measurement, longer duration of diabetes insulin use, and higher systolic blood pressure.

However, microvascular changes consistent with diabetic retinopathy can occur even before the diagnosis of diabetic retinopathy using current definitions. The Diabetes Prevention Program was a multicentered, randomized, controlled clinical trial that enrolled 3234 overweight participants that had elevated blood glucose levels but had not yet met the definitional criteria for diabetes. The study demonstrated that intensive lifestyle changes including a low-fat diet, weight loss, and increased physical activity could reduce the development of type 2 diabetes by 58% compared with placebo and that metformin (850 mg twice daily) lowered diabetes incidence by 31% compared with placebo. It also demonstrated that approximately 8% of these patients who were prediabetic already had diabetic retinopathy.[15]

PATHOGENESIS

The precise processes by which diabetes results in retinopathy are not completely understood; however, damage to the retinal microvasculature is clearly paramount. The molecular mechanism of microvasculature damage is likely multifactorial, with roles for hyperglycemia-induced polyol pathway activation, production of advanced glycation end products, oxidative stress, and activation of the diacylglycerol–protein kinase C (PKC) transcription pathway.

Fig. 1 demonstrates the layers of the retina and the relationship of the retina to the overlying vitreous and the underlying retinal pigment epithelium (RPE). Abnormalities in most of these layers can be seen in diabetic retinopathy.

Vasculature abnormalities are a prominent finding in diabetic retinopathy and can occur anywhere between the nerve fiber layer (NFL) and the outer plexiform layer. Early damage in diabetic retinopathy can be seen by light microscopic evaluation of retinal vessels as a reduction in the number of pericytes surrounding retinal capillary endothelial cells.[16] Microaneurysms are the outpouching of these damaged capillaries. Microaneurysmal leakage likely plays a significant role in DME. Endothelial cell proliferation, deposition of excess basement membrane material, closing of the microaneurysm lumen, and loss of endothelial cells may lead to capillary dropout and ischemia. With progressive damage and capillary nonperfusion, arteriovenous shunts can form. Intraretinal microvascular abnormalities (IRMA) arise in areas of ischemia and can sometimes appear similar to neovascularization except that IRMA does not leak on fluorescein angiography, generally occur deeper in the retina, and are not present on the optic disk.

Cotton wool spots (CWS) are seen in the NFL and under the internal limiting membrane (ILM). They are cytoid bodies and represent stasis of axoplasmic flow in the axons of ganglion cells in the NFL.

Hard exudates are fat-filled, lipoidal histiocytes occurring in the outer plexiform layer. This exudation surrounds damaged retinal vasculature and microaneurysms and may appear in a circinate pattern.

Venous dilatations are the result of abnormalities in the walls of retinal veins. Thickening of the capillary basement membranes and increased constriction at crossing points of retinal arteries and veins are also commonly seen. As the severity of the

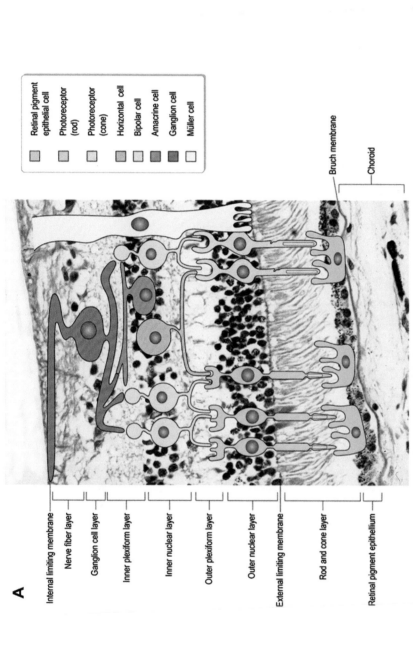

Fig. 1. Layers of the retina and the relationship of the retina to the overlying vitreous and the underlying retinal pigment epithelium. (*From [A]* Herzlich AA, Patel AA, Sauer TC, et al. Chapter 2: retinal anatomy and pathology. Retinal pharmacotherapy. Copyright Elsevier 2010; [B] The eye. Potter's pathology of the fetus, infant and child. Copyright Elsevier 2007.)

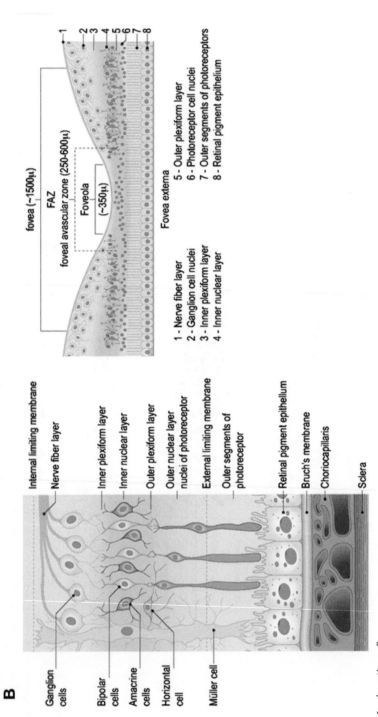

Fig. 1. *(continued)*

retinopathy progresses, beading of the retinal veins resulting from dilated venous walls and saccular aneurysmal dilatation occurs. The appearance of hemorrhages in the retina depends on the layer where the hemorrhage occurs. Intraretinal dot or blot hemorrhages occur in the inner retinal layer but can spread to the outer plexiform layer. They appear as dots because they are contained between the perpendicularly oriented cellular elements. Flame-shaped or splinter intraretinal hemorrhages spread out within the parallel elements of the NFL. Large confluent hemorrhages can involve all of the retinal layers and even break through the ILM into the vitreous space and into the subretinal space.[7]

Thickening of the ILM and posterior vitreous face can be seen in early retinopathy with progressive fibrotic attachment of the ILM to the vitreous as retinopathy advances with fibroblasts, fibrous astrocytes, myofibroblasts, and macrophages present in the ILM and the vitreous in patients with DME.[17]

Retinal neovascularization arises in regions of hypoxia, and it is thought to be mediated by the elaboration of vascular endothelial growth factor (VEGF). New blood vessels commonly arise from retinal venues at the margin of an area of capillary nonperfusion. Fibrovascular proliferation can break through the ILM and onto the surface of the retina and extend into the vitreous space. Rupture of these fragile neovascular vessels can cause extensive hemorrhage into the vitreous. As the fibrovascular process matures, fibrosis can occur on the surface of the retina causing macular distortion. With sufficient contraction, the neurosensory retina can be pulled up of the RPE creating a tractional RD. In extreme cases, the retina can rip, leading to a rhegmatogenous RD.

DIAGNOSIS AND CLASSIFICATION

Despite the fact that the paradigm for treating diabetic retinopathy is moving away from laser photocoagulation (see discussion elsewhere in this article), the classification of retinopathy and, therefore, the timing of treatment and follow-up are still largely based on clinical trials of focal and panretinal laser photocoagulation.

In general, diabetic retinopathy is classified as either nonproliferative (NPDR) or proliferative (PDR) based on the absence or presence of retinal vascular neovascularization. Macular edema can be present independently in either NPDR or PDR and is classified as absent, present, and clinically significant (CSME) or non-clinically significant. Correct classification is important because it gives us information about the preferred intervention and the risk of progression that will determine the appropriate follow-up. Immediate treatment is almost always recommended for macular edema once the threshold for clinical significance has been reached and for PDR once high-risk criteria are met. No treatment is generally recommended for NPDR in the absence of CSME. Classification is based on standard fundus photographs used in the Early Treatment Diabetic Retinopathy Study (ETDRS).[18]

NPDR

Mild NPDR

Patients with mild NPDR have at least one microaneurysm; however, there are fewer intraretinal dot or blot hemorrhages than in the ETDRS standard photograph 2A (**Fig. 2**), and no other retinal abnormalities associated with diabetes are present. Patients with mild NPDR have only a 5% risk of progressing to PDR within 1 year and only a 15% risk of progressing to high-risk PDR necessitating panretinal laser photocoagulation within 5 years.[7]

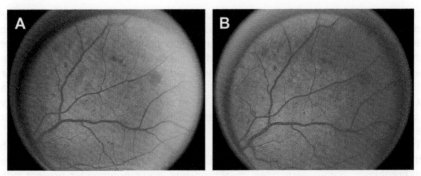

Fig. 2. Stereoscopic pairs of standard photograph 2A of the modified Airlie House classification of diabetic retinopathy illustrates a moderate degree of hemorrhages and microaneurysms. (*From* Aiello LM. Perspectives on diabetic retinopathy. Am J Ophthalmol 2003;136(1):131; with permission.)

Moderate NPDR

Patients with moderate NPDR have more microaneurysms or intraretinal hemorrhages than in the ETDRS standard photograph 2A (see **Fig. 2**) in one field; however, they are present in fewer than 4 quadrants of the retina. NFL infarctions (commonly referred to as CWS or soft exudates), undulations in the caliber of retinal veins (referred to as venous beading [VB]), and IRMA are present but less prominent than in the ETDRS standard photograph 8A (**Fig. 3**). Patients with moderate NPDR have a 12% to 27% risk of progressing to PDR within 1 year and a 33% 5-year risk of reaching the criteria for high-risk PDR.[7]

Severe NPDR

Patients with severe NPDR are defined by having one of the elements of the 4-2-1 rule. They have either 4 quadrants of intraretinal hemorrhages or microaneurysms greater than the ETDRS standard photograph 2A (see **Fig. 2**), 2 quadrants of significant VB, or 1 quadrant of IRMA greater than the ETDRS standard photograph 8A (see **Fig. 3**) and no retinal vascular neovascularization. Patients with severe NPDR have a 52% risk of progressing to PDR within 1 year and a 60% 5-year risk of reaching the criteria for high-risk PDR.[7]

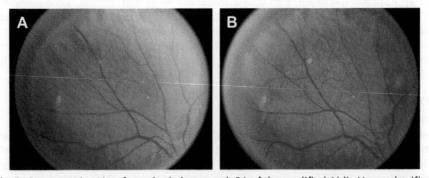

Fig. 3. Stereoscopic pairs of standard photograph 8A of the modified Airlie House classification of diabetic retinopathy illustrates a moderate degree of IRMA. (*From* Aiello LM. Perspectives on diabetic retinopathy. Am J Ophthalmol 2003;136(1):131; with permission.)

Very severe NPDR

Patients with very severe NPDR have at least 2 of the elements of the 4-2-1 rule (defined earlier for severe NPDR) but have no retinal vascular neovascularization. They have a 75% risk of progressing to PDR within 1 year.[7]

PDR

PDR is characterized by neovascularization on the optic disk (NVD) or elsewhere (NVE) on the retina, hemorrhage present within the vitreous or trapped between the interface of the surface of the retina and the posterior margin of the vitreous body (subhyaloid hemorrhage), or fibrovascular proliferation, which can cause pulling on the retina sometimes leading to tractional or rhegmatogenous RD. PDR is defined as either early or high risk. Eyes with early PDR have a 75% 5-year risk of developing high-risk PDR. High-risk PDR is defined by the presence of NVD greater than approximately one-third of the area of the optic disk as defined by the ETDRS reference photograph 10 A (**Fig. 4**), or any NVD associated with vitreous or subhyaloid hemorrhage, or an area of NVE greater than one-half of the area of the optic disk with concomitant vitreous or subhyaloid hemorrhage. Early PDR includes all eyes that meet the criteria for PDR but do not meet the criteria for high risk.[7]

Macular Edema

Damage to the macula can occur at any level of NPDR or PDR. It may involve leakage of serosanguinous fluid from retinal vasculature damaged by diabetes or microaneurysms and result in a collection of intraretinal fluid within the macula causing the macula to become thickened or edematous. This damage may occur in a cystoid (not true cysts because there is no endothelial lining) pattern and may be associated with precipitated lipids sometimes referred to as hard exudates. Macular edema is usually defined as retinal thickening within 2 disk diameters (approximately 3 mm) of the center of the macula. Alternatively, macular damage can be the result of parafoveal capillary nonperfusion and ischemia with or without edema; fibrovascular traction on the macula causing wrinkling, distortion, or detachment of the macula; intraretinal or subhyaloid hemorrhage, which can cause a physical barrier to images reaching the macula; or the formation of macular holes.

CSME

CSME is defined by the ETDRS as macular edema meeting one or more of the following 3 criteria: (1) retinal thickening occurring at or within 500 μm of the center

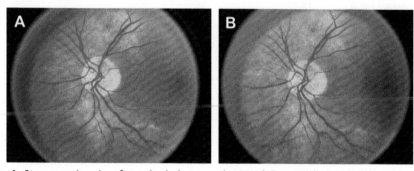

Fig. 4. Stereoscopic pairs of standard photograph 10A of the modified Airlie House classification of diabetic retinopathy illustrates a moderate degree of NVD. (*From* Aiello LM. Perspectives on diabetic retinopathy. Am J Ophthalmol 2003;136(1):131; with permission.)

of the macula; (2) lipid precipitate deposition (hard exudates) with adjacent, associated retinal thickening at or within 500 μm of the center of the macula; or (3) a zone of retinal thickening of at least 1 disk area in size, any part of which is at or within 1 disk diameter (approximately 1.5 mm) of the center of the macula. Identifying CSME is important because patients with CSME were shown to benefit from focal laser photocoagulation in the ETDRS. Visual acuity was not a criterion for defining CSME.

Although recommendations are evolving because of the increased use of intravitreal medications in the treatment of the neovascular and macular edema complications of diabetic retinopathy, recommendations for follow-up are still largely defined by the ETDRS findings regarding the progression of disease. **Table 3** (progression and follow-up recommendations) summarizes the current standard recommendations regarding the appropriate follow-up of patients with various levels of retinopathy.

DIAGNOSTIC MODALITIES FOR EVALUATION OF RETINOPATHY

The mainstay for diagnosis of diabetic retinopathy remains the clinical examination by a qualified examiner; however, additional diagnostic testing may often be helpful. The American Academy of Ophthalmology has developed preferred practice patterns related to the appropriate diagnosis and management of diabetic retinopathy.[19]

Visual acuity measurement with a standard Snellen or ETDRS chart is an easy, low-cost, and useful method of assessing visual function.[20] But visual acuity was not a criterion for determining the need for laser photocoagulation in the ETDRS, and patients with extensive and sight-threatening retinopathy might maintain excellent visual acuity for periods of time.

Slit lamp biomicroscopy of the anterior segment including the cornea, lens, and iris should be performed. In addition, the measurement of the intraocular pressure by any

Table 3
Risk and timing of progression of diabetic retinopathy

Retinopathy Classification	Risk of Progression to		Recommended Follow-up	Treatment
	PDR in 1 y (%)	High-Risk PDR in 5 y (%)		
Mild NPDR	5	15		
(−) CSME			Yearly	No
(+) CSME			3 mo	Yes
Moderate NPDR	12–27	33		
(−) CSME			6 mo	No
(+) CSME			3 mo	Yes
Severe NPDR	52	60		
(−) CSME			4 mo	Rarely
(+) CSME			3 mo	Yes
Very Severe NPDR	75	75		
(−) CSME			3 mo	Occasionally
(+) CSME			3 mo	Yes
Early PDR	—	75		
(−) CSME			2–3 mo	Occasionally
(+) CSME			2–3 mo	Yes
High-Risk PDR	—	—		
(−) CSME			2–3 mo	Yes
(+) CSME			1–2 mo	Yes

of several methods and gonioscopic evaluation of the iris and trabecular structures looking for signs of neovascularization of the iris and angle are necessary to diagnose primary open angle glaucoma, which may be more prevalent in patients with diabetes, and neovascular glaucoma, which is one of the most feared complications of PDR leading, in some cases, to uncontrollable increases in intraocular pressure and blindness. Stereoscopic slit lamp biomicroscopy, with the use of accessory lenses, is the preferred method for evaluating retinopathy of the posterior pole, including the optic disk and macula, as well as the retinal midperiphery.[16] This technique allows for careful evaluation for the presence of macular edema, intraretinal hemorrhages, IRMA, CWS, VB, NVD, and NVE as well as epiretinal membranes and fibrovascular proliferation that can lead to tractional and rhegmatogenous RD. Binocular indirect ophthalmoscopy is used to examine the peripheral retina for NVE, vitreous hemorrhage, and RD. Alternatively, the peripheral retina can be examined with wide-angle or angled-mirror lenses at the slit lamp. Dilation of the pupil is required to adequately assess the retina for the presence of retinopathy because only 50% of eyes have been shown to be accurately graded for retinopathy through undilated pupils.[21] New scanning laser ophthalmoscopic imaging systems may improve visualization of the peripheral retina in undilated eyes.

Ancillary testing, if used appropriately, can enhance the accuracy of diagnosis and improve patient care.[14] Color fundus photography, often with stereoscopic imaging, may be a more reproducible technique than examination at the slit lamp for detecting retinopathy; but clinical examination is frequently superior for detecting macular edema and fine-caliber NVD and NVE. Photographic documentation of a previous examination, however, can be helpful in ascertaining disease progression, response to treatment, and can influence the decision as to whether or not to treat.[22]

Although it is not part of the routine evaluation of patients with diabetes, fluorescein angiography, in which 10% or 25% fluorescein sodium solution is rapidly injected intravenously, can be useful in identifying areas of macular and peripheral capillary nonperfusion; sources of capillary leakage, such as microaneurysms responsible for macular edema; and sometimes in visualizing subtle foci of IRMA and neovascularization. Fluorescein angiography is not needed to diagnose CSME or PDR because both of these are clinical diagnoses[14]; however, it is frequently used as a guide for the treatment CSME.[19] Fluorescein angiography is a very safe procedure; but mild side effects, including nausea and vomiting, are not infrequent, and severe medical complications, including death (approximately 1 per 200 000 patients) can occur.[23] Although adverse effects on the fetus have never been documented, fluorescein angiography is not generally recommended, other than in exceptional circumstances, during pregnancy because fluorescein dye can cross the placental barrier and enter the fetal circulation.[24]

B-scan ultrasonography can be very helpful in diagnosing RD in diabetic eyes with media opacities secondary to corneal clouding, cataracts, and most frequently vitreous hemorrhage.

Ocular coherence tomography (OCT) provides cross-sectional imaging of the retina and macula, the vitreoretinal interface and epiretina, and the subretinal space.[25] Time domain and, more recently, spectral domain instruments allow for high-resolution imaging (<10 μm) and quantification of retinal thickness. OCT's ability to qualitatively and quantitatively assess retinal thickening can frequently be useful in monitoring macular edema and response to treatment as well as identifying areas of vitreoretinal traction that might not be evident by standard clinical examination. OCT is frequently used as a secondary measure during clinical trials; however, OCT measurements of retinal thickness do not always correlate with visual acuity.[26]

CURRENT TREATMENT

Laser photocoagulation for diabetic retinopathy was proposed by Meyer-Schwickerath in 1954 and has remained the mainstay of treatment of both DME and PDR.[27] In 1985, the ETDRS demonstrated that in patients with mild or moderate NPDR, focal laser photocoagulation, either directly to microaneurysms thought to be responsible for the edema or in a grid pattern in the case of more diffuse vascular leakage, could reduce the likelihood of further vision loss in patients with CSME.[28,29] Patients with initial visual acuity worse than 20/40 had twice the likelihood of improvement in vision with laser treatment.

PDR can be treated with panretinal photocoagulation (PRP). The Diabetic Retinopathy Study showed that PRP could reduce the risk of severe vision loss (visual acuity less than 5/200 at 2 consecutive visits) in patients with high-risk PDR.[10,30] Whenever both focal laser treatment of CSME and PRP for neovascularization are needed simultaneously, focal laser is applied first to reduce the likelihood of worsening macular edema caused by the heavier scatter laser. In a recent investigation, no difference in the rate of occurrence or worsening of macular edema was noted whether the PRP was administered in one session or divided into 4 sessions.[31]

Side effects and complications are not rare with laser photocoagulation; however, in most cases, they are not particularly serious, especially when compared with the risk of blindness present without treatment.[32] The most feared complication of focal laser treatment is inadvertent photocoagulation of the fovea. This complication can lead to immediate loss of central vision leaving patients unable to read. This risk can be minimized by properly identifying macular landmarks before the initiation of treatment, but it may also result from accidental movement of either the surgeon or patients. In addition to the usually mild discomfort felt by patients, PRP can cause decreases in peripheral vision, especially when heavy confluent or fill-in laser is needed. Decreases in color and night vision may also be seen following PRP. Transient impairment of central reading vision may also occur but generally resolves over several hours. Persistent loss of acuity may usually resolve over several weeks; but when associated with ischemia or refractory macular edema, it may be permanent. Exudative RD can infrequently occur following PRP, presumably from damage to choroidal vessels causing exudation of fluid through the retinal pigment epithelial barrier into the subretinal space. Vitreous hemorrhage can result from direct photocoagulation treatment of retinal neovascularization.

EMERGING TREATMENTS

Table 4 summarizes the pharmacologic agents used for DME.

Table 4
Pharmacologic agents used for DME

Drug	FDA Approved for Intravitreal Use	FDA Approved for DME
Aflibercept	Yes	No
Bevacizumab	No	No
Dexamethasone (Ozurdex)	Yes	No
Fluocinolone (Retisert, Iluvien)	Yes (Retisert)	No
Infliximab	No	No
Pegaptanib	Yes	No
Ranibizumab	Yes	Yes
Triamcinolone (Triessence)	Yes	No

Diabetic Retinopathy and Inflammatory Modulators

It has become clear over the past several years that inflammation may play a significant role in the progression of diabetic retinopathy and that modulating inflammation may have a role in its treatment. Steroids, nonsteroidal antiinflammatory drugs (NSAIDs), anti-VEGF agents, and anti–tumor necrosis factor (TNF) agents have all been shown to influence the progression of diabetic retinopathy; it is proposed that at least some of this effect is through their antiinflammatory properties. NSAIDs have been demonstrated to prevent progression of retinopathy by inhibiting TNF-alpha.[33]

CORTICOSTEROIDS
Triamcinolone Acetonide

Several studies have demonstrated a benefit to intravitreal triamcinolone acetonide (IVTA) in the treatment of DME.[34–36] Laser photocoagulation was recently compared with1-mg and 4-mg doses of IVTA. Superior visual and anatomic outcomes with laser photocoagulation were reported at both 2[37] and 3[38] years following randomization. However, 4 mg IVTA was associated with better visual outcomes than laser treatment in patients with poor initial visual acuity (20/200 to 20/320) and a reduced risk for progression of retinopathy.[39] Moreover, IVTA may have short-term benefits in patients with PDR in conjunction with panretinal laser photocoagulation[40,41] and may be associated with decreased risks of vitreous hemorrhage following pars plans vitrectomy.[42]

In the United States, there are at least 4 commercially available preparations of IVTA: Kenalog-40, Triesence, Trivaris, and preservative-free triamcinolone acetonide from compounding pharmacies.

Treatment of DME, which is a chronic condition, may require repeated injections, exposing patients to cumulative risks for complications and side effects, such as endophthalmitis, increased intraocular pressure, and cataracts. Additionally, there may be clinically relevant differences between intermittent high-dose administration of corticosteroids and sustained, lose-dose elution. Several extended-release delivery systems have been investigated: Retisert (Bausch & Lomb, Rochester, NY), a surgically implanted device containing fluocinolone acetonide, which received approval by the Food and Drug Administration (FDA) in 2005 for the treatment of chronic, noninfectious posterior uveitis; Iluvien (Alimera Sciences, Alpharetta, GA), an injectable delivery system for fluocinolone acetonide; and Ozurdex (Allergan Inc, Irvine, CA), an injectable sustained delivery system for dexamethasone.

Dexamethasone (Ozurdex)

A novel biodegradable, sustained-released dexamethasone delivery system (Ozurdex) has recently been approved by the FDA for use in macular edema associated with retinal vein occlusions and for noninfectious intermediate and posterior uveitis. A specially designed 22-gauge applicator is used to deliver the implant in a sutureless office-based procedure. Ozurdex (700 µg) has been shown to reduce central retinal thickness as measured by OCT, reduce retinal vascular leakage seen on fluorescein angiography, and improve best-corrected visual acuity (BCVA) in patients with persistent macular edema compared with untreated eyes.[43,44] The beneficial effects may be present within a few days of implantation[45] and were sustained at the 180-day protocol visit.[28] Complications, such as increased intraocular pressure and cataract, may be less frequent with the Ozurdex implant than with repeated intravitreal injections of triamcinolone acetonide.[28,29] In difficult-to-treat eyes that had previous vitrectomy surgery, treatment with Ozurdex led to statistically and clinically significant improvements in both vision and vascular leakage from DME. At present, Ozurdex is approved by the FDA for intravitreal use in noninfectious uveitis and macular edema secondary to retinal vein occlusions. An approval for use in diabetic retinopathy has not been granted yet.

Fluocinolone Acetonide (Retisert, Iluvien)

The Fluocinolone Acetonide in Diabetic Macular Edema (FAME) study investigated the safety and efficacy of a sustained-release fluocinolone acetonide intravitreal implant (Retisert, Iluvien) for the treatment of DME. Fluocinolone acetonide is a soluble, potent steroid and more lipophilic than triamcinolone acetonide or dexamethasone. The FDA has previously approved Retisert for persistent noninfectious posterior uveitis. Retisert is implanted through a pars plana surgical incision and sutured into the sclera in the operating room. It releases fluocinolone for up to 3 years. Iluvien also releases fluocinolone for nearly 3 years, but it is a nonerodible, intravitreal implant that is small enough to be injected through a 25-gauge needle creating a self-sealing wound in an in-office procedure. In a study comparing the 0.59-mg Retisert implant versus standard-of-care laser photocoagulation in patients with persistent or recurrent DME, the fluocinolone implant demonstrated superiority with regard to improved visual acuity and decreased macular edema.[46] Visual acuity improved 3 or more lines in 16.8% of the fluocinolone-implanted eyes at 6 months compared with 1.4% of the standard-of-care eyes ($P = .0012$). At 1 year, there was an improvement of 3 or more lines in 16.4% in the fluocinolone-implanted eyes compared with 8.1% of the standard-of-care eyes ($P = .1191$). By year 2, 31.8% of the fluocinolone-implanted eyes had an improvement of 3 or more lines compared with 9.3% of the standard-of-care eyes ($P = .0016$); and at 3 years, 31.1% of the fluocinolone-implanted eyes had an improvement of 3 or more lines compared with 20.0% of the standard-of-care laser-treated eyes ($P = .1566$). Moreover, the number of Retisert-implanted eyes with no evidence of retinal thickening at the center of the macula was higher than the standard-of-care laser-treated eyes at all time points through 3 years.

However, the side effects were significant. Intraocular pressure of 30 mm Hg or more was recorded in 61.4% of the implanted eyes compared with only 5.8% of the standard-of-care eyes; 33.8% of the Retisert-implanted eyes required surgery for ocular hypertension by 4 years. In addition, more than 90% of Retisert-implanted eyes that had not previously had cataract surgery required cataract extraction by 4 years.

Iluvien is an 0.18-mg fluocinolone acetonide delivery system being evaluated for the treatment of DME in addition to other indications.[47] At present, neither Iluvien nor Retisert is approved for the indication of DME.

PROTEIN KINASE C (PKC) INHIBITION

Ruboxistaurin (RBX) is an orally administered, isoform-selective inhibitor of PKC β that has been shown to have a positive effect in animal models of diabetic retinopathy[48] and improve diabetes-induced retinal hemodynamic abnormalities in patients with diabetes.[49] Two randomized controlled studies and a combined analysis of 2 additional studies have suggested a benefit to oral RBX in terms of reducing the rate of sustained moderate vision loss in patients with diabetes.[50–52] However, these studies did not achieve statistical significance in their primary end points and morphologic analysis of macular anatomy, including occurrence of significant center of macula involvement, OCT-determined center of macula thickness, and need for application of focal photocoagulation did not show a consistent trend in favor of or against

RBX. Additional studies are underway with other oral PKC inhibitors, and there may be a benefit to PKC inhibitors delivered intravitreally.

ANTI-VEGF AGENTS

There are currently 4 major anti-VEGF agents that are available in the United States and have been evaluated in treating DME: pegaptanib sodium (Macugen), ranibizumab (Lucentis), bevacizumab (Avastin), and aflibercept (Eylea)[53]; however, at present, only ranibizumab is approved by the FDA for this indication. Ranibizumab is the Fab fragment of the bevacizumab antibody.

The FDA approved pegaptanib sodium, an aptamer that binds selectively to the 165 isoform of VEGF, in 2004 for the treatment of all subtypes of neovascular age-related macular degeneration.[54] A phase 3, multicenter, randomized study (n = 260) has compared 0.3 mg of intravitreal pegaptanib every 6 weeks with a sham injection for DME. Patients in the study were permitted to receive focal macular laser treatment after study week 18 based on the ETDRS criteria. No significant safety issues were identified, and pegaptanib was found to be superior to sham injection with respect to 2-line visual acuity gains at 1 year (37% [pegaptanib] vs 20% [sham; P = .0047]). The mean BCVA at month 12 was +5.1 letters (pegaptanib) compared with +1.2 letters (sham; $P<.05$). Mean and BCVA at month 24 was +6.1 letters (pegaptanib) compared with 1.3 letters (sham; $P<.01$).[55]

Intravitreal bevacizumab is used off label to treat DME. A short-term level II study by Soheilian and colleagues[56,57] evaluating the visual acuity results of intravitreal bevacizumab alone or combined with intravitreal triamcinolone versus laser photocoagulation for DME found that patients who received bevacizumab injections had significantly better visual acuity outcomes at the 12- and 24-week follow-up compared with patients who received laser photocoagulation.

The Diabetic Retinopathy Clinical Research network (DRCR net) reported a phase II randomized exploratory clinical trial of the short-term effect of intravitreal bevacizumab for DME.[58] Patients in the study who received either 1.25 mg or 2.5 mg of intravitreal bevacizumab at baseline and again at 6 weeks had a greater reduction in retinal thickness measured by OCT at 3 weeks and an approximately 1-line improvement in vision at 12 weeks when compared with patients who had received focal laser photocoagulation. The study failed to demonstrate any short-term benefit by combining bevacizumab with laser photocoagulation.

Several additional studies have also demonstrated anatomic improvement in the morphology of the macula with decreased central retinal thickness in patients receiving 1.25 mg or 2.5 mg of intravitreal bevacizumab compared with laser treatment.[59–61] Most recently, the Bevacizumab or Laser Therapy study has provided support for longer-term usage of bevacizumab for DME.[62] This study (n = 80) compared 2-year results of intravitreal bevacizumab 1.25 mg versus focal macular laser treatment. The median improvement in BCVA was greater for intravitreal bevacizumab (+9 letters; median, 13 treatments) compared with macular laser treatment (+2.5 letters; median, 4 laser treatments; P = .005); however, although mean central macular thickness reduction was slightly greater in the intravitreal bevacizumab group at 24 months (−146 μm) compared with the macular laser treatment group (−118 μm), it was not statistically significant (P = .62).

A phase II prospective, double-masked clinical trial of intravitreal aflibercept demonstrated its benefit compared with macular laser for the treatment of DME.[63] In this study, 221 patients with clinically significant DME involving the central macula were randomized to 1 of 5 treatment protocols: group A, 0.5 mg aflibercept every

4 weeks; group B, 2 mg aflibercept every 4 weeks; group C, 2 mg aflibercept every 4 weeks for 3 months, then every 8 weeks; group D, 2 mg aflibercept every 4 weeks for 3 months, then as needed; and group E, focal/grid laser. At 24 weeks, aflibercept treatment groups had visual acuity improvements between +8.5 and +11.4 ETDRS letters compared with +2.5 letters in the laser group ($P \leq$ .0085 for each treatment group vs laser). The OCT-measured mean central macular thickness was also reduced significantly in the groups treated with aflibercept. Adverse events were no different than with other intravitreal treatment agents.

Multiple studies have demonstrated the safety and efficacy of intravitreal ranibizumab for the treatment of DME. The DRCR net reported that patients treated with 0.5 mg intravitreal ranibizumab with prompt laser (n = 187, +9 ± 12 letters; P<.001) or deferred laser ($\geq$24 weeks; n = 188, +9 ± 12 letters; P<.001) had significantly superior visual acuity outcomes at the 1-year mark than those treated with sham injection plus prompt laser (n = 293, +3 ± 13 letters).[64] These positive effects were maintained at the 2-year follow-up.[65]

The ranibizumab monotherapy or combined with laser versus laser monotherapy for diabetic macular edema (RESTORE) trial[64] (345 patients) reported a 12-month visual acuity improvement of 6.1 ETDRS letters with intravitreal 0.5 mg ranibizumab monthly for 3 months then as needed (group A), a 5.9-letter improvement with 0.5 mg ranibizumab monthly for 3 months then as needed combined with focal laser photocoagulation (group B), compared with a 0.8-letter improvement with focal laser alone (group C). There was a statistically significant difference between both groups A and B compared with group C (P<.0001). In addition, the mean central retinal thickness also decreased significantly in both ranibizumab groups compared with laser alone (group A, −118.7 μm; group B, −128.3 μm; group C, +61.3 μm; P<.001 for both group A and group B).

The RISE (377 patients) and RIDE (382 patients) trials[65] are identical, parallel studies comparing monthly injections of 0.3 mg ranibizumab (group A), 0.5 mg ranibizumab (group B), or sham injection (group C) for the treatment of DME. At 3 months, rescue laser was made available to all patients. In the RISE trial at 24 months, 44.8% of patients (56 of 125) who received 0.3 mg ranibizumab and 39.2% of patients (49 of 125) who received 0.5 mg ranibizumab were able to read at least 15 more letters than at baseline compared with 18.1% of patients (23 of 127) who received sham injections. In the RIDE trial, at 24 months, 33.6% of patients (42 of 125) who received 0.3 mg ranibizumab and 45.7% of patients (58 of 127) who received 0.5 mg ranibizumab were able to read at least 15 more letters than at baseline compared with 12.3% of patients (16 of 130) who received sham injections. The 3-year follow-up results from RISE and RIDE have recently been published.[66] Visual acuity outcomes seen at month 24 were consistent through month 36; the proportions of patients who gained 15 or more letters from baseline at month 36 in the sham, 0.3-mg, and 0.5-mg ranibizumab groups were 19.2%, 36.8%, and 40.2%, respectively, in RIDE and 22.0%, 51.2%, and 41.6%, respectively, in RISE. Central retinal thickness reductions remained stable through 36 months. Patients originally in the sham injection group who ultimately crossed over to 0.5 mg ranibizumab did not achieve the visual acuity improvements seen in the groups originally randomized to intravitreal ranibizumab suggesting that early intervention is preferable to delayed treatment.

The short-term 6-month Ranibizumab for Edema of the Macula in Diabetes (READ-2) study[67] (126 patients) demonstrated that at 6 months patients who had received 0.5 mg of intravitreal ranibizumab at baseline and again at months 1, 3, and 5 had a significantly improved BCVA (+7.24 ETDRS letters; P = .01) compared with patients who had received focal/grid laser at baseline and month 3 if needed or a combination of 0.5 mg ranibizumab and focal/grid laser at baseline and month 3 (group 3). Improvement in visual acuity of 3 lines or more (>15 ETDRS letters) was observed in 22% in the intravitreal ranibizumab–alone group compared with 0% in the laser treatment–alone group (*P* = .002).

The Safety and Efficacy of Ranibizumab in Diabetic Macular Edema (RESOLVE) trial[68] (151 patients) compared 0.3 mg or 0.5 mg intravitreal ranibizumab monthly for 3 months, with dose-doubling allowed after 1 month (group A), with sham injection monthly for 3 months then as needed (group B). All patients were eligible to receive rescue grid laser at 1 year. The BCVA in the ranibizumab group was significantly superior (+10.3 ± 9.1 letters) versus the sham group (−1.4 ± 14.2 letters) (*P*<.0001). A total of 60.8% of the ranibizumab group had 10-letter gains compared with only 18.4% in the sham group (*P*<.0001). A corresponding reduction in central retinal thickness of −194.2 μm was seen in the ranibizumab group versus an increase of 48.4 μm (*P*<.0001) in the sham group. Moreover, a larger proportion of patients in the sham group (34.7) required rescue laser photocoagulation compared with the ranibizumab group (34.7%).

Based on these accumulated data, the FDA has approved the indication of treatment of DME for intravitreal bevacizumab (0.3 mg). The American Diabetes Association has now included intravitreal ranibizumab in its standards of care.[69]

However, treatment with intravitreal bevacizumab is not without significant expense. An analysis of the relative costs and treatment benefits of the various intravitreal anti-VEGF agents as well as other treatment methods for DME has been performed.[70] The cost per line of vision saved at 1 year was $11 372 to $11 609 for ranibizumab compared with $1329 to $2246 for bevacizumab, $3287 for vitrectomy surgery, $3749 for intravitreal triamcinolone, $5099 for laser photocoagulation, $5666 for dexamethasone implant, and $10 500 for pegaptanib. These costs translated to quality-adjusted life-years are $19 251 to $23 119 for ranibizumab compared with $2013 to $4160 for bevacizumab, $5862 for grid photocoagulation, $6246 for intravitreal triamcinolone, $8706 for vitrectomy surgery, $9446 for the dexamethasone implant, and $16 667 for pegaptanib. These costs will clearly increase as treatment and follow-up extend past 1 year.

TUMOR NECROSIS FACTOR (TNF)

TNF is a pleiotropic cytokine that has central importance to the development and homeostasis of the immune system and is a key regulator of cell activation, differentiation, and death.[38] Infliximab (Remicade) is a chimeric monoclonal antibody specific for human TNF that has been demonstrated to be of benefit in the treatment of chronic inflammatory diseases involving the joints, skin, and gut. It has been proposed that abnormal local expression of TNF may be important in the pathogenesis of diabetic vascular damage leading to macular edema and neovascularization[71,72] and that mild subclinical inflammation may influence many of the typical pathologic vascular changes of diabetic retinopathy.[73] It is also possible that high-dose NSAIDs delay the onset of diabetic retinopathy via TNF-alpha suppression. Furthermore, studies in patients with arthritis have shown that anti-TNF therapy decreases vascular permeability and angiogenesis by downregulating VEGF,[74] a key factor in the development and progression of diabetic retinopathy.

A small, randomized, double-blind, placebo-controlled, crossover study has recently shown that short-term intravenous treatment with infliximab could significantly improve BCVA in eyes with advanced-stage sight-threatening DME refractory to standard focal laser treatment with no noted systemic complications.[75] However, because of concerns about systemic toxicity and recent experience with the administration of several drugs intravitreally, a larger, retrospective, multicentered study from the Pan-American Collaborative Retina Study Group reviewing their experience with intravitreal infliximab and adalimumab for the treatment of refractory DME was recently published. This study did not find any visual benefit with intravitreally administered 1 mg or 2 mg of infliximab or 2 mg of adalimumab in eyes with DME that had not responded to focal laser photocoagulation but noted a high rate of severe inflammatory reactions elicited with the 2-mg dose of infliximab.[76] This finding has prompted a call for a moratorium on additional studies of intravitreal anti-TNF agents outside of a well-designed clinical trial.[77]

VITRECTOMY

Vitrectomy surgery has long been the treatment of patients with PDR who have lost vision from tractional and rhegmatogenous RD, epiretinal membranes, and nonclearing vitreous hemorrhages. Vitrectomy for DME was proposed more than 20 years ago. However, because of the high costs of the use of ongoing intravitreal pharmacologic agents, the need for close follow-up when these drugs are used, as well as long-term safety concerns (endophthalmitis, glaucoma, cataract, and so forth) vitrectomy and even peeling of the ILM for DME is being given closer scrutiny.

Vitrectomy for DME was initially described in a series of 10 patients with taut and thickened posterior vitreous hyaloid membranes, with 9 patients having improved vision postoperatively.[78] Studies in animals have shown that vitrectomy surgery to remove the formed vitreous gel and replace it with saline markedly improved the diffusion of oxygen throughout the vitreous cavity.[79] Reports that DME is present in 55% of the eyes of patients with diabetic retinopathy without posterior vitreous separation from the retina (PVD) but only in 20% with PVD[80] and that resolution of DME occurred in 55% of eyes experiencing spontaneous PVDs but in only 25% of eyes that did not develop PVD provide additional rationale to explain the benefit of vitrectomy surgery.[81] Although these studies did not provide proof of the exact mechanisms responsible for these differences, removal of the preretinal vitreous with its low partial pressure of oxygen and substituting the relatively highly oxygenated aqueous that fills the void is a reasonable explanation.

At present, there are no level 1 data proving the benefit of vitrectomy for DME, but a meta-analysis[82] of 37 studies (1881 patients) published since 2002 describing vitrectomy for DME suggests excellent reduction in OCT-measured central macular thickness (weighted average change of −187 μm), following vitrectomy comparing favorably with that achieved by intravitreal injections of anti-VEGF drugs with or without laser photocoagulation (range: −80 μm to −194 μm). These studies also demonstrate that macular edema resolves quickly after vitrectomy and that the effect is long lasting.[83] Studies of eyes that had previously undergone focal laser photocoagulation also demonstrated significant macular thinning after vitrectomy.[84] This finding was true for both retrospective (−242 μm) and prospective (−198 μm) studies.

Unfortunately, although vitrectomy surgery seems to cause rapid and long-lasting resolution of diabetic macular thickening, it is not at all clear whether it produces improvement in visual acuity. This ambiguity may be because in most series, vitrectomy was performed as a salvage procedure on eyes that had persistent and long-lasting edema resistant to other forms of treatment. Permanent and significant structural damage to the macula may have already occurred before undertaking vitrectomy. It is possible that vitrectomy performed earlier in the course of disease, maybe even as first-line therapy, would lead to better visual acuity results.[85]

It is also possible that in the future enzymatic vitreolysis may replace mechanical vitrectomy in some patients. Ocriplasmin (Jetrea, Thrombogenics, Iselin, NJ) has recently been approved by the FDA for enzymatic lysis of symptomatic vitreo-macular adhesions[86]; although there is no specific indication for patients with diabetic macular traction, with or without macular edema (patients with diabetes were excluded from the study), ocriplasmin may have a therapeutic role for selected patients. Vitreosolve (Vitreoretinal Technologies, Inc) is another vitreolytic agent currently in clinical trials for DME and the inhibition of progression of diabetic retinopathy.

DRCR NET

The DRCR net was initiated in 2002 with funding from the National Eye Institute of the NIH as a collaborative network dedicated to facilitating multicenter clinical research of diabetic retinopathy, DME, and associated conditions. The network currently includes more than 100 participating institutions and more than 300 physician investigators.

DRCR Protocol A compared the standard ETDRS technique of focal laser photocoagulation with a new mild macular grid (MMG) strategy for the treatment of clinically significant macular edema. This alternative approach involved the application of mild, widely spaced burns throughout the macula, avoiding the central foveal region. By protocol design, some of the MMG treatment burns were placed in areas of clinically normal retina if the entire retina was not abnormally thickened. These areas could include areas within the macula that were relatively distant from the area of clinically observed thickening. At 12 months after treatment, the MMG technique was found to be less effective at reducing retinal thickening than the standard ETDRS photocoagulation protocol. However, no statistically significant difference was seen in visual acuity outcomes between the two methods of treatment.[87]

DRCR Protocol B evaluated the efficacy and safety of 1-mg and 4-mg doses of intravitreal triamcinolone compared with focal/grid photocoagulation for the treatment of DME. Small previous studies had suggested a role for intravitreal steroids in refractory DME.[88,89] At the 4-month follow-up, the mean visual acuity was better in the 4-mg triamcinolone group than in either the laser group or the 1-mg triamcinolone group. However, by 1 year, no significant differences among groups in the mean visual acuity were seen; from the 16-month through 2-year follow-up, the mean visual acuity was better in the laser group than in the other two groups.[37] Intravitreal triamcinolone acetonide (4 mg) did seem to slightly reduce the risk of progression to PDR but not sufficiently to recommend its use given the cataract and glaucoma side effects.[39] In a separate DRCR protocol (Protocol E), no benefit was seen with peribulbar (adjacent to the eye but not directly into it) triamcinolone with or without laser photocoagulation in patients with DME and relatively good visual acuity (20/40 or better).[90]

DRCR Protocol H, a phase 2 study, suggested that in some patients anti-VEGF treatment with intravitreal bevacizumab (Avastin) may be of benefit in DME. DRCR Protocol T, which is currently underway, is comparing the 3 available anti-VEGF medications bevacizumab, ranibizumab, and aflibercept for DME.

DRCR Protocol I demonstrated that intravitreal ranibizumab (Lucentis) with prompt or deferred laser is more effective compared with prompt laser alone for the treatment of DME involving the central macula. In eyes that have already undergone cataract surgery, intravitreal triamcinolone with prompt laser seems more effective than laser alone; however, it frequently increases the risk of intraocular pressure elevation.[91,92]

DRCR Protocol J showed that one intravitreal triamcinolone injection or 2 ranibizumab injections in conjunction with focal/grid laser for DME and PRP is associated with better visual acuity and decreased macular edema than with laser treatment alone.[93]

Other current DRCR investigations include the following:

Protocol M: Effect of Diabetes Education During Retinal Ophthalmology Visits on Diabetes Control

Protocol N: An Evaluation of Intravitreal Ranibizumab for Vitreous Hemorrhage Due to Proliferative Diabetic Retinopathy

Protocol O: Comparison of Time Domain OCT and Spectral Domain OCT Retinal Thickness Measurement in Diabetic Macular Edema

Protocol P: A Pilot Study in Individuals with Center-Involved DME Undergoing Cataract Surgery

Protocol Q: An Observational Study in Individuals with Diabetic Retinopathy without Center-Involved DME Undergoing Cataract Surgery

Protocol R: A Phase II Evaluation of Topical Non-steroidal Antiinflammatory Agents in Eyes With Non-Central Involved Diabetic Macular Edema

Protocol S: Prompt PRP Compared With Ranibizumab With Deferred PRP for Proliferative Diabetic Retinopathy

Protocol T: A Comparative Effectiveness Study of Intravitreal Aflibercept, Bevacizumab, and Ranibizumab for Diabetic Macular Edema

Protocol V: Treatment (prompt anti-VEGF or prompt focal laser) versus observation for center involved DME in eye with very good visual acuity

The current understanding of all facets of diabetic retinopathy is still imperfect; however, the last several years have shown a tremendous increase in our knowledge of the pathogenesis of the damage that occurs in both NPDR and PDR as well as in our ability to treat their complications. New intravitreal medical treatments are gradually replacing standard laser photocoagulation for the treatment of all forms of diabetic retinopathy; both government- and industry-supported research is yielding exciting new insights. The challenge will be to deliver these new treatments in a cost-effective manner to the increasing number of patients who will need them.

REFERENCES

1. National Society to Prevent Blindness. Operational research department. Vision problems in the US: a statistical analysis. New York: National Society to Prevent Blindness; 1980. p. 146.
2. Patz A, Smith RE. The ETDRS and diabetes 2000. Ophthalmology 1991;98: 739–40.
3. Kahn HA, Hiller R. Blindness caused by diabetic retinopathy. Am J Ophthalmol 1974;78(1):58.
4. Klein R, Klein BE, Moss SE, et al. The Wisconsin epidemiologic study of diabetic retinopathy. VI. Retinal photocoagulation. Ophthalmology 1987;94(7):747.
5. The Diabetes Control and Complications Trial Research Group: The effect of intensive treatment of diabetes on the development and progression of long-term complications in insulin-dependent diabetes mellitus. N Engl J Med 1993;329:977–86.
6. The DCCT Research Group: Effect of intensive diabetes management on macrovascular events and risk factors in the Diabetes Control and Complication Trial. Am J Cardiol 1995;75:894–903.

7. The DCCT Research Group: The relationship of glycemic exposure (HbA1c) to the risk of development and progression of retinopathy in the Diabetes Control and Complications Trial. Diabetes 1995;44:968–83.
8. UK Prospective Diabetes Study Group. Intensive blood-glucose control with sulphonylureas or insulin compared with conventional treatment and risk of complications in patients with type 2 diabetes. UKPDS 33. Lancet 1998;352(9131): 837–53.
9. Klein R, Klein BE, Syrjala SE, et al. Wisconsin Epidemiologic Study of Diabetic Retinopathy. 1. Relationship of diabetic retinopathy to management of diabetes. Preliminary report. In: Friedman EA, L'Esperance FA, editors. Diabetic renal-retinal syndrome. New York: Grune & Stratton; 1982. p. 21–40.
10. Klein R, Klein BE, Davis MD. Is cigarette smoking associated with diabetic retinopathy? Am J Epidemiol 1983;118:228–38.
11. Klein R, Klein BE, Moss SE, et al. The Wisconsin Epidemiologic Study of Diabetic Retinopathy. II. Prevalence and risk of diabetic retinopathy when age at diagnosis is less than 30 years. Arch Ophthalmol 1984;102:520–6.
12. Klein R, Klein BE, Moss SE, et al. The Wisconsin Epidemiologic Study of Diabetic Retinopathy. III. Prevalence and risk of diabetic retinopathy when age at diagnosis is 30 or more years. Arch Ophthalmol 1984;102:527–32.
13. Klein R, Klein BE, Moss SE, et al. The Wisconsin Epidemiologic Study of Diabetic Retinopathy. IV. Diabetic macular edema. Ophthalmology 1984;91:1464–74.
14. Zhang X, Saaddine JB, Chou C, et al. Prevalence of diabetic retinopathy in the United States, 2005-2008. JAMA 2010;304(6):649–56.
15. Diabetes Prevention Program Research Group. The prevalence of retinopathy in impaired glucose tolerance and recent-onset diabetes in the Diabetes Prevention Program. Diabet Med 2007;24:137–44.
16. Yanoff M, Fine BS. Ocular pathology: a text and atlas. Philadelphia: Harper and Row; 1982.
17. Gandorfer A, Rohleder M, Kampik A. Epiretinal pathology of vitreomacular traction syndrome. Br J Ophthalmol 2002;86:902–9.
18. Early treatment diabetic retinopathy study. Report number 12. Fundus photographic risk factors for progression of diabetic retinopathy. Ophthalmology 1991;98:823–33.
19. American Academy of Ophthalmology Retina Panel. Preferred practice pattern guidelines. Diabetic retinopathy. San Francisco (CA): American Academy of Ophthalmology; 2008 (4th printing 2012). Available at: www.aao.org/ppp.
20. Early Treatment Diabetic Retinopathy Study Research Group. Early photocoagulation for diabetic retinopathy. ETDRS report number 9. Ophthalmology 1991; 98:766–85.
21. Klein R, Klein BE, Neider MW, et al. Diabetic retinopathy as detected using ophthalmoscopy, a nonmydriatic camera and a standard fundus camera. Ophthalmology 1985;92:485–91.
22. Rosberger DF, Schachat AP, Bressler SB, et al. Availability of color fundus photographs from previous visit affects practice patterns for patients with diabetes mellitus. Arch Ophthalmol 1998;116(12):1607.
23. Yannuzzi LA, Rohrer KT, Tindel LJ, et al. Fluorescein angiography complication survey. Ophthalmology 1986;93:611–7.
24. Sunness JS. The pregnant woman's eye. Surv Ophthalmol 1988;32:219–39.
25. McDonald HR, Williams GA, Scott IU, et al. Laser scanning imaging for macular disease: a report by the American Academy of Ophthalmology. Ophthalmology 2001;114:1221–8.

26. Browning DJ, Glassman AR, Aiello LP, et al. Relationship between ocular coherence tomography-measured central retinal thickness and visual acuity in diabetic macular edema. Ophthalmology 2007;114:525–36.
27. Röttinger EM, Heckemann R, Scherer E, et al. Radiation therapy of choroidal metastases from breast cancer. Albrecht Von Graefes Arch Klin Exp Ophthalmol 1976;200(3):243–50.
28. ETDRS Research Group. Photocoagulation for diabetic macular edema. Arch Ophthalmol 1985;103:1796–806.
29. Bressler NM, Rosberger DF. Photocoagulation for diabetic retinopathy and other causes of retinal neovascularization. In: Gottsch J, Stark W, Goldberg M, editors. Ophthalmic surgery. London: Oxford University Press; 1999. p. 361–73.
30. Diabetic Retinopathy Study Research Group. Indications for photocoagulation treatment of diabetic retinopathy: diabetic retinopathy study report number 14. Int Ophthalmol Clin 1987;27:239–53.
31. Diabetic Retinopathy Clinical Research Network, Brucker AJ, Qin H, et al. Observational study of the development of diabetic macular edema following panretinal (scatter) photocoagulation given in 1 or 4 sittings. Arch Ophthalmol 2009;127(2):132–40.
32. Bressler NB, Rosberger D. Complications of photocoagulation. In: Gottsch J, Stark W, Goldberg M, editors. Ophthalmic surgery. Oxford University Press; 1999. p. 361–73 p. 390–3.
33. Joussen AM. Nonsteroidal anti-inflammatory drugs prevent early diabetic retinopathy via TNF-a suppression. FASEB J 2002;16:438.
34. Gillies MC, Simpson JM, Gaston C, et al. Five-year results of a randomized trial with open label extension of triamcinolone acetonide for refractory diabetic macular edema. Ophthalmology 2009;116(11):2182–7.
35. Lam DS, Chan CK, Mohamed S, et al. Prospective randomized trial of different doses of intravitreal triamcinolone for diabetic macular edema. Br J Ophthalmol 2007;91(2):199–203.
36. Kim JE, Pollack JS, Miller DG, et al, ISIS Study Group. ISIS-DME: a prospective, randomized, dose escalation intravitreal steroid injection study for refractory diabetic macular edema. Retina 2008;28(5):735–40.
37. Diabetic Retinopathy Clinical Research Network. A randomized trial comparing intravitreal triamcinolone acetonide and focal/grid photocoagulation for diabetic macular edema. Ophthalmology 2008;115(9):1447–9, 1449.e1–10.
38. Beck RW, Edwards AR, Aiello LP, et al, Diabetic Retinopathy Clinical Research Network (DRCR.net). Three-year follow-up of a randomized trial comparing focal/grid photocoagulation and intravitreal triamcinolone for diabetic macular edema. Arch Ophthalmol 2009;127(3):245–51.
39. Bressler NM, Edwards AR, Beck RW, et al, for the Diabetic Retinopathy Clinical Research Network. Exploratory analysis of diabetic retinopathy progression through 3 years in a randomized clinical trial that compares intravitreal triamcinolone acetonide with focal/grid photocoagulation. Arch Ophthalmol 2009;127(12):1566–71.
40. Zacks DN, Johnson MW. Combined intravitreal injection of triamcinolone acetonide and panretinal photocoagulation for concomitant diabetic macular edema and proliferative diabetic retinopathy. Retina 2005;25(2):135–40.
41. Margolis R, Singh RP, Bhatnagar P, et al. Intravitreal triamcinolone as adjunctive treatment to laser panretinal photocoagulation for concomitant proliferative diabetic retinopathy and clinically significant macular oedema. Acta Ophthalmol 2008;86(1):105–10.

42. Faghihi H, Taheri A, Farahvash MS, et al. Intravitreal triamcinolone acetonide injection at the end of vitrectomy for diabetic vitreous hemorrhage: a randomized, clinical trial. Retina 2008;28(9):1241–6.
43. Haller JA, Kuppermann BD, Blumenkranz MS, et al. Randomized controlled trial of an intravitreous dexamethasone drug delivery system in patients with diabetic macular edema. Arch Ophthalmol 2010;128(3):289–96.
44. Kuppermann BD, Blumenkranz MS, Haller JA, et al, Dexamethasone DDS Phase II Study Group. Randomized controlled study of an intravitreous dexamethasone drug delivery system in patients with persistent macular edema. Arch Ophthalmol 2007;125(3):309–17.
45. Zucchiatti I, Lattanzio R, Querques G, Querques L, Del Turco C, Cascavilla ML, Bandello F. Intravitreal dexamethasone implant in patients with persistent diabetic macular edema. Ophthalmologica 2012;228:117–22.
46. Pearson PA, Comstock TL, Ip M, et al. Fluocinolone acetonide intravitreal implant for diabetic macular edema: a 3-year multicenter, randomized, controlled clinical trial. Ophthalmology 2011;118:1580–7.
47. Kane FE, Burdan J, Cutino A. Iluvien: a new sustained delivery technology for posterior eye disease. Expert Opin Drug Deliv 2008;5(9):1039–46.
48. Aiello LP, Bursell SE, Clermont A, et al. Vascular endothelial growth factor-induced retinal permeability is mediated by protein kinase C in vivo and suppressed by an orally effective beta-isoform-selective inhibitor. Diabetes 1997; 46:1473–80.
49. Aiello LP, Clermont A, Arora V, et al. Inhibition of PKC beta by oral administration of ruboxistaurin is well tolerated and ameliorates diabetes-induced retinal hemodynamic abnormalities in patients. Invest Ophthalmol Vis Sci 2006;47:86–92.
50. The PKC-DRS Study Group. The effect of ruboxistaurin on visual loss in patients with moderately severe to very severe nonproliferative diabetic retinopathy: initial results of the Protein Kinase C beta Inhibitor Diabetic Retinopathy Study (PKC-DRS) multicenter, randomized clinical trial. Diabetes 2005;54:2188–97.
51. The PKC-DRS2 Study Group. The effect of ruboxistaurin on visual loss in patients with diabetic retinopathy. Ophthalmology 2006;113:2221–30.
52. Sheetz MJ, Aiello LP, Davis MD, et al. The effect of oral PKC beta inhibitor ruboxistaurin on vision loss in two phase 3 studies. Invest Ophthalmol Vis Sci 2013;54: 1750–7.
53. Ho AC, Scott IU, Kim SJ, et al. Anti–vascular endothelial growth factor pharmacotherapy for diabetic macular edema: a report by the American Academy of Ophthalmology. Ophthalmology 2012;119:2179–88.
54. U.S. Food and Drug Administration new drug application (NDA) number: 21–756. Approved labeling. Macugen (pegaptanib sodium injection).
55. Sultan MB, Zhou D, Macugen 1013 Study Group, et al. A phase 2/3, multicenter, randomized, double-masked, 2-year trial of pegaptanib sodium for the treatment of diabetic macular edema. Ophthalmology 2011;118:1107–18.
56. Soheilian M, Ramezani A, Bijanzadeh B, et al. Intravitreal bevacizumab (Avastin) injection alone or combined with triamcinolone versus macular photocoagulation as primary treatment of diabetic macular edema. Retina 2007;27:1187–95.
57. Soheilian M, Ramezani A, Obudi A, et al. Randomized trial of intravitreal bevacizumab alone or combined with triamcinolone versus macular photocoagulation in diabetic macular edema. Ophthalmology 2009;116:1142–50.
58. Diabetic Retinopathy Clinical Research Network. A phase II randomized clinical trial of intravitreal bevacizumab for diabetic macular edema. Ophthalmology 2007;114:1860–7.

59. Solaiman KA, Diab MM, Abo-Elenin M. Intravitreal bevacizumab and/or macular photocoagulation as a primary treatment for diffuse diabetic macular edema. Retina 2011;30:1638–45.
60. Arevalo JF, Sanchez JG, Pan-American Collaborative Retina Study Group (PA-CORES), et al. Primary intravitreal bevacizumab for diffuse diabetic macular edema: the Pan-American Collaborative Retina Study Group at 24 months. Ophthalmology 2009;116:1488–97.
61. Haritoglou C, Kook D, Neubauer A, et al. Intravitreal bevacizumab (Avastin) therapy for persistent diffuse diabetic macular edema. Retina 2006;26:999–1005.
62. Rajendram R, Fraser-Bell S, Kaines A, et al. A 2-year prospective randomized controlled trial of intravitreal bevacizumab or laser therapy (BOLT) in the management of diabetic macular edema: 24-month data: report 3. Arch Ophthalmol 2012;130(8):972–9.
63. Do DV, Schmidt-Erfurth U, Gonzalez VH, et al. The DA VINCI Study: phase 2 primary results of VEGF Trap-Eye in patients with diabetic macular edema. Ophthalmology 2011;118:1819–26.
64. Mitchell P, Bandello F, RESTORE Study Group, et al. The RESTORE Study: ranibizumab monotherapy or combined with laser versus laser monotherapy for diabetic macular edema. Ophthalmology 2011;118:615–25.
65. Nguyen QD, Brown DM, Marcus DM, et al, RISE and RIDE Research Group. Ranibizumab for diabetic macular edema: results from 2 phase III randomized trials: RISE and RIDE. Ophthalmology 2012;119:789–801.
66. Brown DM, Nguyen QD, Marcus DM. Long-term outcomes of ranibizumab therapy for diabetic macular edema: the 36-month results from two phase III trials: RISE and RIDE. Ophthalmology 2013;120(10):2013–22.
67. Nguyen QD, Shah SM, READ-2 Study Group, et al. Primary end point (six months) results of the Ranibizumab for Edema of the mAcula in Diabetes (READ-2) study. Ophthalmology 2009;116:2175–81.
68. Massin P, Bandello F, Garweg JG, et al. Safety and efficacy of ranibizumab in diabetic macular edema (RESOLVE Study): a 12-month, randomized, controlled, double-masked, multicenter phase II study. Diabetes Care 2010;33:2399–405.
69. American Diabetes Association. Standards of medical care in diabetes—2013. Diabetes Care 2013;36:S11–66.
70. Smiddy WE. Economic considerations of macular edema therapies. Ophthalmology 2011;118:1827–33.
71. Limb GA, Webster L, Soomro H, et al. Platelet expression of tumour necrosis factor-α (TNF-α), TNF receptors and intercellular adhesion molecule-1 (ICAM-1) in patients with proliferative diabetic retinopathy. Clin Exp Immunol 1999;118:213–8.
72. Limb GA, Hollifield RD, Webster L, et al. Soluble TNF receptors in vitreoretinal proliferative disease. Invest Ophthalmol Vis Sci 2001;42:1586–91.
73. Adamis AP, Berman AJ. Immunological mechanisms in the pathogenesis of diabetic retinopathy. Semin Immunopathol 2008;30:65–84.
74. Cañete JD, Pablos JL, Sanmartí R, et al. Antiangiogenic effects of anti-tumor necrosis factor α therapy with infliximab in psoriatic arthritis. Arthritis Rheum 2004;50:1636–41.
75. Sfikakis PP, Grigoropolous V, Emfietzoglou I, et al. Infliximab for diabetic macular edema refractory to laser photocoagulation: a randomized, double-blind, placebo-controlled, crossover, 32-week study. Diabetes Care 2010;33:1523–8.
76. Wu L, Hernadez-Bogantes E, Roca J, et al. Intravitreal tumor necrosis factor inhibitors in the treatment of refractory diabetic macular edema: a pilot study

from the Pan American Collaborative Retina Study Group. Retina 2011;31:
298–303.

77. Pulido JS, Pulido JE, Michet CJ, et al. More questions than answers: a call for a
moratorium on the use of intravitreal infliximab outside of a well-designed trial.
Retina 2010;30:1–5.

78. Lewis H, Abrams GW, Blumenkranz MS, et al. Vitrectomy for diabetic macular
traction and edema associated with posterior hyaloidal traction. Ophthalmology
1992;99:753–9.

79. Gisladottir S, Loftsson T, Stefansson E. Diffusion characteristics of vitreous hu-
mour and saline solution follow the Stokes Einstein equation. Graefes Arch
Clin Exp Ophthalmol 2009;247:1677–84.

80. Nasrallah FP, Jalkh AE, VanCoppenrolle F, et al. The role of the vitreous in diabetic macular edema. Ophthalmology 1988;95:1335–9.

81. Hikichi T, Fujio N, Akiba Y, et al. Association between the short-term natural history of diabetic macular edema and the vitreomacular relationship in type 2 diabetes mellitus. Ophthalmology 1997;104:473–8.

82. Landers MB, Kon Graveren VA, Stewart MW. Early vitrectomy for DME: does it
have a roll? Retin Physician 2013;10:46–53.

83. Kumagai K, Furukawa M, Ogino N, et al. Long-term follow-up of vitrectomy for
diffuse nontractional diabetic macular edema. Retina 2009;29:464–72.

84. Browning DJ, Fraser CM, Powers ME. Comparison of the magnitude and time
course of macular thinning induced by different interventions for diabetic macular edema: implications for sequence of application. Ophthalmology 2006;113:
1713–9.

85. Kimura T, Kiryu J, Nishiwaki H, et al. Efficacy of surgical removal of the internal
limiting membrane in diabetic cystoid macular edema. Retina 2005;25:454–61.

86. Stalmans P, Benz MS, Gandorfer A, et al. Enzymatic vitreolysis with ocriplasmin
for vitreomacular traction and macular holes. N Engl J Med 2012;367:606–15.

87. Writing Committee for the Diabetic Retinopathy Clinical Research Network,
Fong DS, Strauber SF, et al. Comparison of the modified Early Treatment Diabetic Retinopathy Study and mild macular grid laser photocoagulation strategies for diabetic macular edema. Arch Ophthalmol 2007;125(4):469–80.

88. Jonas JB, Sofker A. Intraocular injection of crystalline cortisone as adjunctive
treatment of diabetic macular edema. Am J Ophthalmol 2001;132:425–7.

89. Martidis A, Duker JS, Greenberg PB, et al. Intravitreal triamcinolone for refractory diabetic macular edema. Ophthalmology 2002;109:920–7.

90. Diabetic Retinopathy Clinical Research Network, Chew E, Strauber S, et al. Randomized trial of peribulbar triamcinolone acetonide with and without focal
photocoagulation for mild diabetic macular edema: a pilot study. Ophthalmology 2007;114(6):1190–6.

91. Diabetic Retinopathy Clinical Research Network. Randomized trial evaluating
ranibizumab plus prompt or deferred laser or triamcinolone plus prompt laser
for diabetic macular edema. Ophthalmology 2010;117(6):1064–77.e35.

92. Diabetic Retinopathy Clinical Research Network. Expanded 2-year follow-up of
ranibizumab plus prompt or deferred laser or triamcinolone plus prompt laser
for diabetic macular edema. Ophthalmology 2011;118(4):609–14.

93. Diabetic Retinopathy Clinical Research Network. Randomized trial evaluating
short-term effects of intravitreal ranibizumab or triamcinolone acetonide on macular edema following focal/grid laser for diabetic macular edema in eyes also
receiving panretinal photocoagulation. Retina 2011;31(6):1009–27.

Dermatologic Manifestations of Diabetes Mellitus: A Review

Blair Murphy-Chutorian, BA, MSIV[a], George Han, MD, PhD[b],
Steven R. Cohen, MD, MPH[c],*

KEYWORDS

- Diabetes mellitus • Bullosa diabeticorum • Necrobiosis lipoidica diabeticorum
- Granuloma annulare • Diabetic scleredema • Acanthosis nigricans • Yellow skin
- Periungual erythema

KEY POINTS

- Primer on dermatologic conditions that may serve as markers of impaired glucose metabolism, emphasizing their role in the early identification and management of diabetes mellitus.
- Understand the epidemiology, pathogenesis and treatment of diabetes-associated skin disorders.

INTRODUCTION

Diabetes mellitus is a heterogeneous group of disorders associated with abnormal carbohydrate metabolism. Diabetes affects an estimated 26 million people in the United States, including an estimated 7 million undiagnosed cases.[1] The epidemic is rapidly growing and has been projected to double by 2050.[2] Worldwide, the prevalence of diabetes is approximately 350 million.[3]

Complications of diabetes are the result of metabolic, hormonal, environmental, and genetic factors, manifesting in every organ system. According to various studies, 30% to 91% of diabetic patients experience at least 1 dermatologic complication.[4–6] The numerous cutaneous manifestations of diabetes range widely in severity (from mundane cosmetic concerns to life threatening), in prevalence (relatively common to rare), and in treatment response (responsive to refractory). Many skin manifestations disproportionately affect patients with type 1 or type 2 diabetes mellitus (**Table 1**).

Certain skin manifestations, considered specific cutaneous markers, should prompt studies of glucose metabolism because the risk of diabetes mellitus is high; other

This article originally appeared in Endocrinology and Metabolism Clinics of North America, Vol. 42, Issue 4, December 2013.

[a] University of California, Irvine, Irvine, CA 92697, USA; [b] Albert Einstein College of Medicine, Bronx, NY 10461, USA; [c] Division of Dermatology, Albert Einstein College of Medicine, Montefiore Medical Center, 111 East 210th Street, Bronx, NY 10467, USA

* Corresponding author.
E-mail address: steven.cohen@einstein.yu.edu

Table 1
Skin manifestations demonstrating a disproportionately increased association among 1 of the 2 major types of diabetes

Type 1 Diabetes Mellitus	Type 2 Diabetes Mellitus
Necrobiosis lipoidica diabeticorum	Generalized granuloma annulare
Diabetic bullae	Scleredema diabeticorum
Vitiligo vulgaris	Diabetic dermopathy
Periungual telangiectasia	Acanthosis nigricans
	Acrochordons
	Psoriasis
	Yellow skin and nails

markers are nonspecific for diabetes but are more prevalent among diabetic patients than the general population. Skin findings may be the first sign of a metabolic disturbance caused by undiagnosed diabetes, suboptimal management of known disease, or even a prediabetic state. Skin complications of diabetes can provide clues to current and past metabolic status. Recognition of cutaneous markers enables earlier diagnosis and treatment, which may slow disease progression and ultimately improve the overall prognosis.

This review explores the acute and chronic dermatologic manifestations of diabetes according to the following categories: (1) specific cutaneous markers; (2) nonspecific skin conditions associated with diabetes (**Table 2**); and (3) other dermatologic considerations in the diabetic patient, including complications, primary skin disease associations, infections, and reactions to therapy. The focus is on clinical and histologic presentations, epidemiology, causes, and treatment options.

SPECIFIC CUTANEOUS MARKERS OF DIABETES MELLITUS
Necrobiosis Lipoidica Diabeticorum

Necrobiosis lipoidica (NL) is a chronic, necrotizing, granulomatous skin disease that occurs primarily in individuals with diabetes. It is one of the most disfiguring, disabling, and refractory cutaneous complications of diabetes.[7] NL lesions begin as small, firm, erythematous papules that gradually evolve and enlarge. Typical lesions are well-demarcated, indurated, annular plaques that contain characteristic yellow-brown atrophic centers studded with prominent ectatic vessels, and delimited by narrow, granulomatous, reddish-brown, or violaceous margins (**Fig. 1**). Solitary or

Table 2
Dermatologic manifestations of diabetes by category

Specific Cutaneous Markers	Nonspecific Conditions
Necrobiosis lipoidica	Acrochordons
Generalized granuloma annulare	Yellow skin and nails
Diabetic bullae	Generalized pruritus
Scleredema diabeticorum	Thick skin
Acanthosis nigricans	Rubiosis faciei
Eruptive xanthomatosis	Palmar erythema
Acquired perforating dermatoses	Nailbed erythema
Diabetic dermopathy	Pigmented purpuric dermatoses

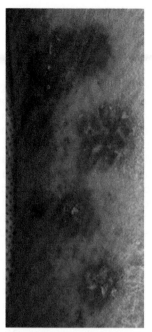

Fig. 1. Necrobiosis lipoidica diabeticorum on the pretibial leg.

multiple lesions are most commonly distributed bilaterally on the lower extremities, particularly the pretibial areas, but may occur on the face, trunk, and upper extremities as well. Distinctive necrobiosis surrounded by palisading granulomas are seen on histopathology.[8]

Although only a small proportion (0.3%–1.6%) of diabetic patients develop NL, it has long been believed that most patients with NL meet criteria for diabetes at some point in their lives.[9,10] In the 1966 seminal study of Muller and Winkelmann,[11] 60% of 171 subjects with NL were found to be diabetic, and another 20% were either glucose intolerant or reported at least 1 parent with diabetes. A strong correlation is consistently reported between NL and diabetes mellitus, although to what degree this association exists has become less clear. A retrospective review in 1999 found only 22% of 65 patients with NL to have or develop diabetes over a 15-year period.[12] Future investigations of a large sample biopsy-proven NL cases are necessary to clarify the relationship.

Diabetes precedes the onset of NL by a mean of 10 years,[9] but can develop concurrently with or later than NL. Therefore, patients with NL with normal glucose metabolism should be closely monitored over time for diabetes or insulin resistance.[10] NL in the setting of diabetes is called necrobiosis lipoidica diabeticorum (NLD).

NLD can be asymptomatic or painful and/or pruritic, especially when ulcerated. The sensation of involved skin is often reduced. The reduced innervation of NL lesions raises the possibility that local inflammation causes nerve damage and sensory loss.[13] Ulceration occurs in approximately 35% of lesions, either spontaneously or secondary to trauma.[14,15] Ulcerative lesions may be complicated by secondary infection and, rarely, by development of squamous cell carcinoma.

NLD occurs more frequently in type 1 diabetes but is associated with both types.[7] There is a female predominance (75%–80% of cases) with typical onset in the third to fourth decades of life.[4,14,16] Shall and colleagues[9] found NLD occurred significantly earlier in insulin-dependent patients (mean 22 years) compared with the non–insulin-dependent group (mean 49 years).

The cause of NLD is unknown. Vasculopathy, collagen alterations, immune complex deposition, and inflammatory mechanisms have all been implicated in the pathogenesis of NLD, and may each play a role.[17] Ngo and colleagues[18] challenged the theory that diabetic vascular disease with resulting ischemia was the main causal factor by demonstrating increased blood flow in NLD, including chronic lesions. The investigators suggest that significant evidence points to an inflammatory process, such as an antibody-mediated vasculitis, as a central cause of NLD.

The association between NL and glycemic control is unclear.[19] Until future studies clarify the relationship, tighter glucose control in NLD management is recommended. Treatment of NL is well recognized as problematic and challenging. Responses to therapy vary widely and refractory cases are the rule. There is no satisfactory universal approach to treatment. Topical and intralesional steroids, calcineurin inhibitors, compression therapy, and psoralen with ultraviolet A (PUVA) are the most frequently used modalities.[14]

There are seemingly endless reports describing successful treatments for NLD in isolated cases or case series, including. antithrombotics and platelet inhibitors (pentoxyfilline, dipyridamole, acetylsalicylic acid), heparin, topical tretinoin, topical tacrolimus, cyclosporine, systemic glucocorticoid, ticlopidine, nicotinamide, clofazimine, mycophenalate mofetil, fumaric acid esters, antimalarials, local excision with skin grafting, compression, photodynamic therapy, and CO_2 laser therapy.[7,8,15,20–31] In addition, topical granulocyte colony-stimulating factor,[32] intralesional tumor necrosis factor (TNF)-alpha inhibitors (infliximab[33] and etanercept[27]), intravenous infliximab,[22,34] and systemic colchicine[35] have demonstrated efficacy in severe refractory cases of ulcerative NL.

No single drug has shown consistent efficacy, and regardless of the modality, NL lesions tend to relapse on cessation of therapy. Without intervention, spontaneous resolution is observed in about 13% to 19% of cases of NL after 6 to 12 years.[10] Healing with persistent scarring, atrophy, and disfigurement is customary.[21] The physical and emotional toll of NLD all too frequently translates as disability and decreased quality of life.[20]

Generalized Granuloma Annulare

Granuloma annulare (GA) is a rare, necrobiotic, inflammatory disorder of unknown cause. Five clinical variants of GA include localized, subcutaneous, perforating, generalized, and arcuate dermal erythema forms. The association between GA and diabetes has been controversial because so many studies have combined data from all clinical variants. It is now accepted that only the generalized form shows consistent and significant correlation with diabetes across most studies.[36–38] Like NLD, the prevalence of GA among diabetics is only 0.3%; however, 21% to 77% of patients with generalized GA have diabetes (predominantly type 2 diabetes).[36,37] All other variants of GA, including the most common, localized GA, are not associated with diabetes.[10,39,40]

Generalized GA initially appears as multiple, small, firm, skin-colored or red dermal papules that tend to be symmetrically distributed on the distal extremities and sun-exposed areas of the trunk.[39,41] Individual lesions gradually expand and centrally involute, forming annular rings with raised borders (**Fig. 2**). The resemblance to NLD is striking but GA lacks epidermal atrophy and yellow discoloration.[42] The eruption is typically asymptomatic but can be pruritic. It is curious that up to 33% of cases of

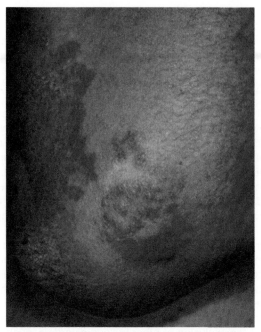

Fig. 2. Generalized granuloma annulare with involvement of upper and lower extremities bilaterally.

generalized GA are atypical presentations with nonannular, mostly coalescing papules.[43]

Generalized GA is twice as common among women and occurs at any age with an approximate mean of 50 years.[43,44] Postulated to be an immunologic disorder, GA is most likely a type IV delayed hypersensitivity reaction.[36,45] Prolonged exposure to high glucose levels may contribute to the development of generalized GA.[39,44]

The histopathology shows lymphohistiocytic granulomatous inflammation of the dermis and collagen degeneration. Colloidal iron stain reveals abundant deposition of mucin. The presence of mucin and the absence of increased plasma cells helps to histologically distinguish GA from NL.

Unlike localized disease, the course of generalized GA is often protracted and seldom resolves spontaneously. Diabetic patients in particular suffer persistent and relapsing courses, with poor long-term outcomes.[36] Although there are no standard treatment guidelines, first-line options comprise ultraviolet A-1 (UVA-1), oral psoralen (8-methoxypsoralen) and PUVA, systemic retinoids, and dapsone. By comparison, second-line therapies rely mostly on anecdotal reports and small case series that include photodynamic therapy, cryotherapy, topical, intralesional, and systemic corticosteroids, chlorambucil, pentoxifylline, antimalarials, cyclosporine, fumaric esters, potassium iodide, niacinamide, etanercept, infliximab, adalimumab, and efalizumab.[36,40,46,47] New cases of generalized GA should be screened for diabetes.

Diabetic Bullae

Diabetic bullae (DB), or bullosa diabeticorum, is a rare, noninflammatory, bullous disorder characterized by tense, painless, bullae that develop abruptly on normal-appearing skin, typically on the distal lower extremities, and less often involving the hand or forearm (**Fig. 3**).[48,49] Acute episodes are likely to occur during sleep and without preceding trauma. The blisters evolve rapidly (as quickly as 15 minutes has been reported[50]) and may become more flaccid, and sometimes uncomfortable, as they enlarge. Solitary or multiple blisters range from a few millimeters to several centimeters in diameter filled with clear, sterile, serous fluid unless complicated by secondary hemorrhage or infection.[51,52]

By definition, all patients with DB have diabetes mellitus, most commonly insulin-dependent; however the low frequency of 0.5% among diabetics may be higher than reported.[50,52] DB is most often encountered in the setting of long-standing, type 1 diabetes with late complications, such as neuropathy, nephropathy, and retinopathy.[50,53–55] DB has been described in type 2 diabetes as well. The predilection for men is reportedly 2:1. The age of onset averages 50 to 70 years, but DB has been documented in teenagers to people in their eighth decade. One study found 29 of 35 (83%) DB eruptions were correlated with highly varying blood glucose levels.[50]

Despite the poorly understood cause of DB, numerous mechanisms have been proposed, including minor trauma-induced blister formation, hypoglycemia or highly fluctuating blood glucose levels, microangiopathy, neuropathy, alterations in calcium or magnesium metabolism, UV exposure, an autoimmune phenomenon, and vascular insufficiency. None provides an adequate explanation.[40,50,53,54]

There are no specific tests for DB. The diagnosis is based on characteristic findings, clinical course, and the exclusion of other bullous disorders, such as drug eruption, immunobullous disease, and porphyria cutanea tarda. The index of suspicion should be high in the setting of negative direct immunofluorescence testing and the absence of urinary uroporphyrins. Histologic examination may aid diagnosis in certain cases.[48,50]

The microscopic findings in DB reveal 2 major groups with different levels of cleavage, suggesting different stages of development or even separate pathogenetic mechanisms.[53] The first and most common group shows intraepidermal or subepidermal cleavage at the level of the lamina lucida, without acantholysis. These lesions usually resolve spontaneously without scarring and reepithelialize early. By contrast, in the second type, cleavage is below the dermoepidermal junction with destruction of anchoring fibrils.[46,53] This type heals with scarring and atrophy.

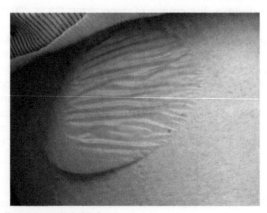

Fig. 3. Diabetic bullae on medial thigh.

Although most DB heal in 2 to 6 weeks without treatment, the course is not always smooth.[53] Secondary infection or ulceration, particularly associated with blisters on the foot, may lead to osteomyelitis, large areas of necrosis and scarring, as well as toe amputation. Healing may be as long as 2 years.[50] Surprisingly, peripheral perfusion tends to be adequate for healing, despite the occurrence of DB in diabetic patients with other late complications.[50] Even with complete resolution of DB, bullae frequently recur.[48]

Treatment of DB is focused on skin protection and preventing secondary infection. Immediate regulation of the blood glucose level has been recommended as a result of the finding that hypoglycemic episodes often precede eruptions. Uncomplicated blisters should be left intact, but sterile aspiration of fluid may prevent rupture in some cases. Ulcerated blisters should be treated with aggressive wound management.[50,53]

Scleredema Diabeticorum

Scleredema diabeticorum, or diabetic scleredema, is a rare chronic connective tissue disorder primarily associated with type 2 diabetes. The condition is characterized by impressive thickening of the reticular dermis affecting the posterior neck, upper back, and shoulders with occasional extension to the face, arms, chest, or abdomen (**Figs. 4** and **5**).[56,57] The involved skin is hard, thick, and indurated, sometimes erythematous, and may have a peau d'orange appearance (**Fig. 6**). Scleredema diabeticorum is usually asymptomatic, but pain and decreased mobility (especially of the back) may be present in severe cases. It is noteworthy that acral skin is always spared.

The prevalence of scleredema ranges from 2.5% to 14% of all diabetic patients.[56,58,59] It is most likely to develop in adults with long-standing diabetes and with poor glycemic control, occurring 10 times more frequently in men.[60]

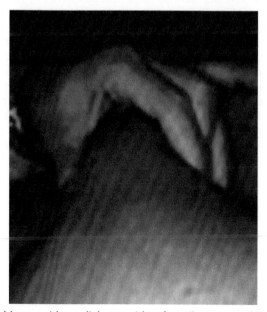

Fig. 4. A 40-year-old man without diabetes with soft easily compressible skin of the shoulder (unaffected).

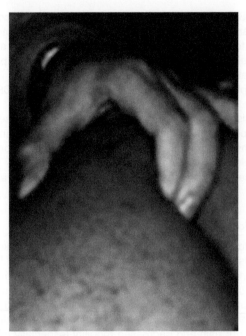

Fig. 5. A 41-year-old man with type 2 diabetes with hard inflexible skin of the shoulder, characteristic of scleredema diabeticorum.

Unequivocal diagnosis of scleredema by histologic examination requires a full thickness excisional biopsy to examine the dermis. The microscopic findings reveal a markedly thickened reticular dermis, thick collagen bundles, and mild infiltrate of mucin in the deeper dermis. Both edema and sclerosis are notably absent.[56] The diagnosis is usually based on history and physical examination.

Scleredema diabeticorum should not be confused with scleredema of Buschke or with systemic scleroderma.[56,61] Despite the similarities between the 2 names, scleredema and scleroderma are unrelated. Scleredema of Buschke and scleredema diabeticorum are frequently used interchangeably in the literature, but these disorders represent 2 distinct subtypes of scleredema. Although the clinical presentations are indistinguishable, scleredema of Buschke occurs in children after a viral or bacterial upper respiratory infection and self-resolves in months.

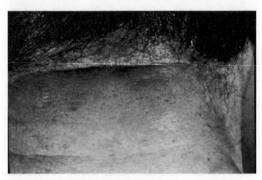

Fig. 6. Scleredema diabeticorum of skin of the neck.

There is no highly effective treatment for scleredema diabeticorum. PUVA seems most effective but other recommended therapies include strict glycemic control with an insulin pump, potent topical and intralesional steroids, penicillamine, intralesional insulin, low-dose methotrexate, prostaglandin E1, and pentoxifylline.[57,62,63] Scleredema incidentally improved in a patient treated with allopurinol for acquired reactive perforating collagenosis.[64] The combination of PUVA and physical therapy may help with mobility in patients with severe diabetic scleredema.[57] Although strict glycemic control does not show consistent therapeutic benefit in scleredema diabeticorum, it is proposed to be an effective preventive measure.

Acanthosis Nigricans

Acanthosis nigricans (AN) is characterized by diffuse, hyperpigmented, light brown to black, velvety to verrucous thickening of intertriginous and flexural areas of the body, particularly in the axilla, groin, and posterior neck (**Fig. 7**). These papillomatous plaques are poorly marginated and cause accentuation of skin markings. As a rule, AN is asymptomatic, but it may be painful, malodorous, or macerated in rare cases.[46] It occurs in all ethnicities, but disproportionately affects Native Americans, nonwhite Hispanics, and African Americans.[65] There are 2 forms of AN, benign and malignant, which share a similar clinical and histologic presentation. Unlike the benign variant, malignant AN is not associated with diabetes. Malignant AN, a rare paraneoplastic syndrome, is associated with an underlying carcinoma, most commonly adenocarcinoma of the stomach.[66,67]

Considered a marker of insulin resistance, benign AN characteristically occurs in the setting of type 2 diabetes mellitus and obesity.[10,16] In a frequently quoted study, 74% of an obese population had AN along with increased plasma insulin levels.[68] Benign AN is also associated with other endocrine abnormalities involving insulin resistance, including polycystic ovarian syndrome, lipodystrophy, acromegaly, Cushing syndrome, Addison disease, thyroid disease, and leprechaunism.[69] Nicotinic acid and other drugs are associated with benign AN, although the exact mechanism is unknown.[46] In addition, AN has been reported as a rare, local, cutaneous side effect of repeated exogenous insulin injections. It is generally accepted that injection site AN is caused by local hyperinsulinemia. Rotating injection sites may help to prevent or reverse the reaction.[70]

The histology of AN shows marked hyperkeratosis, epidermal papillomatosis, and slight, variable acanthosis.[69] There is no change in melanocyte count or melanin content. The hyperpigmentation observed mainly results from a thickened keratin-containing epithelium.[70,71] Diagnosis of AN is usually clinical and warrants screening

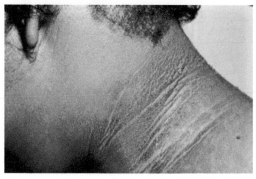

Fig. 7. Acanthosis nigricans on the nape of the neck.

for diabetes and insulin resistance. New onset of AN should prompt an evaluation for underlying malignancy.[72]

ANs is a chronic but reversible condition. Management focuses on treating the underlying cause; skin lesions are mostly of cosmetic concern. In the diabetic patient, weight control, dietary restrictions, and increased physical activity are of primary importance and have been proved to be most effective in controlling AN.[73] Lifestyle modifications may be augmented by various pharmacologic approaches to improve insulin sensitivity and reduce hyperinsulinemia. By contrast, purely dermatologic therapies that do not target hyperinsulinemia are of transient benefit at best. Nonetheless, topical keratolytics (eg, salicylic acid, retinoic acid, and ammonium lactate) and oral isotretinoin can reduce thicker plaques in areas of maceration, decreasing odor and discomfort.[46]

Diabetic Dermopathy

Diabetic dermopathy, also called shin spots or pigmented pretibial patches, is seen in 40% to 50% of diabetic patients.[46,74,75] It is characterized by the eruption of multiple asymptomatic, round, dull red to pink papules or plaques predominantly on the pretibial skin bilaterally but also occurring on the forearms, thighs, and lateral malleoli. Early lesions may be mistaken for dermatophytosis (**Fig. 8**).[76] One to 2 weeks after they appear, these lesions evolve to well-circumscribed, atrophic, brown macules often with fine scale (**Fig. 9**).[77] New lesions may emerge and older ones resolve spontaneously leaving slightly depressed, hyperpigmented areas. It is a dynamic process with lesions of varied stages present at the same time. Shin spots may occasionally be complicated by ulceration.

Diabetic dermopathy is a clinical diagnosis. Because the histopathology is relatively nonspecific, skin biopsy is best avoided. The microscopic findings in new lesions

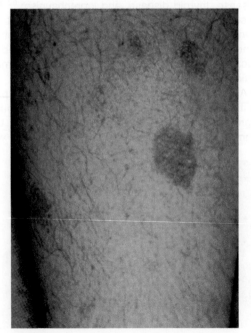

Fig. 8. Early lesions of diabetic dermopathy on the pretibial leg.

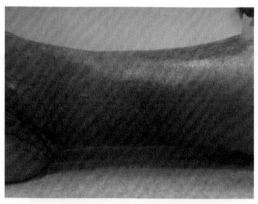

Fig. 9. Pigmented purpura with features of chronic diabetic dermopathy.

show edema of the epidermis and papillary dermis with a mild perivascular lymphohistiocytic infiltrate and hemorrhage. Older lesions feature epidermal atrophy with thickened blood vessels in the papillary dermis, no edema, and scattered hemosiderin deposits. An increase in diastase-resistant material staining positive with periodic acid-Schiff is present in the vessel walls.

Diabetic dermopathy is most commonly identified in diabetic men more than 50 years of age, especially among those with long-standing diabetes and poor glycemic control.[78] Up to 70% of diabetic men aged 60 years and older reportedly have dermopathy[16]; and many of these patients suffer from neuropathy, nephropathy, and retinopathy.[75,79] Dermopathy can also precede the onset of diabetes. Correlations between dermopathy and duration of diabetes or glycemic control have not been found.[80]

The cause of shin spots is unknown. Attempts to explain the pathogenesis have centered on trauma and on microangiopathy with associated capillary changes; however, the literature abounds with evidence to both support and refute these potential factors.[75,77,78,81] Whether dermopathy is specific for diabetes remains controversial.[78,80] It is generally agreed that 4 or more shin spots increase the probability that diabetes is present, warranting an evaluation.[82]

No medical intervention is necessary aside from prevention of secondary infection. Management should address microangiopathic complications and coronary artery disease, because of their association with diabetic dermopathy.[80]

Acquired Perforating Dermatoses

Acquired perforating dermatoses (APD) comprise a group of chronic skin disorders defined histologically by transepidermal perforation and elimination of a connective tissue component of the dermis.[83] Historically, this disorder was classified by the predominant dermal material identified microscopically (such as keratin, collagen, or elastic tissue); hence, the terminology reactive perforating collagenosis, elastosis perforans serpiginosa (EPS), as well as perforating folliculitis and Kyrle disease (**Fig. 10**). The APD group is almost exclusively associated with chronic renal failure, diabetes, and/or hemodialysis (often related to diabetic nephropathy). The skin lesions are highly pruritic, follicular, hyperkeratotic nodules and papules with a central keratin plug that may be described as umbilicated. The eruption is found primarily on the extremities and trunk, less often on the

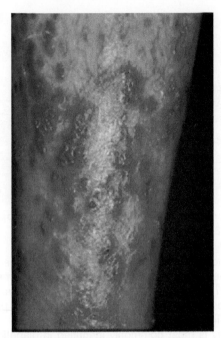

Fig. 10. Kyrle disease affecting the bilateral lower extremities.

head. The papules of EPS are distributed in a distinctive serpiginous pattern. APD undergoes Koebnerization (the development of lesions at sites of trauma) and is typically exacerbated by excoriation.[84] The differential diagnosis of APD includes prurigo nodularis, folliculitis, arthropod bites, multiple keratoacanthomas, psoriasis, and lichen planus.[85]

In a review of 22 patients with APD, Saray and colleagues[86] found almost 73% had chronic renal failure and were on hemodialysis, and 50% had diabetes (91% of the patients with diabetes had chronic renal failure secondary to diabetic nephropathy). Yet, 13.6% of the patients were otherwise in good general health. APD has been associated with other extracutaneous diseases that include but are not limited to malignancy, hepatic disorders, hypothyroidism, AIDS, tuberculosis, atopic dermatitis, and scabies.[83,86]

The pathogenesis is poorly understood. It remains unknown whether the primary abnormality occurs in the dermis or epidermis, and whether the pruritus is an underlying cause or a resultant effect of the skin condition. Proposed theories include (1) metabolic derangements causing an epidermal or dermal alteration; (2) a deposition of some substance not removed by dialysis, which the immune system then perceives as foreign; and (3) microtrauma secondary to scratching or a manifestation of microangiopathy.[83,86–88]

APD in the setting of diabetes is relatively unresponsive to therapy. By avoiding trauma to the area, lesions may resolve slowly. Therefore, symptomatic relief of pruritus is a core treatment strategy. Varying beneficial effects are reported with topical keratolytics, topical and systemic retinoids, allopurinol, PUVA, UVB phototherapy, topical and intralesional corticosteroids, antibiotics (doxycycline), oral antihistamine, cryotherapy, and renal transplantation.[10,83,88,89] Dialysis does not improve the course of the disease.

Eruptive Xanthomatosis

Eruptive xanthomas are uncommon and virtually pathognomonic of hypertriglyceride-mia.[90] They arise suddenly in groups of multiple yellow papules, 1 to 4 mm in diameter, mainly on the extensor surfaces of the extremities and on the buttocks (**Fig. 11**). Eruptive xanthomas often arise as a Koebner phenomenon on pressure points. The papules are surrounded by erythematous halos at their base and may be tender or pruritic.[10] The histopathology shows an accumulation of lipid-laden histiocytic foam cells with a mixed infiltrate of lymphocytes and neutrophils in the dermis.

Approximately one-third of all diabetic patients have serum lipoprotein abnormalities caused by insulinopenia, but the prevalence of xanthomatosis among this population is unclear.[90] The reason for the increased frequency of eruptive xanthomatosis among individuals with diabetes has been well characterized. Because insulin is a stimulating factor critical to the normal activity of lipoprotein lipase, it plays an important role in the metabolism of serum triglycerides and triglyceride-rich lipoproteins. The insulin-deficient state of uncontrolled insulin-dependent diabetes results in the absence of lipoprotein lipase activity.[39] Consequently, the impaired clearance of very-low-density lipoproteins (VLDLs) and chylomicrons leads to a hyperlipemic syndrome, which, if severe enough, can precipitate eruptive xanthomas. Diabetic hyperlipidemia may be accelerated by polyphagia caused by glycosuria.[10,90]

As with so many of the specific cutaneous markers of diabetes, recognizing xanthomatosis may be an essential clue to deteriorating metabolic status. Thus, it cannot be overemphasized that early identification of xanthomatosis can facilitate timely treatment and possible avoidance of more serious manifestations of hyperlipidemia such as atherosclerotic complications and pancreatitis.[91] The diagnosis of eruptive xanthomatosis should prompt further investigation and treatment of hyperglycemia.[92] Xanthomatosis resolves with control of carbohydrate and lipid metabolism, therefore the diabetic patient typically requires just optimized insulin therapy. Statins or fibrates can supplement treatment as tolerated.[93]

NONSPECIFIC SKIN CONDITIONS ASSOCIATED WITH DIABETES
Acrochordons (Skin Tags)

Skin tags are soft fibromas that are particularly common in people with diabetes. These benign, asymptomatic, exophytic growths are observed on the eyelids, neck, axilla, and other skin folds. They may be flesh-colored or, less often, hyperpigmented, and can range from small papules to pedunculated polyps, typically 1 to 6 mm in diameter, with smooth or irregular surfaces.[94–97] There is a slight female predilection, and prevalence increases with age.[39] Although characteristically asymptomatic, skin tags

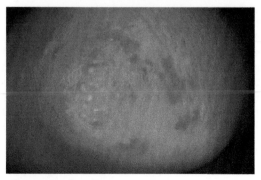

Fig. 11. Eruptive xanthomas on the elbow.

contain nerve cells and therefore may cause discomfort if irritated. Histologic features include a papillarylike dermis consisting of loose collagen fibers and supporting vasculature. The epidermis and dermis are both involved to varying degrees.[39]

Approximately 66% to 75% of patients with skin tags have frank diabetes[46] and more than 80% show impaired carbohydrate metabolism.[95] The association between diabetes and skin tags is likely related to the proliferative effect of hyperinsulinemia on keratinocytes and fibroblasts, similar to the pathogenesis of ANs. Skin tags have also been associated with colonic polyps[98] and human papillomavirus (HPV). One study found HPV DNA in 88% of skin tags.[99]

Data regarding the total number of skin tags per individual and the associated risk of diabetes is controversial.[95,97,100] In a case-control study, researchers observed a positive correlation between the incidence of diabetes or impaired glucose tolerance and the total number of skin tags,[100] however previous studies failed to find such a correlation.[95,97] The discrepancy may be accounted for by differences in the study method. For example, it is possible that a correlation exists only between a very high number of skin tags and diabetes risk. Demir and Demir[95] examined individuals with a lower mean total number of lesions. Of 120 individuals enrolled, 41% had 1 to 3 skin tags and only 31% had 10 or more. In contrast, Rasi and colleagues[100] only included individuals with a minimum of 3 skin tags, and 86.8% of the 104 case subjects had 10 or more skin tags (25.7% had 30+ skin tags). Future studies may help to determine whether there is indeed a statistically significant correlation between number of skin tags and impaired carbohydrate metabolism. Rasi and colleagues[100] found a significantly higher incidence of impaired carbohydrate metabolism in individuals with more than 30 skin tags (52%) than in those with fewer than 30 tags (27.3%).

The only correlation found between anatomic location of skin tags and impaired carbohydrate metabolism was the finding of increased risk of diabetes in inframammary skin tags in women. Treatment of skin tags is medically unnecessary, but cosmetic concerns may be addressed with snip biopsy, laser excision, cryotherapy, or electrodesiccation.[101]

Yellow Skin and Nails

Yellowish skin and nails are described with increased frequency among individuals with diabetes compared with the general population. This finding is asymptomatic and considered benign, but the exact cause has not been elucidated. Carotenoderma has traditionally been proposed as a possible cause, but supporting evidence is weak. Diabetic patients do not have increased levels of serum carotenoids (carotenemia) as previously reported,[102] and the levels of carotenoid in diabetic skin have not actually been reported in the literature. The best explanation for diabetic yellow skin is likely a discoloration caused by certain end products associated with nonenzymatic glycosylation of dermal collagen. One of these end products, 2-(2-furoyl)-4[5]-(2-furanyl)-1H-imidazole, is known to have a characteristic yellow hue.[102] Nonenzymatic glycosylation of proteins occurs only to a minor extent in nondiabetics, but it is stimulated by the hyperglycemic state in diabetes. Many of the skin manifestations of diabetes may be attributable to the glycosylation of proteins. Future biochemical analysis of diabetic skin could lead to better understanding of its yellow hue.

The increased frequency of yellow nails among diabetic patients may be at least partially attributable to an increased prevalence of onychomycosis.

Generalized Pruritus

It is widely accepted that pruritus occurs with a much higher frequency among patients with diabetes than the general population. Poor microcirculation and hypohidrosis causing xerosis were proposed as explanations. A 1986 study by Neilly and colleagues[103] investigated pruritus in diabetes by comparing 300 diabetics and 100 nondiabetic controls. Pruritus vulvae in women was the only type of localized pruritus seen more frequently in patients with diabetes. Although generalized pruritus was found to be more common among people with diabetes than a control population, most cases tended to involve an underlying illness or likely drug reaction that could better explain the itching. Otherwise, cases of generalized pruritus without such an explanation were not significantly more common among diabetics versus controls.[103] Pruritus vulvae is most frequently caused by an infectious process, particularly *Candida*. Therefore, exogenous diabetic drug therapy and pathogens may explain the increased frequency of pruritus in diabetes.[92]

Rubeosis Faciei

Rubeosis faciei has long been described as a common manifestation of diabetes mellitus. The condition is characterized by a chronically flushed face and neck. It tends to be more easily appreciated in Fitzpatrick skin types 1 and 2 because increased melanin can obscure the coloration. The reddish complexion is believed to result from microangiopathic alterations and superficial facial venous dilatation.[104]

The prevalence of rubeosis is unclear and may not be as high as previously believed, or the condition may have become less common.[105] Many review articles from the past several decades have republished data from an Israeli study that found 36 of 61 (59%) hospitalized patients with diabetes had "markedly red faces" and another 21% had "slightly red faces."[106] The only recent data on the prevalence of rubeosis are found in studies that investigated the prevalence of all cutaneous manifestations in individuals with diabetes. All these studies yielded results markedly less than 59%. In Saudi Arabia (2011)[5] and in Pakistan (2005),[6] rubeosis was observed in 3.1% and 7.1% of diabetic outpatients, respectively. Similarly, in 2007, Pavlovic and colleagues[105] reported cutaneous manifestations in 212 young (aged 2–22 years), insulin-dependent, diabetic outpatients in Serbia. Rubeosis faciei was seen in about 7% of cases, compared with none of the nondiabetic controls.

It remains to be determined whether severity of disease, inpatient status, Fitzpatrick skin type, or some other confounding factor can explain the discrepancy in the prevalence of rubeosis among diabetic patients between Gitelson and Wertheimer-Kaplinski[106] and the other studies. Gitelson and Wertheimer-Kaplinski[106] examined hospitalized patients, whereas the other studies enrolled outpatients, and none of the studies (each from different regions of the world) reported Fitzpatrick skin type.

Although rubeosis is a benign condition, it may serve as a clue to the more menacing internal processes of microangiopathy secondary to suboptimal glycemic control. Therefore, thorough patient evaluation for serious complications such as retinopathy is warranted. Treatment of rubeosis faciei is strict diabetic control and avoidance of alcohol, caffeine, and other vasodilators.

Palmar Erythema

Palmar erythema (PE) is believed to be a microvascular complication of both types 1 and 2 diabetes mellitus. This condition is a symmetric, asymptomatic, slightly warm erythema most frequently limited to the thenar and hypothenar eminences. This form of PE differs from normal physiologic mottling that involves the entire palm elicited by factors such as atmospheric temperature, emotional state, elevation of the hand, and pressure on the palm. Although similar to the palmar erythema associated with pregnancy (prevalence >30%), rheumatoid arthritis (prevalence >60%), hepatic disease, thyrotoxicosis, nutritional protein deficiency, smoking, chronic mercury poisoning, drug reactions, and neoplasms of the central nervous system,[107] it differs markedly from the more distal papular erythema of the palms and fingers of systemic lupus erythematosus.[108] The prevalence of PE among diabetic patients does not seem to have been reported in North America, but 2 observational studies in Pakistan have estimated the prevalence of palmar erythema at approximately 4%.[6,109] Like rubeosis faciei and yellow skin, diabetic PE is benign yet may signify an underlying process that calls for therapy.

Nailbed Erythema

Erythema of the proximal nailfold is another reddish color change seen in diabetic skin, and it has been attributed to dilatation of the superficial vascular plexus presenting as periungual telangiectasias (visibly dilated capillaries around the nail bed). Although classically associated with scleroderma and dermatomyositis, periungual telangiectasias are frequently observed among diabetic patients, again representing underlying diabetic microangiopathy.[110]

In 1960, Landau[111] investigated the nailbed vessels of 75 diabetic patients (>40 years of age) using a microscope with a slit lamp, and found that congestion at the venous end of nailbed capillaries was much more common in diabetes compared with healthy controls (65% vs 12%). The periungual capillaries of diabetic patients with this isolated venous portion congestion differs morphologically from those changes seen in connective tissue diseases, where the capillary loops are markedly blunted and attenuated.[110] Although it is usually asymptomatic, nailbed erythema in diabetic patients often presents with associated cuticle changes and tenderness of the fingertip. Nailbed erythema should not be confused with paronychia, which is caused by bacterial or fungal infection.

Pigmented Purpura

Pigmented purpura coexists with diabetic dermopathy (pigmented pretibial patches, shin spots) in about 50% of cases.[112] Pigmented purpura, also called pigmented purpuric dermatoses, is a heterogeneous group of uncommon, idiopathic, progressive skin conditions causing patches of orange to brown, nonblanching pigmentation speckled with 0.3 to 1.0 cm so-called cayenne pepper spots. These asymptomatic lesions are distributed mainly over the lower extremities, especially the pretibial leg (see Fig. 9), with occasional involvement of the ankles and dorsa of the feet,[110,112] and are caused by erythrocyte extravasation from the superficial venous plexus.[112] The deposition of hemosiderin released from red blood cells is responsible for the characteristic color. Pigmented purpura occurs most commonly in elderly diabetic patients, often precipitated by congestive heart failure and, therefore, presenting with lower extremity edema.[110] Of the 6 recognized clinical variants of pigmented purpura, the most common is progressive pigmented dermatosis or Schamberg disease.[113] In the absence of diabetic dermopathy, pigmented purpura is not considered a marker for diabetes.

OTHER DERMATOLOGIC CONSIDERATIONS IN THE DIABETIC PATIENT
Skin Manifestations of Diabetic Vascular Disease

Diabetes mellitus causes both large and small blood vessel disease. Atherosclerosis of vessels in diabetic patients often leads to ischemic changes of the lower extremities that result in classic findings: shiny, hairless, atrophic skin with cold toes and dystrophic nails, pallor on elevation, and mottling on dependence.[39] Large vessel disease contributes to poor wound healing and the frequency and recurrence of cutaneous infections in persons with diabetes, causing increased risk of gangrene and amputation.

Skin Manifestations of Diabetic Neuropathy

The neuropathic manifestations of diabetes can result in changes that affect the skin. Hypohidrosis or anhidrosis can occur as a result of autonomic neuropathy. These changes in perspiration usually affect the lower extremities. They can lead to severe xerosis as well as fissuring of the skin, which provides a portal of entry for pathogens.[92] Vascular dilatation can also result from autonomic neuropathy, manifesting as increased skin temperature and erythema.

Peripheral neuropathy is a common complication of diabetes. Loss of cutaneous sensation usually begins at the distal extremities, especially the fingers and toes. Such sensory deficits often predispose to injury, which is especially dangerous in the diabetic patient with vascular compromise and impaired healing. Chronic foot ulcers (mal perforans) often result from this combination of diabetic complications.

Skin Conditions of the Hands

Multiple skin conditions affecting the hands are seen more commonly among individuals with diabetes than among the general population. These include limited joint mobility, thick dorsal hand skin and finger pebbles, and Dupuytren contracture. Although it is possible for a patient to experience each of these 3 conditions, even concomitantly, they are considered distinct entities.

Limited joint mobility

Limited joint mobility (LJM), or diabetic cheiroarthropathy, has long been recognized as a common finding in diabetes.[114,115] Patients with LJM classically present with mildly restricted extension of the metacarpophalangeal and interphalangeal joints that generally begins with fifth finger involvement and spreads radially.[116–118] The condition is caused by thickening of periarticular connective tissue causing stiffness.[118] The prevalence of LJM in patients with diabetes is estimated to be between 30% and 40%.[116,119–122] In 2013, Rosenbloom[114] demonstrated that, over a 16-year period, LJM was associated with a nearly 4-fold increased risk of microvascular disease. Clearly this physical finding is a warning sign. Long-term diabetic control was positively correlated with LJM such that every unit increase in mean glycated hemoglobin imparted a significant increased risk of development of LJM.

Thick dorsal hand skin and finger pebbles

Nearly one-third of 309 diabetic patients found to have LJM in the study by Rosenbloom and colleagues[122] also had thick, tight, waxy skin of their dorsal hands that could not be tented on examination. Biopsies of the dermis showed marked thickening with accumulated connective tissue. Subsequent studies supported a significant correlation of thick skin with diabetes, and moderate to severe LJM with microvascular complications.[117,122,123] The relationship between thick skin and LJM is somewhat unclear; both can present independently.

A variant of thick skin manifests clinically as finger pebbles, also called pebbling or Huntley papules. These are easily recognizable, multiple, grouped, indurated, noninflammatory micropapules distributed over the extensor surfaces of the fingers and periungual region.[124] Finger papules are most prevalent in type 2 diabetes, and have been reported to affect approximately 75% of diabetics versus 12% of nondiabetic controls.[124,125] Although typically asymptomatic, finger pebbles may be associated with severe dryness and occasional pruritus. For these cases, 12% ammonium lactate reportedly provides some relief. Finger pebbles tend not to respond to topical steroids or moisturizers.[126]

Studies have shown that collagen in the skin of diabetic patients is often less soluble than the collagen of nondiabetic controls and has more ketoamine-linked glucose bound to it.[127,128] The accumulation of collagen is believed to play a major role in the pathogenesis of diabetic thick skin. Two leading theories propose explanations for the abnormal collagen build-up. Hyperglycemic states may promote nonenzymatic glycosylation of collagen, thereby causing increased cross-linking of collagen fibers, which renders the fibers resistant to collagenase degradation and results in abnormal collagen accumulation in tissue.[118,129] The other theory implicates the proliferative effect of excess insulin on collagen.[58] Tight glycemic control seems to aid resolution and prevention of thick skin.[130]

Earlier literature described LJM, diabetic scleredema, and scleredema of Buschke as synonyms. Several investigators have clarified that the 3 are not the same.[61,115]

Dupuytren contracture

Dupuytren contracture (DC), or Dupuytren disease, is a chronic and progressive fibro-proliferative disorder of palmar fascia characterized by nodules of the ventral hand that evolve to cords and fixed flexion contractures, as well as palmar skin tethering caused by shortening of skin-anchoring ligaments (**Fig. 12**).[131–133] DC is estimated to affect approximately 20% of diabetic patients; the prevalence increases with age.[121] Among patients with DC, 13% to 39% have diabetes.[134,135] The pathogenesis of diabetic DC is poorly understood, and DC seems to be independent of glycemic control.[132,136–138]

Digital sclerosis

The finding of LJM in conjunction with thick, waxy, dorsal hand skin is called digital sclerosis. Rosenbloom and Frias[139] described these findings (plus short stature) in association with insulin-dependent diabetes in 1974. A series of investigations that followed led to naming this constellation of findings Rosenbloom syndrome. Much of the literature since that time separates LJM and thick dorsal hand skin as distinct conditions, because they often do not present simultaneously.

Thick Skin

Three distinct forms of thick skin have been identified in diabetes: (1) thick waxy skin of the dorsal hand, (2) scleredema diabeticorum, and (3) subclinical, generalized, thicker-than-average skin. The first 2 have been described earlier. The third type of thick skin of diabetes is believed to be benign and is common. It is asymptomatic and usually goes unnoticed, but is apparent on ultrasonographic measurement of skin

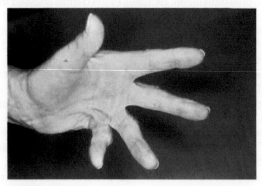

Fig. 12. Dupuytren contracture.

thickness.[140] The thickened skin may occur anywhere on the body, but the skin of the hands and feet are most commonly affected. It is unclear whether the 3 forms of thick skin share a common pathogenesis.

SELECTED CUTANEOUS DISORDERS ASSOCIATED WITH DIABETES
Psoriasis

Psoriasis is a relatively common chronic inflammatory skin disease with systemic manifestations. The worldwide prevalence of psoriasis is estimated to be 1% to 3%.[141] Inflammatory pathways and genetic susceptibility seem to be at the core of the pathologic mechanism. Many risk factors have been associated with psoriasis, including smoking, hypertension, obesity, and insulin resistance.[142] The condition is more frequent and severe in obese patients.[143]

Patients with psoriasis are believed to have a 1.5 times increased risk of developing diabetes compared with the general population, and patients with severe psoriasis may have twice the risk.[144] When adjusted for covariates, Li and colleagues[145] found psoriasis to be associated with an increased risk of type 2 diabetes among patients with psoriasis less than 60 years old.

Psoriasis and type 2 diabetes are independently known to be mediated by many major risk factors in common, such as high body mass index and smoking. Past epidemiologic studies and basic science research provide evidence of some possible links between psoriasis and type 2 diabetes: common immune-mediated inflammatory processes (specifically involving inflammatory cytokines such as interleukin [IL]-6 and TNF), an involvement of leptin and adiponectin, and environmental factors such as smoking.[145,146] The human major histocompatibility (MHC) genomic region at chromosomal position 6p21 has been associated with both psoriasis and diabetes (among 100+ other diseases).[147] Whether this contributes to the pathogenesis of diabetes and/or psoriasis is unclear.

Vitiligo

Vitiligo is an acquired, chronic, depigmenting disorder of the skin characterized by well-demarcated, achromic macules of selectively destroyed melanocytes. The exact cause of vitiligo is still debated, but either a loss of cutaneous melanocytes or a loss of melanocyte function is believed to occur, and this likely involves cell-mediated autoimmunity.[148,149] An estimated 0.1%–2.0% of people worldwide are affected with vitiligo. Dawber[150] observed that patients with type 1 diabetes were significantly more likely to have vitiligo compared with those with type 2 diabetes (3.6% vs 0.4%) and compared with the general population.[151]

CUTANEOUS INFECTIONS

Skin infections are common in those with diabetes mellitus, especially type 2 diabetes. The impaired microcirculation, sensory and autonomic neuropathy, acid-base imbalances, and impaired immune response of diabetes mellitus and its complications predispose diabetic patients to bacterial and fungal infections of the skin that may run an unusually prolonged or recurrent course. Many studies have shown the incidence of cutaneous infections is higher in people with diabetes than in the general population, and that the incidence of infection correlates with mean blood glucose levels.[4,81,152,153] Skin infections may even be the presenting feature of diabetes. The best preventive measure for all skin infections in diabetes is optimal glycemic control beginning as early as possible.

Bacterial

Staphylococcal and β-hemolytic streptococcal infections
The most common bacterial infections in diabetic patients are staphylococcal and β-hemolytic streptococcal infections, causing impetigo, erysipelas, folliculitis, carbuncles, furuncles, styes, and ecthyma.[153] Bacterial infections of the diabetic skin can progress to gangrene and even necrotizing fasciitis, a life-threatening dermatologic emergency. Depending on the severity of the infection, oral or intravenous antibiotics and diabetic control are standards of care. Tissue debridement and aggressive wound care may be required in severe cases.

Corynebacterium minutissimum
Erythrasma is a chronic superficial infection of *Corynebacterium minutissimum* and has an increased prevalence among diabetic patients, especially among obese diabetics. *C minutissimum* occurs as normal skin flora in the general population. It is believed that the increased susceptibility of diabetic patients to *C minutissimum* infection is caused by the ability of these bacteria to ferment glucose. Erythrasma presents as well-demarcated brown to red patches with fine scale, typically distributed over the inner thighs, scrotum, crural area, and fourth web space of the toes. It tends to be asymptomatic but may be pruritic. Under a Wood lamp (UV-A light), erythrasma shows a coral-red fluorescence due to the production of porphyrin by *C minutissimum*. This finding effectively distinguishes erythrasma from *Staphylococcus* intertrigo infection, which often appears identical under room light. Bacterial culture of erythrasma is known to be difficult and is not necessary for diagnosis.

Pseudomonas aeruginosa
Pseudomonas infections of the toe web spaces and colonization of the toenails are more common in diabetes than among the general population. Green discoloration may be visible under the toenail and green fluorescence can be observed under a Wood lamp. Topical antibiotics, or oral ciprofloxacin for more advanced cases, are standard therapy for these superficial infections.

Malignant otitis externa caused by *Pseudomonas aeruginosa* is a rare life-threatening skin infection of the external auditory canal that occurs most frequently in elderly patients with diabetes and is associated with high morbidity and mortality. The infection initially develops as a cellulitis that can progress to chondritis, osteomyelitis, and cerebritis.[4,154] Urgent diagnosis and treatment are essential. Antipseudomonal antibiotic therapy and necrotic tissue debridement should be initiated promptly.[154]

Fungal

Candidiasis (Moniliasis)
Recurrent candidal infections are frequently the presenting manifestation of diabetes. Patients with diabetes are believed to be particularly susceptible to *Candida* because increased glucose concentrations permit the organism to thrive. Candidal infections are often seen in the setting of diabetes include angular stomatitis (classically in young diabetic patients), paronychia of the nailfold, erosio interdigitale blastomycetica (infection of the web space between the third and fourth fingers), thrush, and intertrigo of the skinfolds. Common female-specific candidal skin infections include pruritus vulvae (often accompanying vulvovaginitis) and inframammary infection. Although much less common than female-specific infections, the male-specific infections, balanitis, balanoposthitis, and phimosis, may be an early sign of diabetes in men.[4] The pathogens most frequently implicated include *Candida albicans* and *Candida parapsilosis*.

Candidal infections should be managed with glycemic control and topical antifungals (such as nystatin, clotrimazole, and econazole) or oral fluconazole for more severe or refractory cases.

Dermatophytosis

The dermatophytes are a group of 3 genera of fungi (*Trichophyton*, *Microsporum*, and *Epidermophyton*) that cause hair, skin, and nail infections. Dermatophyte infections of the skin are most frequently caused by *Trichophyton rubrum*. Tinea pedis (dermatophytosis of the foot) is the most prevalent of these infections among both diabetic patients and the general population. Although studies show an increased prevalence of candidal infections among patients with diabetes, the data on dermatophytosis in diabetes is less clear.[155] Obesity poses an additional risk factor for dermatophyte infection of the skin, particularly of the skin folds.[94] Treatment depends on location and severity, and includes topical and systemic antifungals. Treatment of superimposed bacterial infections may be required as well.

Onychomycosis

Onychomycosis, or fungal infection of the nail, is common in diabetes, most often caused by *Candida* or *Trichophyton*. Signs of onychomychosis include yellow discoloration, subungual hyperkeratosis, distal onycholysis, and nail dystrophy (**Fig. 13**). Among 550 diabetic patients, Gupta and colleagues[152] found evidence of fungal infection in 26% versus 6.8% of nondiabetic controls. Onychomycosis has been reported in 50% of patients with type 2 diabetes.[156] The risk of onychomycosis increases with age and with male sex.[152] Nail infections are especially dangerous because they can provide a portal of entry for secondary bacterial infection at the most distal parts of the body, which are exceedingly susceptible to poor wound healing in individuals with diabetes. Patients should be educated about the importance of proper foot and nail care for prevention.

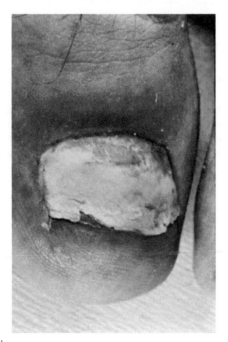

Fig. 13. Onychomycosis.

Mucormycosis

Mucormycosis is a rare life-threatening opportunistic fungal infection that occurs with increased frequency among diabetic patients. The infection is usually caused by *Rhizopus* species, or less often *Mucor* species of Zygomycetes. Typical presenting symptoms include facial or ocular pain and nasal congestion, sometimes with malaise and/or fever. Uncontrolled diabetes, especially with diabetic ketoacidosis, greatly increases the risk of mucormycosis.[157,158] It is believed that the combination of increased availability of glucose, decreased serum pH, and increased expression of host receptors that mediate epithelial cell invasion by *Rhizopus*, enables *Rhizopus* spp. to thrive.[158] Cutaneous mucormycosis begins as a cellulitis that progresses to necrosis. It occurs by introduction of the fungi through abraded skin. The infection causes tissue necrosis, infarction, and thrombosis as hyphae invade blood vessels, and is inevitably fatal without intervention.[157]

Blastomycosis

Blastomycosis, caused by *Blastomyces dermatitidis*, is another noncontagious opportunistic fungal infection that disproportionately affects patients with diabetes. It is endemic to the midwest United States and northwestern Ontario. Lung and skin involvement are most common. Infection usually occurs by inhalation of spores or, less often, by skin contact with spores. Initial symptoms include dry cough, fever, fatigue, and general malaise. Cutaneous presentations of blastomycosis vary, but small crusted pustules that rupture and ulcerate or form nonhealing abscesses are typical. Diagnosis can be achieved through identification of the organism by direct microscopy, culture, histopathology, or serologic tests. Without treatment, blastomycosis eventually causes death. Oral itraconazole or ketoconazole and intravenous amphotericin B are first-line therapies depending on severity.

Increased suspicion for the rare but urgent and life-threatening cutaneous infections of diabetes (mucormycosis, necrotizing fasciitis, and malignant otitis externa) is essential.

CUTANEOUS REACTIONS TO DIABETIC TREATMENT
Insulin

The advent of recombinant insulin preparations has largely done away with once common insulin allergies.[10] Insulin allergy is now seen in less than 1% of patients injecting insulin. Delayed hypersensitivity reactions have been the most common type of allergic reaction, but immediate-local, generalized, and biphasic reactions have also occurred. Treatment options for insulin allergies include antihistamines, the addition of steroid to insulin, desensitization therapy, rotating the injection site, or discontinuation of therapy. Anaphylaxis is extremely rare in insulin allergy.

Lipoatrophy, lipohypertrophy, or a combination of both may occur at the site of insulin injection. The exact cause of lipoatrophy is unknown, but lipohypertrophy may be caused by the lipogenic action of insulin and is best prevented by rotation of injection site.

Oral Hypoglycemic Agents

It is estimated that 1% to 5% of patients treated with a first-generation sulfonylurea, such as chlorpropamide or tolbutamide, experience a cutaneous reaction (most often a maculopapular eruption) within the first 2 months of therapy. Discontinuation usually leads to prompt resolution of the rash. Chlorpropamide causes an alcohol flush reaction, characterized by generalized warmth, erythema, headache, and tachycardia, in 10% to 30% of patients beginning about 15 minutes after consumption of alcohol and lasting for an hour. Susceptibility to this reaction may be inherited autosomal dominantly.[10]

The most common cutaneous reactions to second-generation sulfonylureas, such as glipizide (Glucotrol) and glimepiride (Amaryl), include photosensitivity, urticaria, and pruritus. Metformin (Glucophage) has been reported to cause a psoriasiform drug eruption, erythema multiforme, and leukocytoclastic vasculitis.

SUMMARY

The wide range of dermatologic conditions related to impaired glucose metabolism is important across multiple medical specialties to identify undiagnosed diabetes as early as possible and to better manage patients with known disease. Despite numerous investigations, the exact causes of many cutaneous complications of diabetes remain elusive, due in part to inherent challenges of research in diabetes, a heterogeneous group of conditions affecting patients of widely ranging demographics and often with multiple comorbidities. Much of the data has come from outdated studies and small case series. There have also been off-cited figures pertaining to diabetic skin manifestations for which no primary source seems to exist.

Better understanding of the underlying disease mechanisms, perhaps through advanced biochemical analyses and large-scale studies, could enable more tailored therapies leading to improved treatment outcomes in diabetes. Continued efforts to educate patients and encourage healthy lifestyles are of foremost importance in halting the epidemic of diabetes mellitus and its complications.

REFERENCES

1. Centers for Disease Control and Prevention. In: US Department of Health and Human Services, editor. National diabetes fact sheet: national estimates and general information on diabetes and prediabetes in the United States. Atlanta (GA): Centers for Disease Control and Prevention; 2011.
2. Boyle JP, Thompson TJ, Gregg EW, et al. Projection of the year 2050 burden of diabetes in the US adult population: dynamic modeling of incidence, mortality, and prediabetes prevalence. Popul Health Metr 2010;8:29.
3. Danaei G, Finucane MM, Lu Y, et al, Global Burden of Metabolic Risk Factors of Chronic Diseases Collaborating, Group. National, regional, and global trends in fasting plasma glucose and diabetes prevalence since 1980: systematic analysis of health examination surveys and epidemiological studies with 370 country-years and 2.7 million participants. Lancet 2011;378:31–40.
4. Perez MI, Kohn SR. Cutaneous manifestations of diabetes mellitus. J Am Acad Dermatol 1994;30:519–31 [quiz: 532–4].
5. Shahzad M, Al Robaee A, Al Shobaili HA, et al. Skin manifestations in diabetic patients attending a diabetic clinic in the Qassim region, Saudi Arabia. Med Princ Pract 2011;20:137–41.
6. Mahmood T, Bari A, Agha H. Cutaneous manifestations of diabetes mellitus. Journal of Pakistan Association of Dermatologists 2005;15:227–32.
7. Boyd AS. Tretinoin treatment of necrobiosis lipoidica diabeticorum. Diabetes Care 1999;22:1753–4.
8. Petzelbauer P, Wolff K, Tappeiner G. Necrobiosis lipoidica: treatment with systemic corticosteroids. Br J Dermatol 1992;126:542–5.
9. Shall L, Millard L, Stevens A, et al. Necrobiosis lipoidica: 'the footprint not the footstep'. Br J Dermatol 1990;123:47.

10. Ferringer T, Miller F 3rd. Cutaneous manifestations of diabetes mellitus. Dermatol Clin 2002;20:483–92.

11. Muller SA, Winkelmann RK. Necrobiosis lipoidica diabeticorum. A clinical and pathological investigation of 171 cases. Arch Dermatol 1966;93:272–81.

12. O'Toole EA, Kennedy U, Nolan JJ, et al. Necrobiosis lipoidica: only a minority of patients have diabetes mellitus. Br J Dermatol 1999;140:283–6.

13. Boulton AJ, Cutfield RG, Abouganem D, et al. Necrobiosis lipoidica diabeticorum: a clinicopathologic study. J Am Acad Dermatol 1988;18:530–7.

14. Erfurt-Berge C, Seitz AT, Rehse C, et al. Update on clinical and laboratory features in necrobiosis lipoidica: a retrospective multicentre study of 52 patients. Eur J Dermatol 2012;22:770–5.

15. Suarez-Amor O, Perez-Bustillo A, Ruiz-Gonzalez I, et al. Necrobiosis lipoidica therapy with biologicals: an ulcerated case responding to etanercept and a review of the literature. Dermatology 2010;221:117–21.

16. Sibbald RG, Landolt SJ, Toth D. Skin and diabetes. Endocrinol Metab Clin North Am 1996;25:463–72.

17. Souza AD, El-Azhary RA, Gibson LE. Does pancreas transplant in diabetic patients affect the evolution of necrobiosis lipoidica? Int J Dermatol 2009;48:964–70.

18. Ngo B, Wigington G, Hayes K, et al. Skin blood flow in necrobiosis lipoidica diabeticorum. Int J Dermatol 2008;47:354–8.

19. Cohen O, Yaniv R, Karasik A, et al. Necrobiosis lipoidica and diabetic control revisited. Med Hypotheses 1996;46:348–50.

20. Basaria S, Braga-Basaria M. Necrobiosis lipoidica diabeticorum: response to pentoxiphylline. J Endocrinol Invest 2003;26:1037–40.

21. Rogers C. Necrobiosis lipoidica diabeticorum. Dermatol Nurs 2005;17:301, 307.

22. Kolde G, Muche JM, Schulze P, et al. Infliximab: a promising new treatment option for ulcerated necrobiosis lipoidica. Dermatology 2003;206:180–1.

23. Jelinek T, Nothdurft HD, Rieder N, et al. Cutaneous myiasis: review of 13 cases in travelers returning from tropical countries. Int J Dermatol 1995;34:624–6.

24. Binamer Y, Sowerby L, El-Helou T. Treatment of ulcerative necrobiosis lipoidica with topical calcineurin inhibitor: case report and literature review. J Cutan Med Surg 2012;16:458–61.

25. Buggiani G, Tsampau D, Krysenka A, et al. Fractional CO_2 laser: a novel therapeutic device for refractory necrobiosis lipoidica. Dermatol Ther 2012;25:612–4.

26. Kosaka S, Kawana S. Case of necrobiosis lipoidica diabeticorum successfully treated by photodynamic therapy. J Dermatol 2012;39:497–9.

27. Zeichner JA, Stern DW, Lebwohl M. Treatment of necrobiosis lipoidica with the tumor necrosis factor antagonist etanercept. J Am Acad Dermatol 2006;54:S120–1.

28. Stanway A, Rademaker M, Newman P. Healing of severe ulcerative necrobiosis lipoidica with cyclosporin. Australas J Dermatol 2004;45:119–22.

29. Handfield-Jones S, Jones S, Peachey R. High dose nicotinamide in the treatment of necrobiosis lipoidica. Br J Dermatol 1988;118:693–6.

30. Fjellner B. Treatment of diabetic nebrobiosis with aspirin and dipyridamole [letter to editor]. N Engl J Med 1978;299.

31. Unge G, Tornling G. Treatment of diabetic nebrobiosis with dipyridamole [letter to editor]. N Engl J Med 1978;299.

32. Evans AV, Atherton DJ. Recalcitrant ulcers in necrobiosis lipoidica diabeticorum healed by topical granulocyte-macrophage colony-stimulating factor. Br J Dermatol 2002;147:1023–5.

33. Barde C, Laffitte E, Campanelli A, et al. Intralesional infliximab in noninfectious cutaneous granulomas: three cases of necrobiosis lipoidica. Dermatology 2011; 222:212–6.
34. Hu SW, Bevona C, Winterfield L, et al. Treatment of refractory ulcerative necrobiosis lipoidica diabeticorum with infliximab: report of a case. Arch Dermatol 2009;145:437–9.
35. Schofield C, Sladden MJ. Ulcerative necrobiosis lipoidica responsive to colchicine. Australas J Dermatol 2012;53:e54–7.
36. Dabski K, Winkelmann RK. Generalized granuloma annulare: clinical and laboratory findings in 100 patients. J Am Acad Dermatol 1989;20:39–47.
37. Haim S, Friedman-Birnbaum R, Haim N, et al. Carbohydrate tolerance in patients with granuloma annulare. Study of fifty-two cases. Br J Dermatol 1973;88:447–51.
38. Andersen BL, Verdich J. Granuloma annulare and diabetes mellitus. Clin Exp Dermatol 1979;4:31–7.
39. Huntley AC. The cutaneous manifestations of diabetes mellitus. J Am Acad Dermatol 1982;7:427–55.
40. Levy L, Zeichner JA. Dermatologic manifestation of diabetes. J Diabetes 2012; 4:68–76.
41. Muhlbauer JE. Granuloma annulare. J Am Acad Dermatol 1980;3:217–30.
42. Jabbour SA. Cutaneous manifestations of endocrine disorders: a guide for dermatologists. Am J Clin Dermatol 2003;4:315–31.
43. Dabski K, Winkelmann RK. Generalized granuloma annulare: histopathology and immunopathology. Systematic review of 100 cases and comparison with localized granuloma annulare. J Am Acad Dermatol 1989;20:28–39.
44. Spicuzza L, Salafia S, Capizzi A, et al. Granuloma annulare as first clinical manifestation of diabetes mellitus in children: a case report. Diabetes Res Clin Pract 2012;95:e55–7.
45. Smith MD, Downie JB, DiCostanzo D. Granuloma annulare. Int J Dermatol 1997; 36:326–33.
46. Ahmed I, Goldstein B. Diabetes mellitus. Clin Dermatol 2006;24:237–46.
47. Setterfield J, Huilgol SC, Black MM. Generalised granuloma annulare successfully treated with PUVA. Clin Exp Dermatol 1999;24:458–60.
48. Toonstra J. Bullosis diabeticorum. Report of a case with a review of the literature. J Am Acad Dermatol 1985;13:799–805.
49. Allen GE, Hadden DR. Bullous lesions of the skin in diabetes (bullosis diabeticorum). Br J Dermatol 1970;82:216–20.
50. Larsen K, Jensen T, Karlsmark T, et al. Incidence of bullosis diabeticorum–a controversial cause of chronic foot ulceration. Int Wound J 2008;5:591–6.
51. Anand KP, Kashyap AS. Bullosis diabeticorum. Postgrad Med J 2004;80:354.
52. Lopez PR, Leicht S, Sigmon JR, et al. Bullosis diabeticorum associated with a prediabetic state. South Med J 2009;102:643–4.
53. Lipsky BA, Baker PD, Ahroni JH. Diabetic bullae: 12 cases of a purportedly rare cutaneous disorder. Int J Dermatol 2000;39:196–200.
54. Bernstein JE, Levine LE, Medenica MM, et al. Reduced threshold to suction-induced blister formation in insulin-dependent diabetics. J Am Acad Dermatol 1983;8:790–1.
55. Basarab T, Munn SE, McGrath J, et al. Bullosis diabeticorum. A case report and literature review. Clin Exp Dermatol 1995;20:218–20.
56. Cole GW, Headley J, Skowsky R. Scleredema diabeticorum: a common and distinct cutaneous manifestation of diabetes mellitus. Diabetes Care 1983;6: 189–92.

57. Martin C, Requena L, Manrique K, et al. Scleredema diabeticorum in a patient with type 2 diabetes mellitus. Case Rep Endocrinol 2011;2011:560273.
58. Brik R, Berant M, Vardi P. The scleroderma-like syndrome of insulin-dependent diabetes mellitus. Diabetes Metab Rev 1991;7:120–8.
59. Wilson BE, Newmark JJ. Severe scleredema diabeticorum and insulin resistance. J Am Board Fam Pract 1995;8:55–7.
60. Sattar MA, Diab S, Sugathan TN, et al. Scleroedema diabeticorum: a minor but often unrecognized complication of diabetes mellitus. Diabet Med 1988;5:465–8.
61. Hanna W, Friesen D, Bombardier C, et al. Pathologic features of diabetic thick skin. J Am Acad Dermatol 1987;16:546–53.
62. Seyger MM, van den Hoogen FH, de Mare S, et al. A patient with a severe scleroedema diabeticorum, partially responding to low-dose methotrexate. Dermatology 1999;198:177–9.
63. Ikeda Y, Suehiro T, Abe T, et al. Severe diabetic scleredema with extension to the extremities and effective treatment using prostaglandin E1. Intern Med 1998;37: 861–4.
64. Lee FY, Chiu HY, Chiu HC. Treatment of acquired reactive perforating collagenosis with allopurinol incidentally improves scleredema diabeticorum. J Am Acad Dermatol 2011;65:e115–7.
65. Abraham C, Rozmus CL. Is acanthosis nigricans a reliable indicator for risk of type 2 diabetes in obese children and adolescents? A systematic review. J Sch Nurs 2012;28:195–205.
66. Torley D, Bellus GA, Munro CS. Genes, growth factors and acanthosis nigricans. Br J Dermatol 2002;147:1096–101.
67. Matsuoka LY, Wortsman J, Goldman J. Acanthosis nigricans. Clin Dermatol 1993;11:21–5.
68. Hud JA Jr, Cohen JB, Wagner JM, et al. Prevalence and significance of acanthosis nigricans in an adult obese population. Arch Dermatol 1992;128:941–4.
69. Matsuoka LY, Wortsman J, Gavin JR, et al. Spectrum of endocrine abnormalities associated with acanthosis nigricans. Am J Med 1987;83:719–25.
70. Buzasi K, Sapi Z, Jermendy G. Acanthosis nigricans as a local cutaneous side effect of repeated human insulin injections. Diabetes Res Clin Pract 2011;94: e34–6.
71. Hermanns-Le T, Scheen A, Pierard GE. Acanthosis nigricans associated with insulin resistance: pathophysiology and management. Am J Clin Dermatol 2004;5: 199–203.
72. Katz RA. Treatment of acanthosis nigricans with oral isotretinoin. Arch Dermatol 1980;116:110–1.
73. Kuroki R, Sadamoto Y, Imamura M, et al. Acanthosis nigricans with severe obesity, insulin resistance and hypothyroidism: improvement by diet control. Dermatology 1999;198:164–6.
74. Fleischmajer R, Faludi G, Krol S. Scleredema and diabetes mellitus. Arch Dermatol 1970;101:21–6.
75. Shemer A, Bergman R, Linn S, et al. Diabetic dermopathy and internal complications in diabetes mellitus. Int J Dermatol 1998;37:113–5.
76. Dicken CH, Carrington SG, Winkelmann RK. Generalized granuloma annulare. Arch Dermatol 1969;99:556–63.
77. Melin H. An atrophic circumscribed skin lesion in the lower extremities of diabetics. Acta Med Scand 1964;176(Suppl 423):1–75.
78. Danowski TS, Sabeh G, Sarver ME, et al. Shin spots and diabetes mellitus. Am J Med Sci 1966;251:570–5.

79. Abdollahi A, Daneshpazhooh M, Amirchaghmaghi E, et al. Dermopathy and reti-nopathy in diabetes: is there an association? Dermatology 2007;214:133–6.
80. Morgan AJ, Schwartz RA. Diabetic dermopathy: a subtle sign with grave impli-cations. J Am Acad Dermatol 2008;58:447–51.
81. Yosipovitch G, Hodak E, Vardi P, et al. The prevalence of cutaneous manifesta-tions in IDDM patients and their association with diabetes risk factors and micro-vascular complications. Diabetes Care 1998;21:506–9.
82. Murphy R. The "spotted leg" syndrome. Am J Med Sci 1965;14:10–4.
83. Karpouzis A, Giatromanolaki A, Sivridis E, et al. Acquired reactive perforating collagenosis: current status. J Dermatol 2010;37:585–92.
84. Lynde CB, Pratt MD. Clinical Images: acquired perforating dermatosis: associ-ation with diabetes and renal failure. CMAJ 2009;181:615.
85. Rapini R. Perforating Diseases. In: Bolognia J, Jorizzo J, Rapini R, editors. Dermatology. 3rd edition. London: Mosby Elsevier; 2012. p. 1492–502.
86. Saray Y, Seckin D, Bilezikci B. Acquired perforating dermatosis: clinicopatho-logical features in twenty-two cases. J Eur Acad Dermatol Venereol 2006;20: 679–88.
87. Kawakami T, Saito R. Acquired reactive perforating collagenosis associated with diabetes mellitus: eight cases that meet Faver's criteria. Br J Dermatol 1999;140: 521–4.
88. Maurice PD, Neild GH. Acquired perforating dermatosis and diabetic nephrop-athy–a case report and review of the literature. Clin Exp Dermatol 1997;22: 291–4.
89. Farrell AM. Acquired perforating dermatosis in renal and diabotic patients. Lan-cet 1997;349:895–6.
90. Parker F. Xanthomas and hyperlipidemias. J Am Acad Dermatol 1985;13:1–30.
91. Kala J, Mostow EN. Images in clinical medicine. Eruptive xanthoma. N Engl J Med 2012;366:835.
92. Feingold KR, Elias PM. Endocrine-skin interactions. Cutaneous manifestations of pituitary disease, thyroid disease, calcium disorders, and diabetes. J Am Acad Dermatol 1987;17:921–40.
93. Wani AM, Hussain WM, Fatani MI, et al. Eruptive xanthomas with Koebner phe-nomenon, type 1 diabetes mellitus, hypertriglyceridaemia and hypertension in a 41-year-old man. BMJ Case Rep 2009;2009. http://dx.doi.org/10.1136/bcr.05. 2009.1871.
94. Garcia Hidalgo L. Dermatological complications of obesity. Am J Clin Dermatol 2002;3:497–506.
95. Demir S, Demir Y. Acrochordon and impaired carbohydrate metabolism. Acta Diabetol 2002;39:57–9.
96. Crook MA. Skin tags and the atherogenic lipid profile. J Clin Pathol 2000;53: 873–4.
97. Kahana M, Grossman E, Feinstein A, et al. Skin tags: a cutaneous marker for diabetes mellitus. Acta Derm Venereol 1987;67:175–7.
98. Chobanian SJ, Van Ness MM, Winters C Jr, et al. Skin tags as a marker for adenomatous polyps of the colon. Ann Intern Med 1985;103:892–3.
99. Dianzani C, Calvieri S, Pierangeli A, et al. The detection of human papillomavirus DNA in skin tags. Br J Dermatol 1998;138:649–51.
100. Rasi A, Soltani-Arabshahi R, Shahbazi N. Skin tag as a cutaneous marker for impaired carbohydrate metabolism: a case-control study. Int J Dermatol 2007; 46:1155–9.
101. Scheinfeld NS. Obesity and dermatology. Clin Dermatol 2004;22:303–9.

102. Hoerer E, Dreyfuss F, Herzberg M. Carotenemic, skin colour and diabetes mellitus. Acta Diabetol Lat 1975;12:202–7.
103. Neilly JB, Martin A, Simpson N, et al. Pruritus in diabetes mellitus: investigation of prevalence and correlation with diabetes control. Diabetes Care 1986;9: 273–5.
104. Namazi MR, Jorizzo JL, Fallahzadeh MK. Rubeosis faciei diabeticorum: a common, but often unnoticed, clinical manifestation of diabetes mellitus. ScientificWorldJournal 2010;10:70–1.
105. Pavlovic MD, Milenkovic T, Dinic M, et al. The prevalence of cutaneous manifestations in young patients with type 1 diabetes. Diabetes Care 2007;30:1964–7.
106. Gitelson S, Wertheimer-Kaplinski N. Color of the face in diabetes mellitus; observations on a group of patients in Jerusalem. Diabetes 1965;14:201–8.
107. Serrao R, Zirwas M, English JC. Palmar erythema. Am J Clin Dermatol 2007;8: 347–56.
108. Bravermen I. Skin signs of systemic disease. 3rd edition. Philadelphia: WB Saunders; 1998.
109. Ahmed K, Muhammad Z, Qayum I. Prevalence of cutaneous manifestations of diabetes mellitus. J Ayub Med Coll Abbottabad 2009;21:76–9.
110. Ngo BT, Hayes KD, DiMiao DJ, et al. Manifestations of cutaneous diabetic microangiopathy. Am J Clin Dermatol 2005;6:225–37.
111. Landau J, Davis E. The small blood-vessels of the conjunctiva and nailbed in diabetes mellitus. Lancet 1960;2:731–4.
112. Lithner F. Purpura, pigmentation and yellow nails of the lower extremities in diabetics. Acta Med Scand 1976;199:203–8.
113. Ratnam KV, Su WP, Peters MS. Purpura simplex (inflammatory purpura without vasculitis): a clinicopathologic study of 174 cases. J Am Acad Dermatol 1991; 25:642–7.
114. Rosenbloom AL. Limited joint mobility in childhood diabetes: discovery, description, and decline. J Clin Endocrinol Metab 2013;98:466–73.
115. Jelinek JE. Cutaneous manifestations of diabetes mellitus. J Am Acad Dermatol 1995;32:143–4.
116. Fitzgibbons PG, Weiss AP. Hand manifestations of diabetes mellitus. J Hand Surg Am 2008;33:771–5.
117. Fitzcharles MA, Duby S, Waddell RW, et al. Limitation of joint mobility (cheiroarthropathy) in adult noninsulin-dependent diabetic patients. Ann Rheum Dis 1984;43:251–4.
118. Otto-Buczkowska E, Jarosz-Chobot P. Limited joint mobility syndrome in patients with diabetes. Int J Clin Pract 2012;66:332–3.
119. Jennings AM, Milner PC, Ward JD. Hand abnormalities are associated with the complications of diabetes in type 2 diabetes. Diabet Med 1989;6:43–7.
120. Somai P, Vogelgesang S. Limited joint mobility in diabetes mellitus: the clinical implications. J Musculoskelet Med 2011;28:118–24.
121. Al-Matubsi HY, Hamdan F, Alhanbali OA, et al. Diabetic hand syndromes as a clinical and diagnostic tool for diabetes mellitus patients. Diabetes Res Clin Pract 2011;94:225–9.
122. Rosenbloom AL, Silverstein JH, Lezotte DC, et al. Limited joint mobility in childhood diabetes mellitus indicates increased risk for microvascular disease. N Engl J Med 1981;305:191–4.
123. Collier A, Matthews DM, Kellett HA, et al. Change in skin thickness associated with cheiroarthropathy in insulin dependent diabetes mellitus. Br Med J (Clin Res Ed) 1986;292:936.

124. Huntley AC. Finger pebbles: a common finding in diabetes mellitus. J Am Acad Dermatol 1986;14:612–7.
125. Cabo H, Woscoff A, Casas JG. Cutaneous manifestations of diabetes mellitus. J Am Acad Dermatol 1995;32:685.
126. Libecco JF, Brodell RT. Finger pebbles and diabetes: a case with broad involvement of the dorsal fingers and hands. Arch Dermatol 2001;137:510–1.
127. Schnider SL, Kohn RR. Effects of age and diabetes mellitus on the solubility and nonenzymatic glucosylation of human skin collagen. J Clin Invest 1981;67:1630–5.
128. Hamlin CR, Kohn RR, Luschin JH. Apparent accelerated aging of human collagen in diabetes mellitus. Diabetes 1975;24:902–4.
129. Seibold JR, Uitto J, Dorwart BB, et al. Collagen synthesis and collagenase activity in dermal fibroblasts from patients with diabetes and digital sclerosis. J Lab Clin Med 1985;105:664–7.
130. Lieberman LS, Rosenbloom AL, Riley WJ, et al. Reduced skin thickness with pump administration of insulin. N Engl J Med 1980;303:940–1.
131. Michou L, Lermusiaux JL, Teyssedou JP, et al. Genetics of Dupuytren's disease. Joint Bone Spine 2012;79:7–12.
132. Noble J, Heathcote JG, Cohen H. Diabetes mellitus in the aetiology of Dupuytren's disease. J Bone Joint Surg Br 1984;66:322–5.
133. Renard E, Jacques D, Chammas M, et al. Increased prevalence of soft tissue hand lesions in type 1 and type 2 diabetes mellitus: various entities and associated significance. Diabete Metab 1994;20:513–21.
134. Starkman HS, Gleason RE, Rand LI, et al. Limited joint mobility (LJM) of the hand in patients with diabetes mellitus: relation to chronic complications. Ann Rheum Dis 1986;45:130–5.
135. Lennox IA, Murali SR, Porter R. A study of the repeatability of the diagnosis of Dupuytren's contracture and its prevalence in the Grampian region. J Hand Surg Br 1993;18:258–61.
136. Arkkila PE, Kantola IM, Viikari JS. Dupuytren's disease: association with chronic diabetic complications. J Rheumatol 1997;24:153–9.
137. Arkkila PE, Kantola IM, Viikari JS, et al. Dupuytren's disease in type 1 diabetic patients: a five-year prospective study. Clin Exp Rheumatol 1996;14:59–65.
138. Sherry DD, Rothstein RR, Petty RE. Joint contractures preceding insulin-dependent diabetes mellitus. Arthritis Rheum 1982;25:1362–4.
139. Grgic A, Rosenbloom AL, Weber FT, et al. Joint contracture - Common manifestation of diabetes mellitus. J Pediatr 1976;88(4):584–8.
140. Huntley AC, Walter RM Jr. Quantitative determination of skin thickness in diabetes mellitus: relationship to disease parameters. J Med 1990;21:257–64.
141. Arunachalam M, Dragoni F, Colucci R, et al. Non-segmental vitiligo and psoriasis comorbidity - a case-control study in Italian patients. J Eur Acad Dermatol Venereol 2013. [Epub ahead of print].
142. Cohen JD, Bournerias I, Buffard V, et al. Psoriasis induced by tumor necrosis factor-alpha antagonist therapy: a case series. J Rheumatol 2007;34:380–5.
143. Farias MM, Achurra P, Boza C, et al. Psoriasis following bariatric surgery: clinical evolution and impact on quality of life on 10 patients. Obes Surg 2012;22:877–80.
144. Cheng J, Kuai D, Zhang L, et al. Psoriasis increased the risk of diabetes: a meta-analysis. Arch Dermatol Res 2012;304:119–25.
145. Li W, Han J, Hu FB, et al. Psoriasis and risk of type 2 diabetes among women and men in the United States: a population-based cohort study. J Invest Dermatol 2012;132:291–8.

146. Takahashi N, Takasu S. A close relationship between type 1 diabetes and vitamin A-deficiency and matrix metalloproteinase and hyaluronidase activities in skin tissues. Exp Dermatol 2011;20:899–904.

147. Shiina T, Inoko H, Kulski JK. An update of the HLA genomic region, locus information and disease associations: 2004. Tissue Antigens 2004;64:631–49.

148. Richetta A, D'Epiro S, Salvi M, et al. Serum levels of functional T-regs in vitiligo: our experience and mini-review of the literature. Eur J Dermatol 2013;23(2): 154–9.

149. Forschner T, Buchholtz S, Stockfleth E. Current state of vitiligo therapy–evidence-based analysis of the literature. J Dtsch Dermatol Ges 2007;5:467–75.

150. Dawber RP. Vitiligo in mature-onset diabetes mellitus. Br J Dermatol 1968;80: 275–8.

151. Gould IM, Gray RS, Urbaniak SJ, et al. Vitiligo in diabetes mellitus. Br J Dermatol 1985;113:153–5.

152. Gupta AK, Konnikov N, MacDonald P, et al. Prevalence and epidemiology of toenail onychomycosis in diabetic subjects: a multicentre survey. Br J Dermatol 1998;139:665–71.

153. Meurer M, Szeimies RM. Diabetes mellitus and skin diseases. Curr Probl Dermatol 1991;20:11–23.

154. Grandis R, Branstetter B, Yu V. The changing face of malignant (necrotising) external otitis: clinical, radiological, and anatomic correlations. Lancet Infect Dis 2004;4:34–9.

155. Lugo-Somolinos A, Sanchez JL. Prevalence of dermatophytosis in patients with diabetes. J Am Acad Dermatol 1992;26:408–10.

156. Gulcan A, Gulcan E, Oksuz S, et al. Prevalence of toenail onychomycosis in patients with type 2 diabetes mellitus and evaluation of risk factors. J Am Podiatr Med Assoc 2011;101:49–54.

157. Petrikkos G, Skiada A, Lortholary O, et al. Epidemiology and clinical manifestations of mucormycosis. Clin Infect Dis 2012;54(Suppl 1):S23–34.

158. Casqueiro J, Casqueiro J, Alves C. Infections in patients with diabetes mellitus: a review of pathogenesis. Indian J Endocrinol Metab 2012;16(Suppl 1):S27–36.

Diabetic Neuropathy

Aaron I. Vinik, MD, PhD*, Marie-Laure Nevoret, MD,
Carolina Casellini, MD, Henri Parson, PhD

KEYWORDS

- Diabetic nephropathy • Painful neuropathy • Diabetes mellitus • Pregabalin

KEY POINTS

- Diabetic neuropathy (DN) is the most common and troublesome complication of diabetes mellitus, leading to the greatest morbidity and mortality and resulting in a huge economic burden for diabetes care.
- Diabetic peripheral neuropathy has been recently defined as a symmetric, length-dependent sensorimotor polyneuropathy attributable to metabolic and microvascular alterations as a result of chronic hyperglycemia exposure (diabetes) and cardiovascular risk covariates.
- Both the clinical assessment and treatment options are multifactorial. Patients with DN should be screened for autonomic neuropathy, as there is a high degree of coexistence of the 2 complications.
- Two drugs have been approved for neuropathic pain in the United States, pregabalin and duloxetine, but neither of these has afforded complete relief, even when used in combination.

INTRODUCTION

Diabetic neuropathy (DN) is the most common and troublesome complication of diabetes mellitus (DM), leading to the greatest morbidity and mortality and resulting in a huge economic burden for diabetes care.[1,2] It is the most common form of neuropathy in the developed countries of the world, accounts for more hospitalizations than all the other diabetic complications combined, and is responsible for 50% to 75% of nontraumatic amputations.[2,3] DN is a set of clinical syndromes that affect distinct regions of the nervous system, singly or combined. It may be silent and go undetected while exercising its ravages; or it may present with clinical symptoms and signs that, although nonspecific and insidious with slow progression, also mimic those seen in many other diseases. DN is, therefore, diagnosed by exclusion. Unfortunately both endocrinologists and nonendocrinologists have not been trained to recognize the condition, and even when DN is symptomatic, less than one-third of physicians recognize the cause or discuss this with their patients.[4]

This article originally appeared in Endocrinology and Metabolism Clinics of North America, Volume 42, Issue 4, December 2013.
Internal Medicine, Strelitz Diabetes Center, Eastern Virginia Medical School, 855 West Brambleton Avenue, Norfolk, VA 23510, USA
* Corresponding author.
E-mail address: VinikAI@evms.edu

The true prevalence is not known, and reports vary from 10% to 90% in diabetic patients, depending on the criteria and methods used to define neuropathy.[2,3,5,6] Twenty-five percent of patients attending a diabetes clinic volunteered symptoms; 50% were found to have neuropathy after a simple clinical test such as the ankle jerk or vibration perception test; and almost 90% tested positive to sophisticated tests of autonomic function or peripheral sensation.[7] Neurologic complications occur equally in type 1 and type 2 DM and additionally in various forms of acquired diabetes.[6] The major morbidity associated with somatic neuropathy is foot ulceration, the precursor of gangrene and limb loss. Neuropathy increases the risk of amputation 1.7-fold, 12-fold if there is deformity (itself a consequence of neuropathy), and 36-fold if there is a history of previous ulceration.[8] Each year 96,000 amputations are performed on diabetic patients in the United States, yet up to 75% of them are preventable.[3] Globally there is an amputation every 30 seconds. DN also has a tremendous impact on patients' quality of life (QOL) predominantly by causing weakness, ataxia, and incoordination, predisposing to falls and fractures.[9] Once autonomic neuropathy sets in, life can become dismal and the mortality rate can approximate 25% to 50% within 5 to 10 years.[10,11]

SCOPE OF THE PROBLEM

Diabetic peripheral neuropathy (DPN) is a common late complication of diabetes. It results in a variety of syndromes for which there is no universally accepted classification. Such neuropathies are generally subdivided into focal/multifocal neuropathies, including diabetic amyotrophy, and symmetric polyneuropathies, including sensorimotor polyneuropathy (DSPN). The latter is the most common type, affecting about 30% of diabetic patients in hospital care and 25% of those in the community.[12,13] DPN has been recently defined as a symmetric, length-dependent sensorimotor polyneuropathy attributable to metabolic and microvascular alterations as a result of chronic hyperglycemia exposure (diabetes) and cardiovascular risk covariates.[14] Its onset is generally insidious, and without treatment the course is chronic and progressive. The loss of small-fiber–mediated sensation results in the loss of thermal and pain perception, whereas large-fiber impairment results in loss of touch and vibration perception. Sensory-fiber involvement may also result in "positive" symptoms, such as paresthesias and pain. Nonetheless, up to 50% of neuropathic patients can be asymptomatic. DPN can be associated with the involvement of the autonomic nervous system (ie, diabetic autonomic neuropathy that rarely causes severe symptoms),[15,16] but in its cardiovascular form is definitely associated with at least a 3-fold increased risk for mortality.[17–19] More recently, diabetic autonomic neuropathy or even autonomic imbalance between the sympathetic and the parasympathetic nervous systems has been implicated as a predictor of cardiovascular risk.[18,19]

EPIDEMIOLOGY OF NEUROPATHIC PAIN

Neuropathic pain is not uncommon, but may be correctable in some instances. Perhaps a little recognized fact is that mononeuritis and entrapments are 3 times as common as DPN, and fully one-third of the diabetic population has some form of entrapment[20] which, when recognized, is readily amenable to intervention.[21] Even more impressive is the mounting evidence that even with impaired glucose tolerance (IGT), patients may experience pain.[22–24] In the general population (region of Augsburg, Southern Germany), the prevalence of painful peripheral neuropathy was 13.3% in the diabetic subjects, 8.7% in those with IGT, 4.2% in those with impaired fasting glucose (IFG), and 1.2% in those with normal glucose tolerance (NGT).[25] Among survivors of myocardial infarction (MI) from the Augsburg MI Registry, the prevalence of neuro-pathic pain was 21% in the patients with diabetes, 14.8% in those with IGT, 5.7% in those with IFG, and 3.7% in those with NGT.[24] Thus, subjects with macrovascular disease appear to be prone to neuropathic pain. The most important risk factors of DSPN and neuropathic pain in these surveys were age, obesity, and low physical activity while the predominant comorbidity was peripheral arterial disease, highlighting the paramount role of cardiovascular risk factors and diseases in prevalent DSPN.

CLASSIFICATION OF DIABETIC NEUROPATHIES

Fig. 1 and **Table 1** describe the different forms of diabetic neuropathies. It is important to be aware that different forms of DN often coexist in the same patient (eg, distal pol-yneuropathy and carpal tunnel syndrome).

PATHOGENESIS OF DIABETIC NEUROPATHIES

Causative factors include persistent hyperglycemia, microvascular insufficiency, oxidative and nitrosative stress, defective neurotropism, and autoimmune-mediated nerve destruction. **Fig. 2** summarizes the current view of the pathogenesis of DN.[12] Detailed discussion of the different theories is beyond the scope of this article, and there are several excellent recent reviews. However, DN is a heterogeneous group of conditions with widely varying pathology, suggesting differences in pathogenic mech-anisms for the different clinical syndromes. Recognition of the clinical homolog of these pathologic processes is the first step in achieving the appropriate form of intervention.

CLINICAL PRESENTATION

The spectrum of clinical neuropathic syndromes described in patients with DM in-cludes dysfunction of almost every segment of the somatic peripheral and autonomic nervous system.[26] Each syndrome can be distinguished by its pathophysiologic, ther-apeutic, and prognostic features.

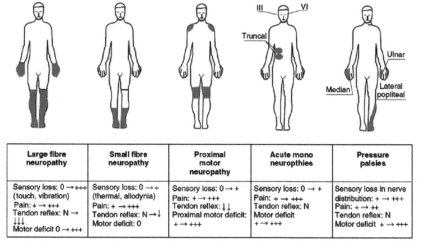

Large fibre neuropathy	Small fibre neuropathy	Proximal motor neuropathy	Acute mono neuropthies	Pressure palsies
Sensory loss: 0 →+++ (touch, vibration) Pain: + → +++ Tendon reflex: N → ↓↓↓ Motor deficit 0 → +++	Sensory loss: 0 →+ (thermal, allodynia) Pain: + → +++ Tendon reflex: N→↓ Motor deficit: 0	Sensory loss: 0 → + Pain: + → +++ Tendon reflex: ↓↓ Proximal motor deficit: + → +++	Sensory loss: 0 → + Pain: + → +++ Tendon reflex: N Motor deficit + → +++	Sensory loss in nerve distribution: + → +++ Pain: + → ++ Tendon reflex: N Motor deficit + → +++

Fig. 1. Clinical manifestations of small-fiber and large-fiber neuropathies. N, normal. (*From* Vinik AI, Mehrabyan A. Diabetic neuropathies. Med Clin N Am 2004;88:947–99; with permission.)

Table 1
Distinguishing characteristics of mononeuropathies, entrapment syndromes, and distal symmetric polyneuropathy

Feature	Mononeuropathy	Entrapment Syndrome	Neuropathy
Onset	Sudden	Gradual	Gradual
Pattern	Single nerve but may be multiple	Single nerve exposed to trauma	Distal symmetric poly neuropathy
Nerves involved	CN III, VI, VII, ulnar, median, peroneal	Median, ulnar, peroneal, medial, and lateral plantar	Mixed, motor, sensory, autonomic
Natural history	Resolves spontaneously	Progressive	Progressive
Distribution of sensory loss	Area supplied by the nerve	Area supplied beyond the site of entrapment	Distal and symmetric. "Glove and stocking" distribution

Abbreviation: CN, cranial nerves.

Focal and Multifocal Neuropathies

Focal neuropathies comprise focal-limb neuropathies and cranial neuropathies. Focal-limb neuropathies are usually due to entrapment, and mononeuropathies must be distinguished from these entrapment syndromes (see **Fig. 1**).[27,28] Mononeuropathies often occur in the older population; they have an acute onset, are associated with pain, and have a self-limiting course resolving in 6 to 8 weeks. Mononeuropathies

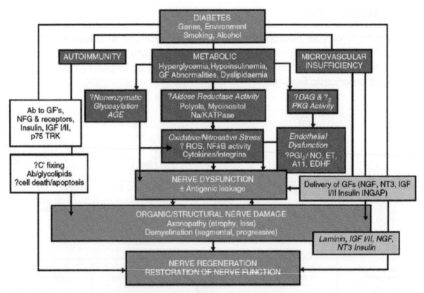

Fig. 2. Pathogenesis of diabetic neuropathies. Ab, antibody; AGE, advance glycation end products; ATPase, adenosine triphosphatase; C′, complement; DAG, diacylglycerol; EDHF, endothelium-derived hyperpolarizing factor; ET, endothelin; GF, growth factor; IGF, insulin-like growth factor; NFkB, nuclear factor κB; NGF, nerve growth factor; NO, nitric oxide; NT3, neurotropin 3; PGI₂, prostaglandin I₂; PKC, protein kinase C; ROS, reactive oxygen species; TRK, tyrosine kinase. (*From* Vinik A, Ullal J, Parson HK, et al. Diabetic neuropathies: clinical manifestations and current treatment options. Nat Clin Pract Endocrinol Metab 2006;2:269–81; with permission.)

can involve the median (5.8% of all diabetic neuropathies), ulnar (2.1%), radial (0.6%), and common peroneal nerves.[29] Cranial neuropathies in diabetic patients are extremely rare (0.05%) and occur in older individuals with a long duration of diabetes.[30] Entrapment syndromes start slowly, and will progress and persist without intervention. Carpal tunnel syndrome occurs 3 times as frequently in diabetics as in healthy populations,[31] and is found in up to one-third of patients with diabetes. Its increased prevalence in diabetes may be related to repeated undetected trauma, metabolic changes, and/or accumulation of fluid or edema within the confined space of the carpal tunnel.[28] The diagnosis is confirmed by electrophysiologic studies. Treatment consists of rest, aided by placement of a wrist splint in a neutral position to avoid repetitive trauma. Anti-inflammatory medications and steroid injections are sometimes useful. Surgery should be considered if weakness appears and medical treatment fails.[16,27]

Proximal Motor Neuropathy (Diabetic Amyotrophy) and Chronic Demyelinating Neuropathies

For many years proximal neuropathy has been considered a component of DN. Its pathogenesis was ill understood,[32] and its treatment was neglected with the anticipation that the patient would eventually recover, albeit over a period of some 1 to 2 years and after suffering considerable pain, weakness, and disability. The condition has several synonyms including diabetic amyotrophy and femoral neuropathy. It can be clinically identified based on the occurrence of these common features: (1) it primarily affects the elderly (50–60 years old) with type 2 DM; (2) onset can be gradual or abrupt; (3) it presents with severe pain in the thighs, hips, and buttocks, followed by significant weakness of the proximal muscles of the lower limbs with inability to rise from the sitting position (positive Gower maneuver); (4) it can start unilaterally and then spread bilaterally; (5) it often coexists with distal symmetric polyneuropathy; and (6) it is characterized by muscle fasciculation, either spontaneous or provoked by percussion. Pathogenesis is not yet clearly understood, although immune-mediated epineurial microvasculitis has been demonstrated in some cases. The condition is now recognized as being secondary to a variety of causes unrelated to diabetes, but which have a greater frequency in patients with diabetes than in the general population. It includes patients with chronic inflammatory demyelinating polyneuropathy (CIDP), monoclonal gammopathy, circulating GM1 antibodies, and inflammatory vasculitis.[30,31,33,34]

Treatment options include: intravenous immunoglobulin for CIDP,[35] plasma exchange for monoclonal gammopathy of unknown significance, steroids and azathioprine for vasculitis, and withdrawal of drugs or other agents that may have caused vasculitis. It is important to divide proximal syndromes into these 2 subcategories, because the CIDP variant responds dramatically to intervention,[36,37] whereas amyotrophy runs its own course over months to years. Until more evidence is available, they should be considered separate syndromes.

Diabetic Truncal Radiculoneuropathy

Diabetic truncal radiculoneuropathy affects middle-aged to elderly patients and has a predilection for males. Pain is the most important symptom, and occurs in a girdle-like distribution over the lower thoracic or abdominal wall. It can be unilaterally or bilaterally distributed. Motor weakness is rare. Resolution generally occurs within 4 to 6 months.

Rapidly Reversible Hyperglycemic Neuropathy

Reversible abnormalities of nerve function may occur in patients with recently diagnosed or poorly controlled diabetes. These disorders are unlikely to be caused by structural abnormalities, as recovery soon follows restoration of euglycemia. Rapidly reversible hyperglycemic neuropathy usually presents with distal sensory symptoms, and whether these abnormalities result in an increased risk of developing chronic neuropathies in the future remains unknown.[16,38]

Generalized Symmetric Polyneuropathy

Acute sensory neuropathy

Acute sensory (painful) neuropathy is considered by some investigators a distinctive variant of distal symmetric polyneuropathy. The syndrome is characterized by severe pain, cachexia, weight loss, depression, and, in males, erectile dysfunction. It occurs predominantly in male patients and may appear at any time in the course of both type 1 and type 2 DM. Conditions such as Fabry disease, amyloidosis, human immunodeficiency virus (HIV) infection, heavy-metal poisoning (such as arsenic), and excess alcohol consumption should be excluded.[39]

Acute sensory neuropathy is usually associated with poor glycemic control, but may also appear after sudden improvement of glycemia, and has been associated with the onset of insulin therapy, being termed insulin neuritis on occasions.[40] Although the pathologic basis has not been determined, one hypothesis suggests that changes in blood glucose flux produce alterations in epineurial blood flow, leading to ischemia. Other investigators relate this syndrome to diabetic lumbosacral radiculoplexus neuropathy (DLRPN) and propose an immune-mediated mechanism.[41]

The key in the management of this syndrome is achieving stability of blood glucose.[40] Most patients also require medication for neuropathic pain.[42] The natural history of this disease is resolution of symptoms within 1 year.[43]

Chronic Sensorimotor Neuropathy or Distal Symmetric Polyneuropathy

Clinical presentation and pain characteristics

DPN is probably the most common form of the diabetic neuropathies.[16,41] It is seen in both type 1 and type 2 DM with similar frequency, and may be already present at the time of diagnosis of type 2 DM.[44] A population survey reported that 30% of type 1 and 36% to 40% of type 2 diabetic patients experienced neuropathic symptoms.[45] Several studies have also suggested that IGT may lead to polyneuropathy, reporting rates of IGT in patients with chronic idiopathic polyneuropathies between 30% and 50%.[46–49] Studies using skin and nerve biopsies have shown progressive reduction in peripheral nerve fibers from the time of the diagnosis of diabetes or even in earlier prediabetic stages (IGT and metabolic syndrome).[50,51] Sensory symptoms are more prominent than motor symptoms and usually involve the lower limbs; these include pain, paresthesias, hyperesthesias, deep aching, burning, and sharp stabbing sensations similar to but less severe than those described in acute sensory neuropathy. In addition, patients may experience negative symptoms such as numbness in the feet and legs, leading in time to painless foot ulcers and subsequent amputations if the neuropathy is not promptly recognized and treated. Unsteadiness is also frequently seen, owing to abnormal proprioception and muscle sensory function.[52,53] Alternatively, some patients may be completely asymptomatic, and signs may be only discovered by a detailed neurologic examination.

On physical examination a symmetric stocking-like distribution of sensory abnormalities in both lower limbs is usually seen. In more severe cases the hands may be involved. All sensory modalities can be affected, particularly vibration, touch, and position perceptions (large $A\alpha/\beta$ fiber damage); and pain, with abnormal heat and cold temperature perception (small thinly myelinated $A\delta$ and unmyelinated C fiber damage) (Fig. 3). Deep tendon reflexes may be absent or reduced, especially in the lower

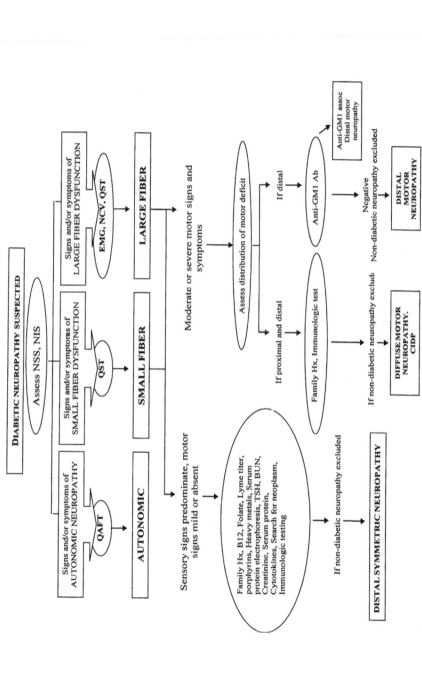

Fig. 3. Evaluation of the patient suspected of having DPN. A diagnostic algorithm for assessment of neurologic deficit and classification of neuropathic syndromes. B12, vitamin B$_{12}$; BUN, blood urea nitrogen; CIDP, chronic inflammatory demyelinating polyneuropathy; EMG, electromyogram; Hx, history; MGUS, monoclonal gammopathy of unknown significance; NCV, nerve conduction velocity studies; NIS, neurologic impairment score (sensory and motor evaluation); NSS, neurologic symptom score; QAFT, quantitative autonomic function tests; QST, quantitative sensory tests.

extremities. Mild muscle wasting may be seen, but severe weakness is rare and should raise the question of a possible nondiabetic origin of the neuropathy.[6,16,41] DPN is frequently accompanied by autonomic neuropathy (see later discussion). It is important to remember that all patients with DPN are at increased risk of neuropathic complications such as foot ulceration and Charcot neuroarthropathy.

Pain associated with a peripheral nerve injury has several distinct clinical characteristics. Some describe bees stinging through the socks, whereas others talk of walking on hot coals. The pain, worse at night, keeps the patient awake and is associated with sleep deprivation.[9] Patients volunteer allodynia (pain due to a stimulus that does not normally cause pain, eg, stroking) or pain from normal stimuli, such as the touch of bedclothes, and may have hyperesthesias (increased sensitivity to touch) or hyperalgesia (increased sensitivity to painful stimuli). These symptoms may be paradoxic, with differences in sensation to one or other modality of stimulation. Unlike animal models of DPN, the pain is spontaneous and does not need provocation. It has a glove-and-stocking distribution. Pain usually occurs at rest and improves with ambulation, in contrast to osteoarthritic pain, which is worsened with ambulation and decreased with rest. Pain may persist over several years, causing considerable disability and impaired QOL in some patients, whereas it remits partially or completely in others despite further deterioration in small-fiber function. Pain exacerbation or even acute onset of pain tends to be associated with sudden metabolic changes, insulin neuritis, short duration of pain or diabetes, or preceding weight loss, and has less severe or no sensory loss, and normal strength and reflexes.

By contrast, the nociceptive pain of inflammatory arthritis does not have these qualities. It is localized to the joints, starts with morning stiffness, and improves as the day wears on.[54] Fasciitis pain is localized to the fascia; entrapment produces pain in a dermatome; and claudication is made worse by walking.

Clinical manifestations of small-fiber neuropathies (see **Fig. 1**):

- Small thinly myelinated Aδ and unmyelinated C fibers are affected
- Prominent symptoms with burning, superficial, or lancinating pain often accompanied by hyperalgesia, dysesthesia, and allodynia
- Progression to numbness and hypoalgesia (disappearance of pain may not necessarily reflect nerve recovery but rather nerve death, and progression of neuropathy must be excluded by careful examination)
- Abnormal cold and warm thermal sensation
- Abnormal autonomic function with decreased sweating, dry skin, impaired vasomotion and skin blood flow, with cold feet
- Intact motor strength and deep tendon reflexes
- Negative findings from nerve conduction velocity (NCV) studies
- Loss of cutaneous nerve fibers on skin biopsies
- Can be diagnosed clinically by reduced sensitivity to 1.0 g Semmes-Weinstein monofilament and prickling pain perception using the Wartenberg wheel or similar instrument
- Patients are at higher risk of foot ulceration and subsequent gangrene and amputations

Clinical manifestations of large-fiber neuropathies (see **Fig. 1**):

- Large myelinated, rapidly conducting Aα/β fibers are affected and may involve sensory and/or motor nerves
- Prominent signs with sensory ataxia (waddling like a duck), wasting of small intrinsic muscles of feet and hands, with hammertoe deformities and weakness of hands and feet

- Abnormal deep tendon reflexes
- Impaired vibration perception (often the first objective evidence), light touch, and joint position perception
- Shortening of the Achilles tendon with pes equinus
- Symptoms may be minimal: sensation of walking on cotton, pain is deep-seated and gnawing in quality, "like a toothache" in the foot, floors feeling "strange," inability to turn the pages of a book, or inability to discriminate among coins; in some patients with severe distal muscle weakness, inability to stand on the toes or heels
- Abnormal NCV findings
- Increased skin blood flow with hot feet
- Patients are at higher risk of falls, fractures, and development of Charcot neuroarthropathy
- Most patients with DPN, however, have a "mixed" variety of neuropathy with both large and small nerve-fiber damage

Diagnostic assessment of DPN

Because of the lack of agreement on the definition and diagnostic assessment of neuropathy, several consensus conferences were convened to overcome the current problems, the most recent of which has redefined the minimal criteria for the diagnosis of typical DSPN as summarized here.[14] **Tables 2** and **3** provide information on the appropriate testing for each nerve fiber type and its function.

Toronto classification of distal symmetric diabetic polyneuropathies[14]:

1. *Possible DSPN*. The presence of symptoms or signs of DSPN may include the following: symptoms—decreased sensation, positive neuropathic sensory symptoms (eg, "asleep numbness," prickling or stabbing, burning or aching pain) predominantly in the toes, feet, or legs; or signs—symmetric decrease of distal sensation or unequivocally decreased or absent ankle reflexes.
2. *Probable DSPN*. The presence of a combination of symptoms and signs of neuropathy including any 2 or more of the following: neuropathic symptoms, decreased distal sensation, or unequivocally decreased or absent ankle reflexes.
3. *Confirmed DSPN*: The presence of an abnormality of nerve conduction and a symptom or symptoms, or a sign or signs, of neuropathy confirm DSPN. If nerve conduction is normal, a validated measure of small-fiber neuropathy (SFN) (with class 1 evidence) may be used. To assess for the severity of DSPN, several approaches can be recommended: for example, the graded approach outlined

Table 2
Examination: bedside sensory tests

Sensory Modality	Nerve Fiber	Instrument	Associated Sensory Receptors
Vibration	Aβ (large)	128 Hz tuning fork	Ruffini corpuscle mechanoreceptors
Pain (pinprick)	C (small)	Neuro-tips	Nociceptors for pain and warmth
Pressure	Aβ, Aα (large)	1 g and 10 g monofilament	Pacinian corpuscle
Light touch	Aβ, Aα (large)	Wisp of cotton	Meissner corpuscle
Cold	Aδ (small)	Cold tuning fork	Cold thermoreceptors

Table 3
Advanced objective testing for diabetic neuropathy

Neurologic Test	Type of Neuropathy	Measurement	Advantages
Quantitative sensory testing	Small- and large-fiber neuropathies	Assessment of sensory deficits	Uses controlled quantifiable stimuli with standard procedures
Skin biopsy and intraepidermal nerve fiber (IENF) density	Small-fiber neuropathy	Small-caliber sensory nerves including somatic unmyelinated IENFs, dermal myelinated nerve fibers, and autonomic nerve fibers	Quantitates small epidermal nerve fibers through various antibody staining
Corneal confocal microscopy	Small-fiber neuropathy	Detects small nerve fiber loss in the cornea	Noninvasive technique that correlates with neuropathy severity
Contact heat evoked potentials	Small-fiber neuropathy	Uses nociceptive heat as a stimulus that is recorded through electroencephalographic readings	Detects small-fiber neuropathy in the absence of other indices
Sudomotor function	Distal small-fiber neuropathy	Assesses the sweat response by analyzing sweat production or sweat chloride concentrations	Detects early neurophysiologic abnormalities in peripheral autonomic function
Nerve conduction studies	Small- and large-fiber neuropathy	Measure the ability of the nerves to conduct an electrical stimulus	Standardized universal technique that is well documented and recommended

above; various continuous measures of sum scores of neurologic signs, symptoms, or nerve test scores; scores of function of activities of daily living; or scores of predetermined tasks or of disability.

4. *Subclinical DSPN.* The presence of no signs or symptoms of neuropathy are confirmed with abnormal nerve conduction or a validated measure of SFN (with class 1 evidence). Definitions 1, 2, or 3 can be used for clinical practice, and definitions 3 or 4 can be used for research studies.

5. *Small-fiber neuropathy (SFN).* SFN should be graded as follows: (1) possible: the presence of length-dependent symptoms and/or clinical signs of small-fiber damage; (2) probable: the presence of length-dependent symptoms, clinical signs of small-fiber damage, and normal sural nerve conduction; and (3) definite: the presence of length-dependent symptoms, clinical signs of small-fiber damage, normal sural nerve conduction, and altered intraepidermal nerve-fiber (IENF) density at the ankle and/or abnormal thermal thresholds at the foot.

The diagnosis of DSPN should rest on the findings of the clinical and neurologic examinations; that is, the presence of neuropathic symptoms (positive and negative, sensory and motor) and signs (sensory deficit, allodynia and hyperalgesia, motor weakness, absence of reflexes).[55]

1. Symptoms alone have poor diagnostic accuracy in predicting the presence of polyneuropathy.
2. Signs are better predictors than symptoms.
3. Multiple signs are better predictors than a single sign.
4. Relatively simple examinations are as accurate as complex scoring systems.

Thus, both symptoms and signs should be assessed. The following findings should alert the physician to consider causes for DSPN other than diabetes and referral for a detailed neurologic workup: (1) pronounced asymmetry of the neurologic deficits, (2) predominant motor deficits, mononeuropathy, or cranial nerve involvement, (3) rapid development or progression of the neuropathic impairments, (4) progression of the neuropathy despite optimal glycemic control, (5) symptoms from the upper limbs, (6) family history of nondiabetic neuropathy, and (7) a diagnosis of DSPN cannot be ascertained by clinical examination.[56]

Conditions Mimicking Diabetic Neuropathy

There are several conditions that can be mistaken for painful DN: intermittent claudication, whereby the pain is exacerbated by walking; Morton neuroma, whereby the pain and tenderness are localized to the intertarsal space and are elicited by applying pressure with the thumb in the appropriate intertarsal space; osteoarthritis, whereby the pain is confined to the joints, made worse with joint movement or exercise, and associated with morning stiffness that improves with ambulation; radiculopathy, whereby the pain originates in the shoulder, arm, thorax, or back, and radiates into the legs and feet; Charcot neuropathy, whereby the pain is localized to the site of the collapse of the bones of the foot, and the foot is hot rather than cold as occurs in neuropathy; plantar fasciitis, whereby there is shooting or burning in the heel with each step and there is exquisite tenderness in the sole of the foot; and tarsal tunnel syndrome, whereby the pain and numbness radiate from beneath the medial malleolus to the sole and are localized to the inner side of the foot. These conditions contrast with the pain of DPN, which is bilateral, symmetric, covers the whole foot and particularly the dorsum, and is worse at night, interfering with sleep.

The most important differential diagnoses from the general medicine perspective include neuropathies caused by alcohol abuse, uremia, hypothyroidism, vitamin B_{12} deficiency, peripheral arterial disease, cancer, inflammatory and infectious diseases, and neurotoxic drugs.[57]

A good medical history is essential to exclude other causes of neuropathy: a history of trauma, cancer, unexplained weight loss, fever, substance abuse, or HIV infection suggests that an alternative source should be sought. As recommended for all patients with distal symmetric polyneuropathy, screening laboratory tests may be considered in selected patients with DSPN, serum B_{12} with its metabolites and serum protein immunofixation electrophoresis being those with the highest yield of abnormalities.[58]

Clinical Assessment Tools for Diabetic Neuropathy

Clinical assessment should be standardized using validated scores for both the severity of symptoms and the degree of neuropathic deficits which are sufficiently reproducible. These assessments would include the Michigan Neuropathy Screening Instrument (MNSI)[59]; the Neuropathy Symptom Score for neuropathic symptoms; and the Neuropathy Disability Score or the Neuropathy Impairment Score (NIS) for neuropathic deficits.[5] The Neurologic Symptom Score has 38 items that capture symptoms of muscle weakness, sensory disturbances, and autonomic dysfunction. The neurologic history and examination should be performed initially and then with all subsequent visits. These questionnaires are useful for patient follow-up and to assess response to treatment. As discussed earlier, the exclusive presence of neuropathic symptoms without deficits is not sufficient to diagnose DSPN. Therefore, early stages of DSPN or painful small-fiber neuropathy with or without minimal deficits can only be verified using more sophisticated tests such as thermal thresholds or skin biopsy.

Objective Devices for the Diagnosis of Neuropathy

The neurologic examination should focus on the lower extremities and should always include an accurate foot inspection for deformities, ulcers, fungal infection, muscle wasting, hair distribution or loss, and the presence or absence of pulses. Sensory modalities should be assessed using simple handheld devices (touch by cotton wool or soft brush; vibration by 128-Hz tuning fork; pressure by the Semmes-Weinstein 1-g and 10-g monofilament; pinprick by Wartenberg wheel, Neurotip, or temperature by cold and warm objects) (level of evidence Ia/A).[60] Finally, the Achilles reflexes should be tested (see **Table 2**).[61,62]

More sophisticated testing of DN can be conducted according to the findings of the clinical neurologic examination. These tests and indications for their use are described in **Table 2**. Some are readily available in the clinical setting, whereas others are still confined to the research environment.

Summary of Clinical Assessment of DPN

A detailed clinical examination is the key to the diagnosis of DPN. The last position statement of the American Diabetes Association recommends that all patients with diabetes be screened for DN at diagnosis in type 2 DM and 5 years after diagnosis in type 1 DM. DN screening should be repeated annually and must include sensory examination of the feet and ankle reflexes.[61] One or more of the following can be used to assess sensory function: pinprick (using the Wartenberg wheel or similar instrument), temperature, vibration perception (using 128-Hz tuning fork), or 1-g and 10-g monofilament pressure perception at the distal halluces. Combinations of more than 1 test have more than 87% sensitivity in detecting DPN.[61,63] Longitudinal studies have shown that these simple tests are good predictors of risk for foot ulcer.[64] Numerous composite scores to evaluate clinical signs of DN, such as the NIS, are currently available. In combination with symptom scores, these are useful in documenting and monitoring neuropathic patients in the clinic.[65] The feet should always be examined in detail to detect ulcers, calluses, and deformities, and footwear must be inspected at every visit.

It is widely recognized that neuropathy per se can affect the QOL of the diabetic patient. Several instruments have been developed and validated to assess QOL in DN. The NeuroQoL measures patients' perceptions of the impact of neuropathy and foot ulcers.[66] The Norfolk QOL questionnaire for DN is a validated tool addressing specific symptoms and the impact of functions of large, small, and autonomic nerve fibers.

The diagnosis of DPN is mainly a clinical one, with the aid of specific diagnostic tests according to the type and severity of the neuropathy. However, other nondiabetic causes of neuropathy must always be excluded, depending on the clinical findings (vitamin B_{12} deficiency, hypothyroidism, uremia, CIDP, and so forth) (see **Fig. 3**).

TREATMENT OF DIABETIC POLYNEUROPATHIES

Treatment of DN should be targeted toward several different aspects: first, treatment of specific underlying pathogenic mechanisms; second, treatment of symptoms and improvement in QOL; and third, prevention of progression and treatment of complications of neuropathy (see **Fig. 1**, **Tables 6** and **7**).[67]

Treatment of Specific Underlying Pathogenic Mechanisms

Glycemic and metabolic control

Several long-term prospective studies have assessed the effects of intensive diabetes therapy on the prevention and progression of chronic diabetic complications. Studies in type 1 diabetic patients show that intensive diabetes therapy retards but does not completely prevent the development of DSPN. In the DCCT/EDIC cohort, the benefits of former intensive insulin treatment persisted for 13 to 14 years after DCCT closeout and provided evidence of a durable effect of prior intensive treatment on polyneuropathy and cardiac autonomic neuropathy ("hyperglycemic memory") (Ia/A).[68,69]

By contrast, in type 2 diabetic patients, who represent the vast majority of people with diabetes, the results were largely negative. The UK Prospective Diabetes Study (UKPDS) showed a lower rate of impaired vibration perception threshold (VPT) (>25 V) after 15 years for intensive therapy (IT) versus conventional therapy (CT) (31% vs 52%). However, the only additional time point at which VPT reached a significant difference between IT and CT was the 9-year follow-up, whereas the rates after 3, 6, and 12 years did not differ between the groups. Likewise, the rates of absent knee and ankle reflexes as well as the heart-rate responses to deep breathing did not differ between the groups.[70] In the ADVANCE study of 11,140 patients with type 2 DM randomly assigned to either standard glucose control or intensive glucose control, the relative risk reduction (95% confidence interval [CI]) for new or worsening neuropathy for intensive versus standard glucose control after a median of 5 years of follow-up was −4 (−10 to 2), without a significant difference between the groups.[71]

In the Steno 2 Study,[72] intensified multifactorial risk intervention including intensive diabetes treatment, angiotensin-converting enzyme inhibitors, antioxidants, statins, aspirin, and smoking cessation in patients with microalbuminuria showed no effect on DSPN after 7.8 (range: 6.9–8.8) years and again at 13.3 years, after the patients were subsequently followed for a mean of 5.5 years. However, the progression of cardiac autonomic neuropathy (CAN) was reduced by 57%. Thus, there is no evidence that intensive diabetes therapy or a target-driven intensified intervention aimed at multiple risk factors favorably influences the development or progression of DSPN as opposed to CAN in type 2 diabetic patients. However, the Steno study used only vibration detection, which measures exclusively the changes in large-fiber function.

Oxidative stress

Several studies have shown that hyperglycemia causes oxidative stress in tissues that are susceptible to complications of diabetes, including peripheral nerves. **Fig. 2** presents our current understanding of the mechanisms and potential therapeutic pathways for oxidative stress–induced nerve damage. Studies show that hyperglycemia induces an increased presence of markers of oxidative stress, such as superoxide and peroxynitrite ions, and that antioxidant defense moieties are reduced in patients with DPN.[73] Advanced glycation end products (AGE) are the result of nonenzymatic addition of glucose or other saccharides to proteins, lipids, and nucleotides. In diabetes, excess glucose accelerates AGE generation, which leads to intracellular and extracellular protein cross-linking and protein aggregation.

Therapies known to reduce oxidative stress are therefore recommended. Therapies that are under investigation include aldose reductase inhibitors, α-lipoic acid, γ-linolenic acid, benfotiamine, and protein kinase C inhibitors (**Table 4**).

Table 4
Oxidative stress therapeutic targets

Therapy	Mechanism	Clinical Improvements
Aldose reductase inhibitors (ARIs)	Reduce the flux of glucose through the polyol pathway, inhibiting tissue accumulation of sorbitol and fructose	Neuropathy symptoms, nerve conduction velocity, and vibration perception
α-Lipoic acid	Antioxidant properties and thiol-replenishing redox-modulating properties	Microcirculation and reversal of neuropathy symptoms
γ-Linolenic acid	—	Clinical and eletrophysiologic tests
Benfotiamine	Transketolase activator that reduces tissue advanced glycation end products	Conduction velocity in peroneal nerve and vibratory perception when combined with vitamin B_6/B_{12}
Protein kinase C inhibitors	Decrease production of vasoconstrictive, angiogenic, and chemotactic cytokines	Neuropathy symptoms and nerve conduction velocity
Methylcobolamin, methylfolate, and pyridoxal phosphate	Reduction of peroxynitrite and superoxide and restoration of glutathione levels to normal. Also restore the coupling of endogenous nitric acid synthase, reducing nitrosative and oxidative stress and therefore improving microvascular function	Reduce nerve damage, may also improve sensory nerve conduction and skin nerve fiber density

Growth factors

There is increasing evidence that there is a deficiency of nerve growth factor (NGF) in diabetes, as well as the dependent neuropeptides substance P and calcitonin gene-related peptide (CGRP), and that this contributes to the clinical perturbations in small-fiber function.[74] Clinical trials with NGF have not been successful but are subject to certain caveats with regard to design; however, NGF still holds promise for sensory and autonomic neuropathies.[75] The pathogenesis of DN includes loss of vasa nervorum, so it is likely that appropriate application of vascular endothelial growth factor (VEGF) would reverse the dysfunction. Introduction of the VEGF gene into the muscle of DM animal models improved nerve function.[76] There are ongoing VEGF gene studies with transfection of the gene into the muscle in humans. INGAP peptide comprises the core active sequence of Islet Neogenesis-Associated Protein (INGAP), a pancreatic cytokine that can induce new islet formation and restore euglycemia in diabetic rodents. Tam and colleagues[77] showed significant improvement in thermal hypoalgesia in diabetic mice after a 2-week treatment with INGAP peptide; humans have shown an increase in C-peptide secretion in type 1 DM patients and improvement in glycemic control in type 2 DM patients.[78] Nonetheless, information about its effect on DPN is still lacking. Finally, human trials are ongoing with human hepatocyte growth factor (HGF), which has been shown to be a potent angiogenic, antiapoptotic, and neurotropic factor. Because of the multiplicity of its actions, HGF is an intriguing candidate for targeting the complex pathogenesis of DN.[79–84]

Immune therapy

Several different autoantibodies in human sera have been reported that can react with epitopes in neuronal cells and have been associated with DN. The authors have reported a 12% incidence of a predominantly motor form of neuropathy in patients with diabetes associated with monosialoganglioside antibodies (anti-GM1 antibodies).[85] Perhaps the clearest link between autoimmunity and neuropathy has been the demonstration of an 11-fold increased likelihood of CIDP, multiple motor polyneuropathy, vasculitis, and monoclonal gammopathies in diabetes.[86] New data, however, support a predictive role of the presence of antineuronal antibodies on the later development of neuropathy, suggesting that these antibodies may not be innocent bystanders but neurotoxins.[87,88] There may be select cases, particularly those with autonomic neuropathy, evidence of antineuronal autoimmunity, and CIDP, that may benefit from intravenous immunoglobulin or large dose steroids.[36]

Treatment of Symptoms and Improvement in QOL

Pain, QOL, and comorbidities in diabetic neuropathy

Pain is the reason for 40% of patient visits in a primary care setting, and about 20% of these have had pain for longer than 6 months.[89] Chronic pain may be nociceptive, which occurs as a result of disease or damage to tissue wherein there is no abnormality in the nervous system. By contrast, experts in the neurology and pain community define neuropathic pain as "pain arising as a direct consequence of a lesion or disease affecting the somatosensory system."[90] Persistent neuropathic pain interferes significantly with QOL, impairing sleep and recreation; it also significantly affects emotional well-being, and is associated with, if not the cause of, depression, anxiety, loss of sleep, and noncompliance with treatment.[91] Painful diabetic peripheral neuropathy (PDPN) is a clinical problem that is difficult to manage, and patients with PDPN are more apt to seek medical attention than those with other types of DN. Two population-based studies showed that neuropathic pain is associated with a greater psychological burden than nociceptive pain,[92] and is considered to be more severe than other pain types. Early recognition of psychological problems is critical to the management of pain, and physicians need to go beyond the management of pain per se if they are to achieve success. Patients may also complain of decreased physical activity and mobility, increased fatigue, and negative effects on their social lives. Providing significant pain relief markedly improves QOL measures, including sleep and vitality.[9,93] Pathway analysis has shown that drugs that relieve pain may do so directly or indirectly via effects on sleep, depression, and anxiety, and an algorithm is provided for appropriate selection based on the comorbidities (**Fig. 4**).[94,95]

Castro and Daltro[96] studied 400 patients with depression, anxiety, and sleep disturbances. Two-thirds of depressed patients and three-quarters of anxious patients had pain, but the most impressive finding was that more than 90% of sleep-deprived patients had experienced pain. As a corollary, Gore and colleagues[97] showed that with increasing pain severity there was a linear increase in Hospital Anxiety and Depression Scales (HADS) pain and depression scores. The impact of depression complicated diabetes management, increased length of hospital stays, and almost doubled the yearly cost of diabetes management from $7000 to $11,000.[98] Moreover, Gupta and colleagues[99] showed that higher scores for anxiety, depression, and sleep disturbances predicted the development of pain.

Several studies have consistently found that neuropathic pain has a negative impact on global health-related QOL. A systematic review of 52 studies in patients with 1 out of 6 different disorders associated with neuropathic pain, including PDPN, established

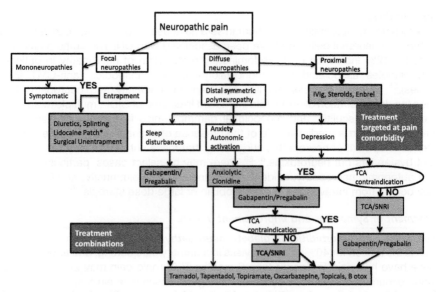

Fig. 4. Treatment algorithm: neuropathic pain after exclusion of nondiabetic etiology and stabilization of glycemic control. (*Adapted from* Vinik A. The approach to the management of the patient with neuropathic pain. J Clin Endocrinol Metab 2010;95:4802–811; and Vinik, A. Management of the Patient with Neuropathic Pain. In: Wartofsky L, editor. A clinical approach to endocrine and metabolic diseases, Vol 2. Chevy Chase (MD): The Endocrine Society, 2012. p. 177–94; with permission.)

that neuropathic pain impairs physical and emotional functioning, role functioning (including participation in gainful employment), sleep, and, to a lesser degree, social functioning. In addition, there is also evidence suggesting an association between neuropathic pain and depression, as for other types of pain.[91,100] The impact of pain on QOL in PDPN has recently been shown in 1111 patients: physical and mental QOL were significantly more impaired in patients with PDPN than in both diabetic patients without neuropathy and those with non-PDPN.[22] The nature of pain may also be important, as Daousi and colleagues[101] have reported significantly poorer QOL in patients with PDPN than in diabetic patients with non-neuropathic pain.

The diagnostic workup

Because of its complexity the presentation of pain poses a diagnostic dilemma for the clinician, who needs to distinguish between neuropathic pain arising as a direct consequence of a lesion or disease of the somatosensory system, and nociceptive pain that is due to trauma, inflammation, or injury. It is imperative to try to establish the nature of any predisposing factor, including the pathogenesis of the pain, if one is to be successful in its management. Management of neuropathic pain requires a sound relationship between patient and physician, with an emphasis on a positive outlook and encouragement that there is a solution, using patience and targeted pain-centered strategies that deal with the underlying disorder rather than the usual Band-Aid prescription of drugs approved for general pain, which do not address the disease process. The inciting injury may be focal or diffuse and may involve single or, more likely, multiple mechanisms such as metabolic disturbances encompassing hyperglycemia, dyslipidemia, glucose fluctuations, or intensification of therapy with insulin. On the other hand, the injury might embrace autoimmune mechanisms, neurovascular insufficiency, deficient neurotropism, oxidative and nitrosative stress, and inflammation.[12,42] Because pain syndromes in diabetes may be focal or diffuse, proximal or distal, acute or chronic, each has its own pathogenesis, and the treatment must be tailored to the underlying disorder if the outcome is to be successful. The presence of diabetes must be established if this has not already been done.

The diagnosis of neuropathic pain

The diagnosis of neuropathic pain, as opposed to pain from causes other than neuropathy, is first and foremost made by careful history taking. Patients should be queried at the time of an office visit as to whether they are experiencing tingling, burning, or pain at rest in their feet. A positive response warrants further investigation and screening for PDPN. Somatosensory, motor, and autonomic bedside evaluation can be done and is complemented by use of one of the pain screening tools (Douleur Neuropathique en 4 questions [DN4], Pain DETECT, and so forth).[102] The physician should ensure that all the features of pain such as distribution, quality, severity, timing, associated symptoms, and exacerbating and relieving factors (if any) are recorded. In particular, the presence of numbness, burning, tingling, lightning pain, stabbing, and prickling should be recorded, as is done in the Norfolk QOL tool (Ia/A),[9] the Neuropathy Total Symptom Score-6 questionnaire (NTSS-6),[103] and the Pain DETECT.[102] Secondly, pain intensity and quality should be assessed, using pain intensity scales (Visual Analog Scale or NRS) (Ia/A)[104] and pain questionnaires (Brief Pain Inventory [BPI], Neuropathic Pain Symptom Inventory [NPSI]). Several tools and questionnaires have been developed to quantify the impact of pain on sleep, mood, and QOL, mainly to be used in clinical trials. In clinical practice the BPI Interference scale, the Profile of Moods, or the HADS can provide a simple measure of the impact of pain on QOL. Responses to treatment by self-reporting using a diary can record the course of painful symptoms and their impact on daily life (Ia/A).[105] These reports are also most useful for outcomes measures in clinical trials on drugs used for pain relief. Validated scoring systems for symptoms and signs are available in the form of questionnaires or checklists, such as the Neuropathy Symptom Score and the MNSI questionnaire for symptoms, and the MNSI and the Neuropathy Disability Score for signs (Ia/A).[59,106]

Definition of neuropathic pain

A definition of peripheral neuropathic pain in diabetes, adapted from a definition proposed by the International Association for the Study of Pain,[90] is "pain arising as a direct consequence of abnormalities in the peripheral somatosensory system in people with diabetes."[14] A grading system for the degree of certainty of the diagnosis of neuropathic pain has been proposed. It is based on 4 simple criteria, namely:

1. Whether the pain has a distinct neuroanatomical distribution
2. Whether the history of the patient suggests the presence or absence of a lesion or disease of the peripheral or central somatosensory system
3. Whether either of these findings is supported by at least 1 confirmatory test
4. Whether there is an abnormality of nerve conduction[90]

Degree of certainty is defined according to the number of criteria met: 1 to 4 (definite neuropathic pain); 1 and 2 plus 3 or 4 (probable neuropathic pain); or only 1 and 2 (possible neuropathic pain). There is no consensus on their diagnostic validity, because neuropathic pain is a composite of pain and other sensory symptoms associated with nerve injury. For example, sensory deficits, abnormal spontaneous or induced sensations such as paresthesias (eg, tingling), spontaneous attacks of electric shock-like sensations, and allodynia preclude a simple definition (see later discussion).

Distinction between nociceptive and non-nociceptive pain

Several tools have been developed to differentiate non-nociceptive stimuli (allodynia), increased pain sensitivity to stimuli (hyperalgesia),[107] and summation, which is progressive worsening of pain caused by repeated mild noxious stimuli (IIb/B).[102] Several self-administered questionnaires have been developed, validated, translated, and subjected to cross-cultural adaptation to both diagnose and distinguish neuropathic as opposed to non-neuropathic pain (Leeds Assessment of Neuropathic Symptoms and Signs Pain Scale, DN4, Neuropathic Pain Questionnaire, Pain DETECT, and ID-Pain).[102,108–113] Others assess pain quality and intensity (assessment questionnaires such as the Short-Form McGill Pain Questionnaire, the BPI, and the NPSI) (III/B).[108,114,115]

According to IMMPACT (Initiative on Methods, Measurement and Pain Assessment in Clinical Trials), the following pain characteristics should be evaluated to assess the efficacy and effectiveness of chronic pain treatment[116]:

1. Pain intensity measured on a 0 to 10 numerical rating scale (NRS)
2. Physical functioning assessed by the Multidimensional Pain Inventory (MPI) and BPI Interferences scale
3. Emotional functioning, assessed by the Beck Depression Inventory and Profile of Mood states
4. Patient rating of overall improvement, assessed by the Patient Global Impression of Change (PGI-C) (III/B)

Laboratory tests to evaluate neuropathic pain

Because neuropathic pain is subjective there are no tests that can objectively quantify this in humans, meaning that the results of laboratory tests become useful only in the context of a comprehensive clinical examination.

Late laser-evoked potentials (Aδ-LEPs) are the easiest and most reliable neurophysiologic tools for assessing nociceptive Aδ-fiber pathway function, useful in both peripheral and central neuropathic pain, with the limitation of very low availability (IIb/B).[117] The morphologic study of cutaneous nerve fibers using skin biopsy and IENF density assessment is regarded as a reproducible marker of small-fiber sensory pathology, but is still not widely available. Functional neuroimaging techniques, such as positron emission tomography for the central nervous system and functional magnetic resonance (MR) imaging for both central and peripheral nervous systems (MR neurography), have been used mainly for research purposes to evaluate the central mechanisms of pain in chronic pain conditions or to visualize intraneural and extraneural lesions of peripheral nerves (IV/C).[118]

Contact heat-evoked potential stimulation (CHEPS) was introduced to study nociceptive pathways by using a contact thermode that rapidly increases skin temperature. The CHEPS device delivers rapid heat pulses to selectively stimulate Aδ and C fibers while simultaneously recording cerebral evoked potentials. Several groups have established CHEPS as a clinically feasible approach to examine the physiology of thermonociceptive nerves. CHEPS is a noninvasive technique that can objectively evaluate small-fiber dysfunction. It has been shown that patients with sensory neuropathy of differing etiology have lower CHEPS amplitudes, which correlates with IENF densities.[119–121] Chao and colleagues[122] evaluated 32 type 2 diabetic patients with painful neuropathy. CHEP amplitudes were reduced in diabetic patients compared with age- and sex-matched control subjects, and abnormal CHEP patterns (reduced amplitude or prolonged latency) were noted in 81.3% of these patients. The CHEP amplitude was the most significant parameter correlated with IENF density ($P = .003$) and pain perception to contact heat stimuli ($P = .019$) on multiple linear regression models. The authors' group evaluated 31 healthy controls and 30 patients with type 2 DM and DPN using neurologic examination, NCV, autonomic function tests, quantitative sensory tests (QST), and CHEPS. CHEPS amplitudes were significantly reduced in the DPN group at the lower back (44.93 ± 6.5 vs 23.87 ± 3.36 μV; $P<.01$), lower leg (15.87 ± 1.99 vs 11.68 ± 1.21 μV; $P<.05$), and dorsal forearm (29.89 ± 8.86 vs 14.96 ± 1.61 μV; $P<.05$). Pooled data from both groups showed that amplitudes and latencies at different sites significantly correlated with clinical neurologic scores, NCV, QST, and autonomic function.

Evaluation of pain intensity is essential for monitoring response to therapy. There are several symptom-based screening tools such as the NTSS-6, BPI, QOL-DN, SF-36, Visual Analog Scale for Pain Intensity, Neuro-QOL, and Norfolk Neuropathy Symptoms Score (Ia/A). With the visual analog scale the patient marks the intensity of their pain on a scale from 0 to 10, allowing an assessment of the response to intervention. Simultaneously, the patient should complete a QOL tool such as the Norfolk QOL-DN, which needs to include comorbidities such as anxiety, depression, and sleep interference (Ia/A).

PHARMACOLOGIC THERAPEUTIC MODALITIES FOR DIABETIC NEUROPATHIC PAIN
Treatment Based on Pathogenic Concepts of Pain

Painful symptoms in DSPN may constitute a considerable management problem. The efficacy of a single therapeutic agent is not the rule, and simple analgesics are usually inadequate to control the pain. There is agreement that patients should be offered the available therapies in a stepwise fashion (Ia/A).[123–126] Effective pain treatment considers a favorable balance between pain relief and side effects without implying a maximum effect. The following general considerations in the pharmacotherapy of neuropathic pain require attention.

- The appropriate and effective drug has to be tried and identified in each patient by carefully titrating the dose based on efficacy and side effects.
- Lack of efficacy should be judged only after 2 to 4 weeks of treatment using an adequate dose.
- Because the evidence from clinical trials suggests only a maximum response of approximately 50% for any monotherapy, analgesic combinations may be useful.
- Potential drug interactions have to be considered, given the frequent use of polypharmacy in diabetic patients.

The relative benefit of an active treatment over a control in clinical trials is usually expressed as the relative risk, the relative risk reduction, or the odds ratio (OR). However, to estimate the extent of a therapeutic effect (ie, pain relief) that can be translated into clinical practice, it is useful to apply a simple measure that serves the physician to select the appropriate treatment for the individual patient. Such a practical measure is the number needed to treat (NNT); that is, the number of patients that need to be treated with a particular therapy to observe a clinically relevant effect or adverse event in one patient. The OR, NNT, and number needed to harm (NNH) for the individual agents used in the treatment of painful DN are given in **Table 5**. Usually drugs with NNTs exceeding 6 for 50% or greater pain relief are regarded as showing limited efficacy. However, some investigators have cautioned against using NNT estimates because of the lack of homogeneity in treatment therapies, mechanisms of action, pain syndromes, and outcome measures.[127]

The growing knowledge about the neural and pharmacologic basis of neuropathic pain is likely to have important treatment implications, including development and

Table 5
Odds ratios for efficacy and withdrawal, numbers needed to treat (NNT), and numbers needed to harm (NNH)

Drug Class	Odds Ratio: Efficacy	Odds Ratio: Withdrawal (Secondary to Adverse Event)	NNT	NNH
Tricyclics	22.2 (5.8–84.7)	2.3 (0.6–9.7)	1.5–3.5	2.7–17.0
Duloxetine	2.6 (1.6–4.8)	2.4 (1.1–5.4)	5.7–5.8	15.0
Traditional anticonvulsants	5.3 (1.8–16.0)	1.5 (0.3–7.0)	2.1–3.2	2.7–3.0
New-generation anticonvulsants	3.3 (2.3–4.7)	3.0 (1.75–5.1)	2.9–4.3	26.1
Opioids	4.3 (2.3–7.8)	4.1 (1.2–14.2)	2.6–3.9	9.0

Data from Vinik A. The approach to the management of the patient with neuropathic pain. J Clin Endocrinol Metab 2010;95:4802–11.

refinement of a symptom-/mechanism-based approach to neuropathic pain and implementation of novel treatment strategies using the newer antiepileptic agents, which may address the underlying neurophysiologic aberrations in neuropathic pain, allowing the clinician to increase the likelihood of effective management. The neuropharmacology of pain is also becoming better understood. For example, recent data suggest that γ-aminobutyric acid (GABA), voltage-gated sodium channels, and glutamate receptors may be involved in the pathophysiology of neuropathic pain. Many of the newer agents have significant effects on these neurophysiologic mechanisms. Hyperglycemia may be a factor in lowering the pain threshold. Pain is often worse with wide glycemic excursions. Paradoxically, acute onset of pain may appear soon after initiation of therapy with insulin or oral agents.[128] By contrast, it has been reported that a striking amelioration of symptoms can occur with continuous subcutaneous insulin administration, which may reduce the amplitude of excursions of blood glucose.[128] This dichotomy is not well explained. There is a sequence in DN, beginning when Aδ and C nerve fiber function is intact and there is no pain. With damage to C fibers there is sympathetic sensitization, and peripheral autonomic symptoms are interpreted as painful. Topical application of clonidine causes antinociception by blocking emerging pain signals at the peripheral terminals via α2-adrenoceptors,[129] in contrast with the central actions of clonidine on control of blood pressure. With the death of C fibers there is nociceptor sensitization. Aδ fibers conduct all varieties of peripheral stimuli such as touch and these are interpreted as painful (eg, allodynia). With time there is reorganization at the cord level and the patient experiences cold hyperalgesia and, ultimately, even with the death of all fibers, pain is registered in the cerebral cortex whereupon the syndrome becomes chronic without the need for peripheral stimulation. Disappearance of pain may not necessarily reflect nerve recovery but rather nerve death. When patients volunteer the loss of pain, progression of the neuropathy must be excluded by careful examination.

A summary of The Toronto Consensus Panel on Diabetic Neuropathy guidelines,[130] American Academy of Neurology (AAN) recommendations,[131] and treatment options for symptomatic PDPN are shown in **Tables 6–8**.[130–132]

α-Lipoic acid

According to a meta-analysis comprising 1258 patients, infusions of α-lipoic acid (600 mg/d intravenously) ameliorated neuropathic symptoms and deficits after 3 weeks.[133] In a multicenter, randomized, double-masked, parallel-group clinical trial

Table 6
Treatment options for symptomatic diabetic polyneuropathy pain-dosing and side effects

Drug Class	Drug	Dose	Side Effects
Tricyclics (mg)	Amitriptyline	50–150 QHS	Somnolence, dizziness, dry mouth, tachycardia,
	Nortriptyline	50–150 QHS	Constipation, urinary retention, blurred vision
	Imipramine	25–150 QHS	Confusion
	Desipramine	25–150 QHS	
SSRIs (mg)	Paroxetine	40 QD	Somnolence, dizziness, sweating, nausea, anorexia
	Citalopram	40 QD	Diarrhea, impotence, tremor
SNRIs (mg)	Duloxetine	60 QD	Nausea, somnolence, dizziness, anorexia
Anticonvulsants (mg)	Gabapentin	300–1200 TID	Somnolence, dizziness, confusion, ataxia
	Pregabalin	50–150 TID	Somnolence, confusion, edema, weight gain
	Carbamazepine/ oxcarbazepine	Up to 200 QID	Dizziness, somnolence, nausea, leukopenia
	Topiramate	Up to 400 QD	Somnolence, dizziness, ataxia, tremor
Opioids (mg)	Tramadol	50–100 BID	Nausea, constipation, HA, somnolence
	Oxycodone CR	10–30 BID	Somnolence, nausea, constipation, HA
Topical	Capsaicin	0.075% QID	Local irritation
	Lidocaine	0.04% QD	Local irritation
Injection	Botulinum toxin		None

Abbreviations: BID, twice daily; QD, once daily; QHS, every night at bedtime; QID, 4 times daily; TID, 3 times daily.
  Data from Vinik A. The approach to the management of the patient with neuropathic pain. J Clin Endocrinol Metab 2010;95:4802–11.

(NATHAN 1), 460 diabetic patients with DSPN were randomly assigned to oral treatment with α-lipoic acid 600 mg (n = 233) or placebo (n = 227). After 4 years of treatment, NIS, but not NCV, was improved, and the drug was well tolerated throughout the trial.[134] A response analysis of clinically meaningful improvement and progression in

Table 7
Treatment algorithm for painful diabetic peripheral neuropathy (The Toronto Consensus Panel on Diabetic Neuropathy)

	Painful Diabetic Neuropathy		
First line	α2-δ agonist (pregabalin or gabapentin)	SNRI (duloxetine)	TCA
If pain control is inadequate and considering contraindications			
Second line	TCA or SNRI	TCA or α2-δ agonist (pregabalin or gabapentin)	SNRI or α2-δ agonist (pregabalin or gabapentin)
If pain control is still inadequate			
Third line	Add opioid agonist as combination therapy		

Abbreviations: SNRI, serotonin noradrenaline reuptake inhibitor; TCA, tricyclic antidepressant.
  Modified from Tesfaye S, Vileikyte L, Rayman G, et al. Painful diabetic peripheral neuropathy: consensus recommendations on diagnosis, assessment and management. Diabetes Metab Res Rev 2011;27:629–38.

Table 8
Tailoring treatment to the patient (The Toronto Consensus Panel on Diabetic Neuropathy)

Comorbidities	Contraindication
Glaucoma	TCAs
Orthostatic hypotension	TCAs
Cardiovascular disease	TCAs
Hepatic disease	Duloxetine
Edema	Pregabalin, gabapentin
Unsteadiness and falls	TCAs
Weight gain	TCAs, pregabalin, gabapentin
Other factors: Cost	Duloxetine, pregabalin

Modified from Tesfaye S, Vileikyte L, Rayman G, et al. Painful diabetic peripheral neuropathy: consensus recommendations on diagnosis, assessment and management. Diabetes Metab Res Rev 2011;27:629–38.

the NIS and NIS of the lower limbs (NIS-LL) by at least 2 points showed that the rates of clinical responders were significantly higher and the rates of clinical progressors were lower with α-lipoic acid when compared with placebo for NIS (P = .013) and NIS-LL (P = .025).

Adrenergic blockers

When there is ongoing damage to the nerves the patient initially experiences pain of the burning, lancinating, dysesthetic type often accompanied by hyperalgesia and allodynia. Because the peripheral sympathetic nerve fibers are also small unmyelinated C fibers, sympathetic blocking agents (clonidine) may improve the pain.

Topical capsaicin

C fibers use the neuropeptide substance P as their neurotransmitter, and depletion of axonal substance P (through the use of capsaicin) will often lead to amelioration of the pain. Prolonged application of capsaicin depletes stores of substance P, and possibly other neurotransmitters, from sensory nerve endings. This process reduces or abolishes the transmission of painful stimuli from the peripheral nerve fibers to the higher centers.[135] Several studies have demonstrated significant pain reduction and improvement in QOL in diabetic patients with painful neuropathy after 8 weeks of treatment with capsaicin cream 0.075%.[136] It has been pointed out that a double-blind design is not feasible for topical capsaicin because of the transient local hyperalgesia (usually mild burning sensation in >50% of the cases) it may produce as a typical adverse event. Treatment should be restricted to a maximum of 8 weeks, as during this period no adverse effect on sensory function (due to the mechanism of action) was noted in diabetic patients. The 8% capsaicin patch (Qutenza), which is effective in post-herpetic neuralgia,[137] is contraindicated in painful DN because of desensitization of nociceptive sensory nerve endings, which may theoretically increase the risk of diabetic foot ulcers (IIb/B).

Lidocaine

A multicenter, randomized, open-label, parallel-group study with a drug washout phase of up to 2 weeks and a comparative phase of 4-week treatment periods of 5% lidocaine (n = 99) versus pregabalin (n = 94) showed that lidocaine was as effective as pregabalin in reducing pain and was free of side effects.[138] This form of therapy may be most useful in self-limited forms of neuropathy. If successful, therapy can be continued with oral mexiletine. This class of compounds targets the pain caused by hyperexcitability of superficial, free nerve endings.[139]

Opioids and NMDA-receptor antagonists

Tramadol is a centrally acting weak opioid analgesic for treating moderate to severe pain. Tramadol was shown to be better than placebo in a randomized controlled trial[140] of only 6 weeks' duration, but a subsequent follow-up study suggested that symptomatic relief could be maintained for at least 6 months.[141] Side effects are relatively common and similar to other opioid-like drugs, but the development of tolerance and dependence during long-term tramadol treatment is uncommon and its abuse liability appears to be low.[140] Another spinal cord target for pain relief is the excitatory glutaminergic N-methyl-D-aspartate (NMDA) receptor. Blockade of NMDA receptors is believed to be one mechanism by which dextromethorphan exerts analgesic efficacy.[142] The NMDA receptors play an important role in central sensitization of neuropathic pain. Their use, however, has not been widespread, in part because of their dose-limiting side effects (Ia/A).[143]

Severe and refractory pain may require administration of strong opioids such as oxycodone. Although few data are available on combination treatment, combinations of different substance classes have to be used in patients with pain resistant to monotherapy. Several add-on trials have demonstrated significant pain relief and improvement in QOL following treatment with controlled-release oxycodone, a pure μ-agonist in patients with painful DSPN whose pain is not adequately controlled on standard treatment with antidepressants and anticonvulsants.[144,145] Recent recommendations have emphasized the need for clinical skills in risk assessment and management as a prerequisite to the safe and effective prescribing of opioids.[126]

Tapentadol is a novel centrally active analgesic with a dual mode of action: μ-opioid receptor agonist and norepinephrine reuptake inhibitor. The efficacy and tolerability of tapentadol extended release (ER) were evaluated using pooled data from 2 randomized-withdrawal, placebo-controlled, phase 3 trials of similar design in patients with moderate to severe PDPN. With placebo (n = 343) and tapentadol ER (n = 360), respectively, mean (SD) pain intensity scores were 3.48 (2.02) and 3.67 (1.85) at the start of the double-blind maintenance phase and 4.76 (2.52) and 3.77 (2.19) at week 12. Mean (SD) changes from the start to week 12 were 1.28 (2.41) and 0.08 (1.87), indicating that pain intensity worsened with placebo but was relatively unchanged with tapentadol ER. Tapentadol has recently been approved by the Food and Drug Administration for the treatment of PDPN. For the Toronto Consensus Panel on Diabetic Neuropathy recommendations, the reader is referred to **Table 7**.[130] Of note is that the tapentadol publications postdated the AAN and the Toronto Consensus Panel recommendations.

Antidepressants

Antidepressants are now emerging as the first line of agents in the treatment of chronic neuropathic pain.[123] Clinical trials have focused on interrupting pain transmission using antidepressant drugs that inhibit the reuptake of norepinephrine or serotonin. This central action accentuates the effects of these neurotransmitters in activation of endogenous pain-inhibitory systems in the brain that modulate pain-transmission cells in the spinal cord.[146] Putative mechanisms of pain relief by antidepressants include the inhibition of norepinephrine and/or serotonin reuptake at synapses of central descending pain control systems, and the antagonism of NMDA receptors that mediate hyperalgesia and allodynia.

Tricyclic antidepressants

Imipramine, amitriptyline, and clomipramine induce a balanced reuptake inhibition of both norepinephrine and serotonin, whereas desipramine is a relatively selective norepinephrine inhibitor. The NNT (CI) for at least 50% pain relief by tricyclic antidepressants (TCAs) in painful neuropathies is 2.1 (1.9–2.6). The NNH in patients with neuropathic pain for one drop-out of the study due to adverse events is 16 (11–26).[124] The starting dose of amitriptyline should be 25 mg (10 mg in frail patients) taken as a single nighttime dose 1 hour before sleep. It should be increased by 25 mg at weekly intervals until pain relief is achieved or adverse events occur. The maximum dose is usually 150 mg per day.

The use of TCAs is limited by relatively high rates of adverse events and several contraindications (see **Tables 6** and **8**).

Selective serotonin reuptake inhibitors

Because of the relatively high rates of adverse effects and several contraindications of TCAs, it has been reasoned that patients who do not tolerate them because of adverse events could alternatively be treated with selective serotonin reuptake inhibitors (SSRIs). SSRIs specifically inhibit presynaptic reuptake of serotonin but not norepinephrine, and, unlike the tricyclics, they lack the postsynaptic receptor-blocking effects and quinidine-like membrane stabilization. However, only weak effects on neuropathic pain were observed after treatment with fluoxetine, paroxetine, citalopram, and escitalopram. The NNT (CI) for at least 50% pain relief by SSRIs in painful neuropathies is 6.8 (3.9–27).[124] Because of these limited-efficacy data, SSRIs have not been licensed for the treatment of neuropathic pain (IIb/B).

Serotonin noradrenaline reuptake inhibitors

Because SSRIs have been found to be less effective than TCAs, recent interest has focused on antidepressants with dual selective inhibition of serotonin and noradrenaline, such as duloxetine and venlafaxine. Serotonin noradrenaline reuptake inhibitors (SNRIs) relieve pain by increasing the synaptic availability of 5-hydroxytryptamine and noradrenaline in the descending pathways that are inhibitory to pain impulses. A further advantage of duloxetine is that it has antidepressant effects in addition to the analgesic effects in DN. Adverse events are usually mild to moderate, and transient (see **Table 6**). To minimize them the starting dose should be 30 mg/d for 4 to 5 days. Nonetheless, physicians must be aware about the possibility of orthostatic hypotension during the first week of treatment on the 30-mg dose. In contrast to TCAs and some anticonvulsants, duloxetine does not cause weight gain, but a small increase in fasting blood glucose may occur.[147]

Venlafaxine Venlafaxine is another SNRI that has mixed action on catecholamine uptake. At lower doses, it inhibits serotonin uptake and at higher doses it inhibits norepinephrine uptake.[148] The ER version of venlafaxine was found to be superior to placebo in diabetic neuropathic pain in nondepressed patients at doses of 150 to 225 mg daily, and when added to gabapentin there was improved pain, mood, and QOL.[149] Duloxetine, but not venlafaxine, has been licensed in the United States for the treatment of painful DN (Ia/A). See **Table 7** for the Toronto Consensus Panel on Diabetic Neuropathy recommendations.[130]

Antiepileptic Drugs

Antiepileptic drugs (AEDs) have a long history of effectiveness in the treatment of neuropathic pain.[150] Principal mechanisms of action include sodium channel blockade (felbamate, lamotrigine, oxcarbazepine, topiramate, zonisamide), potentiation of

GABA activity (tiagabine, topiramate), calcium channel blockade (felbamate, lamotrigine, topiramate, zonisamide), antagonism of glutamate at NMDA receptors (felbamate) or AMPA (α-amino-3-hydroxy-5-methyl-4-isoxazole propionic acid) receptors (felbamate, topiramate), and mechanisms of action as yet to be fully determined (gabapentin, pregabalin, levetiracetam).[151] An understanding of the mechanisms of action of the various drugs leads to the concept of "rational polytherapy," whereby drugs with complementary mechanisms of action can be combined for synergistic effect. For example, one might choose a sodium-channel blocker such as lamotrigine to be used with a glutamate antagonist such as felbamate. Furthermore, a single drug may possess multiple mechanisms of action, perhaps increasing its likelihood of success (eg, topiramate). If pain is divided according to its derivation from different types of nerve fiber (eg, Aδ vs C fiber), spinal cord or cortical, then different types of pain should respond to different therapies.

The evidence supporting the use of AEDs for the treatment of PDPN continues to evolve.[148] Patients who have failed to respond to 1 AED may respond to another or to 2 or more drugs in combination (Ia/A).[152]

Calcium-channel modulators (gabapentin and pregabalin)
Five types of voltage-gated calcium channels have been identified, and the L and N types of channels have a role to play in the neuromodulation of sensory neurons of the spinal cord. Gabapentin and pregabalin are medications that bind at the $\alpha2$-δ subunits of the channels. Unlike traditional calcium-channel antagonists, they do not block calcium channels but modulate their activity and sites of expression. The exact mechanism of action of this group of agents on neuromodulation has yet to be clearly defined (IIb/B).

Gabapentin Gabapentin is an anticonvulsant structurally related to GABA, a neurotransmitter that plays a role in pain transmission and modulation. In an 8-week multicenter dose-escalation trial including 165 diabetic patients with painful neuropathy, 60% of the patients on gabapentin (3600 mg/d achieved in 67%) had at least moderate pain relief compared with 33% on placebo. The NNT (CI) for at least 50% pain relief by gabapentin in painful neuropathies is 6.4 (4.3–12). Because of this relatively high NNT and publication bias toward unpublished negative trials,[153] the overall level of evidence in favor of gabapentin in painful DSPN is weak. Gabapentin has the additional benefit of improving sleep.[154] Side effects are listed in **Table 6**; over the long term, it is also known to produce weight gain.[155] Combination therapy has been examined using gabapentin and morphine, indicating slight superiority of the combination (Ia/B).[145]

Pregabalin Pregabalin is a more specific $\alpha2$-δ ligand with a 6-fold higher binding affinity than gabapentin. Four clinical studies evaluated the efficacy of pregabalin,[156–159] all of which found that it relieved pain, but the effect size was small relative to placebo, reducing pain by 11% to 13% on the 11-point Likert scale in 3 of them. A large dose-dependent effect (24%–50%) reduction in Likert pain scores compared with placebo was observed in the fourth study.[159] The NNT from these studies for a 50% reduction in pain was 4 at 600 mg/d.[156–159] QOL measures, social functioning, mental health, bodily pain, and vitality improved, and sleep interference decreased, and all changes were significant. The most frequent side effects for 150 to 600 mg/d are dizziness (22.0%), somnolence (12.1%), peripheral edema (10.0%), headache (7.2%), and weight gain (5.4%).[160] The evidence supporting a favorable effect in painful DN is more solid, and dose titration is considerably easier for pregabalin than for gabapentin (Ia/A).[131]

Sodium-channel blockers (carbamazepine, oxcarbazepine, lancosamide)

Voltage-gated sodium channels are crucial determinants of neuronal excitability and signaling. After nerve injury, hyperexcitability and spontaneous firing develop at the site of injury and also in the dorsal root ganglion cell bodies. This hyperexcitability results at least partly from accumulation of sodium channels at the site of injury.[161] Carbamazepine and oxcarbazepine are most effective against the "lightning" pain produced by such spontaneous neuronal firing.[162]

Although carbamazepine has been widely used for treating neuropathic pain, it cannot be recommended in painful DN, owing to very limited data. Its successor drug, oxcarbazepine, as well as other sodium-channel blockers such as valproate, mexiletine, topiramate, and lamotrigine, showed only marginal efficacy and have not been licensed for the treatment of painful DN.

Topiramate

Although topiramate failed in 3 clinical trials owing to the use of the wrong end point,[163] it has been shown to successfully reduce pain and induce nerve regeneration.[164,165] Topiramate has the added advantages of causing weight loss and improving the lipoprotein profile, both of which are particularly useful in overweight type 2 diabetic patients.

In summary, 2 drugs have been approved for neuropathic pain in the United States, pregabalin and duloxetine. A recent meta-analysis, in which duloxetine was compared indirectly with pregabalin and gabapentin for the treatment of PDPN, concluded that these 2 agents have comparable efficacy and tolerability.[166] Some studies have analyzed health care costs in patients with PDPN treated with pregabalin, duloxetine, or other commonly used drugs. In general all show similar results, with a good cost-effective profile for both drugs.[167–169]

The response rates to analgesic monotherapy in painful diabetic DSPN are only around 50%. Therefore, combination pharmacotherapy is required in patients who have only partial response or in whom the drug cannot be further titrated because of intolerable side effects. A recent trial showed that the combination of nortriptyline and gabapentin at the maximum tolerated dose was more effective than either monotherapy, despite a lower maximum tolerable dose compared with monotherapy.[170] Appropriate analgesic combinations include antidepressants with anticonvulsants, or each of these with opioids. Some patients may even require a triple combination of these drug classes. The ORs for efficacy and withdrawal from medications are given in **Table 5**.

Based on evidence from clinical trials for the various pharmacologic agents (efficacy and safety) for painful DPN, the Toronto Consensus Panel on Diabetic Neuropathy recommended that a TCA, SNRI, or α2-δ agonist (calcium-channel modulator) should be considered for first-line treatments (see **Table 7**). Based on trial data, duloxetine would be the preferred SNRI and pregabalin would be the preferred α2-δ agonist. If pain is inadequately controlled, depending on contraindications (see **Table 8**) these first-line agents can be combined, although this is not backed by trial evidence. If pain is still inadequately controlled, opioids such as tramadol and oxycodone might be added in a combination treatment.[130]

Natural Products

Metanx

Metanx is a product for management of endothelial dysfunction, containing L-methylfolate, pyridoxal 5'-phosphate, and methylcobalamin. Metanx ingredients counteract endothelial nitric oxide synthase uncoupling and oxidative stress in vascular endothelium and peripheral nerves. A 24-week placebo-controlled trial on the effects of

Metanx on patients with established DN was presented at the American Association of Clinical Endocrinologists annual meeting in 2011. The NTSS-6, which includes numbness, tingling, aching, burning, lancinating pain, and allodynia, improved significantly at week 16 (P = .013 vs placebo) and week 24 (P = .033). Moreover, there were significant improvements in the mental health component of the SF-36 Role Emotional, Social Function, and Vitality. This response occurred with adverse events of less than 2%, mainly rash and gastrointestinal upset, which was no greater than occurred with placebo.[171,172]

Botulinum toxin
Botulinum toxin has been tried for trigeminal neuralgia[173] and has been shown to have long-lasting antinociceptive effects in carpal tunnel syndrome, with no electrophysiologic restoration.[174]

NONPHARMACOLOGIC TREATMENT OF PAINFUL DIABETIC NEUROPATHY

Because there is no entirely satisfactory pharmacotherapy for painful DN, nonpharmacologic treatment options should always be considered. A recent systematic review assessed the evidence from rigorous clinical trials and meta-analyses of complementary and alternative therapies for treating neuropathic and neuralgic pain. Data on the following complementary and alternative medicine treatments were identified: acupuncture, electrostimulation, herbal medicine, magnets, dietary supplements, imagery, and spiritual healing. The conclusion was that the evidence is not fully convincing for most complementary and alternative medicine modalities in relieving neuropathic pain. The evidence can be classified as encouraging and warrants further study for cannabis extract, magnets, carnitine, and electrostimulation (III/C).[175]

Psychological Support

A psychological component to pain should not be underestimated. Hence, an explanation to the patient that even severe pain may remit, particularly in poorly controlled patients with acute painful neuropathy or in those painful symptoms precipitated by intensive insulin treatment, is justified. Addressing the concerns and anxieties of patients with neuropathic pain is essential for their successful management.[176]

Physical Measures

The temperature of the painful neuropathic foot may be increased because of arteriovenous shunting. Cold-water immersion may reduce shunt flow and relieve pain. Allodynia may be relieved by wearing silk pajamas or the use of a bed cradle. Patients who describe painful symptoms on walking as comparable to walking on pebbles may benefit from the use of comfortable footwear.[176]

GUIDELINES FOR THE TREATMENT OF PAINFUL NEUROPATHY

Fig. 4 is an algorithm that the authors use for the management of painful neuropathy in diabetes. The identification of neuropathic pain as being focal or diffuse dictates the initial course of action. Focal neuropathic pain is best treated with diuretics to reduce edema in the canal, with splinting and surgery to release entrapment. Diffuse neuropathies are treated with medical therapy and, in a majority of cases, need multidrug therapy. Essential to the evaluation is the identification of the comorbidities and the choice of drugs that can serve dual actions: for example, pregabalin improves sleep and pain by both direct and indirect pathways, whereas duloxetine may reduce the depression and anxiety that accompany pain. Immune-mediated neuropathies are treated with intravenous immunoglobulin, steroids, or other immunomodulators. When single agents fail, combinations of drugs with different mechanisms of action are in order.

DIABETIC CARDIAC AUTONOMIC NEUROPATHY
Pathogenesis

The etiology of cardiovascular autonomic dysfunction seen early after the diagnosis of diabetes is not well understood. Hyperglycemia increases protein glycation and causes a gradual accumulation of AGEs in body tissues. These AGEs form on intracellular and extracellular proteins, lipids, and nucleic acids in complex arrangements that lead to cross-linking. The authors hypothesize that in metabolic syndrome and diabetes there is a constant increase in low-grade inflammation mediated by a large cadre of exogenous and endogenous ligands in combination with the central and autonomic nervous systems. Thus, the loss of autonomic control with reduction of parasympathetic activity, which is the hallmark of loss of autonomic balance in diabetes, initiates a cascade of inflammatory responses which, if continued unabated, will culminate in considerable morbidity and mortality.

Epidemiology of CAN

Establishing the prevalence of CAN has been hampered by heterogeneous and inadequate diagnostic criteria and population selection. A recent Consensus Panel on Diabetic Neuropathy, after extensive review of the literature, concluded that the prevalence of confirmed CAN in unselected people with type 1 and type 2 DM is approximately 20%, but can be as high as 65% with increasing age and diabetes duration. Clinical correlates or risk markers for CAN are age, diabetes duration, glycemic control, microvascular complications (peripheral polyneuropathy, retinopathy, and nephropathy), hypertension, and dyslipidemia. Established risk factors for CAN are glycemic control in type 1 DM, and a combination of hypertension, dyslipidemia, obesity, and glycemic control in type 2 DM.[177]

CAN is a significant cause of morbidity and mortality associated with a high risk of cardiac arrhythmias and sudden death, possibly related to silent myocardial ischemia. Results from the Action to Control Cardiovascular Risk in Diabetes (ACCORD) trial confirmed that individuals with baseline CAN were 1.55 to 2.14 times as likely to die as individuals without CAN.[68] Furthermore, CAN in the presence of peripheral neuropathy was the highest predictor of mortality from cardiovascular disease (ie, hazard ratio 2.95, $P<.008$). Indeed, combining indices of autonomic dysfunction have been shown to be associated with the risk of mortality.[178–180]

Clinical Manifestations

CAN has been linked to resting tachycardia, postural hypotension, exercise intolerance, enhanced intraoperative or perioperative cardiovascular liability, increased incidence of asymptomatic ischemia, MI, and decreased rate of survival after myocardial infarction.

Resting tachycardia

Whereas abnormalities in heart-rate variability (HRV) are early findings of CAN, resting tachycardia and a fixed heart rate are characteristic late findings in diabetic patients with vagal impairment. A blunted heart-rate response to adenosine receptor agonists was described in both patients with diabetes and patients with metabolic syndrome, and was attributed to earlier stages of CAN.[181] The prognostic value of resting heart rate is a useful tool for cardiovascular risk stratification and as a therapeutic target in high-risk patients.[18,19,177]

Exercise intolerance

Diabetic patients who are likely to have CAN should be tested for cardiac stress before undertaking an exercise program. Patients with CAN need to rely on their perceived exertion, not heart rate, to avoid hazardous levels of intensity of exercise.

Intraoperative cardiovascular lability

Perioperative cardiovascular morbidity and mortality are increased 2- to 3-fold in patients with diabetes, manifested as greater declines in heart rate and blood pressure during induction of anesthesia; a greater need for vasopressor support[182]; and more severe intraoperative hypothermia with consequent impaired wound healing.[183] Preoperative cardiovascular autonomic screening of diabetic patient may help anesthesiologists identify those at greater risk of intraoperative complications.[17]

Orthostatic hypotension

Orthostatic hypotension is defined as a decrease in blood pressure (ie, >20 mm Hg for systolic or >10 mm Hg for diastolic) in response to postural change, from supine to standing.[184] In patients with diabetes, orthostatic hypotension is usually a result of damage to the efferent sympathetic vasomotor fibers, particularly in the splanchnic vasculature.[185] Patients may present with light-headedness and presyncopal symptoms, or may remain asymptomatic despite significant drops in blood pressure. Orthostatic symptoms can also be misjudged as hypoglycemia and can be aggravated by several drugs, including vasodilators, diuretics, phenothiazines, and particularly TCAs and insulin.[17]

Diagnosis and Staging of CAN

Methods of CAN assessment in clinical practice include assessment of symptoms and signs, cardiovascular autonomic reflex tests (CARTs) based on heart rate and blood pressure, and ambulatory blood pressure monitoring (ABPM).[177]

Screening for autonomic dysfunction should be performed at the diagnosis of type 2 DM and 5 years after the diagnosis of type 1 DM, particularly in patients at greater risk because of a history of poor glycemic control, cardiovascular risk factors, DPN, and macroangiopathic or microangiopathic diabetic complications.

The Toronto Consensus Panel on Diabetic Neuropathy has concluded the following regarding diagnosis of CAN (**Table 9**):

- The following CARTs are the gold standard for clinical autonomic testing: heart-rate response to deep breathing, standing, and Valsalva maneuver, and blood-pressure response to standing (class II evidence).
- These CARTs are sensitive, specific, reproducible, easy to perform, safe, and standardized (classes II and III).
- The Valsalva maneuver is not advisable in the presence of proliferative retinopathy and when there is an increased risk of retinal hemorrhage (class N).
- CARTs are subject to several confounding or interfering factors (class III).
- Age is the most relevant factor affecting heart-rate tests (class I).
- A definite diagnosis of CAN and CAN staging requires more than 1 heart-rate test and the orthostatic hypotension test (class III).

Staging of CANs is based on the number of abnormal test results:

- The presence of 1 abnormal cardiovagal test result identifies the condition of possible or early CAN, to be confirmed over time.

Table 9
Cardiovascular autonomic tests and suggested indications for their use

Test	Clinical Diagnosis	Research	End Point in Clinical Trials
Heart rate cardiovascular tests	Yes	Yes	Yes
Orthostatic hypotension test	Yes	Yes	No (low sensitivity)
QT interval	Yes (additional information and risk stratification)	Yes	No (low sensitivity)
Ambulatory blood pressure monitoring for dipping status (ABPM)	Yes (risk stratification)	Yes	No (low sensitivity)
HRV time and frequency domain indices	Yes (additional information and risk stratification)	Yes	Yes
Baroreflex sensitivity measures	No (early additional information and risk stratification but low availability)	Yes	Yes
Scintigraphic studies	No (low availability, limited standardization)	Yes	Yes
Muscle sympathetic nerve activity	No (low availability, limited data in cardiovascular autonomic neuropathy)	Yes	Possible (used in lifestyle intervention trials in obesity)
Catecholamine assessment	No (low availability)	Yes	Possible (used in lifestyle intervention trials in obesity)

Abbreviation: HRV, heart-rate variability.
Reproduced from Spallone V, Ziegler D, Freeman R, et al. Cardiovascular autonomic neuropathy in diabetes: clinical impact, assessment, diagnosis, and management. Diabetes Metab Res Rev 2011;27:639–53.

- At least 2 abnormal cardiovagal results are required for a definite or confirmed diagnosis of CAN.
- The presence of orthostatic hypotension in addition to heart-rate test abnormalities identifies severe or advanced CAN (level B).
- CARTs allow CAN staging from early to advanced involvement (level C).
- Progressive stages of CAN are associated with increasingly worse prognosis (level B).

Treatment of Autonomic Dysfunction

Intervention studies have documented the protective effects of glycemic control on autonomic function in type 1 diabetic patients (DCCT trial). In the Steno memorial trial, Gaede and colleagues[72,186] showed that a multifactorial strategy aimed at lifestyle change with pharmacologic correction of hyperglycemia, hypertension, dyslipidemia, and microalbuminuria in type 2 diabetic patients reduces abnormalities in autonomic function by 68%.

The Toronto Consensus Panel on Diabetic Neuropathy concluded the following in relation to CAN treatment:

- Intensive diabetes therapy retards the development of CAN in type 1 DM (level A).

Table 10
Diagnosis and management of autonomic dysfunction

Symptoms	Assessment Modalities	Management
Resting tachycardia, exercise intolerance, early fatigue and weakness with exercise	HRV, respiratory HRV, MUGA thallium scan, ^{123}I MIBG scan	Graded supervised exercise, β-blockers, ACE inhibitors
Postural hypotension, dizziness, light-headedness, weakness, fatigue, syncope, tachycardia/bradycardia	HRV, blood pressure measurement lying and standing	Mechanical measures, clonidine, midodrine, octreotide, erythropoietin, pyridostigmine
Hyperhidrosis	Sympathetic/parasympathetic balance	Clonidine, amitriptyline, trihexyphenidyl, propantheline, or scopolamine, botulinum toxin, glycopyrrolate

Abbreviations: ACE, angiotensin-converting enzyme; HRV, heart-rate variability; MIBG, metaiodo-benzylguanidine; MUGA, multigated acquisition.
Reproduced from Vinik AI, Suwanwalaikorn S, Stansberry KB, et al. Quantitative measurement of cutaneous perception in diabetic neuropathy. Muscle Nerve 1995;18:574–84.

- Intensive multifactorial cardiovascular risk intervention retards the development and progression of CAN in type 2 DM (level B).
- Lifestyle intervention might improve HRV in prediabetes (level B) and diabetes (level B).
- Symptomatic orthostatic hypotension might be improved by nonpharmacologic measures (level B), and by midodrine (level A) and/or fludrocortisone (level B).

Specific assessment modalities and therapeutic interventions for CAN are detailed in **Table 10**.

Diabetic CAN is a serious complication found in one-quarter of type 1 and one-third of type 2 diabetic patients. It is associated with increased mortality and silent myocardial ischemia, and with a poor prognosis. Symptoms usually occur with advanced disease, and screening of diabetic patients for CAN is essential. The CARTs are the gold standard. Restoration of autonomic balance is possible and has been shown with therapeutic lifestyle changes, increased physical activity, and diabetes treatment (β-adrenergic blockers and potent antioxidants, such as α-lipoic acid). There are exciting new prospects for pathogenesis-oriented intervention.

SUMMARY

DN is the most common and troublesome complication of DM, leading to the greatest morbidity and mortality and resulting in a huge economic burden for diabetes care. It results in a variety of syndromes for which there is no universally accepted classification, and may even be asymptomatic for years while progressing insidiously. DPN has been recently defined as a symmetric, length-dependent sensorimotor polyneuropathy attributable to metabolic and microvascular alterations as a result of chronic hyperglycemia exposure (diabetes) and cardiovascular risk covariates. Both the clinical assessment and treatment options are multifactorial, as detailed herein. Patients with DN should be screened for autonomic neuropathy, as there is a high degree of coexistence of the 2 complications.

Painful neuropathy is an important complication of diabetes. Pathogenesis is multifactorial and requires attention to detailed management if one is to achieve success. Two drugs, pregabalin and duloxetine, have been approved for neuropathic pain in the United States, but neither of these have afforded complete relief, even when used in combination. Indeed, a sobering view is that few drugs achieve a greater than 30% reduction in pain in more than 50% of patients, dictating a need to use more than 1 drug with different mechanisms of action. There is a great need to understand pathogenic mechanisms more fully, particularly the differences in origin of peripheral and central pain. One needs to be aware of the conditions that masquerade as painful neuropathy and the treatment directed toward the underlying disorder as suggested in the algorithm provided. Treatment of peripheral neuropathic pain conditions can benefit from further understanding of the impact of pain response on QOL, activities in daily life, and sleep. As Winston Churchill said, "We need to go from failure to failure without losing our enthusiasm and ultimately we will succeed..."

REFERENCES

1. Vinik AI, Mitchell BD, Leichter SB, et al. Epidemiology of the complications of diabetes. In: Leslie RD, Robbins DC, editors. Diabetes: clinical science in practice. Cambridge (United Kingdom): Cambridge University Press; 1995. p. 221–87.
2. Holzer SE, Camerota A, Martens L, et al. Costs and duration of care for lower extremity ulcers in patients with diabetes. Clin Ther 1998;20:169–81.
3. Caputo GM, Cavanagh PR, Ulbrecht JS, et al. Assessment and management of foot disease in patients with diabetes. N Engl J Med 1994;331:854–60.
4. Herman WH, Kennedy L. Underdiagnosis of peripheral neuropathy in type 2 diabetes. Diabetes Care 2005;28:1480–1.
5. Young MJ, Boulton AJ, MacLeod AF, et al. A multicenter study of the prevalence of diabetic peripheral neuropathy in the United Kingdom hospital clinic population. Diabetologia 1993;36:150–4.
6. Dyck PJ, Kratz KM, Karnes JL, et al. The prevalence by staged severity of various types of diabetic neuropathy, retinopathy, and nephropathy in a population-based cohort: The Rochester Diabetic Neuropathy Study. Neurology 1993;43:817–24.
7. Vinik A. Diabetic neuropathy: pathogenesis and therapy. Am J Med 1999; 107(2B):17S–26S.
8. Armstrong DG, Lavery LA, Harkless LB. Validation of a diabetic wound classification system. The contribution of depth, infection, and ischemia to risk of amputation. Diabetes Care 1998;21:855–9.
9. Vinik EJ, Hayes RP, Oglesby A, et al. The development and validation of the Norfolk QOL-DN, a new measure of patients' perception of the effects of diabetes and diabetic neuropathy. Diabetes Technol Ther 2005;7:497–508.
10. Levitt NS, Stansberry KB, Wychanck S, et al. Natural progression of autonomic neuropathy and autonomic function tests in a cohort of IDDM. Diabetes Care 1996;19:751–4.
11. Rathmann W, Ziegler D, Jahnke M, et al. Mortality in diabetic patients with cardiovascular autonomic neuropathy. Diabet Med 1993;10:820–4.
12. Vinik A, Ullal J, Parson HK, et al. Diabetic neuropathies: clinical manifestations and current treatment options. Nat Clin Pract Endocrinol Metab 2006;2:269–81.
13. Sadosky A, McDermott AM, Brandenburg NA, et al. A review of the epidemiology of painful diabetic peripheral neuropathy, postherpetic neuralgia, and less commonly studied neuropathic pain conditions. Pain Pract 2008;8:45–56.

14. Tesfaye S, Boulton AJ, Dyck PJ, et al. Diabetic neuropathies: update on definitions, diagnostic criteria, estimation of severity, and treatments. Diabetes Care 2010;33:2285–93.
15. Ziegler D. Painful diabetic neuropathy: treatment and future aspects. Diabetes Metab Res Rev 2008;24(Suppl 1):S52–7.
16. Boulton AJ, Malik RA, Arezzo JC, et al. Diabetic somatic neuropathies. Diabetes Care 2004;27:1458–86.
17. Vinik AI, Ziegler D. Diabetic cardiovascular autonomic neuropathy. Circulation 2007;115:387–97.
18. Vinik AI, Maser RE, Ziegler D. Neuropathy: the crystal ball for cardiovascular disease? Diabetes Care 2010;33:1688–90.
19. Vinik AI, Maser RE, Ziegler D. Autonomic imbalance: prophet of doom or scope for hope? Diabet Med 2011;28:643–51.
20. Dieleman JP, Kerklaan J, Huygen FJ, et al. Incidence rates and treatment of neuropathic pain conditions in the general population. Pain 2008;137:681–8.
21. Cornblath DR, Vinik A, Feldman E, et al. Surgical decompression for diabetic sensorimotor polyneuropathy. Diabetes Care 2007;30:421–2.
22. Ziegler D, Rathmann W, Dickhaus T, et al. Prevalence of polyneuropathy in pre-diabetes and diabetes is associated with abdominal obesity and macroangiopathy: the MONICA/KORA Augsburg Surveys S2 and S3. Diabetes Care 2008;31: 464–9.
23. Smith AG, Russell J, Feldman EL, et al. Lifestyle intervention for pre-diabetic neuropathy. Diabetes Care 2006;29:1294–9.
24. Ziegler D, Rathmann W, Meisinger C, et al. Prevalence and risk factors of neuropathic pain in survivors of myocardial infarction with pre-diabetes and diabetes. The KORA Myocardial Infarction Registry. Eur J Pain 2009;13:582–7.
25. Ziegler D, Rathmann W, Dickhaus T, et al. Neuropathic pain in diabetes, prediabetes and normal glucose tolerance: the MONICA/KORA Augsburg Surveys S2 and S3. Pain Med 2009;10:393–400.
26. Vinik AI, Holland MT, LeBeau JM, et al. Diabetic neuropathies. Diabetes Care 1992;15:1926–75.
27. Vinik A, Mehrabyan A. Diabetic neuropathies. Med Clin North Am 2004;88: 947–99.
28. Vinik A, Mehrabyan A, Colen L, et al. Focal entrapment neuropathies in diabetes. Diabetes Care 2004;27:1783–8.
29. Wilbourn AJ. Diabetic entrapment and compression neuropathies. In: Dyck PJ, Thomas PK, editors. Diabetic neuropathy. Toronto: WB Saunders; 1999. p. 481–508.
30. Watanabe K, Hagura R, Akanuma Y, et al. Characteristics of cranial nerve palsies in diabetic patients. Diabetes Res Clin Pract 1990;10:19–27.
31. Perkins B, Olaleye D, Bril V. Carpal tunnel syndrome in patients with diabetic polyneuropathy. Diabetes Care 2002;25:565–9.
32. Llewelyn JG, Thomas PK, King RH. Epineurial microvasculitis in proximal diabetic neuropathy. J Neurol 1998;245:159–65.
33. Vinik AI, Pittenger GL, Milicevic Z, et al. Autoimmune mechanisms in the pathogenesis of diabetic neuropathy. In: Eisenbarth RG, editor. Molecular mechanisms of endocrine and organ specific autoimmunity. 1st edition. Georgetown, Texas: Landes Company; 1998. p. 217–51.
34. Steck AJ, Kappos L. Gangliosides and autoimmune neuropathies: classification and clinical aspects of autoimmune neuropathies. J Neurol Neurosurg Psychiatry 1994;57(Suppl):26–8.

35. Ayyar DR, Sharma KR. Chronic inflammatory demyelinating polyradiculoneuropathy in diabetes mellitus. Curr Diab Rep 2004;4:409–12.
36. Krendel DA, Costigan DA, Hopkins LC. Successful treatment of neuropathies in patients with diabetes mellitus. Arch Neurol 1995;52:1053–61.
37. Barada A, Reljanovic M, Milicevic Z, et al. Proximal diabetic neuropathy—response to immunotherapy. Diabetes 1999;48(Suppl 1):A148.
38. Boulton AJ, Malik RA. Diabetic neuropathy. Med Clin North Am 1998;82:909–29.
39. Thomas PK. Classification, differential diagnosis, and staging of diabetic peripheral neuropathy. Diabetes 1997;46(Suppl 2):S54–7.
40. Oyibo SO, Prasad YD, Jackson NJ, et al. The relationship between blood glucose excursions and painful diabetic peripheral neuropathy: a pilot study. Diabet Med 2002;19:870–3.
41. Sinnreich M, Taylor BV, Dyck PJ. Diabetic neuropathies. Classification, clinical features, and pathophysiological basis. Neurologist 2005;11:63–79.
42. Vinik A. Management of the patient with neuropathic pain. In: Wartofsky L, editor. Endocrine Society; 2012. p. 177–94 J Clin Endocrinol Metab 2010;95:4802–11 [reprint].
43. Archer AG, Watkins PJ, Thomas PK, et al. The natural history of acute painful neuropathy in diabetes mellitus. J Neurol Neurosurg Psychiatry 1983;46:491–9.
44. Partanen J, Niskanen L, Lehtinen J, et al. Natural history of peripheral neuropathy in patients with non-insulin-dependent diabetes mellitus. N Engl J Med 1995;333:89–94.
45. Harris M, Eastman R, Cowie C. Symptoms of sensory neuropathy in adults with NIDDM in the U.S. population. Diabetes Care 1993;16:1446–52.
46. Singleton JR, Smith AG, Bromberg MB. Painful sensory polyneuropathy associated with impaired glucose tolerance. Muscle Nerve 2001;24:1225–8.
47. Singleton JR, Smith AG, Bromberg MB. Increased prevalence of impaired glucose tolerance in patients with painful sensory neuropathy. Diabetes Care 2001;24:1448–53.
48. Novella SP, Inzucchi SE, Goldstein JM. The frequency of undiagnosed diabetes and impaired glucose tolerance in patients with idiopathic sensory neuropathy. Muscle Nerve 2001;24:1229–31.
49. Sumner C, Sheth S, Griffin J, et al. The spectrum of neuropathy in diabetes and impaired glucose tolerance. Neurology 2003;60:108–11.
50. Pittenger GL, Ray M, Burcus NI, et al. Intraepidermal nerve fibers are indicators of small-fiber neuropathy in both diabetic and nondiabetic patients. Diabetes Care 2004;27:1974–9.
51. Dyck PJ, Lais A, Karnes JL, et al. Fiber loss is primary and multifocal in sural nerves in diabetic polyneuropathy. Ann Neurol 1986;19:425–39.
52. Cavanagh PR, Simoneau GG, Ulbrecht JS. Ulceration, unsteadiness, and uncertainty: the biomechanical consequences of diabetes mellitus. J Biomech 1993;26(Suppl 1):23–40.
53. Katoulis EC, Ebdon-Parry M, Lanshammar H, et al. Gait abnormalities in diabetic neuropathy. Diabetes Care 1997;20:1904–7.
54. Vinik AI, Strotmeyer ES, Nakave AA, et al. Diabetic neuropathy in older adults. Clin Geriatr Med 2008;24:407–35.
55. England JD, Gronseth GS, Franklin G, et al. Distal symmetric polyneuropathy: a definition for clinical research: report of the American Academy of Neurology, the American Association of Electrodiagnostic Medicine, and the American Academy of Physical Medicine and Rehabilitation. Neurology 2005;64:199–207.

56. Ziegler D, Hidvegi T, Gurieva I, et al. Efficacy and safety of lacosamide in painful diabetic neuropathy. Diabetes Care 2010;33:839–41.
57. Young RJ, Ewing DJ, Clarke BF. Chronic and remitting painful diabetic polyneuropathy. Correlations with clinical features and subsequent changes in neurophysiology. Diabetes Care 1988;11:34–40.
58. England JD, Gronseth GS, Franklin G, et al. Practice Parameter: evaluation of distal symmetric polyneuropathy: role of autonomic testing, nerve biopsy, and skin biopsy (an evidence-based review). Report of the American Academy of Neurology, American Association of Neuromuscular and Electrodiagnostic Medicine, and American Academy of Physical Medicine and Rehabilitation. Neurology 2009;72:177–84.
59. Feldman EL, Stevens MJ, Thomas PK, et al. A practical two-step quantitative clinical and electrophysiological assessment for the diagnosis and staging of diabetic neuropathy. Diabetes Care 1994;17:1281–9.
60. Haanpaa ML, Backonja MM, Bennett MI, et al. Assessment of neuropathic pain in primary care. Am J Med 2009;122:S13–21.
61. Boulton AJ, Vinik AI, Arezzo JC, et al. Diabetic neuropathies: a statement by the American Diabetes Association. Diabetes Care 2005;28:956–62.
62. Boulton AJ, Gries FA, Jervell JA. Guidelines for the diagnosis and outpatient management diabetic peripheral neuropathy. Diabet Med 1998;15:508–14.
63. Vinik AI, Suwanwalaikorn S, Stansberry KB, et al. Quantitative measurement of cutaneous perception in diabetic neuropathy. Muscle Nerve 1995;18:574–84.
64. Abbott CA, Carrington AL, Ashe H, et al. The North-West Diabetes Foot Care Study: incidence of, and risk factors for, new diabetic foot ulceration in a community-based patient cohort. Diabet Med 2002;19:377–84.
65. Dyck PJ, Melton LJ III, O'Brien PC, et al. Approaches to improve epidemiological studies of diabetic neuropathy: insights from the Rochester Diabetic Neuropathy Study. Diabetes 1997;46(Suppl 2):S5–8.
66. Vileikyte L, Peyrot M, Bundy C, et al. The development and validation of a neuropathy- and foot ulcer-specific quality of life instrument. Diabetes Care 2003; 26:2549–55.
67. Cameron NE, Eaton SE, Cotter MA. Vascular factors and metabolic interactions in the pathogenesis of diabetic neuropathy. Diabetologia 2001;44:1973–88.
68. Albers JW, Herman WH, Pop-Busui R, et al. Effect of prior intensive insulin treatment during the Diabetes Control and Complications Trial (DCCT) on peripheral neuropathy in type 1 diabetes during the Epidemiology of Diabetes Interventions and Complications (EDIC) Study. Diabetes Care 2010;33:1090–6.
69. Pop-Busui R, Low PA, Waberski BH, et al. Effects of prior intensive insulin therapy on cardiac autonomic nervous system function in type 1 diabetes mellitus: The Diabetes Control and Complications Trial/Epidemiology of Diabetes Interventions and Complications study (DCCT/EDIC). Circulation 2009;119: 2886–93.
70. Intensive blood-glucose control with sulphonylureas or insulin compared with conventional treatment and risk of complications in patients with type 2 diabetes (UKPDS 33). UK Prospective Diabetes Study (UKPDS) Group. Lancet 1998;352: 837–53.
71. The ADVANCE Collaborative Group. Intensive blood glucose control and vascular outcomes in patients with type 2 diabetes. N Engl J Med 2008;358: 2560–72.
72. Gaede P, Lund-Andersen H, Parving HH, et al. Effect of a multifactorial intervention on mortality in type 2 diabetes. N Engl J Med 2008;358:580–91.

73. Ziegler D, Sohr CG, Nourooz-Zadeh J. Oxidative stress and antioxidant defense in relation to the severity of diabetic polyneuropathy and cardiovascular autonomic neuropathy. Diabetes Care 2004;27:2178–83.
74. Pittenger G, Vinik A. Nerve growth factor and diabetic neuropathy. Exp Diabesity Res 2003;4:271–85.
75. Vinik AI. Treatment of diabetic polyneuropathy (DPN) with recombinant human nerve growth factor (rhNGF). Diabetes 1999;48(Suppl 1):A54–5.
76. Rivard A, Silver M, Chen D, et al. Rescue of diabetes-related impairment of angiogenesis by intramuscular gene therapy with adeno-VEGF. Am J Pathol 1999;154:355–63.
77. Tam J, Rosenberg L, Maysinger D. INGAP peptide improves nerve function and enhances regeneration in streptozotocin-induced diabetic C57BL/6 mice. FASEB J 2004;18:1767–9.
78. Dungan KM, Buse JB, Ratner RE. Effects of therapy in type 1 and type 2 diabetes mellitus with a peptide derived from islet neogenesis associated protein (INGAP). Diabetes Metab Res Rev 2009;25:558–65.
79. Bussolino F, Di Renzo MF, Ziche M, et al. Hepatocyte growth factor is a potent angiogenic factor which stimulates endothelial cell motility and growth. J Cell Biol 1992;119:629–41.
80. Nakagami H, Kaneda Y, Ogihara T, et al. Hepatocyte growth factor as potential cardiovascular therapy. Expert Rev Cardiovasc Ther 2005;3:513–9.
81. Matsumoto K, Nakamura T. Emerging multipotent aspects of hepatocyte growth factor. J Biochem 1996;119:591–600.
82. Jayasankar V, Woo YJ, Pirolli TJ, et al. Induction of angiogenesis and inhibition of apoptosis by hepatocyte growth factor effectively treats postischemic heart failure. J Card Surg 2005;20:93–101.
83. Hashimoto N, Yamanaka H, Fukuoka T, et al. Expression of HGF and cMet in the peripheral nervous system of adult rats following sciatic nerve injury. Neuroreport 2001;12:1403–7.
84. Ajroud-Driss S, Christiansen M, Allen JA, et al. Phase 1/2 open-label dose-escalation study of plasmid DNA expressing two isoforms of hepatocyte growth factor in patients with painful diabetic peripheral neuropathy. Mol Ther 2013;21(6):1279–86.
85. Milicevic Z, Newlon PG, Pittenger GL, et al. Anti-ganglioside GM1 antibody and distal symmetric "diabetic polyneuropathy" with dominant motor features. Diabetologia 1997;40:1364–5.
86. Sharma K, Cross J, Farronay O, et al. Demyelinating neuropathy in diabetes mellitus. Arch Neurol 2002;59:758–65.
87. Granberg V, Ejskjaer N, Peakman M, et al. Autoantibodies to autonomic nerves associated with cardiac and peripheral autonomic neuropathy. Diabetes Care 2005;28:1959–64.
88. Vinik AI, Anandacoomaraswamy D, Ullal J. Antibodies to neuronal structures: innocent bystanders or neurotoxins? Diabetes Care 2005;28:2067–72.
89. Mantyselka P, Ahonen R, Kumpusalo E, et al. Variability in prescribing for musculoskeletal pain in Finnish primary health care. Pharm World Sci 2001;23:232–6.
90. Treede RD, Jensen TS, Campbell JN, et al. Neuropathic pain: redefinition and a grading system for clinical and research purposes. Neurology 2008;70:1630–5.
91. Jensen MP, Chodroff MJ, Dworkin RH. The impact of neuropathic pain on health-related quality of life: review and implications. Neurology 2007;68:1178–82.

92. Bouhassira D, Lanteri-Minet M, Attal N, et al. Prevalence of chronic pain with neuropathic characteristics in the general population. Pain 2008;136:380–7.
93. Vinik E, Paulson J, Ford-Molvik S, et al. German-Translated Norfolk Quality of Life (QOL-DN) identifies the same factors as the English version of the tool and discriminates different levels of neuropathy severity. J Diabetes Sci Technol 2008;2:1075–86.
94. Vinik AI, Casellini CM. Guidelines in the management of diabetic nerve pain: clinical utility of pregabalin. Diabetes Metab Syndr Obes 2013;6:57–78.
95. Vinik A, Emir B, Raymond C, et al. The relationship between pain relief and improvements in patient function/quality of life in patients with painful diabetic peripheral neuropathy or post-herpetic neuralgia treated with pregabalin. Clin Ther 2013;35(5):612–23.
96. Castro MM, Daltro C. Sleep patterns and symptoms of anxiety and depression in patients with chronic pain. Arq Neuropsiquiatr 2009;67:25–8.
97. Gore M, Brandenburg NA, Dukes E, et al. Pain severity in diabetic peripheral neuropathy is associated with patient functioning, symptom levels of anxiety and depression, and sleep. J Pain Symptom Manage 2005;30:374–85.
98. Boulanger L, Zhao Y, Foster TS, et al. Impact of comorbid depression or anxiety on patterns of treatment and economic outcomes among patients with diabetic peripheral neuropathic pain. Curr Med Res Opin 2009;25:1763–73.
99. Gupta A, Silman J, Ray D, et al. The role of psychosocial factors in predicting the onset of chronic widespread pain: results from a prospective population-based study. Rheumatology 2007;46:666–71.
100. O'Connor AB. Neuropathic pain: quality-of-life impact, costs and cost effectiveness of therapy. Pharmacoeconomics 2009;27:95–112.
101. Daousi C, MacFarlane IA, Woodward A, et al. Chronic painful peripheral neuropathy in an urban community: a controlled comparison of people with and without diabetes. Diabet Med 2004;21:976–82.
102. Bennett MI, Attal N, Backonja MM, et al. Using screening tools to identify neuropathic pain. Pain 2007;127:199–203.
103. Bastyr E, Zhang D, Bril V, The MBBQ Study Group. Neuropathy Total symptom Score-6 Questionnaire (NTSS-6) is a valid instrument for assessing the positive symptoms of diabetic peripheral neuropathy (DPN). Diabetes 2002; 51:A199.
104. Scholz J, Mannion RJ, Hord DE, et al. A novel tool for the assessment of pain: validation in low back pain. PLoS Med 2009;6:e1000047.
105. Spallone V, Morganti R, D'Amato C, et al. Clinical correlates of painful diabetic neuropathy and relationship of neuropathic pain with sensorimotor and autonomic nerve function. Eur J Pain 2011;15(2):153–60.
106. Young RJ. Structural functional interactions in the natural history of diabetic polyneuropathy: a key to the understanding of neuropathic pain? Diabet Med 1993; 10(Suppl 2):89S–90S.
107. Loeser JD, Treede RD. The Kyoto protocol of IASP basic pain terminology. Pain 2008;137:473–7.
108. Bouhassira D, Attal N, Fermanian J, et al. Development and validation of the neuropathic pain symptom inventory. Pain 2004;108:248–57.
109. Bennett MI, Smith BH, Torrance N, et al. The S-LANSS score for identifying pain of predominantly neuropathic origin: validation for use in clinical and postal research. J Pain 2005;6:149–58.
110. Krause S, Backonja M. Development of a neuropathic pain questionnaire. Clin J Pain 2003;19:306–14.

111. Bouhassira D, Attal N, Alchaar H, et al. Comparison of pain syndromes associated with nervous or somatic lesions and development of a new neuropathic pain diagnostic questionnaire (DN4). Pain 2005;114:29–36.

112. Freyhagen R, Baron R, Gockel U. Pain detect: a new screening questionnaire to detect neuropathic components in patients with back pain. Curr Med Res Opin 2006;22:1911–20.

113. Portenoy R. Development and testing of a neuropathic pain screening questionnaire: ID pain. Curr Med Res Opin 2006;22:1555–65.

114. Dworkin RH, Turk DC, Revicki DA, et al. Development and initial validation of an expanded and revised version of the Short-form McGill Pain Questionnaire (SF-MPQ-2). Pain 2009;144:35–42.

115. Daut RL, Cleeland CS, Flanery RC. Development of the Wisconsin Brief Pain Questionnaire to assess pain in cancer and other diseases. Pain 1983;17:197–210.

116. Dworkin RH, Turk DC, Wyrwich KW, et al. Interpreting the clinical importance of treatment outcomes in chronic pain clinical trials: IMMPACT recommendations. J Pain 2008;9:105–21.

117. Cruccu G, Truini A. Tools for assessing neuropathic pain. PLoS Med 2009;6: e1000045.

118. Stephenson DT, Arneric SP. Neuroimaging of pain: advances and future prospects. J Pain 2008;9:567–79.

119. Chao CC, Hsieh SC, Tseng MT, et al. Patterns of contact heat evoked potentials (CHEP) in neuropathy with skin denervation: correlation of CHEP amplitude with intraepidermal nerve fiber density. Clin Neurophysiol 2008;119:653–61.

120. Atherton DD, Facer P, Roberts KM, et al. Use of the novel Contact Heat Evoked Potential Stimulator (CHEPS) for the assessment of small fibre neuropathy: correlations with skin flare responses and intra-epidermal nerve fibre counts. BMC Neurol 2007;7:21.

121. Casanova-Molla J, Grau-Junyent JM, Morales M, et al. On the relationship between nociceptive evoked potentials and intraepidermal nerve fiber density in painful sensory polyneuropathies. Pain 2011;152:410–8.

122. Chao CC, Tseng MT, Lin YJ, et al. Pathophysiology of neuropathic pain in type 2 diabetes: skin denervation and contact heat-evoked potentials. Diabetes Care 2010;33:2654–9.

123. Finnerup NB, Otto M, McQuay HJ, et al. Algorithm for neuropathic pain treatment: an evidence based proposal. Pain 2005;118:289–305.

124. Finnerup NB, Sindrup SH, Jensen TS. The evidence for pharmacological treatment of neuropathic pain. Pain 2010;150:573–81.

125. Dworkin RH, O'Connor AB, Backonja M, et al. Pharmacologic management of neuropathic pain: evidence-based recommendations. Pain 2007;132:237–51.

126. Dworkin RH, O'Connor AB, Audette J, et al. Recommendations for the pharmacological management of neuropathic pain: an overview and literature update. Mayo Clin Proc 2010;85:S3–14.

127. Edelsberg J, Oster G. Summary measures of number needed to treat: how much clinical guidance do they provide in neuropathic pain? Eur J Pain 2009; 13:11–6.

128. Said G, Bigo A, Ameri A, et al. Uncommon early-onset neuropathy in diabetic patients. J Neurol 1998;245:61–8.

129. Dogrul A, Uzbay IT. Topical clonidine antinociception. Pain 2004;111:385–91.

130. Tesfaye S, Vileikyte L, Rayman G, et al. Painful diabetic peripheral neuropathy: consensus recommendations on diagnosis, assessment and management. Diabetes Metab Res Rev 2011;27:629–38.

131. Bril V, England J, Franklin GM, et al. Evidence-based guideline: treatment of painful diabetic neuropathy: report of the American Academy of Neurology, the American Association of Neuromuscular and Electrodiagnostic Medicine, and the American Academy of Physical Medicine and Rehabilitation. Neurology 2011;76:1758–65.
132. Vinik A. The approach to the management of the patient with neuropathic pain. J Clin Endocrinol Metab 2010;95:4802–11.
133. Ziegler D, Nowak H, Kempler P, et al. Treatment of symptomatic diabetic poly-neuropathy with the antioxidant alpha-lipoic acid: a meta-analysis. Diabet Med 2004;21:114–21.
134. Ziegler D, Low PA, Boulton AJ. Antioxidant treatment with alpha-lipoic acid in diabetic polyneuropathy: a 4-year randomized double-blind trial (NATHAN 1). Diabetologia 2011;50:S63.
135. Rains C, Bryson HM. Topical capsaicin. A review of its pharmacological proper-ties and therapeutic potential in post-herpetic neuralgia, diabetic neuropathy and osteoarthritis. Drugs Aging 1995;7:317–28.
136. Mason L, Moore RA, Derry S, et al. Systematic review of topical capsaicin for the treatment of chronic pain. BMJ 2004;328:991.
137. Backonja M, Wallace MS, Blonsky ER, et al. NGX-4010, a high-concentration capsaicin patch, for the treatment of postherpetic neuralgia: a randomised, double-blind study. Lancet Neurol 2008;7:1106–12.
138. Baron R, Mayoral V, Leijon G, et al. Efficacy and safety of combination therapy with 5% lidocaine medicated plaster and pregabalin in post-herpetic neuralgia and diabetic polyneuropathy. Curr Med Res Opin 2009;25:1677–87.
139. Jarvis B, Coukell AJ. Mexiletine. A review of its therapeutic use in painful dia-betic neuropathy. Drugs 1998;56:691–707.
140. Harati Y, Gooch C, Swenson M, et al. Double-blind randomized trial of tramadol for the treatment of the pain of diabetic neuropathy. Neurology 1998;50:1842–6.
141. Harati Y, Gooch C, Swenson M, et al. Maintenance of the long-term effective-ness of tramadol in treatment of the pain of diabetic neuropathy. J Diabetes Complications 2000;14:65–70.
142. Nelson KA, Park KM, Robinovitz E, et al. High-dose oral dextromethorphan versus placebo in painful diabetic neuropathy and postherpetic neuralgia. Neurology 1997;48:1212–8.
143. Sang CN. NMDA-receptor antagonists in neuropathic pain: experimental methods to clinical trials. J Pain Symptom Manage 2000;19:S21–5.
144. Watson CP, Moulin D, Watt-Watson J, et al. Controlled-release oxycodone re-lieves neuropathic pain: a randomized controlled trial in painful diabetic neurop-athy. Pain 2003;105:71–8.
145. Gilron I, Bailey JM, Tu D, et al. Morphine, gabapentin, or their combination for neuropathic pain. N Engl J Med 2005;352:1324–34.
146. Max M, Lynch S, Muir J. Effects of desipramine, amitriptyline and fluoxetine on pain in diabetic neuropathy. N Engl J Med 1992;326:1250–6.
147. Hardy T, Sachson R, Shen S, et al. Does treatment with duloxetine for neuro-pathic pain impact glycemic control? Diabetes Care 2007;30:21–6.
148. Sansone RA, Sansone LA. Pain, pain, go away: antidepressants and pain man-agement. Psychiatry (Edgmont) 2008;5:16–9.
149. Simpson DA. Gabapentin and venlafaxine for the treatment of painful diabetic neuropathy. J Clin Neuromuscul Dis 2001;3:53–62.
150. Blom S. Trigeminal neuralgia: its treatment with a new anticonvulsant drug (g-32883). Lancet 1962;21:839–40.

151. LaRoche SM, Helmers SL. The new antiepileptic drugs: scientific review. JAMA 2004;291:605–14.
152. Dworkin RH, Backonja M, Rowbotham MC, et al. Advances in neuropathic pain: diagnosis, mechanisms, and treatment recommendations. Arch Neurol 2003;60: 1524–34.
153. Landefeld CS, Steinman MA. The Neurontin legacy—marketing through misinformation and manipulation. N Engl J Med 2009;360:103–6.
154. Backonja M, Beydoun A, Edwards KR, et al. Gabapentin for the symptomatic treatment of painful neuropathy in patients with diabetes mellitus: a randomized controlled trial. JAMA 1998;280:1831–6.
155. DeToledo JC, Toledo C, DeCerce J, et al. Changes in body weight with chronic, high-dose gabapentin therapy. Ther Drug Monit 1997;19:394–6.
156. Lesser H, Sharma U, LaMoreaux L, et al. Pregabalin relieves symptoms of painful diabetic neuropathy: a randomized controlled trial. Neurology 2004;63: 2104–10.
157. Richter RW, Portenoy R, Sharma U, et al. Relief of painful diabetic peripheral neuropathy with pregabalin: a randomized, placebo-controlled trial. J Pain 2005;6:253–60.
158. Rosenstock J, Tuchman M, LaMoreaux L, et al. Pregabalin for the treatment of painful diabetic peripheral neuropathy: a double-blind, placebo-controlled trial. Pain 2004;110:628–38.
159. Freynhagen R, Strojek K, Griesing T, et al. Efficacy of pregabalin in neuropathic pain evaluated in a 12-week, randomised, double-blind, multicentre, placebo-controlled trial of flexible- and fixed-dose regimens. Pain 2005;115:254–63.
160. Freeman R, Durso-Decruz E, Emir B. Efficacy, safety, and tolerability of pregabalin treatment for painful diabetic peripheral neuropathy: findings from seven randomized, controlled trials across a range of doses. Diabetes Care 2008; 31:1448–54.
161. Kalso E. Sodium channel blockers in neuropathic pain. Curr Pharm Des 2005; 11:3005–11.
162. Dogra S, Beydoun S, Mazzola J, et al. Oxcarbazepine in painful diabetic neuropathy: a randomized, placebo-controlled study. Eur J Pain 2005;9:543–54.
163. Vinik AI. Diabetic neuropathies: endpoints in clinical research studies. In: LeRoith D, Vinik AI, editors. Contemporary endocrinology: controversies in treating diabetes: clinical and research aspects. Totowa (NJ): Humana Press; 2008. p. 135–56.
164. Pittenger G, Mehrabyan A, Simmons K, et al. Small fiber neuropathy is associated with the metabolic syndrome. Metab Syndr Relat Disord 2005;3:113–21.
165. Raskin P, Donofrio PD, Rosenthal NR, et al. Topiramate vs placebo in painful diabetic neuropathy: analgesic and metabolic effects. Neurology 2004;63: 865–73.
166. Quilici S, Chancellor J, Lothgren M, et al. Meta-analysis of duloxetine vs. pregabalin and gabapentin in the treatment of diabetic peripheral neuropathic pain. BMC Neurol 2009;9:6–19.
167. Burke J, Sanchez R, Joshi A, et al. Health care costs in patients with painful diabetic peripheral neuropathy prescribed pregabalin or duloxetine. Pain Pract 2012;12:209–18.
168. De Salas-Cansado M, Perez C, Saldana MT, et al. An economic evaluation of pregabalin versus usual care in the management of community-treated patients with refractory painful diabetic peripheral neuropathy in primary care settings. Prim Care Diabetes 2012;6:303–12.

169. Bellows BK, Dahal A, Jiao T, et al. A cost-utility analysis of pregabalin versus du-loxetine for the treatment of painful diabetic neuropathy. J Pain Palliat Care Pharmacother 2012;26:153–64.
170. Gilron I, Bailey JM, Tu D, et al. Nortriptyline and gabapentin, alone and in combination for neuropathic pain: a double-blind, randomised controlled crossover trial. Lancet 2009;374:1252–61.
171. Thethi TK, Fonseca VA, Lavery LA, et al. Metanx in Type 2 Diabetes with Peripheral Neuropathy, A Randomized Trial. Am J Med 2013;126(2):141–9.
172. Vinik AJ. A medicinal food provides food for thought in managing diabetic neuropathy. Am J Med 2013;126(2):95–6.
173. Piovesan EJ, Teive HG, Kowacs PA, et al. An open study of botulinum-A toxin treatment of trigeminal neuralgia. Neurology 2005;65:1306–8.
174. Tsai CP, Liu CY, Lin KP, et al. Efficacy of botulinum toxin type A in the relief of carpal tunnel syndrome: a preliminary experience. Clin Drug Investig 2006;26:511–5.
175. Pittler MH, Ernst E. Complementary therapies for neuropathic and neuralgic pain: systematic review. Clin J Pain 2008;24:731–3.
176. Tesfaye S. Painful diabetic neuropathy. Aetiology and nonpharmacological treatment. In: Veves A, editor. Clinical management of diabetic neuropathy. Totowa (NJ): Humana Press; 1998. p. 369–86.
177. Spallone V, Ziegler D, Freeman R, et al. Cardiovascular autonomic neuropathy in diabetes: clinical impact, assessment, diagnosis, and management. Diabetes Metab Res Rev 2011;27:639–53.
178. Maser RE, Mitchell BD, Vinik AI, et al. The association between cardiovascular autonomic neuropathy and mortality in individuals with diabetes: a meta-analysis. Diabetes Care 2003;26:1895–901.
179. Ziegler D, Zentai CP, Perz S, et al. Prediction of mortality using measures of cardiac autonomic dysfunction in the diabetic and nondiabetic population: the MONICA/KORA Augsburg Cohort Study. Diabetes Care 2008;31:556–61.
180. Lykke JA, Tarnow L, Parving HH, et al. A combined abnormality in heart rate variation and QT corrected interval is a strong predictor of cardiovascular death in type 1 diabetes. Scand J Clin Lab Invest 2008;68:654–9.
181. Hage FG, Iskandrian AE. Cardiovascular imaging in diabetes mellitus. J Nucl Cardiol 2011;18:959–65.
182. Burgos LG, Ebert TJ, Assiddao C, et al. Increased intraoperative cardiovascular morbidity in diabetics with autonomic neuropathy. Anesthesiology 1989;70:591–7.
183. Kitamura A, Hoshino T, Kon T, et al. Patients with diabetic neuropathy are at risk of a greater intraoperative reduction in core temperature. Anesthesiology 2000;92:1311–8.
184. The definition of orthostatic hypotension, pure autonomic failure, and multiple system atrophy. J Auton Nerv Syst 1996;58:123–4.
185. Low PA, Walsh JC, Huang CY, et al. The sympathetic nervous system in diabetic neuropathy. A clinical and pathological study. Brain 1975;98:341–56.
186. Gaede P, Vedel P, Parving HH, et al. Intensified multifactorial intervention in patients with type 2 diabetes mellitus and microalbuminuria: the Steno type 2 randomized study. Lancet 1999;353:617–22.

Relationships Between Diabetes and Cognitive Impairment

Suzanne M. de la Monte, MD, MPH[a,b,c,d,*]

KEYWORDS

- Diabetes • Insulin resistance • Cognitive impairment • Neurodegeneration
- Alzheimer disease • Insulin sensitizers • Obesity

KEY POINTS

- Alzheimer disease is a neurodegenerative disease associated with impairments in glucose metabolism and insulin resistance in the brain.
- Many of the molecular and biochemical defects in Alzheimer disease are identical to those in either type 1 or type 2 diabetes mellitus as well as other insulin-resistance disease states.
- Peripheral insulin-resistance disease states, including diabetes, obesity, and nonalcoholic fatty liver disease, are associated with cognitive impairment and can exacerbate Alzheimer disease, (ie, cause it to progress).
- Therapeutic measures used for diabetes show efficacy in the early and moderate stages of Alzheimer disease.
- Endocrinologists and diabetologists should play a larger role in the early detection and monitoring of cognitive impairment in obese and/or diabetic patients.

INTRODUCTION

Like most organ systems throughout the body, the brain requires insulin and insulinlike growth factors (IGFs) to maintain energy metabolism, cell survival, and homeostasis. In addition, insulin and IGFs support neuronal plasticity and cholinergic functions,

This article originally appeared in Endocrinology and Metabolism Clinics of North America, Volume 43, Issue 1, March 2014.

The author has no competing interests.

Funding sources are grants AA-11431 and AA-12908 from the National Institutes of Health.

[a] Department of Pathology (Neuropathology), Rhode Island Hospital, Warren Alpert Medical School of Brown University, Providence, RI, USA; [b] Department of Neurology, Rhode Island Hospital, Warren Alpert Medical School of Brown University, Providence, RI, USA; [c] Department of Neurosurgery, Rhode Island Hospital, Warren Alpert Medical School of Brown University, Providence, RI, USA; [d] Department of Medicine, Rhode Island Hospital, Warren Alpert Medical School of Brown University, Providence, RI, USA
* Pierre Galletti Research Building, Rhode Island Hospital, 55 Claverick Street, 4th Floor, Room 419, Providence, RI 02903.
E-mail address: Suzanne_DeLaMonte_MD@Brown.edu

Clinics Collections 1 (2014) 341–363
http://dx.doi.org/10.1016/j.ccol.2014.08.018

which are needed for learning, memory, and myelin maintenance. Impairments in insulin and IGF signaling, caused by receptor resistance or ligand deficiency, disrupt energy balance and disable networks that support a broad range of brain functions. Over the past several years, evidence that impairment in brain insulin and IGF signaling mediates cognitive impairment and neurodegeneration has grown, particularly in relation to mild cognitive impairment and Alzheimer disease (AD). Although amyloid deposits and phospho-tau–associated neuronal cytoskeletal lesions account for some AD-associated brain abnormalities, they do not explain the prominent and well-documented deficits in brain metabolism that begin very early in the course of the disease. Metabolic derangements in AD are similar to those in both type 1 type and 2 diabetes mellitus. However, the consequences of insulin/IGF receptor resistance and ligand deficiency include cognitive impairment and neurodegeneration caused by deficits in signaling through progrowth, proplasticity, and prosurvival pathways.

How brain insulin/IGF resistance and deficiency develop is not completely understood. Although a considerable number of studies have linked the recently increased rates of AD to other insulin resistance states, including obesity, type 2 diabetes mellitus (T2DM), nonalcoholic fatty liver disease (NAFLD), and metabolic syndrome, it is important to realize that most cases of sporadic (nonfamilial) AD arise with no evidence of peripheral insulin-resistance disease. This review focuses on how peripheral insulin-resistance diseases, including diabetes mellitus, contribute to cognitive impairment and neurodegeneration. The working hypothesis is that peripheral insulin resistance promotes or exacerbates cognitive impairment and neurodegeneration by causing brain insulin resistance. Mechanistically, insulin resistance with dysregulated lipid metabolism leads to increased inflammation, cytotoxic lipid production, oxidative and endoplasmic reticulum (ER) stress, and worsening of insulin resistance. Some investigators are researching the role of cytotoxic ceramides that can promote inflammation, oxidative stress, and insulin resistance. Ceramides generated in liver or visceral fat can leak into peripheral blood because of local cellular injury or death, cross the blood-brain barrier, and initiate or propagate a cascade of neurodegeneration mediated by brain insulin resistance, inflammation, stress, and cell death (**Fig. 1**). These concepts help delineate the strategies needed to detect, monitor, treat, and prevent AD as well as other major insulin-resistance diseases.

INSULIN SIGNALING
The Master Hormone

Insulin is a 5800 Da, 51 amino acid polypeptide, composed of A (21 residues) and B (30 residues) chains linked by disulfide bonds. Banting, Best and others are credited for discovering insulin in pancreatic secretions,[1,2] and later it was shown that it reversed hyperglycemia.[3] Nearly 30 years later, methods to stabilize insulin, prolong its actions, and delay its absorption emerged; 50 years after its discovery, 99% pure insulin, free of proinsulin and other islet polypeptides, was produced.[4] Genetic engineering and yeast fermentation technology have enabled human insulin to be efficiently produced on a large scale.[5] The field continues to evolve, with some of the latest advances directed toward replacing injectable insulin with an oral form[6] and optimizing approaches for intranasal delivery of insulin to treat diabetes or cognitive impairment (see later discussion).[7–9]

Insulin-Stimulated Effects

The main targets of insulin stimulation include skeletal muscle, adipose tissue, and liver, although virtually all organs, tissues, and cell types are responsive to insulin.

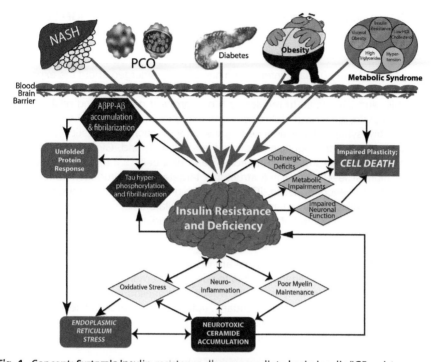

Fig. 1. Concept: Systemic Insulin-resistance diseases mediate brain insulin/IGF resistance and neurodegeneration. In T2DM, nonalcoholic steatohepatitis (NASH), visceral obesity, and metabolic syndrome, dysregulated lipid metabolism causes oxidative stress and increased levels of toxic lipids, such as ceramides, which can cross the blood-brain barrier to promote brain insulin resistance. The molecular and biochemical consequences of brain insulin resistance are nearly identical to those in non–central nervous system organs and tissues (ie, oxidative stress, inflammation, ER stress, metabolic impairments, and local accumulations of neurotoxic lipids, [eg, ceramides]). However, the structural consequences are that the brain undergoes atrophy with progressive cell loss, white matter fiber and myelin degeneration, and synaptic disconnection, leading to impairments in learning and memory. Ultimately, a self-reinforcing cycle of neurodegeneration gets established, making it impossible to halt neurodegeneration by one mechanism. Instead, multipronged efforts must be used, including treatment of systemic insulin-resistance diseases. AβPP, amyloid-beta precursor protein; HDL, high-density lipoprotein; PCO, polycystic ovarian syndrome.

Insulin regulates glucose uptake and utilization by cells and free fatty acid levels in peripheral blood. Free fatty acids are substrates for generating complex lipids. In skeletal muscle, insulin stimulates glucose uptake by inducing translocation of the glucose transporter protein, GLUT4, from the Golgi to the plasma membrane.[10] In liver, insulin stimulates lipogenesis and triglyceride storage and inhibits gluconeogenesis. In adipose tissue, insulin decreases lipolysis and fatty acid efflux.[11] These prometabolic effects of insulin on glucose and free fatty acid disposal help to maintain energy balance.

IGFs

Insulin is closely related to IGF-1, which is also referred to as *somatomedin C* or *mechano growth factor*.[12,13] IGF-1 regulates growth during development and exerts anabolic effects on mature organs and tissues. IGF-1 contains 70 amino acids

(7649 Da) in a single chain with 3 intramolecular disulfide bridges.[12,13] IGF-1 and IGF-2 are abundantly produced in liver and regulated by IGF-binding proteins.[14]

Insulin and IGF Signaling in the Brain

Within the last 15 to 20 years, information has steadily emerged about the expression and function of insulin and IGF polypeptides and receptors in the brain. It is now known that insulin and IGF signal to regulate a broad array of neuronal and glial activities, including growth, survival, metabolism, gene expression, protein synthesis, cytoskeletal assembly, synapse formation, neurotransmitter function, and plasticity,[15,16] which are needed to support cognitive function. Insulin, IGF-1, and IGF-2 polypeptide and receptor genes are expressed in neurons[15] and glial cells[17,18] throughout the brain; but their highest levels are within structures targeted by neurodegeneration.[15,19,20] Since genes that encode insulin, IGFs, and insulin-like peptides and their receptors have been identified in human, rodent, and drosophila brains,[21] related signaling networks allow for local control of diverse functions, including energy metabolism.

Insulin and IGF Signal Transduction

Brain insulin/IGF signaling mechanisms are virtually the same as in other organs. The networks are activated by ligand binding to specific receptors and subsequent activation of receptor tyrosine kinases and downstream signaling through insulin receptor substrate (IRS) proteins. The attendant activation of phosphoinositol-3-kinase (PI3K)-Akt and extracellular mitogen-activated protein kinase and the inhibition of glycogen synthase kinase 3β (GSK-3β) promote growth, survival, metabolism, and plasticity and inhibit apoptosis.[20]

INSULIN RESISTANCE AND NEURODEGENERATION
Insulin Resistance and its Consequences

Insulin resistance is classically defined as the state in which high levels of circulating insulin (hyperinsulinemia) are associated with hyperglycemia. The concept has broadened to include organ- and tissue-related impairments in insulin signaling associated with reduced activation of the pathways. As a result, progressively higher levels of ligand are needed to achieve normal insulin actions.[10] However, sustained high levels of insulin can cause insulin resistance,[22] thereby worsening and possibly broadening tissue involvement. Furthermore, hyperinsulinemia impairs insulin secretion from β cells in pancreatic islets, yielding hybrid states of both insulin resistance and insulin deficiency.[22]

Long-term consequences of insulin resistance include cellular energy failure (lack of fuel), elevated plasma lipids, and hypertension. In addition, chronic hyperinsulinemia vis-à-vis normoglycemia predicts future development of diabetes mellitus.[23] Insulin resistance is an independent predictor of serious diseases, including cerebrovascular and cardiovascular disease, hypertension, and malignancy.[24–28] Insulin resistance is now front and center stage because of its link to obesity, T2DM, NAFLD, metabolic syndrome, polycystic ovarian disease, age-related macular degeneration, and AD epidemics (**Fig. 2**).

AD Occurrence and Clinical Diagnosis

AD is the most common cause of dementia in North America. Sporadic AD has no clear genetic transmission and accounts for more than 90% of the cases. In contrast, familial (heritable) AD accounts for 5% to 10% of all cases. Over the past few decades, sporadic AD has become epidemic, raising questions about environmental and lifestyle mediators of cognitive impairment and neurodegeneration.[29] Although the clinical diagnosis of AD is based on criteria set by the National Institute of Neurologic

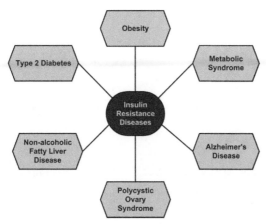

Fig. 2. Spectrum of insulin-resistance diseases affecting different primary target organs. Overlap among these diseases occurs frequently, and rates have increased with the obesity epidemic.

and Communicative Disorders and Stroke, the Alzheimer's Disease and Related Disorders Association, and the *Diagnostic and Statistical Manual of Mental Disorders* (Fourth Edition),[30] neuroimaging and a few biomarker panels have facilitated the detection of early brain metabolic derangements in AD.[31]

AD Neuropathology

Neuropathologic hallmarks of AD include neuronal loss, abundant accumulations of abnormal, hyperphosphorylated cytoskeletal proteins in neuronal perikarya and dystrophic fibers, and increased expression and abnormal processing of amyloid-beta precursor protein (AβPP), leading to AβPP-Aβ peptide deposition in neurons, plaques, and vessels. A definitive diagnosis of AD requires more-than-normal aging densities of neurofibrillary tangles, neuritic plaques, and AβPP-Aβ deposits in the brain but particularly in corticolimbic structures (**Figs. 3–5**). The pathognomonic molecular abnormalities that correspond with these dementia-associated structural lesions include accumulations of insoluble aggregates of abnormally phosphorylated and ubiquitinated tau, and neurotoxic AβPP-Aβ as oligomers, fibrillar aggregates, or plaques. Secreted neurotoxic AβPP-Aβ oligomers inhibit synaptic plasticity, learning, and memory via impairments in hippocampal long-term potentiation.[32]

AD is a Metabolic Disease with Brain Insulin/IGF Resistance

For the better part of the last 3 decades, AD research was largely focused on the pathogenic roles of hyperphosphorylated tau and AβPP-Aβ, despite hints that insulin resistance and metabolic dysfunction were important factors.[33,34] With the wealth of data collected over the past 8 to10 years, it is fair to state that AD should be regarded as a metabolic disease that is mediated by brain insulin and IGF resistance.[35,36] This concept is supported by the findings that AD shares many features in common with systemic insulin-resistance diseases. For example, reduced insulin-stimulated growth and survival signaling, increased oxidative stress, proinflammatory cytokine activation, mitochondrial dysfunction, and impaired energy metabolism all occur in peripheral insulin-resistance diseases as well as in AD (**Table 1**).[20,37,38] In the early stages of disease, AD is marked by reductions in cerebral glucose utilization[39–41]; as AD progresses, brain metabolic derangements,[42,43] including impairments in insulin

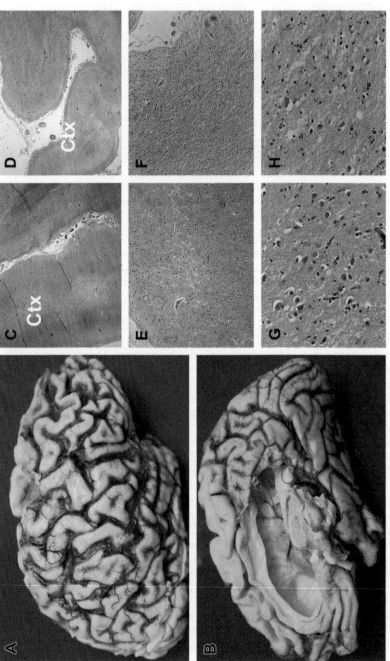

Fig. 3. Human brain with severe AD showing extreme atrophy of the cortex with thinning of gyri *(tan curvy hill-like structures)* and widening of sulci *(grooves between gyri)*. (A) Lateral surface of right hemisphere–frontal lobe to right, parietal is toward the middle, occipital to left, and temporal at the base. (B) Same half-brain as in (A) showing medial surface with frontal pole to the left, occipital on the right. Frontal, parietal, and temporal lobes are markedly atrophic. (C, E, G) Represent histologic images of the left temporal lobe and (D, F, H) represent the right temporal lobe shown at low (C, D), medium (E, F) and high (G, H) magnifications to illustrate more severe atrophy of the cortex (Ctx) with extensive replacement of neurons in the right compared with left temporal lobe. Note absence (loss) of large neuronal cell bodies in (H) compared with (G). Both sides are severely damaged; but asymmetry is not uncommon, meaning that neurodegeneration does not arise in all brain regions or progress in both hemispheres at the same time ([C–H] Luxol fast blue, hematoxylin-eosin, original magnifications: C, D = ×20; E, F = ×100; G, H = ×400).

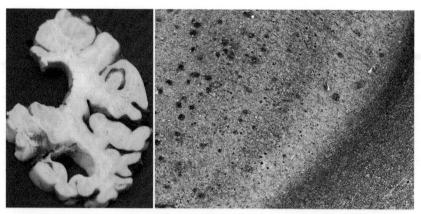

Fig. 4. Left: Coronal section through the right cerebral hemisphere showing extreme atrophy of the hippocampus, thalamus, and white matter, with compensatory enlargement of the ventricles. Right: Histologic section through the hippocampus stained to illustrate abundant senile plaques and neurofibrillary tangles replacing the normal architecture (Bielschowsky silver impregnation) (original magnification ×100).

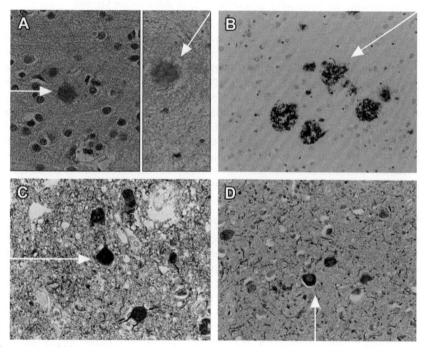

Fig. 5. Typical histopathologic lesions in AD. Arrows point to the following: (*A*) dense core plaques in cerebral cortex (*Congo red*); (*B*) amyloid precursor protein-amyloid beta (AβPP-Aβ) immunoreactivity in cortical plaques; (*C*) phospho-tau immunoreactive neurofibrillary tangles accumulated in cortical neurons; and (*D*) ubiquitin immunostained neurofibrillary tangles in neurons. Fine dotlike and linear structures in the background neutrophil of (*C, D*) represent dystrophic neuritis. Immunoreactivity was detected with biotinylated secondary antibody, horseradish peroxidase conjugated streptavidin, and diaminobenzidine (brown precipitate). Background structures were stained with hematoxylin (original magnifications: *A, C, D* = ×200; *B* = ×100).

Table 1
Mechanisms and consequences of cellular injury and degeneration in insulin-resistance diseases

Mediator of Injury	Mechanisms and Consequences of Injury
Inflammation	Activation of proinflammatory cytokines
Stress	ER, oxidative, and nitrosative stress; DNA, RNA, protein damage and adduct formation
Cell injury/death	Activation of proapoptosis pathways
Metabolic deficiencies	Dysregulated lipid metabolism, lipid peroxidation
Mitochondrial dysfunction	Reduced ATP production, increased reactive oxygen species
Vascular	Stress and mechanical injuy, ischemic tissue damage, end-organ hypertensive injury with microhemorrhages and toxin exposure

signaling, insulin-responsive gene expression, glucose utilization, and energy production, and stress worsen.[35,36,44]

Brain Insulin and IGF Resistance and Deficiency in AD-Human Studies

Human postmortem studies have convincingly shown that brain insulin resistance with reduced activation of receptors and downstream neuronal survival and plasticity mechanisms are consistent and fundamental abnormalities in AD.[35,36,44] Importantly, IGF-1 and IGF-2 networks were also found to be impaired,[35,36] meaning that their crosstalk functions were also deficient. Deficits in brain insulin and IGF signaling worsen as AD progresses,[35] along with declines in brain energy production, gene expression, and plasticity.[33] One of the most important realizations from these studies was that nearly all of the critical features of AD, including the activation of the kinases responsible for aberrant phosphorylation of tau and formation of neurofibrillary tangles, dystrophic neuritic plaques and neutrophil threads, AβPP and accumulation and toxicity, oxidative and endoplasmic reticulum stress, mitochondrial dysfunction, and cholinergic dyshomeostasis, can be explained by brain insulin/IGF resistance.

Does AD = Type 3 Diabetes?

Although the term type 3 diabetes is controversial, it serves to inform that the fundamental abnormalities in AD are quite similar to those present in type 1 and type 2 diabetes, except the primary target is the brain.[35,36] Like type 1 diabetes (T1DM) in which insulin deficiency is the underlying problem, in AD, neuronal expression of insulin polypeptide gene and insulin levels in brain and cerebrospinal fluid (CSF) are reduced.[34–36] As in T2DM, which has insulin resistance at its core, early AD is marked by insulin resistance and desensitization of insulin receptors in the brain; as AD progresses, these deficits worsen. In essence, AD can be regarded as a brain form of diabetes that has elements of both insulin resistance (T2DM) and insulin deficiency (T1DM). Although T1DM and T2DM can be associated with cognitive impairment and drive the onset or worsen the clinical course of AD, it is important to know that AD often occurs in people who do not have diabetes mellitus (**Table 2**). The notion that AD is a diabetes-type metabolic disease that is mediated by brain insulin and IGF resistance is further supported by human and experimental studies showing neuroprotective effects of glucagonlike peptide-1,[45] IGF-1,[46] and caloric restriction[47] with respect to brain aging and insulin resistance.

Table 2			
Comparison of T1DM, T2DM, and type 3 diabetes			
Target Effects	**T1DM**	**T2DM**	**Type 3 Diabetes**
Insulin ligand	Reduced	Increased	Reduced
Insulin receptor	Unaffected or increased	Reduced activation	Reduced activation and expression
Glucose utilization	Decreased	Decreased	Decreased
Primary targets	Pancreas, (brain)	Skeletal muscle, adipose tissue, vessels	Brain: neurons, white matter
Secondary targets	Brain, retina, blood vessels, kidneys, skin, peripheral and autonomic nerves	Brain, blood vessels, kidneys, peripheral and autonomic nerves, retina, skin	Brain satiety centers with increased proneness to obesity

The inclusion of AD within the spectrum of insulin-resistance diseases opens doors for endocrinologists and specifically diabetologists to detect disease earlier in patients with overlapping organ-system involvement and also helps design and monitor the effects of treatment. The wealth of clinical, translational, and basic science data accrued by experts in the field could be extended to AD to accelerate the development of programs to better control and possibly cure AD. Similarly, the clustering of other insulin-resistance diseases, such as metabolic syndrome, NAFLD, and polycystic ovarian disease, under one analytical roof could lead to better management of these diseases and also increase the likelihood that their causes could be found.

Experimental Evidence that Type 3 Diabetes = Sporadic AD

Experimental intracerebroventricular injections of streptozotocin, a prodiabetes drug, produce deficits in brain energy metabolism,[48] impairments in spatial learning and memory, brain insulin resistance, brain insulin deficiency, and AD-type neurodegeneration but not diabetes mellitus.[48,49] In contrast, intraperitoneal or intravenous administration of streptozotocin causes diabetes mellitus with mild hepatic steatosis and modest degrees of neurodegeneration.[50,51] Therefore, these experiments unequivocally demonstrate that brain diabetes (type 3) can occur independent of T1DM and T2DM and vice versa (**Fig. 6**).

Because streptozotocin is a nitrosamine-related toxin, which may be highly relevant to its overall effects, the specific consequences of brain insulin and IGF resistance are not tested by models generated with this and related compounds. To address this point, further studies were performed using small interfering RNA (siRNA) duplex molecules to silence insulin or IGF receptor expression in the brain.[52] This approach avoided the genotoxic and nitrosative damage produced by streptozotocin.[50] The inhibition of brain insulin and IGF receptor expression with siRNA molecules was found to be sufficient to cause cognitive impairment and hippocampal degeneration with AD-type impairments in protein and gene expression.[52] However, the phenotype was mild compared with the effects of streptozotocin. Therefore, oxidative and nitrosative damage may also be needed to produce a model that is entirely reflective of sporadic AD in humans.

Metabolic Deficits in AD: the Starving Brain

Insulin and IGF signaling regulate glucose utilization and ATP production in the brain. In AD, deficits in cerebral glucose utilization and metabolism occur early and before

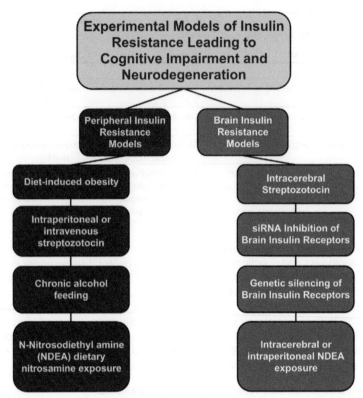

Fig. 6. Experimental models of peripheral and brain insulin resistance that lead to neurodegeneration. siRNA, small interfering RNA.

cognitive decline.[53] Therefore, impairments in brain insulin signaling are probably pivotal to AD pathogenesis.[36] Oxidative stress stemming from insulin resistance or other superimposed diseases can damage mitochondria, further impairing electron transport and ATP production. In addition, oxidative stress activates proinflammatory networks that cause organelle dysfunction; disinhibits proapoptosis mechanisms; stimulates AβPP expression[54] and cleavage to neurotoxic fibrils[55]; and activates GSK-3β, which promotes tau phosphorylation (**Table 3**).[15,35,56]

The glucose transporter 4 (GLUT4) mediates glucose uptake in the brain,[57] which is abundantly expressed along with insulin receptors in the medial temporal lobe and other targets of AD.[15,20] Insulin stimulates GLUT4 mRNA expression and GLUT4 protein trafficking from the Golgi to the plasma membrane where it engages in glucose uptake. In AD, because GLUT4 expression is preserved,[36] deficits in brain glucose utilization and energy metabolism vis-à-vis brain insulin/IGF resistance could be mediated in part by functional impairments in GLUT4 (ie, posttranslational mechanisms responsible for GLUT4 trafficking to the plasma membrane).

Chronic Ischemic Cerebral Microvascular Disease

Cerebral microvascular disease is a consistent feature of AD, and recognized mediator of cognitive impairment (**Fig. 7**). Postmortem studies demonstrated similar degrees of dementia in people with severe classical AD and those with moderate AD plus chronic ischemic encephalopathy. The ischemic injury mainly consists of

Table 3
Role of insulin resistance or insulin deficiency in the molecular and pathologic features of AD

Alzheimer Pathology	Role of Insulin Resistance/Deficiency
Phospho-tau neuronal cytoskeletal lesions	Increased activation of GSK-3β caused by inhibition of insulin signaling and increased oxidative stress
Amyloid pathology	Formation of toxic amyloid-beta soluble oligomeric fibrils
Cell injury/death	Activation of proapoptosis pathways; inhibition of prosurvival mechanisms; increased endoplasmic reticulum, oxidative, and nitrosative stress; macromolecular adducts
Impaired glucose utilization	Reduced glucose uptake, impaired GLUT4 function, reduced signaling downstream of the insulin receptor through IRS, PI3K, and Akt
Impaired learning and memory	Inhibition of growth pathways needed for synapse formation and remodeling, reduced cholinergic and other neurotransmitter functions, impaired neurogenesis
Microvascular disease	Hyperinsulinemia in T2DM, possibly local insulin resistance
White matter atrophy	Cerebral microvascular disease, inhibition of myelin maintenance by oligodendrocytes
Cholinergic functional deficits	Inhibition of choline acetyltransferase expression, which is regulated by insulin/IGF-1
Mitochondrial dysfunction	Oxidative stress-induced DNA damage leading to reduced ATP production and increased levels of reactive oxygen species
Neuroinflammation	Activation of proinflammatory cytokines

multifocal small infarcts and leukoaraiosis (ie, extensive white matter fiber attrition with pallor of myelin staining) and prominent cerebral microvascular disease (see **Fig. 7**; **Fig. 8**).[58] T2DM and hypertension cause microvascular disease throughout the body, including the brain. Evidence that microvascular disease contributes to neurodegeneration was suggested by the finding that the medial temporal lobe, which houses the hippocampus, undergoes progressive atrophy with advancing stages of T2DM.[59] Perhaps the regular finding of chronic ischemic leukoencephalopathy (white matter atrophy and fiber degeneration) with microvascular disease in AD is just another manifestation of brain diabetes. It is noteworthy that besides the impairments in brain glucose metabolism, white matter atrophy is one of the earliest abnormalities in AD.[60]

Hyperinsulinemia causes progressive injury to microvessels. Chronic microvascular injury is characterized by reactive proliferation of endothelial cells, thickening of the intima, fibrosis of the media, and narrowing of the lumens. Mural scarring reduces vascular compliance and compromises blood flow and nutrient delivery, particularly in periods of high metabolic demand. Moreover, weakened and damaged blood vessels are leaky and permeable to toxins,[61,62] which together could contribute to increased frequencies of microhemorrhage and perivascular white matter tissue loss in T2DM and AD. Therefore, hyperinsulinemia ultimately produces a state of chronic hypoperfusion with toxic/metabolic/ischemic tissue degeneration in the brain. These pathologic processes have not received adequate attention, and their mechanistic links to cognitive impairment in diabetes and AD are only in the rudimentary stages of investigation.

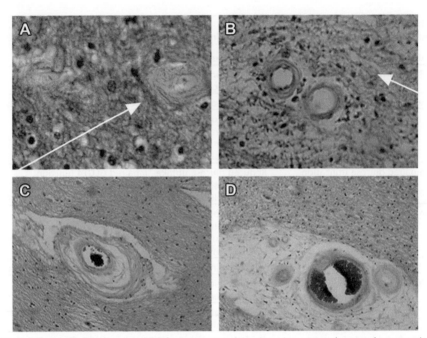

Fig. 7. Microvascular disease contributes to cognitive impairment and neurodegeneration in AD. (A) Arteriolosclerosis and capillary sclerosis are associated with fibrotic thickening of vessel walls and extreme narrowing of the lumens (arrow). (B) Arteriosclerosis results in chronic ischemic injury with rarefaction of white matter fibers (loss of dense Luxol fast blue myelin staining in vicinity of blood vessels [arrow]). Note fibrosis of vessel walls and perivascular microhemorrhages in center. These abnormalities reflect increased stiffness and reduce vascular compliance, together with weakness and leakiness of vascular walls. (C) Marked fibrotic thickening and damage to vessel wall caused by destruction (clearing) of the media. Tissue surrounding vessel in center is lost. Adjacent myelin is stained blue (Luxol fast blue). (D) Large area of perivascular tissue loss and further pallor adjacent to lacunar infarct. Note small vessels with tiny lumens and rigid fibrotic vessels in the middle of the perivascular lacunar infarct ([A–D] Luxol fast blue, hematoxylin-eosin).

BRAIN METABOLIC DERANGEMENTS IN OTHER NEURODEGENERATIVE DISEASES

Advances in neuroimaging, including positron emission tomography, magnetic resonance imaging (MRI), functional MRI, and magnetic spectroscopy, together with molecular and biochemical biomarkers have helped demonstrate the common themes surrounding disease mechanisms among clinically and pathologically diverse sets of neurodegenerative diseases.[63–65] For example, like AD, other major neurodegenerative diseases are associated with deficits in brain metabolism. Parkinson-dementia with Lewy bodies (DLB), frontotemporal lobar dementia, motor neuron disease, and multiple systems atrophy are all associated with brain accumulations of misfolded ubiquitinated proteins (often cytoskeletal) and increased levels of oxidative stress, neuroinflammation, autophagy, mitochondrial dysfunction, apoptosis, and necrosis.[66–70] Parkinson disease (PD) has epidemiologic links to diabetes mellitus,[45] and experimental PD is associated with insulin resistance in the basal ganglia.[71] Finally, impairments in insulin and IGF signaling exist in human brains with PD or DLB, although the nature and distribution of abnormalities differ from those in AD.[72] Therefore, many sporadic human neurodegenerative diseases could potentially be

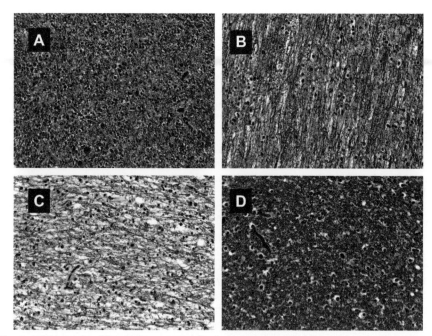

Fig. 8. White matter fiber loss in AD. Myelin is produced by oligodendrocytes, which are insulin and IGF-1 responsive. Insulin resistance impairs oligodendrocyte function. In AD, brain insulin/IGF-1 resistance develop early in the course of neurodegeneration, and the earliest abnormalities include impairments in glucose metabolism and white matter atrophy. White matter from the (*A*) anterior frontal, (*B*) posterior frontal, (*C*) parietal, and (*D*) occipital lobes (Luxol fast blue). The normal appearance of staining is depicted in (*D*), an area least affected by AD. The pink coloration in (*A, B*) reflect loss of myelin and myelinated fibers. The extreme pallor of myelin staining in (*C*) corresponds to the severity of neurodegeneration and extensive fiber loss.

approached from diagnostic and therapeutic perspectives through knowledge gained in endocrinology and specifically diabetology.

UNDERLYING CAUSES OF BRAIN INSULIN RESISTANCE IN AD
Aging

Insulin and IGF resistance increase with aging, whereas longevity is associated with the preservation of insulin/IGF responsiveness.[73–75] Furthermore, evidence suggests that chronic stress over a lifespan damages cells because of excessive signaling through insulin/IGF-1 receptors.[76] Correspondingly, neuronal overexpression of IRS2 leads to increased fat mass, insulin resistance, and glucose intolerance with aging.[77] These findings suggest that chronic overuse of insulin/IGF signaling networks, which occurs with hyperinsulinemia and insulin resistance, accelerates aging.

Declines in growth hormone levels and metabolism also promote aging because of the anabolic deficiencies that accelerate metabolic dysfunction.[78] Because growth hormone deficiency promotes obesity[79] and obesity promotes insulin resistance and hyperinsulinemia, aging-associated declines in growth hormone could be a cause of insulin resistance.[80] Because this concept is broadly applicable to insulin resistance–related degenerative diseases, efforts should be made to improve our understanding of cellular aging, with the goal of preventing or delaying the onset of neurodegeneration.

Arguments could be made that insulin resistance, cognitive impairment, and AD are inevitable consequences of aging[81] because aging-associated chronic low-grade inflammation[82,83] causes insulin resistance.[83,84] Because inflammation and insulin resistance increase oxidative stress, over time, reactive oxygen species and advanced glycation end-products accumulate, driving mitochondrial dysfunction, DNA damage, and cell death cascades,[80] which are pivotal to aging-associated cognitive impairment and brain atrophy.

On the other hand, opposing arguments offer an alternative perspective and suggest that other intrinsic host factors, lifetime exposures, and lifestyle choices dictate the quality of aging and propensity to develop insulin-resistance diseases. An excellent example of this phenomenon exists with respect to postpolio syndrome, in which people who recovered from childhood poliomyelitis exhibit high rates of motor neuron disease as middle-aged adults.[85,86] During childhood, recovery from poliomyelitis was enabled by the vigorous regenerative and reparative activities of the youthful plastic central nervous system (CNS). However, with aging, the regenerative capacity of the CNS declines. Individuals develop postpolio motor neuron disease because the underlying previously damaged motor neuron system gets exposed, resulting in significant weakness caused by denervation myopathy.[87,88] In contrast, aging of the previously undamaged CNS results in mild weakness and reduced mobility; this suggests that chronic enrichment and protection of neuronal circuitry may be required to maintain excellent brain function throughout the normal human lifespan.

Lifestyle Choices and Aging

Obesity, T2DM, NAFLD/nonalcoholic steatohepatitis (NASH), metabolic syndrome, and AD have grown in prevalence to epidemic proportions in many societies.[29,89,90] In recent years, countries throughout the world have witnessed rapid increases in the prevalence rates of insulin-resistance diseases and their consequences in nonaged individuals, including adolescents and children.[81] These trends have been linked to obesity and sedentary lifestyles. Because the spectra of insulin resistance–related diseases are nearly identical across different age groups, it could be argued that certain lifestyles, habits, and behaviors cause disease by accelerating aging. By the same token, lifestyle modifications could potentially retard aging and defer or prevent aging-associated insulin-resistance diseases, including neurodegeneration.

Obesity and Cognitive Impairment

Obesity significantly increases the risk for cognitive impairment and leads to brain insulin resistance because of the disruption of homeostatic mechanisms.[11,91–93] Concerns about obesity's effects on the brain arose from studies showing an increased risk for mild cognitive impairment (MCI) or AD-type dementia in individuals with glucose intolerance, deficits in insulin secretion, T2DM, obesity/dyslipidemic disorders, or NASH.[20,94–96] Other studies correlated obesity with deficits in executive function[96,97] and eventual development of AD.[98] These concepts were confirmed in experimental animal models of diet-induced obesity with T2DM.[47,91,99,100] Perhaps the most convincing evidence that obesity contributes to cognitive impairment was provided by studies showing that weight-loss reversal of insulin resistance improves cognitive performance[101,102] and neuropsychiatric function[103] and that adherence to Mediterranean diets reduces metabolic risk for AD.[104]

T2DM

The molecular and biochemical abnormalities in AD mimic the effects of T2DM on skeletal muscle and NASH on liver. Epidemiologic and longitudinal studies demonstrated increased risks for MCI or AD in people with glucose intolerance, T2DM, obesity/dyslipidemic disorders, or deficits in insulin secretion.[105–107] More recently, investigators linked increased rates of cognitive impairment to chronic hyperglycemia,[108] which precedes the diagnosis of T2DM. Similarly, postmortem studies revealed that peripheral insulin resistance contributes to cognitive impairment and AD progression,[109,110] whereas experimental studies showed that diet-induced obesity with T2DM leads to deficits in spatial learning and memory,[99] brain atrophy with brain insulin resistance, neuroinflammation, oxidative stress, and deficits in cholinergic function.[91,111]

NAFLD/NASH

Several studies have shown that cognitive impairment and neuropsychiatric dysfunction occur with steatohepatitis caused by obesity, alcohol abuse, chronic hepatitis C virus infection, Reyes syndrome, or nitrosamine exposure.[111–114] Mechanistically, steatohepatitis (ie, inflammation with fatty liver disease) increases ER stress, oxidative damage, mitochondrial dysfunction, and lipid peroxidation, which together drive hepatic insulin resistance.[93] Hepatic insulin resistance dysregulates lipid metabolism and promotes lipolysis,[115] which increases the production of toxic lipids, including ceramides, which further impair insulin signaling, mitochondrial function, and cell viability.[93,116,117] Liver disease worsens as ER stress and mitochondrial dysfunction exacerbate insulin resistance,[11] lipolysis, and ceramide accumulation.[118–120]

Experimental models of NAFLD with T2DM and visceral obesity are associated with brain atrophy, neurodegeneration, and cognitive impairment.[56,91,100,111,114] In humans with NASH, the rates of neuropsychiatric disease, including depression and anxiety,[121] and the risks for developing cognitive impairment[122] are increased. In fact, cognitive impairment and neuropsychiatric dysfunction correlate more with steatohepatitis and insulin resistance than obesity or T2DM.[123,124] Therefore, the potential roles of steatohepatitis and hepatic insulin resistance in relation to neurodegeneration must be considered. To this end, the author and colleagues hypothesized that increased levels of cytotoxic ceramides generated in liver (or visceral adipose tissue) could cause neurodegeneration.[56,100,111,114] In humans and experimental models with steatohepatitis, ceramide gene expression and ceramide levels are increased regardless of the cause.[19,20,91,125–128] Correspondingly, CNS exposures to cytotoxic ceramides cause AD-type molecular and biochemical abnormalities in vitro[129,130] and cognitive-motor deficits, brain insulin resistance, oxidative stress, metabolic dysfunction, and neurodegeneration with features similar to AD in vivo.[128] Ex vivo treatment of frontal lobe slice cultures with long-chain ceramide-containing plasma from obese rats with steatohepatitis produces neurotoxic responses with impairments in viability and mitochondrial function.[125] This concept illustrates how peripheral insulin-resistance diseases might cause or contribute to cognitive impairment and neurodegeneration.

Metabolic Syndrome

Metabolic syndrome is a cluster of disease processes that pivots around insulin resistance, visceral obesity, hypertension, and dyslipidemia.[131] Metabolic syndrome increases the risk for coronary artery disease, atherosclerosis, and T2DM and is frequently associated with NAFLD/NASH, proinflammatory and prothrombotic states, and sleep apnea.[131] Studies have linked peripheral insulin resistance,[132] visceral obesity,[133] and metabolic syndrome[134–136] to brain atrophy, cognitive impairment, and declines in executive function. These associations sound an alarm in light of the recent increases in the prevalence of metabolic syndrome among adults and children.[137] If T2DM, obesity, metabolic syndrome, and NAFLD/NASH could actually be demonstrated to serve as cofactors in the pathogenesis and progression of neurodegeneration, then aggressive efforts would be needed to treat and prevent the full spectrum of systemic insulin-resistance diseases. Accordingly, antihyperglycemic or insulin sensitizer agents have already been shown to reduce AD clinical manifestations and pathology.[56,138–143]

SUMMARY

Brain insulin/IGF resistance initiates a cascade of progressive oxidative stress, neuroinflammation, impaired cell survival, mitochondrial dysfunction, dysregulated lipid metabolism, and ER stress. Continued compromise of neuronal and glial functions causes cognitive impairment and the eventual development of neurodegeneration. Because many of the molecular and cellular abnormalities in AD exist in systemic/peripheral insulin resistance, such as in obesity, T2DM, and NAFLD/NASH, common mechanisms of insulin and IGF resistance should be investigated. By regarding these clinically diverse diseases as fundamentally related on molecular, biochemical, and perhaps etiologic bases, their clustering beneath an umbrella term of *insulin resistance spectrum disorders* could accelerate the discovery of new treatments and improve the understanding of disease pathogenesis and progression.

REFERENCES

1. Best CH, Scott DA. The preparation of insulin. J Biol Chem 1923;57:709–23.
2. Roth J, Qureshi S, Whitford I, et al. Insulin's discovery: new insights on its ninetieth birthday. Diabetes Metab Res Rev 2012;28(4):293–304.
3. Gilchrist JA, Best CH, Banting FG. Observations with insulin on Department of Soldiers' Civil Re-Establishment Diabetics. Can Med Assoc J 1923;13(8): 565–72.
4. Gualandi-Signorini AM, Giorgi G. Insulin formulations–a review. Eur Rev Med Pharmacol Sci 2001;5(3):73–83.
5. Heinemann L, Richter B. Clinical pharmacology of human insulin. Diabetes Care 1993;16(Suppl 3):90–100.
6. Dave N, Hazra P, Khedkar A, et al. Process and purification for manufacture of a modified insulin intended for oral delivery. J Chromatogr A 2008;1177(2):282–6.
7. Freiherr J, Hallschmid M, Frey WH 2nd, et al. Intranasal insulin as a treatment for Alzheimer's disease: a review of basic research and clinical evidence. CNS Drugs 2013;27(7):505–14.
8. Ott V, Benedict C, Schultes B, et al. Intranasal administration of insulin to the brain impacts cognitive function and peripheral metabolism. Diabetes Obes Metab 2012;14(3):214–21.
9. Plum MB, Sicat BL, Brokaw DK. Newer insulin therapies for management of type 1 and type 2 diabetes mellitus. Consult Pharm 2003;18(5):454–65.
10. Zeyda M, Stulnig TM. Obesity, inflammation, and insulin resistance–a minireview. Gerontology 2009;55(4):379–86.
11. Capeau J. Insulin resistance and steatosis in humans. Diabetes Metab 2008; 34(6 Pt 2):649–57.

12. Dai Z, Wu F, Yeung EW, et al. IGF-IEc expression, regulation and biological function in different tissues. Growth Horm IGF Res 2010;20(4):275–81.
13. Matheny RW Jr, Nindl BC, Adamo ML. Minireview: mechano-growth factor: a putative product of IGF-I gene expression involved in tissue repair and regeneration. Endocrinology 2010;151(3):865–75.
14. Kuemmerle JF. Insulin-like growth factors in the gastrointestinal tract and liver. Endocrinol Metab Clin North Am 2012;41(2):409–23, vii.
15. de la Monte SM, Wands JR. Review of insulin and insulin-like growth factor expression, signaling, and malfunction in the central nervous system: relevance to Alzheimer's disease. J Alzheimers Dis 2005;7(1):45–61.
16. D'Ercole AJ, Ye P. Expanding the mind: insulin-like growth factor I and brain development. Endocrinology 2008;149(12):5958–62.
17. Freude S, Schilbach K, Schubert M. The role of IGF-1 receptor and insulin receptor signaling for the pathogenesis of Alzheimer's disease: from model organisms to human disease. Curr Alzheimer Res 2009;6(3):213–23.
18. Zeger M, Popken G, Zhang J, et al. Insulin-like growth factor type 1 receptor signaling in the cells of oligodendrocyte lineage is required for normal in vivo oligodendrocyte development and myelination. Glia 2007;55(4):400–11.
19. de la Monte SM, Longato L, Tong M, et al. The liver-brain axis of alcohol-mediated neurodegeneration: role of toxic lipids. Int J Environ Res Public Health 2009;6(7):2055–75.
20. de la Monte SM, Longato L, Tong M, et al. Insulin resistance and neurodegeneration: roles of obesity, type 2 diabetes mellitus and non-alcoholic steatohepatitis. Curr Opin Investig Drugs 2009;10(10):1049 60.
21. Gronke S, Clarke DF, Broughton S, et al. Molecular evolution and functional characterization of Drosophila insulin-like peptides. PLoS Genet 2010;6(2): e1000857.
22. Shanik MH, Xu Y, Skrha J, et al. Insulin resistance and hyperinsulinemia: is hyperinsulinemia the cart or the horse? Diabetes Care 2008;31(Suppl 2):S262–8.
23. Dankner R, Chetrit A, Shanik MH, et al. Basal-state hyperinsulinemia in healthy normoglycemic adults is predictive of type 2 diabetes over a 24-year follow-up: a preliminary report. Diabetes Care 2009;32(8):1464–6.
24. Garcia RG, Rincon MY, Arenas WD, et al. Hyperinsulinemia is a predictor of new cardiovascular events in Colombian patients with a first myocardial infarction. Int J Cardiol 2011;148(1):85–90.
25. Kasai T, Miyauchi K, Kajimoto K, et al. The adverse prognostic significance of the metabolic syndrome with and without hypertension in patients who underwent complete coronary revascularization. J Hypertens 2009;27(5): 1017–24.
26. Agnoli C, Berrino F, Abagnato CA, et al. Metabolic syndrome and postmenopausal breast cancer in the ORDET cohort: a nested case-control study. Nutr Metab Cardiovasc Dis 2010;20(1):41–8.
27. Faulds MH, Dahlman-Wright K. Metabolic diseases and cancer risk. Curr Opin Oncol 2012;24(1):58–61.
28. Colonna SV, Douglas Case L, Lawrence JA. A retrospective review of the metabolic syndrome in women diagnosed with breast cancer and correlation with estrogen receptor. Breast Cancer Res Treat 2012;131(1):325–31.
29. de la Monte SM, Neusner A, Chu J, et al. Epidemiological trends strongly suggest exposures as etiologic agents in the pathogenesis of sporadic Alzheimer's disease, diabetes mellitus, and non-alcoholic steatohepatitis. J Alzheimers Dis 2009;17(3):519–29.

30. Cummings JL. Definitions and diagnostic criteria. 3rd edition. London: Informa UK Limited; 2007.
31. Gustaw-Rothenberg K, Lerner A, Bonda DJ, et al. Biomarkers in Alzheimer's disease: past, present and future. Biomark Med 2010;4(1):15–26.
32. Walsh DM, Klyubin I, Fadeeva JV, et al. Naturally secreted oligomers of amyloid beta protein potently inhibit hippocampal long-term potentiation in vivo. Nature 2002;416(6880):535–9.
33. Frolich L, Blum-Degen D, Bernstein HG, et al. Brain insulin and insulin receptors in aging and sporadic Alzheimer's disease. J Neural Transm 1998;105(4–5): 423–38.
34. Hoyer S. Glucose metabolism and insulin receptor signal transduction in Alzheimer disease. Eur J Pharmacol 2004;490(1–3):115–25.
35. Rivera EJ, Goldin A, Fulmer N, et al. Insulin and insulin-like growth factor expression and function deteriorate with progression of Alzheimer's disease: link to brain reductions in acetylcholine. J Alzheimers Dis 2005;8(3):247–68.
36. Steen E, Terry BM, Rivera EJ, et al. Impaired insulin and insulin-like growth factor expression and signaling mechanisms in Alzheimer's disease–is this type 3 diabetes? J Alzheimers Dis 2005;7(1):63–80.
37. de la Monte SM. Therapeutic targets of brain insulin resistance in sporadic Alzheimer's disease. Front Biosci (Elite Ed) 2012;E4:1582–605.
38. de la Monte SM, Re E, Longato L, et al. Dysfunctional pro-ceramide, ER stress, and insulin/IGF signaling networks with progression of Alzheimer's disease. J Alzheimers Dis 2012;30(0):S217–29.
39. Caselli RJ, Chen K, Lee W, et al. Correlating cerebral hypometabolism with future memory decline in subsequent converters to amnestic pre-mild cognitive impairment. Arch Neurol 2008;65(9):1231–6.
40. Mosconi L, Pupi A, De Leon MJ. Brain glucose hypometabolism and oxidative stress in preclinical Alzheimer's disease. Ann N Y Acad Sci 2008;1147:180–95.
41. Langbaum JB, Chen K, Caselli RJ, et al. Hypometabolism in Alzheimer-affected brain regions in cognitively healthy Latino individuals carrying the apolipoprotein E epsilon4 allele. Arch Neurol 2010;67(4):462–8.
42. Hoyer S, Nitsch R. Cerebral excess release of neurotransmitter amino acids subsequent to reduced cerebral glucose metabolism in early-onset dementia of Alzheimer type. J Neural Transm 1989;75(3):227–32.
43. Hoyer S, Nitsch R, Oesterreich K. Predominant abnormality in cerebral glucose utilization in late-onset dementia of the Alzheimer type: a cross-sectional comparison against advanced late-onset and incipient early-onset cases. J Neural Transm Park Dis Dement Sect 1991;3(1):1–14.
44. Talbot K, Wang HY, Kazi H, et al. Demonstrated brain insulin resistance in Alzheimer's disease patients is associated with IGF-1 resistance, IRS-1 dysregulation, and cognitive decline. J Clin Invest 2012;122(4):1316–38.
45. Salcedo I, Tweedie D, Li Y, et al. Neuroprotective and neurotrophic actions of glucagon-like peptide-1: an emerging opportunity to treat neurodegenerative and cerebrovascular disorders. Br J Pharmacol 2012;166(5):1586–99.
46. Piriz J, Muller A, Trejo JL, et al. IGF-I and the aging mammalian brain. Exp Gerontol 2011;46(2–3):96–9.
47. Mattson MP. The impact of dietary energy intake on cognitive aging. Front Aging Neurosci 2010;2:5.
48. Weinstock M, Shoham S. Rat models of dementia based on reductions in regional glucose metabolism, cerebral blood flow and cytochrome oxidase activity. J Neural Transm 2004;111(3):347–66.

49. Lester-Coll N, Rivera EJ, Soscia SJ, et al. Intracerebral streptozotocin model of type 3 diabetes: relevance to sporadic Alzheimer's disease. J Alzheimers Dis 2006;9(1):13–33.
50. Bolzan AD, Bianchi MS. Genotoxicity of streptozotocin. Mutat Res 2002; 512(2–3):121–34.
51. Koulmanda M, Qipo A, Chebrolu S, et al. The effect of low versus high dose of streptozotocin in cynomolgus monkeys (Macaca fascilularis). Am J Transplant 2003;3(3):267–72.
52. de la Monte SM, Tong M, Bowling N, et al. si-RNA inhibition of brain insulin or insulin-like growth factor receptors causes developmental cerebellar abnormalities: relevance to fetal alcohol spectrum disorder. Mol Brain 2011;4:13.
53. Hoyer S. Causes and consequences of disturbances of cerebral glucose metabolism in sporadic Alzheimer disease: therapeutic implications. Adv Exp Med Biol 2004;541:135–52.
54. Chen GJ, Xu J, Lahousse SA, et al. Transient hypoxia causes Alzheimer-type molecular and biochemical abnormalities in cortical neurons: potential strategies for neuroprotection. J Alzheimers Dis 2003;5(3):209–28.
55. Tsukamoto E, Hashimoto Y, Kanekura K, et al. Characterization of the toxic mechanism triggered by Alzheimer's amyloid-beta peptides via p75 neurotrophin receptor in neuronal hybrid cells. J Neurosci Res 2003;73(5):627–36.
56. de la Monte SM, Tong M, Lester-Coll N, et al. Therapeutic rescue of neurodegeneration in experimental type 3 diabetes: relevance to Alzheimer's disease. J Alzheimers Dis 2006;10(1):89–109.
57. Gonzalez-Sanchez JL, Serrano-Rios M. Molecular basis of insulin action. Drug News Perspect 2007;20(8):527–31.
58. Etiene D, Kraft J, Ganju N, et al. Cerebrovascular pathology contributes to the heterogeneity of Alzheimer's disease. J Alzheimers Dis 1998;1(2):119–34.
59. Korf ES, White LR, Scheltens P, et al. Brain aging in very old men with type 2 diabetes: the Honolulu-Asia Aging Study. Diabetes Care 2006;29(10): 2268–74.
60. de la Monte SM. Quantitation of cerebral atrophy in preclinical and end-stage Alzheimer's disease. Ann Neurol 1989;25(5):450–9.
61. Kincaid-Smith P. Hypothesis: obesity and the insulin resistance syndrome play a major role in end-stage renal failure attributed to hypertension and labelled 'hypertensive nephrosclerosis'. J Hypertens 2004;22(6):1051–5.
62. Matsumoto H, Nakao T, Okada T, et al. Insulin resistance contributes to obesity-related proteinuria. Intern Med 2005;44(6):548–53.
63. O'Brien JT. Role of imaging techniques in the diagnosis of dementia. Br J Radiol 2007;80(Spec No 2):S71–7.
64. Poljansky S, Ibach B, Hirschberger B, et al. A visual [18F]FDG-PET rating scale for the differential diagnosis of frontotemporal lobar degeneration. Eur Arch Psychiatry Clin Neurosci 2011;261(6):433–46.
65. Teune LK, Bartels AL, de Jong BM, et al. Typical cerebral metabolic patterns in neurodegenerative brain diseases. Mov Disord 2010;25(14):2395–404.
66. Nijholt DA, De Kimpe L, Elfrink HL, et al. Removing protein aggregates: the role of proteolysis in neurodegeneration. Curr Med Chem 2011;18(16):2459–76.
67. Uehara T. Accumulation of misfolded protein through nitrosative stress linked to neurodegenerative disorders. Antioxid Redox Signal 2007;9(5):597–601.
68. Hol EM, Fischer DF, Ovaa H, et al. Ubiquitin proteasome system as a pharmacological target in neurodegeneration. Expert Rev Neurother 2006;6(9): 1337–47.

69. Kahle PJ, Haass C. How does parkin ligate ubiquitin to Parkinson's disease? EMBO Rep 2004;5(7):681–5.
70. Turner BJ, Atkin JD. ER stress and UPR in familial amyotrophic lateral sclerosis. Curr Mol Med 2006;6(1):79–86.
71. Morris JK, Seim NB, Bomhoff GL, et al. Effects of unilateral nigrostriatal dopamine depletion on peripheral glucose tolerance and insulin signaling in middle aged rats. Neurosci Lett 2011;504(3):219–22.
72. Tong M, Dong M, de la Monte SM. Brain insulin-like growth factor and neurotrophin resistance in Parkinson's disease and dementia with Lewy bodies: potential role of manganese neurotoxicity. J Alzheimers Dis 2009;16(3):585–99.
73. Sato N, Takeda S, Uchio-Yamada K, et al. Role of insulin signaling in the interaction between Alzheimer disease and diabetes mellitus: a missing link to therapeutic potential. Curr Aging Sci 2011;4(2):118–27.
74. Holzenberger M. Igf-I signaling and effects on longevity. Nestle Nutr Workshop Ser Pediatr Program 2011;68:237–45 [discussion: 246–9].
75. Schuh AF, Rieder CM, Rizzi L, et al. Mechanisms of brain aging regulation by insulin: implications for neurodegeneration in late-onset Alzheimer's disease. ISRN Neurol 2011;2011:306905.
76. Valentini S, Cabreiro F, Ackerman D, et al. Manipulation of in vivo iron levels can alter resistance to oxidative stress without affecting ageing in the nematode C. elegans. Mech Ageing Dev 2012;133(5):282–90.
77. Zemva J, Udelhoven M, Moll L, et al. Neuronal overexpression of insulin receptor substrate 2 leads to increased fat mass, insulin resistance, and glucose intolerance during aging. Age (Dordr) 2012;35(5):1881–97.
78. Castilla-Cortazar I, Garcia-Fernandez M, Delgado G, et al. Hepatoprotection and neuroprotection induced by low doses of IGF-II in aging rats. J Transl Med 2011;9:103.
79. Luque RM, Lin Q, Cordoba-Chacon J, et al. Metabolic impact of adult-onset, isolated, growth hormone deficiency (AOiGHD) due to destruction of pituitary somatotropes. PloS One 2011;6(1):e15767.
80. Srikanth V, Westcott B, Forbes J, et al. Methylglyoxal, cognitive function and cerebral atrophy in older people. J Gerontol A Biol Sci Med Sci 2012;68(1):68–73.
81. Williamson R, McNeilly A, Sutherland C. Insulin resistance in the brain: an old-age or new-age problem? Biochem Pharmacol 2012;84(6):737–45.
82. Oxenkrug G. Interferon-gamma - inducible inflammation: contribution to aging and aging-associated psychiatric disorders. Aging Dis 2011;2(6):474–86.
83. Horrillo D, Sierra J, Arribas C, et al. Age-associated development of inflammation in Wistar rats: effects of caloric restriction. Arch Physiol Biochem 2011; 117(3):140–50.
84. Cai D, Liu T. Inflammatory cause of metabolic syndrome via brain stress and NF-kappaB. Aging (Albany NY) 2012;4(2):98–115.
85. Birk TJ. Poliomyelitis and the post-polio syndrome: exercise capacities and adaptation–current research, future directions, and widespread applicability. Med Sci Sports Exerc 1993;25(4):466–72.
86. Jubelt B, Cashman NR. Neurological manifestations of the post-polio syndrome. Crit Rev Neurobiol 1987;3(3):199–220.
87. Gordon T, Hegedus J, Tam SL. Adaptive and maladaptive motor axonal sprouting in aging and motoneuron disease. Neurol Res 2004;26(2):174–85.
88. Dalakas MC. Pathogenetic mechanisms of post-polio syndrome: morphological, electrophysiological, virological, and immunological correlations. Ann N Y Acad Sci 1995;753:167–85.

89. Chiang DJ, Pritchard MT, Nagy LE. Obesity, diabetes mellitus, and liver fibrosis. Am J Physiol Gastrointest Liver Physiol 2011;300(5):G697–702.

90. Vernon G, Baranova A, Younossi ZM. Systematic review: the epidemiology and natural history of non-alcoholic fatty liver disease and non-alcoholic steatohepatitis in adults. Aliment Pharmacol Ther 2011;34(3):274–85.

91. Lyn-Cook LE Jr, Lawton M, Tong M, et al. Hepatic ceramide may mediate brain insulin resistance and neurodegeneration in type 2 diabetes and non-alcoholic steatohepatitis. J Alzheimers Dis 2009;16(4):715–29.

92. de la Monte SM, Wands JR. Alzheimer's disease is type 3 diabetes: evidence reviewed. J Diabetes Sci Technol 2008;2(6):1101–13.

93. Kraegen EW, Cooney GJ. Free fatty acids and skeletal muscle insulin resistance. Curr Opin Lipidol 2008;19(3):235–41.

94. Luchsinger JA, Reitz C, Patel B, et al. Relation of diabetes to mild cognitive impairment. Arch Neurol 2007;64(4):570–5.

95. Craft S. Insulin resistance and Alzheimer's disease pathogenesis: potential mechanisms and implications for treatment. Curr Alzheimer Res 2007;4(2):147–52.

96. Lokken KL, Boeka AG, Austin HM, et al. Evidence of executive dysfunction in extremely obese adolescents: a pilot study. Surg Obes Relat Dis 2009;5(5):547–52.

97. Gunstad J, Paul RH, Cohen RA, et al. Elevated body mass index is associated with executive dysfunction in otherwise healthy adults. Compr Psychiatry 2007;48(1):57–61.

98. Yaffe K. Metabolic syndrome and cognitive decline. Curr Alzheimer Res 2007;4(2):123–6.

99. Winocur G, Greenwood CE. Studies of the effects of high fat diets on cognitive function in a rat model. Neurobiol Aging 2005;26(Suppl 1):46–9.

100. Moroz N, Tong M, Longato L, et al. Limited Alzheimer-type neurodegeneration in experimental obesity and Type 2 diabetes mellitus. J Alzheimers Dis 2008;15(1):29–44.

101. Baker LD, Frank LL, Foster-Schubert K, et al. Aerobic exercise improves cognition for older adults with glucose intolerance, a risk factor for Alzheimer's disease. J Alzheimers Dis 2010;22(2):569–79.

102. Baker LD, Frank LL, Foster-Schubert K, et al. Effects of aerobic exercise on mild cognitive impairment: a controlled trial. Arch Neurol 2010;67(1):71–9.

103. Bryan J, Tiggemann M. The effect of weight-loss dieting on cognitive performance and psychological well-being in overweight women. Appetite 2001;36(2):147–56.

104. Gu Y, Luchsinger JA, Stern Y, et al. Mediterranean diet, inflammatory and metabolic biomarkers, and risk of Alzheimer's disease. J Alzheimers Dis 2010;22(2):483–92.

105. Martins IJ, Hone E, Foster JK, et al. Apolipoprotein E, cholesterol metabolism, diabetes, and the convergence of risk factors for Alzheimer's disease and cardiovascular disease. Mol Psychiatry 2006;11(8):721–36.

106. Pasquier F, Boulogne A, Leys D, et al. Diabetes mellitus and dementia. Diabetes Metab 2006;32(5 Pt 1):403–14.

107. Whitmer RA. Type 2 diabetes and risk of cognitive impairment and dementia. Curr Neurol Neurosci Rep 2007;7(5):373–80.

108. Crane PK, Walker R, Hubbard RA, et al. Glucose levels and risk of dementia. N Engl J Med 2013;369(6):540–8.

109. Nelson PT, Smith CD, Abner EA, et al. Human cerebral neuropathology of type 2 diabetes mellitus. Biochim Biophys Acta 2008;1792(5):454–69.

110. Janson J, Laedtke T, Parisi JE, et al. Increased risk of type 2 diabetes in Alzheimer disease. Diabetes 2004;53(2):474–81.

111. Tong M, Longato L, de la Monte SM. Early limited nitrosamine exposures exacerbate high fat diet-mediated type2 diabetes and neurodegeneration. BMC Endocr Disord 2010;10(1):4.

112. Perry W, Hilsabeck RC, Hassanein TI. Cognitive dysfunction in chronic hepatitis C: a review. Dig Dis Sci 2008;53(2):307–21.

113. Weiss JJ, Gorman JM. Psychiatric behavioral aspects of comanagement of hepatitis C virus and HIV. Curr HIV/AIDS Rep 2006;3(4):176–81.

114. Tong M, Neusner A, Longato L, et al. Nitrosamine exposure causes insulin resistance diseases: relevance to type 2 diabetes mellitus, non-alcoholic steatohepatitis, and Alzheimer's disease. J Alzheimers Dis 2009;17(4):827–44.

115. Kao Y, Youson JH, Holmes JA, et al. Effects of insulin on lipid metabolism of larvae and metamorphosing landlocked sea lamprey, Petromyzon marinus. Gen Comp Endocrinol 1999;114(3):405–14.

116. Holland WL, Summers SA. Sphingolipids, insulin resistance, and metabolic disease: new insights from in vivo manipulation of sphingolipid metabolism. Endocr Rev 2008;29(4):381–402.

117. Langeveld M, Aerts JM. Glycosphingolipids and insulin resistance. Prog Lipid Res 2009;48(3–4):196–205.

118. Kaplowitz N, Than TA, Shinohara M, et al. Endoplasmic reticulum stress and liver injury. Semin Liver Dis 2007;27(4):367–77.

119. Malhi H, Gores GJ. Molecular mechanisms of lipotoxicity in nonalcoholic fatty liver disease. Semin Liver Dis 2008;28(4):360–9.

120. Sundar-Rajan S, Srinivasan V, Balasubramanyam M, et al. Endoplasmic reticulum (ER) stress & diabetes. Indian J Med Res 2007;125(3):411–24.

121. Elwing JE, Lustman PJ, Wang HL, et al. Depression, anxiety, and nonalcoholic steatohepatitis. Psychosom Med 2006;68(4):563–9.

122. Felipo V, Urios A, Montesinos E, et al. Contribution of hyperammonemia and inflammatory factors to cognitive impairment in minimal hepatic encephalopathy. Metab Brain Dis 2011;27(1):51–8.

123. Schmidt KS, Gallo JL, Ferri C, et al. The neuropsychological profile of alcohol-related dementia suggests cortical and subcortical pathology. Dement Geriatr Cogn Disord 2005;20(5):286–91.

124. Kopelman MD, Thomson AD, Guerrini I, et al. The Korsakoff syndrome: clinical aspects, psychology and treatment. Alcohol Alcohol 2009;44(2):148–54.

125. de la Monte SM. Triangulated mal-signaling in Alzheimer's disease: roles of neurotoxic ceramides, ER stress, and insulin resistance reviewed. J Alzheimers Dis 2012;30:S231–49.

126. de la Monte SM, Tong M, Lawton M, et al. Nitrosamine exposure exacerbates high fat diet-mediated type 2 diabetes mellitus, non-alcoholic steatohepatitis, and neurodegeneration with cognitive impairment. Mol Neurodegener 2009; 4:54.

127. de la Monte SM, Tong M, Nguyen V, et al. Ceramide-mediated insulin resistance and impairment of cognitive-motor functions. J Alzheimers Dis 2010;21(3): 967–84.

128. Tong M, de la Monte SM. Mechanisms of ceramide-mediated neurodegeneration. J Alzheimers Dis 2009;16(4):705–14.

129. Alessenko AV, Bugrova AE, Dudnik LB. Connection of lipid peroxide oxidation with the sphingomyelin pathway in the development of Alzheimer's disease. Biochem Soc Trans 2004;32(Pt 1):144–6.

130. Adibhatla RM, Hatcher JF. Altered lipid metabolism in brain injury and disorders. Subcell Biochem 2008;49:241–68.
131. Kassi E, Pervanidou P, Kaltsas G, et al. Metabolic syndrome: definitions and controversies. BMC Med 2011;9:48.
132. Tan ZS, Beiser AS, Fox CS, et al. Association of metabolic dysregulation with volumetric brain magnetic resonance imaging and cognitive markers of subclinical brain aging in middle-aged adults: the Framingham Offspring Study. Diabetes Care 2011;34(8):1766–70.
133. Debette S, Beiser A, Hoffmann U, et al. Visceral fat is associated with lower brain volume in healthy middle-aged adults. Ann Neurol 2010;68(2):136–44.
134. Hassenstab JJ, Sweat V, Bruehl H, et al. Metabolic syndrome is associated with learning and recall impairment in middle age. Dement Geriatr Cogn Disord 2010;29(4):356–62.
135. Frisardi V, Solfrizzi V, Capurso C, et al. Is insulin resistant brain state a central feature of the metabolic-cognitive syndrome? J Alzheimers Dis 2010;21(1): 57–63.
136. Yates KF, Sweat V, Yau PL, et al. Impact of metabolic syndrome on cognition and brain: a selected review of the literature. Arterioscler Thromb Vasc Biol 2012; 32(9):2060–7.
137. Burns JM, Honea RA, Vidoni ED, et al. Insulin is differentially related to cognitive decline and atrophy in Alzheimer's disease and aging. Biochim Biophys Acta 2012;1822(3):333–9.
138. Benedict C, Hallschmid M, Schmitz K, et al. Intranasal insulin improves memory in humans: superiority of insulin aspart. Neuropsychopharmacology 2007;32(1): 239–43.
139. Craft S, Baker LD, Montine TJ, et al. Intranasal insulin therapy for Alzheimer disease and amnestic mild cognitive impairment: a pilot clinical trial. Arch Neurol 2011;69(1):29–38.
140. Holscher C. Incretin analogues that have been developed to treat type 2 diabetes hold promise as a novel treatment strategy for Alzheimer's disease. Recent Pat CNS Drug Discov 2010;5(2):109–17.
141. Krikorian R, Eliassen JC, Boespflug EL, et al. Improved cognitive-cerebral function in older adults with chromium supplementation. Nutr Neurosci 2010;13(3): 116–22.
142. Reger MA, Watson GS, Green PS, et al. Intranasal insulin improves cognition and modulates {beta}-amyloid in early AD. Neurology 2008;70(6):440–8.
143. Luchsinger JA. Type 2 diabetes, related conditions, in relation and dementia: an opportunity for prevention? J Alzheimers Dis 2010;20(3):723–36.

Effects of Antipsychotic Medications on Appetite, Weight, and Insulin Resistance

Chao Deng, PhD

KEYWORDS

- Antipsychotic • Appetite • Obesity • Weight gain • Insulin resistance
- Glucose dysregulation

KEY POINTS

- Although some atypical antipsychotic drugs, particularly olanzapine and clozapine, have more severe weight-gain side effects, all antipsychotics, including typical antipsychotics currently used clinically, may cause some degree of weight gain.
- There are time-dependent changes in weight gain associated with antipsychotic medication, with development of a 3-stage time course; in particular, rapid weight gain in the initial stage is a good indicator for a long-term outcome of weight gain and obesity.
- Accumulated data suggest that increasing appetite and food intake, as well as delayed satiety signaling, are key behavioral changes related to weight gain/obesity induced by antipsychotics.
- Antipsychotics may induce insulin resistance, glucose dysregulation, and even type 2 diabetes mellitus independent of weight gain and adiposity.
- There are also time-dependent changes for insulin and glucose dysregulation associated with antipsychotic medication.
- Current evidence from clinical trials in first-episode psychotic patients shows that typical antipsychotics such as haloperidol have a relatively high risk for weight gain/obesity and glucometabolic side effects.
- Monitoring weight gain is important but insufficient. Periodic monitoring of blood sugar may also be required during antipsychotic therapy, particularly for drugs with high diabetic liabilities such as olanzapine and clozapine.
- There are marked individual variations in weight gain and other metabolic side effects associated with antipsychotics. For example, irrespective of the antipsychotic drug some patients lose weight, some maintain weight, and some gain weight.

Continued

This article originally appeared in Endocrinology and Metabolism Clinics of North America, Volume 42, Issue 3, September 2013.

Funding Sources: This study was supported by a Project grant (APP1044624) from the National Health and Medical Research Council (NHMRC), Australia.

Conflicts of Interest: None.

Antipsychotic Research Laboratory, School of Health Sciences, Illawarra Health and Medical Research Institute, University of Wollongong, Northfields Avenue, Wollongong, New South Wales 2522, Australia

E-mail address: chao@uow.edu.au

http://dx.doi.org/10.1016/j.ccol.2014.08.019

Continued

- Mechanisms for antipsychotic-related weight gain, insulin resistance, and glucose dysregulation have yet to be elucidated. Current results suggest that antagonistic effects of atypical antipsychotics on serotonin 5-HT_{2C} and histamine H_1 receptors play an important role in weight-gain/obesity side effects, whereas muscarinic M_3 receptors have been identified as most closely linked with diabetic side effects. However, blockade of dopamine D_2 receptors may be a common mechanism for these metabolic side effects in both atypical and typical antipsychotics.

INTRODUCTION

Mental disorders are the greatest overall cause of disability.[1] Antipsychotic drugs (APDs) are the most widely prescribed medications and are used frequently to control various mental disorders such as schizophrenia, bipolar disorder, dementia, major depression, Tourette syndrome, eating disorders, and even substance abuse.[2,3] Unfortunately, APDs may cause some serious side effects, including extrapyramidal and metabolic side effects. Since typical APDs were introduced into clinics in the 1950s their side effects of increasing body weight have been reported, but have gained less attention because these drugs often have worse and problematic extrapyramidal side effects.[4] In the 1980s and 1990s, clozapine, olanzapine, and other atypical APDs with reduced extrapyramidal side effects were widely introduced into psychiatric clinics, and currently form the first line of APD treatment.[5,6] Unfortunately, atypical APDs, particularly clozapine and olanzapine, cause serious metabolic side effects, such as substantial weight gain, intra-abdominal obesity, hyperlipidemia, insulin resistance, hyperglycemia, and type 2 diabetes mellitus (T2DM).[7–10] These adverse effects are a major risk for cardiovascular disease, stroke, and premature death (by 20–30 years).[7,11] In addition to medical consequences, weight gain and obesity can lead to noncompliance with medication, which is a primary problem for the treatment of schizophrenia because cessation of APD treatment dramatically (up to 5-fold) increases the relapse rate for these patients.[12,13] Given that the majority of patients with psychiatric disorders face chronic, even life-long, treatment with APDs, the risks of weight gain, obesity, and other metabolic symptoms are major considerations for individual APD maintenance treatment. This review focuses on the effects of APDs on weight gain, appetite, insulin resistance, and glucose dysregulation, as well as relevant underlying mechanisms that may be help to prevent and treat weight gain/obesity and other metabolic side effects caused by APD therapy.

WEIGHT GAIN AND OBESITY INDUCED BY ANTIPSYCHOTICS
Weight-Gain/Obesity Side Effects: Typical Versus Atypical APDs

It had been reported since the 1950s that treatment with some typical APDs (such as chlorpromazine) is associated with weight gain; however, many psychiatrists still hold believe that atypical APDs are associated with significant weight gain and obesity side effects, whereas typical APDs are not.[14] For example, the commonly used typical APD, haloperidol, was once believed to have a minimal weight-gain side effect.[14] However, a recent report on the European First-Episode Schizophrenia Trial (EUFEST) has clearly shown that 1 year of treatment with haloperidol caused clinically significant weight gain (≥7% from baseline) in 53% of patients, with an average weight gain of 7.3 kg.[15] A dramatic weight gain (9.56 kg) was also observed in another study of first-episode patients after 1 year treatment with haloperidol.[16] Therefore, while certain atypical APDs (such as olanzapine and clozapine) might lead to greater weight gain, typical APDs could also lead to significant weight and other metabolic changes in patients.

Underestimation of weight-gain and obesity side effects has also been the case for atypical APDs. In 2005, the National Institutes of Health–funded CATIE (The Clinical Antipsychotic Trials of Intervention Effectiveness) study reported the effects of the atypical APDs olanzapine, quetiapine, risperidone, and ziprasidone on body weight over an 18-months period in chronic schizophrenia patients who had an average of more than 14 years' APD medication history.[17] The CATIE study found that olanzapine treatment caused significant weight gain ($\geq$7% from baseline) in a higher proportion of patients (30%) than quetiapine (16%), risperidone (14%), and ziprasidone (7%). Patients treated with olanzapine also gained more weight (average addition 0.9 kg [2 lb] per month) than patients treated with quetiapine (average addition 0.23 kg [0.5 lb] per month) and risperidone (average addition 0.18 kg [0.4 lb] per month), whereas ziprasidone-treated patients lost body weight (average loss 0.14 kg [−0.3 lb] per month).[17] However, the subsequent EUFEST and CAFE (Comparison of Atypical Antipsychotics for First Episode) studies showed that these atypical APDs caused more severe weight gain in first-episode schizophrenia patients.[15,18] The CAFE study reported that after a 12-week treatment, significant weight gain ($\geq$7% body weight) occurred in a large number of first-episode schizophrenia patients treated with olanzapine (59.8%), compared with risperidone (32.5%) and quetiapine (29.2%). Furthermore, after 52 weeks' treatment, 80% of olanzapine-treated patients gained at least 7% body weight (with an average 1.76 kg [3.88 lb] per month), compared with 57.6% of risperidone-treated (with an average 1.28 kg [2.81 lb] per month) and 50% of quetiapine-treated (with an average 1.29 kg [2.85 lb] per month) patients.[18] The EUFEST study confirmed that after 12 months of treatment, olanzapine caused the most significant weight gain in first-episode schizophrenia (in 86% of patients with an average 1.16 kg [2.56 lb] per month) compared with quetiapine (in 65% of patients with an average 0.88 kg [1.94 lb] per month), amisulpride (in 63% of patients with an average [1.78 lb] per month), and ziprasidone (in 37% of patients with an average 0.4 kg [0.88 lb] per month).[15] In another study of first-episode patients, dramatic weight gain was observed in olanzapine (average 12.02 kg), risperidone (8.99 kg), and haloperidol (9.56 kg) treatment after 1 year.[16] It is interesting that ziprasidone and amisulpride have been widely regarded as atypical APDs with low weight gain risk in previous studies[10]; ziprasidone was even found to cause weight loss in the CATIE study.[17] Therefore, it is worth exploring why a lesser weight-gain side effect was observed in the CATIE study. The main difference between these studies was that subjects in the CATIE study had a chronic APD medication history (average >14 years) in comparison with first-episode patients without previous APD medication in the EUFEST and CAFE studies.[15,17,18] These clinical trials indicate that previous studies on patients with chronic schizophrenia may have underestimated the magnitude of weight-gain/obesity side effects associated with APDs. Furthermore, although mean weight gain and the incidence of clinically significant weight gain may vary between APDs, olanzapine and clozapine have the highest risk; accumulated evidence indicates that both typical and atypical APDs have more weight-gain and other metabolic side effects than placebo-level effects.[9,10,15]

Time Course of APD-Induced Weight Gain/Obesity

Although various APDs cause weight gain at different magnitudes, both typical and atypical APDs exhibit a similar temporal course of weight gain that includes

3 stages: stage 1, an early acceleration stage in which APDs induce a rapid increase in body weight within the first few months of treatment (eg, about 3 months for clozapine, olanzapine, risperidone, and haloperidol); stage 2, a middle stage in which body weight continues to increase at a much steadier rate for a period of at least a year or longer; and stage 3, further treatment that leads to a plateau of weight gain, representing a possible "ceiling effect" of APDs, in which patients will maintain the heavier weight with ongoing APD treatment.[19,20] For example, patients with first-episode psychosis treated with olanzapine or haloperidol gained weight rapidly during the first 12 weeks (mean ± standard deviation [SD]: olanzapine, 9.2 ± 5.31 kg; haloperidol, 3.7 ± 4.9 kg), then continued to gain weight until a plateau was reached (olanzapine, 15.5 ± 9.6 kg; haloperidol, 7.1 ± 6.7 kg) at approximately 1 year, after which weight gain remained at this high level (olanzapine, 15.4 ± 10.0 kg; haloperidol, 7.5 ± 9.2 kg) up to the end of 2 years.[20] The changes in body mass index (BMI; calculated as weight in kilograms divided by height in meters squared, ie, kg/m^2) during the 2-year study period followed a pattern similar to that for weight gain; in the olanzapine group the mean BMI increased from 23.6 ± 4.8 (mean ± SD) at baseline to 26.4 ± 4.6 at 12 weeks, 28.8 ± 4.5 at 1 year, and 28.3 ± 4.0 at 2 years, compared with the haloperidol group's increase from 23.9 ± 4.5 at baseline to 24.8 ± 4.1 at 12 weeks, 26.2 ± 4.3 at 1 year, and 26.6 ± 4.4 at 2 years.[20] Several long-term studies indicate that some APDs may take a much longer time to reach the plateau.[19,21,22] This temporal course is well mimicked in an animal model of olanzapine-induced weight gain.[23,24] Although the final weight plateau is often reached after several years, accumulated evidence indicates that rapid weight gain in the first few weeks (Stage 1) of APD treatment is a strong indicator for the long-term outcome of weight gain and obesity.[25–27] Therefore, although the time course of weight gain has been observed to have a similar pattern in various APDs, the exact time course of weight gain induced by a specific APD still remains a topic of further research.

Are Weight-Gain and Obesity Side Effects of APD Dose Dependent?

To date, the possible relationship between APD dosages and associated weight gain has not been systematically investigated. Simon and colleagues[28] reviewed publications between 1975 and 2008, and suggested that olanzapine and clozapine appear to have dose-dependent and serum concentration–dependent weight-gain side effects. For example, Perry and colleagues[29] reported associations of weight gain with both olanzapine dosages and plasma concentrations. More recently, in an 8-week, randomized clinical trial of olanzapine, 10-, 20-, and 40-mg (oral) doses in 634 patients with schizophrenia or schizoaffective disorder, a significant dose-related change in weight gain was found, which suggested that higher than standard doses of olanzapine may be associated with greater weight gain compared with standard doses.[30] This finding was supported by a study into long-acting olanzapine injection, in which clear dose-dependent changes of weight gain were observed; a high dose (300 mg every 2 weeks) had a higher weight gain than medium (405 mg every 4 weeks) and low (150 mg every 2 weeks) doses in schizophrenia patients.[31] Risperidone-induced weight gain could be dose related to some extent but data are contradictory, and no study has assessed risperidone serum concentrations in association with weight gain.[28] Current evidence indicates that other APDs including aripiprazole, amisulpride, quetiapine, sertindole, and ziprasidone have no dose-related metabolic effects; however, no study has assessed serum concentrations of these APDs.[28] Therefore, prescribing the lowest possible effective doses, at least for clozapine, olanzapine, and risperidone, will be helpful in minimizing their weight-gain side effects.

EFFECTS OF ANTIPSYCHOTIC MEDICATION ON APPETITE AND FOOD INTAKE

Theoretically, gain in body weight results from an imbalance between energy intake and energy expenditure, whereby overeating and/or less energy expenditure (such as decreasing resting metabolism and activity) may contribute to overweight and obesity. Over the past 15 years, accumulated data from both clinical and animal studies suggest that increasing appetite and food intake, as well as delayed satiety signaling, are key behavioral changes related to APD-induced weight gain/ obesity.[32–34] On the other hand, there is less understanding of to what extent changes of resting metabolism rate and activity/sedation affect weight gain associated with APD medication, although current evidence suggests that they may play an important role in the development of APD-induced weight gain.[19,35,36]

Altered eating behaviors have been reported in several clinical studies with treatment involving various APDs. Gothelf and colleagues[37] first reported that increased food intake, but not resting energy expenditure and physical activity, was associated with olanzapine-induced weight gain in schizophrenia patients. A randomized double-blind study found that both clozapine and olanzapine were associated with food craving and binge eating over the 6-week treatment period.[38] Compared with those taking clozapine, patients receiving olanzapine tended to have higher rates of food craving (olanzapine 48.9% vs clozapine 23.3%) and binge eating (olanzapine 16.7% vs clozapine 8.9%), which also occurred earlier (1 week vs 3 weeks for binge eating).[38] In another study[33] eating behavior in patients treated with atypical APDs (clozapine, olanzapine, risperidone, quetiapine, or ziprasidone) were also compared with healthy controls by recording appetite sensation before and after a standardized breakfast using visual analog scales. The investigators found that: (1) atypical APD-treated patients showed greater adiposity and a higher degree of hunger following the standardized breakfast; and (2) patients had significantly higher cognitive dietary restraint, disinhibition, and susceptibility to hunger than controls. The patients treated with atypical APDs were also more reactive to external eating cues.[34] Furthermore, a recent study reported that, consistent with the significant increase in body weight, food consumption, and disinhibited eating, 1 week of treatment with olanzapine enhanced both the anticipatory and consummatory reward response to food rewards in the brain's reward circuitry, including the inferior frontal cortex, striatum, and anterior cingulate cortex, but decreased activation in the brain region (the lateral orbital frontal cortex) believed to inhibit feeding behavior.[39]

These clinical findings are confirmed in animal studies where APD-induced hyperphagia is repeatedly found in animal models of APD-induced weight gain.[23,40–43] Furthermore, recently olanzapine has been found to selectively increase rats' response to sucrose pellets in an operant conditioning without affecting free-feeding intake of sucrose; by contrast, sibutramine (a noradrenaline/serotonin reuptake inhibitor and a weight-reducing agent) prevented the increase of rats' response to sucrose pellets induced by olanzapine.[44] It has been well established that the hypothalamic arcuate nucleus plays a crucial role in appetite and energy homeostasis through activation of 2 distinct populations of anorexigenic and orexigenic neurons: neurons that express appetite inhibiting cocaine- and amphetamine-related transcript (CART) and pro-opiomelanocortin (POMC), and neurons that express appetite-stimulating agouti-related peptide (AgRP) and neuropeptide Y (NPY).[45] Using the animal model for olanzapine-induced weight gain, it has been revealed that olanzapine elevated the expression of appetite-stimulating AgRP and NPY, and decreased appetite-inhibiting POMC.[46,47] These results suggest that patients treated with APDs may develop abnormal eating behaviors in response to altered appetite sensations and increased susceptibility to hunger, which may lead to a positive energy balance and contribute to gain in body weight.

INSULIN RESISTANCE, GLUCOSE DYSREGULATION, AND DIABETES ASSOCIATED WITH ANTIPSYCHOTIC MEDICATION
Effects of Atypical APDs

Validated evidence over the past 20 years has indicated that APD medication significantly increases the risk of insulin resistance, glucose dysregulation, and the development of T2DM.[5,48,49] Although patients with psychiatric disorders such as schizophrenia have been observed to have an increased risk of developing diabetes regardless of antipsychotics, suggesting that the disease itself may be a predisposing risk factor,[50–52] APD medication has been widely recognized as a main contributor in these metabolic disorders.[7,48,49] An analysis of the US Food and Drug Administration Adverse Event database also showed that adjusted report ratios for T2DM were the following: olanzapine 9.6 (95% confidence interval [CI] 9.2–10.0), risperidone 3.8 (95% CI 3.5–4.1), quetiapine 3.5 (95% CI 3.2–3.9), clozapine 3.1 (95% CI 2.9–3.3), ziprasidone 2.4 (95% CI 2.0–2.9), aripiprazole 2.4 (95% CI 1.9–2.9), and haloperidol 2.0 (95% CI 1.7–2.3), which suggests differential risks of diabetes across various APDs.[53]

Owing to relatively short trial periods, many clinical trials have not been able to capture most new cases of diabetes; however, numerous studies have shown strong relationships between APDs and indicators of insulin resistance and glucose dysregulation.[48,54] In the CATIE study of patients with chronic schizophrenia, compared with baseline the fasting blood glucose (FBG) level was most elevated with olanzapine (15.0 ± 2.8 mg/dL; mean $\pm$ standard error), followed by quetiapine (6.8 ± 2.5 mg/dL), risperidone (6.7 ± 2.0 mg/dL), perphenazine (5.2 ± 2.0 mg/dL), and ziprasidone (2.3 ± 3.9 mg/dL).[17] The EUFEST study has reported a similar incidence rate of hyperglycemia among various APDs after 1 year of treatment with haloperidol (18%), amisulpride (21%), olanzapine (30%), quetiapine (22%) and ziprasidone (22%), with a significant increase of fasting insulin level (haloperidol 2.0 ± 1.4 mU/L, amisulpride 8.6 ± 3.1 mU/L, olanzapine 2.5 ± 3.9 mU/L, quetiapine 2.1 ± 1.2 mU/L, and ziprasidone 0.1 ± 2.0 mU/L).[15] Chronically elevated insulin levels and concurrent hyperglycemia are consistent with insulin resistance, and may indicate T2DM.[55] In fact, numerous clinical studies have reported that chronic APD treatment increases insulin resistance. Using the homeostasis model assessment index for insulin resistance (HOMA-IR), chronic (8 weeks to 5 months) treatment with olanzapine, clozapine, and risperidone has been repeatedly reported to significantly increase the HOMA-IR,[56–61] although risperidone was normally observed to have a lesser effect on HOMA-IR.[58,60,61] Furthermore, patients with chronic olanzapine treatment also showed a greater decrease in insulin sensitivity during an oral glucose tolerance test than those treated with risperidone.[61] Using a frequently sampled intravenous glucose tolerance test and minimal model analysis, significant insulin resistance and impairment of glucose effectiveness were reported in nonobese patients chronically treated with clozapine and olanzapine, but with a lesser effect in patients treated with risperidone and quetiapine.[62,63] Recently, a 2-step euglycemic, hyperinsulinemic clamp procedure has been used to assess changes in insulin sensitivity in nondiabetic patients with schizophrenia or schizoaffective disorder treated with olanzapine or risperidone, whereby olanzapine and risperidone treatment caused a decrement in insulin sensitivity.[59] These results were confirmed in numerous animal studies using the HOMA-IR or euglycemic/hyperinsulinemic clamp procedures: chronic treatment with olanzapine and clozapine caused insulin resistance, a reduction in insulin sensitivity, and glucose dysregulation.[64–68]

Effects of Typical APDs Using Haloperidol as an Example

Although over the past 15 years the metabolic side effects of atypical APDs have attracted most attention, there is evidence that treatment with some typical APDs also increases the risk of insulin resistance, glucose dysregulation, and T2DM.[11,49,69,70] Since they were introduced to clinics in the 1950s, chlorpromazine and thioridazine have been repeatedly reported to cause abnormal glucose tolerance, insulin resistance, and even T2DM.[70–76] Although, on the other hand, it was generally believed that haloperidol did not increase the risk of insulin resistance and T2DM,[49] recent evidence from clinical trials in first-episode patients showed that haloperidol may have a higher risk than originally thought. As discussed earlier, the EUFEST study has reported that 1 year of treatment with haloperidol has an incidence rate of hyperglycemia and increased fasting insulin levels similar to that of the atypical APDs olanzapine and quetiapine.[15] Another randomized, double-blind trial in patients with first-episode schizophrenia also found that both FBG and 2-hour postprandial blood glucose (PPBG) levels were significantly increased by a 6-week treatment with haloperidol (FBG, 6.8 ± 14.1/dL, mean $\pm$ SD; PPBG, 6.7 ± 12.6 mg/dL), olanzapine, (FBG, 6.6 ± 12.7 mg/dL; PPBG, 21.5 ± 32.2 mg/dL), and risperidone (FBG, 4.3 ± 12.5 mg/dL; PPBG, 21.0 ± 23.4 mg/dL), with a similar incidence rate of diabetes induced by APD treatment (haloperidol 9.7%, olanzapine 11.4%, risperidone 9.1%) by World Health Organization criteria.[69] A 1-year treatment of haloperidol in drug-naïve first-episode patients showed a similarly increased insulin level and HOMA-IR in comparison with olanzapine and risperidone.[77] Analyzing data from the Italian Health Search Database also showed that, in initially nondiabetic and APD-free patients, the diabetic risk ratios were 12.4% (95% CI 6.3–24.5) for haloperidol, 18.7% (95% CI 8.2–42.8) for risperidone, 20.4% (95% CI 6.9–60.3) for olanzapine, and 33.7% (95% CI 9.2–123.6) for quetiapine, with no significant difference between various drug groups.[78] These findings were confirmed by a large population-based study conducted in Denmark, which included 345,937 patients treated with an APD and 1,426,488 unexposed control subjects. A significantly higher relative risk compared with the general population was observed in drug-naïve patients treated with olanzapine (1.35, 95% CI 1.18–1.54), risperidone (1.24, 95% CI 1.09–1.40), sertindole (9.53, 95% CI 1.34–67.63), perphenazine (1.60, 95% CI 1.45–1.77), ziprasidone (3.09, 95% CI 1.54–6.17), and haloperidol (1.32, 95% CI 1.17–1.49), but not in patients treated with aripiprazole, amisulpride, or quetiapine.[79] These results suggest that treatment with haloperidol, like chlorpromazine and thioridazine, is associated an increased risk of glucose and insulin dysregulation.

Indirect Effects of APD-Induced Weight Gain and Obesity Versus Direct Effects of APDs on Insulin Resistance and Glucose Dysregulation

Given the well-established association between obesity and insulin resistance and hyperglycemia, APD-induced dysregulation of glucose homeostasis has been frequently linked to the high propensity of these drugs for weight gain and obesity. For example, many studies have found the increased HOMA-IR induced by chronic treatment of olanzapine, clozapine, or risperidone to be correlated with weight gain and adiposity.[58,77,80] Weight gain and adiposity were also found to be significantly correlated with changes in insulin sensitivity in patients following a 12-week treatment with olanzapine and risperidone.[59] In 2010, Kim and colleagues[81] reported that BMI contributed one-quarter to one-third of the variance in insulin resistance in olanzapine-treated patients. However, growing evidence has demonstrated that treatment with APDs, particularly short-term treatment, can directly affect insulin resistance and glucose homeostasis independent of weight gain.[82] In fact, clinical studies have shown impaired glucose regulation without weight gain in some schizophrenia patients treated with APDs.[83] Insulin resistance has also been reported to be induced by olanzapine treatment within days without any weight gain.[84,85] Diabetic ketoacidosis has been reported in patients in early treatment with various APDs and without weight gain.[86] In APD-naïve schizophrenia patients, 2 weeks' treatment of olanzapine decreased insulin secretory response to a hyperglycemic challenge, which suggests that olanzapine might directly impair pancreatic β-cell function.[87] Data from animal studies also showed that acute treatment, even a single acute dose, of olanzapine, risperidone, or clozapine can cause hyperglycemia and hyperinsulinemia, impair insulin sensitivity, and induce insulin resistance.[66,88–91] An in vitro study also showed that olanzapine and clozapine can directly decrease glucose-stimulated insulin secretion from pancreatic β cells.[92] Furthermore, olanzapine and clozapine can significantly decrease the insulin-stimulated glucose transport rate by about 40% in 3T3-L1 adipocytes, whereas clozapine and risperidone reduced the insulin-stimulated glucose transport rate by about 40% in primary cultured rat adipocytes.[93] Therefore, these typical APDs may directly induce insulin resistance by directly impairing insulin-responsive glucose resistance in adipocytes.[93]

Time Course of APD-Induced Insulin Dysregulation

Although a growing body of evidence has shown that short-term/acute APD treatment decreases fasting plasma insulin levels and attenuates glucose-stimulated insulin response,[87,88,91,92,94] as already discussed, chronic treatment is associated with hyperinsulinemia, insulin resistance, and T2DM.[49,59,95] The apparent conflict in reports between chronic and short-term APD treatment may be reconciled by a hypothesis of time-dependent changes of APD-induced insulin dysregulation. This hypothesis is supported by a recent report that found time-dependent changes of glucose-stimulated insulin response in individuals with schizophrenia: decreased insulin levels during the first 2 weeks of olanzapine treatment compared with their baseline levels, followed by a return to baseline levels after 4 weeks of treatment, and increased insulin response following 8 weeks of olanzapine treatment.[96] In another study in schizophrenia patients who started or switched to a different APD for 3 months, a time-dependent worsening of plasma glucose levels was observed in subjects taking clozapine, olanzapine, and quetiapine.[97] A recent animal study also demonstrated that acute treatment of rats with olanzapine showed both glucose dysregulation and insulin resistance; however, rats treated intermittently with olanzapine (once per week) showed a marked worsening in both glucose dysregulation and insulin resistance over the course of a 10-week treatment.[67] The mechanisms underlying this time-dependent change in APD-induced insulin and glucose dysregulation have not been investigated, however.

NEUROPHARMACOLOGIC MECHANISMS FOR APD-INDUCED WEIGHT GAIN AND GLUCOMETABOLIC SIDE EFFECTS

In contrast to typical APDs (such as haloperidol) that are largely potent and selective D_2 antagonists, atypical APDs have binding affinities for various neurotransmitter receptors, such as dopamine D_2, serotonin $5-HT_{2A}$ and $5-HT_{2C}$, adrenergic α_{1-2}, muscarinic M_1 and M_3, and histamine H_1 receptors.[98] Among these receptors, dopamine D_2 and $5-HT_2$ receptors play critical roles in the therapeutic effects of atypical APDs.[99,100]

Accumulated evidence has revealed that the antagonistic properties of 5-HT_{2C} and H_1 receptors are involved in APD-induced weight gain.[32,101,102] In fact, among APDs, clozapine and olanzapine have the highest affinities for 5-HT_{2C} and H_1 receptors, and have the highest risk of weight-gain/obesity side effects.[36,98,103] Therefore, the neuropharmacologic mechanisms reviewed here are mainly from studies on olanzapine and clozapine. It is worth noting that because of the variations in receptor-binding profiles between different APDs, the mechanisms underlying the weight gain and glucometabolic side effects might not be exactly the same between various APDs.

Over the past 30 years the 5-HT receptor has been revealed to regulate appetite and body weight, mainly through acting at the hypothalamic 5-HT_{2C} receptors.[104] In fact, 5-HTergic neurons project to the hypothalamic POMC neurons that coexpress 5-HT_{2C} receptors, and 5-HT has been found to influence appetite by activating anorexigenic POMC neurons and melanocortin-4 receptors.[104] Considering the finding that olanzapine decreases expression of POMC in animal studies,[46,47] APDs may therefore increase appetite by inhibiting POMC neurons through the 5-HT_{2C} receptors. It is interesting that 5-HT_{2C} agonists reduce food intake by advancing satiety, and these effects are reversed by 5-HT_{2C} antagonists.[105,106] These results suggest that blockade of 5-HT_{2C} receptors could possibly be the mechanism for the clinical findings showing that treatment with both clozapine and olanzapine could induce food craving and binge eating in patients.[38] Furthermore, the role of 5-HT_{2C} in APD-induced weight gain was confirmed by an animal study, which showed that the initial (5 days) increase in weight gain and food intake associated with olanzapine treatment could be mimicked by combining a 5-HT_{2C} antagonist (SB243213) with haloperidol, but not by an H_1 antagonist alone or in combination with haloperidol.[107] However, there is clear evidence that 1-week and 12-week treatment with olanzapine reduces the expression of hypothalamic H_1 receptors, and H_1 receptor changes have been correlated with increased food intake and weight gain in rats.[24] Olanzapine and clozapine have been reported to activate the hypothalamic adenosine monophosphate-activated protein kinase (AMPK) pathway via H_1 receptors to increase food intake and gain in body weight.[108] Olanzapine has also been reported to regulate feeding behavior in rats by modulating histaminergic neurotransmission.[109] The role of the H_1 receptor in APD-induced weight gain has also been supported by findings that cotreatment of betahistine (an H_1 agonist and an H_3 antagonist) can significantly reduce olanzapine-induced weight gain in both schizophrenia patients and animals.[110–112] It has also been postulated that different neural mechanisms are responsible for the 3 stages of weight gain induced by APDs.[19]

APD affinity for the muscarinic M_3 receptor has been identified as most closely linked to its diabetic side effects,[113–115] and can even be used to predict its diabetogenic liability.[113] Consistently, olanzapine and clozapine, 2 of the APDs associated with a high risk of insulin resistance, glucose dysregulation, and diabetic side effects, possess the highest M_3 receptor-binding affinity.[116] M_3 receptors play a crucial role in the regulation of insulin secretion through both the peripheral and central cholinergic pathways.[117] An in vitro study has shown that olanzapine and clozapine can impair cholinergic-stimulated insulin secretion.[92] A recent animal study found that a single subcutaneous injection of darifenacin (a selective M_3 muscarinic antagonist) significantly decreased insulin response to glucose challenge in comparison with controls.[118] M_3 receptors are widely expressed in the hypothalamic arcuate nucleus and ventromedial nucleus, and the dorsal vagal complex of the brainstem, brain regions well documented for their role in insulin and glucagon secretion and glucose homeostasis.[119,120] Recently, Weston-Green[121] found that a 2-week treatment with olanzapine decreased fasting insulin levels and correlated with an increase in

M_3 receptor-binding density in the arcuate nucleus, ventromedial nucleus, and dorsal vagal complex. In addition, acute central treatment with olanzapine via intracerebroventricular infusion induced hepatic insulin resistance and increased hypothalamic AMPK expression.[122] Results from the 2 studies suggest that olanzapine may block M_3 receptor signaling pathways in the brain, thus affecting insulin production and insulin resistance. Therefore, APDs may act through both peripheral and central M_3 antagonism to impair compensatory insulin response, resulting in diabetes.

Since the introduction of APDs in the 1950s, binding at dopamine D_2 receptors (antagonism or partial agonism) remains the only mechanism common to the therapeutic efficacy of all APDs.[100] There is evidence that both atypical and typical APDs can cause weight gain and other metabolic side effects. In particular, recent clinical data from studies in first-episode patients demonstrated haloperidol (a potent and selective D_2 antagonist) to be associated with weight gain, insulin resistance, and glucose dysregulation, as already discussed; it is therefore reasonable to propose D_2 receptors as a possible common mechanism underlying these side effects. Although it has been the subject of fewer investigations, there is some evidence supporting the involvement of D_2 receptors in APD-induced weight gain, insulin resistance, and glucose dysregulation. As discussed earlier, only treatment using a $5-HT_{2C}$ antagonist combined with haloperidol can mimic olanzapine-induced weight gain.[107] A relationship between a functional promoter region polymorphism in *DRD2* and weight gain induced by olanzapine and risperidone has been reported in first-episode schizophrenia.[123] Dopamine and D_2 receptors are key components of the reward system controlling the desire for food and, hence, regulation of body weight.[124] A previous study by the author's group[125] found that D_2 receptor density in the rostral part of the caudate putamen in obese mice was significantly lower compared with that in lean mice. It is well established that blockade of dopamine D_2 receptor activity in the mesolimbic and nigrostriatal pathways is the common mechanism of APD action,[100,126] and that these are also key pathways for food reward.[127] In fact, reduced striatal activation was detected by functional magnetic resonance imaging during reward anticipation, owing to appetite-provoking cues in chronic schizophrenia under APD treatment.[128] Therefore, APDs may increase appetite and food intake by acting on dopamine D_2–mediated reward.[127] It is interesting that D_2-like receptors are also expressed in pancreatic β cells, which function to inhibit glucose-stimulated insulin secretion,[129] and permanent lack of D_2 receptor–mediated inhibition (such as in D_2 knockout mice *Drd2*$^{-/-}$) eventually results in glucose intolerance.[130] It has been reported that a single subcutaneous injection of raclopride (a D_2/D_3 selective antagonist) can enhance insulin secretion and marginally decrease insulin sensitivity.[118] Therefore, this may provide a mechanism to explain why chronic treatment of some typical APDs (such as haloperidol) leads to glucose dysregulation, hyperinsulinemia, and, eventually, diabetes.

SUMMARY

Over the past 20 years it has been established that treatment with atypical APDs is associated with serious weight gain, obesity, and other metabolic side effects such as insulin resistance, glucose dysregulation, and T2DM; however, the metabolic side effects associated with some typical APDs are possibly underestimated. Emerging evidence over the past 5 to 6 years from the studies in first-episode psychotic and drug-naïve patients show that some commonly used typical APDs (such as haloperidol) may also cause significant weight gain, insulin resistance, glucose dysregulation, and even T2DM, particularly under chronic treatment. In fact, although some atypical APDs, particularly clozapine and olanzapine, have a higher liability than others in inducing metabolic side effects, current evidence indicates that all APDs have more weight gain and other metabolic side effects than placebo-level effects.

It is worth noting that variations in weight gain and other metabolic side effects are observed not only among APDs; marked individual variations have also been observed in all reported clinical studies and, irrespective of the APD, some subjects lose weight, some maintain weight, and some gain weight.[15,17] It is also noteworthy that not all weight gain is detrimental. For those patients who are underweight before APD treatment, possibly reflecting that their psychotic illness has caused them to neglect themselves, weight gain associated with APD is beneficial if the medication results in these individuals returning to a premorbid and healthy weight.[131] This individual variation could be related to both genetic and nongenetic factors (such as gender, age, and initial body weight/BMI).[132,133] Although there is no reliable biomarker for the prediction of weight gain, several studies have identified female gender, younger age, and a low BMI before the first APD treatment as risk factors for APD-induced weight gain and obesity.[133–136] A diagnosis of undifferentiated schizophrenia or schizophrenia spectrum disorder was also identified as a possible predictor for APD-induced weight gain.[133,136] As APD-induced weight gain has a time-dependent development, and particularly because rapid weight gain in the first few weeks of APD treatment is a good indicator for a long-term outcome of weight gain and obesity,[19,27] weight monitoring during the early phase of APD therapy is crucial for prevention of this serious side effect. Because insulin resistance and glucose dysregulation may develop independently of weight gain, monitoring only weight gain is not sufficient, and periodic monitoring of blood sugar may also be required during APD therapy, particularly for drugs with high diabetic liabilities such as olanzapine and clozapine. Although current evidence suggests that multiple neurotransmitter receptors such as $5-HT_{2C}$, histamine H_1, and muscarinic M_3 (and possibly also dopamine D_2 receptors) are involved in weight gain/obesity and insulin and glucose dysregulation associated with APDs, one important issue that needs to be investigated is how these neurotransmitter systems interact during the time-dependent development of these side effects. An improved understanding of the mechanisms underlying the time-dependent development of these metabolic side effects could help in designing better strategies to prevent and treat these devastating side effects and their associated cardiovascular disease, stroke, and premature death.

REFERENCES

1. Murray CJ, Lopez AD. The Global Burden of Disease: a comprehensive assessment of mortality and disability from diseases, injuries and risk factors in 1990 and projected to 2020. Cambridge (MA): Harvard School of Public Health; 1996.
2. Lambert T. Managing the metabolic adverse effects of antipsychotic drugs in patients with psychosis. Australian Prescriber 2011;34(4):97–9.
3. Newcomer J. Second-generation atypical antipsychotics and metabolic effects. a comprehensive literature review. CNS Drugs 2005;19:1–93.
4. Hasan A, Wobrock T, Reich-Erkelenz D, et al. Treatment of first-episode schizophrenia: pharmacological and neurobiological aspects. Drug Discov Today 2011;8(1–2):31–5.
5. Vohora D. Atypical antipsychotic drugs: current issues of safety and efficacy in the management of schizophrenia. Curr Opin Investig Drugs 2007;8(7): 531–8.

6. Asenjo Lobos C, Komossa K, Rummel-Kluge C, et al. Clozapine versus other atypical antipsychotics for schizophrenia. Cochrane Database Syst Rev 2010;(11):CD006633.

7. Stahl SM, Mignon L, Meyer JM. Which comes first: atypical antipsychotic treatment or cardiometabolic risk? Acta Psychiatr Scand 2009;119(3):171–9.

8. Lambert MT, Copeland LA, Sampson N, et al. New-onset type-2 diabetes associated with atypical antipsychotic medications. Prog Neuropsychopharmacol Biol Psychiatry 2006;30(5):919–23.

9. Allison D, Mentore J, Heo M, et al. Antipsychotic-induced weight gain: a comprehensive research synthesis. Am J Psychiatry 1999;156(11):1686–96.

10. Correll CU, Lencz T, Malhotra AK. Antipsychotic drugs and obesity. Trends Mol Med 2011;17(2):97–107.

11. Newcomer JW. Metabolic considerations in the use of antipsychotic medications: a review of recent evidence. J Clin Psychiatry 2007;68(Suppl 1):20–7.

12. Robinson D, Woerner MG, Alvir JMJ, et al. Predictors of relapse following response from a first episode of schizophrenia or schizoaffective disorder. Arch Gen Psychiatry 1999;56(3):241–7.

13. Weiden PJ, Mackell JA, McDonnell DD. Obesity as a risk factor for antipsychotic noncompliance. Schizophr Res 2004;66(1):51–7.

14. Nasrallah HA. Folie en masse! It's so tempting to drink the Kool-Aid. Curr Psychiatr 2011;10(3):12–6.

15. Kahn RS, Fleischhacker WW, Boter H, et al. Effectiveness of antipsychotic drugs in first-episode schizophrenia and schizophreniform disorder: an open randomised clinical trial. Lancet 2008;371(9618):1085–97.

16. Perez-Iglesias R, Vazquez-Barquero JL, Amado JA, et al. Effect of antipsychotics on peptides involved in energy balance in drug-naive psychotic patients after 1 year of treatment. J Clin Psychopharmacol 2008;28(3):289–95.

17. Lieberman JA, Stroup TS, McEvoy JP, et al. Effectiveness of antipsychotic drugs in patients with chronic schizophrenia. N Engl J Med 2005;353(12):1209–23.

18. Patel JK, Buckley PF, Woolson S, et al. Metabolic profiles of second-generation antipsychotics in early psychosis: findings from the CAFE study. Schizophr Res 2009;111(1–3):9–16.

19. Pai N, Deng C, Vella S-L, et al. Are there different neural mechanisms responsible for three stages of weight gain development in anti-psychotic therapy: temporally based hypothesis. Asian J Psychiatr 2012;5(4):315–8.

20. Zipursky RB, Gu H, Green AI, et al. Course and predictors of weight gain in people with first-episode psychosis treated with olanzapine or haloperidol. Br J Psychiatry 2005;187:537–43.

21. Henderson DC, Cagliero E, Gray C, et al. Clozapine, diabetes mellitus, weight gain, and lipid abnormalities: a five-year naturalistic study. Am J Psychiatry 2000;157(6):975–81.

22. Gentile S. Long-term treatment with atypical antipsychotics and the risk of weight gain: a literature analysis. Drug Saf 2006;29(4):303–19.

23. Huang X-F, Han M, Huang X, et al. Olanzapine differentially affects 5-HT2A and 2C receptor mRNA expression in the rat brain. Behav Brain Res 2006;171(2): 355–62.

24. Han M, Deng C, Burne TH, et al. Short- and long-term effects of antipsychotic drug treatment on weight gain and H1 receptor expression. Psychoneuroendocrinology 2008;33(5):569–80.

25. Bai YM, Lin C-C, Chen J-Y, et al. Association of initial antipsychotic response to clozapine and long-term weight gain. Am J Psychiatry 2006;163(7):1276–9.

26. Kinon BJ, Kaiser CJ, Ahmed S, et al. Association between early and rapid weight gain and change in weight over one year of olanzapine therapy in patients with schizophrenia and related disorders. J Clin Psychopharmacol 2005;25(3):255–8.

27. Case M, Treuer T, Karagianis J, et al. The potential role of appetite in predicting weight changes during treatment with olanzapine. BMC Psychiatry 2010; 10:72.

28. Simon V, van Winkel R, De Hert M. Are weight gain and metabolic side effects of atypical antipsychotics dose dependent? A literature review. J Clin Psychiatry 2009;70(7):1041–50.

29. Perry PJ, Argo TR, Carnahan RM, et al. The association of weight gain and olanzapine plasma concentrations. J Clin Psychopharmacol 2005;25(3): 250–4.

30. Citrome L, Stauffer VL, Chen L, et al. Olanzapine plasma concentrations after treatment with 10, 20, and 40 mg/d in patients with schizophrenia: an analysis of correlations with efficacy, weight gain, and prolactin concentration. J Clin Psychopharmacol 2009;29(3):278–83.

31. Kane JM, Detke HC, Naber D, et al. Olanzapine long-acting injection: a 24-week, randomized, double-blind trial of maintenance treatment in patients with schizophrenia. Am J Psychiatry 2010;167(2):181–9.

32. Deng C, Weston-Green K, Huang XF. The role of histaminergic H1 and H3 receptors in food intake: a mechanism for atypical antipsychotic-induced weight gain? Prog Neuropsychopharmacol Biol Psychiatry 2010;34(1):1–4.

33. Blouin M, Tremblay A, Jalbert M-E, et al. Adiposity and eating behaviors in patients under second generation antipsychotics. Obesity 2008;16(8):1780–7.

34. Sentissi O, Viala A, Bourdel MC, et al. Impact of antipsychotic treatments on the motivation to eat: preliminary results in 153 schizophrenic patients. Int Clin Psychopharmacol 2009;24(5):257–64.

35. Cuerda C, Merchan-Naranjo J, Velasco C, et al. Influence of resting energy expenditure on weight gain in adolescents taking second-generation antipsychotics. Clin Nutr 2011;30(5):616–23.

36. Coccurello R, Moles A. Potential mechanisms of atypical antipsychotic-induced metabolic derangement: clues for understanding obesity and novel drug design. Pharmacol Ther 2010;127(3):210–51.

37. Gothelf D, Falk B, Singer P, et al. Weight gain associated with increased food intake and low habitual activity levels in male adolescent schizophrenic inpatients treated with olanzapine. Am J Psychiatry 2002;159(6):1055–7.

38. Kluge M, Schuld A, Himmerich H, et al. Clozapine and olanzapine are associated with food craving and binge eating: results from a randomized double-blind study. J Clin Psychopharmacol 2007;27(6):662–6.

39. Mathews J, Newcomer JW, Mathews JR, et al. Neural correlates of weight gain with olanzapine. Arch Gen Psychiatry 2012;69(12):1226–37.

40. Cooper GD, Goudie AJ, Halford JC. Acute effects of olanzapine on behavioural expression including the behavioural satiety sequence in female rats. J Psychopharmacol 2010;24(7):1069–78.

41. Thornton-Jones Z, Neill JC, Reynolds GP. The atypical antipsychotic olanzapine enhances ingestive behaviour in the rat: a preliminary study. J Psychopharmacol 2002;16(1):35–7.

42. Minet-Ringuet J, Even PC, Guesdon B, et al. Effects of chronic neuroleptic treatments on nutrient selection, body weight, and body composition in the male rat under dietary self-selection. Behav Brain Res 2005;163(2):204–11.

43. Weston-Green K, Huang X-F, Deng C. Olanzapine treatment and metabolic dysfunction: a dose response study in female Sprague Dawley rats. Behav Brain Res 2011;217(2):337–46.
44. van der Zwaal EM, Janhunen SK, Luijendijk MC, et al. Olanzapine and sibutramine have opposing effects on the motivation for palatable food. Behav Pharmacol 2012;23(2):198–204.
45. Schwartz MW, Woods SC, Porte D, et al. Central nervous system control of food intake. Nature 2000;404(6778):661–71.
46. Ferno J, Varela L, Skrede S, et al. Olanzapine-induced hyperphagia and weight gain associate with orexigenic hypothalamic neuropeptide signaling without concomitant AMPK phosphorylation. PLoS One 2011;6(6):e20571.
47. Weston-Green K, Huang X-F, Deng C. Alterations to melanocortinergic, GABAergic and cannabinoid neurotransmission associated with olanzapine-induced weight gain. PLoS One 2012;7(3):e33548.
48. Allison DB, Newcomer JW, Dunn AL, et al. Obesity among those with mental disorders: a National Institute of Mental Health meeting report. Am J Prev Med 2009;36(4):341–50.
49. De Hert M, Detraux J, van Winkel R, et al. Metabolic and cardiovascular adverse effects associated with antipsychotic drugs. Nat Rev Endocrinol 2012;8(2): 114–26.
50. Henderson DC. Atypical antipsychotic-induced diabetes mellitus: how strong is the evidence? CNS Drugs 2002;16(2):77–89.
51. Meyer JM, Stahl SM. The metabolic syndrome and schizophrenia. Acta Psychiatr Scand 2009;119(1):4–14.
52. Davoodi N, Kalinichev M, Korneev SA, et al. Hyperphagia and increased meal size are responsible for weight gain in rats treated sub-chronically with olanzapine. Psychopharmacology (Berl) 2009;203(4):693–702.
53. Baker RA, Pikalov A, Tran Q-V, et al. Atypical antipsychotic drugs and diabetes mellitus in the US Food and Drug Administration Adverse Event database: a systematic Bayesian signal detection analysis. Psychopharmacol Bull 2009; 42(1):11–31.
54. Simpson GM, Weiden P, Pigott T, et al. Six-month, blinded, multicenter continuation study of ziprasidone versus olanzapine in schizophrenia. Am J Psychiatry 2005;162(8):1535–8.
55. Ahrén B. Autonomic regulation of islet hormone secretion—Implications for health and disease. Diabetologia 2000;43(4):393–410.
56. Rettenbacher MA, Hummer M, Hofer A, et al. Alterations of glucose metabolism during treatment with clozapine or amisulpride: results from a prospective 16-week study. J Psychopharmacol 2007;21(4):400–4.
57. Ebenbichler CF, Laimer M, Eder U, et al. Olanzapine induces insulin resistance: results from a prospective study. J Clin Psychiatry 2003;64(12):1436–9.
58. Wu R-R, Zhao J-P, Zhai J-G, et al. Sex difference in effects of typical and atypical antipsychotics on glucose-insulin homeostasis and lipid metabolism in first-episode schizophrenia. J Clin Psychopharmacol 2007;27(4): 374–9.
59. Hardy TA, Henry RR, Forrester TD, et al. Impact of olanzapine or risperidone treatment on insulin sensitivity in schizophrenia or schizoaffective disorder. Diabetes Obes Metab 2011;13(8):726–35.
60. Sato Y, Yasui-Furukori N, Furukori H, et al. A crossover study on the glucose metabolism between treatment with olanzapine and risperidone in schizophrenic patients. Exp Clin Psychopharmacol 2010;18(5):445–50.

61. Smith RC, Lindenmayer J-P, Davis JM, et al. Effects of olanzapine and risperidone on glucose metabolism and insulin sensitivity in chronic schizophrenic patients with long-term antipsychotic treatment: a randomized 5-month study. J Clin Psychiatry 2009;70(11):1501–13.

62. Henderson DC, Cagliero E, Copeland PM, et al. Glucose metabolism in patients with schizophrenia treated with atypical antipsychotic agents: a frequently sampled intravenous glucose tolerance test and minimal model analysis. Arch Gen Psychiatry 2005;62(1):19–28.

63. Henderson DC, Copeland PM, Borba CP, et al. Glucose metabolism in patients with schizophrenia treated with olanzapine or quetiapine: a frequently sampled intravenous glucose tolerance test and minimal model analysis. J Clin Psychiatry 2006;67(5):789–97.

64. Coccurello R, Brina D, Caprioli A, et al. 30 days of continuous olanzapine infusion determines energy imbalance, glucose intolerance, insulin resistance, and dyslipidemia in mice. J Clin Psychopharmacol 2009;29(6):576–83.

65. Chintoh AF, Mann SW, Lam TK, et al. Insulin resistance following continuous, chronic olanzapine treatment: an animal model. Schizophr Res 2008;104(1–3): 23–30.

66. Albaugh VL, Henry CR, Bello NT, et al. Hormonal and metabolic effects of olanzapine and clozapine related to body weight in rodents. Obesity 2006;14(1): 36–51.

67. Boyda HN, Procyshyn RM, Tse L, et al. Intermittent treatment with olanzapine causes sensitization of the metabolic side-effects in rats. Neuropharmacology 2012;62(3):1391 400.

68. Boyda HN, Tse L, Procyshyn RM, et al. Preclinical models of antipsychotic drug-induced metabolic side effects. Trends Pharmacol Sci 2010;31(10):484–97.

69. Saddichha S, Manjunatha N, Ameen S, et al. Diabetes and schizophrenia—effect of disease or drug? Results from a randomized, double-blind, controlled prospective study in first-episode schizophrenia. Acta Psychiatr Scand 2008; 117(5):342–7.

70. Park S, Hong SM, Lee JE, et al. Chlorpromazine exacerbates hepatic insulin sensitivity via attenuating insulin and leptin signaling pathway, while exercise partially reverses the adverse effects. Life Sci 2007;80(26):2428–35.

71. Amamoto T, Kumai T, Nakaya S, et al. The elucidation of the mechanism of weight gain and glucose tolerance abnormalities induced by chlorpromazine. J Pharm Sci 2006;102(2):213–9.

72. Lorenzen J, Remvig J. Diabetes mellitus in a psychotic patient with recovery during chlorpromazine therapy. Dan Med Bull 1957;4(4):134–6.

73. Schwarz L, Munoz R. Blood sugar levels in patients treated with chlorpromazine. Am J Psychiatry 1968;125(2):253–5.

74. Meltzer HY, Perry E, Jayathilake K. Clozapine-induced weight gain predicts improvement in psychopathology. Schizophr Res 2003;59(1):19–27.

75. Amdisen A. Diabetes mellitus as a side effect of treatment with tricyclic neuroleptics. Acta Psychiatr Scand 1964;40(Suppl 180):411–4.

76. Price WA, Giannini AJ. Thioridazine and diabetes. J Clin Psychiatry 1983;44(12): 469.

77. Perez-Iglesias R, Mata I, Pelayo-Teran JM, et al. Glucose and lipid disturbances after 1 year of antipsychotic treatment in a drug-naive population. Schizophr Res 2009;107(2–3):115–21.

78. Sacchetti E, Turrina C, Parrinello G, et al. Incidence of diabetes in a general practice population: a database cohort study on the relationship with

haloperidol, olanzapine, risperidone or quetiapine exposure. Int Clin Psycho-pharmacol 2005;20(1):33–7.

79. Kessing LV, Thomsen AF, Mogensen UB, et al. Treatment with antipsychotics and the risk of diabetes in clinical practice. Br J Psychiatry 2010;197(4): 266–71.

80. Tschoner A, Engl J, Rettenbacher M, et al. Effects of six second generation antipsychotics on body weight and metabolism—risk assessment and results from a prospective study. Pharmacopsychiatry 2009;42(1):29–34.

81. Kim SH, Nikolics L, Abbasi F, et al. Relationship between body mass index and insulin resistance in patients treated with second generation antipsychotic agents. J Psychiatr Res 2010;44(8):493–8.

82. Guenette MD, Giacca A, Hahn M, et al. Atypical antipsychotics and effects of adrenergic and serotonergic receptor binding on insulin secretion in-vivo: an animal model. Schizophr Res 2013;146(1–3):162–9.

83. Newcomer JW, Haupt DW, Fucetola R, et al. Abnormalities in glucose regulation during antipsychotic treatment of schizophrenia. Arch Gen Psychiatry 2002; 59(4):337–45.

84. Koller EA, Doraiswamy PM. Olanzapine-associated diabetes mellitus. Pharmacotherapy 2002;22(7):841–52.

85. Laimer M, Ebenbichler CF, Kranebitter M, et al. Olanzapine-induced hyperglycemia: role of humoral insulin resistance-inducing factors. J Clin Psychopharmacol 2005;25(2):183–5.

86. Guenette M, Hahn M, Cohn T, et al. Atypical antipsychotics and diabetic ketoacidosis: a review. Psychopharmacology (Berl) 2013;226(1):1–12.

87. Chiu CC, Chen KP, Liu HC, et al. The early effect of olanzapine and risperidone on insulin secretion in atypical-naive schizophrenic patients. J Clin Psychopharmacol 2006;26(5):504–7.

88. Houseknecht KL, Robertson AS, Zavadoski W, et al. Acute effects of atypical antipsychotics on whole-body insulin resistance in rats: implications for adverse metabolic effects. Neuropsychopharmacology 2007;32(2):289–97.

89. Chintoh AF, Mann SW, Lam L, et al. Insulin resistance and secretion in vivo: effects of different antipsychotics in an animal model. Schizophr Res 2009; 108(1–3):127–33.

90. Boyda HN, Tse L, Procyshyn RM, et al. A parametric study of the acute effects of antipsychotic drugs on glucose sensitivity in an animal model. Prog Neuropsychopharmacol Biol Psychiatry 2010;34(6):945–54.

91. Girault EM, Alkemade A, Foppen E, et al. Acute peripheral but not central administration of olanzapine induces hyperglycemia associated with hepatic and extra-hepatic insulin resistance. PLoS One 2012;7(8):e43244.

92. Johnson DE, Yamazaki H, Ward KM, et al. Inhibitory effects of antipsychotics on carbachol-enhanced insulin secretion from perfused rat islets: role of muscarinic antagonism in antipsychotic-induced diabetes and hyperglycemia. Diabetes 2005;54(5):1552–8.

93. Vestri HS, Maianu L, Moellering DR, et al. Atypical antipsychotic drugs directly impair insulin action in adipocytes: effects on glucose transport, lipogenesis, and antilipolysis. Neuropsychopharmacology 2007;32(4):765–72.

94. Chintoh AF, Mann SW, Lam L, et al. Insulin resistance and decreased glucose-stimulated insulin secretion after acute olanzapine administration. J Clin Psychopharmacol 2008;28(5):494–9.

95. Lambert TJ, Chapman LH. Diabetes, psychotic disorders and antipsychotic therapy: a consensus statement. Med J Aust 2005;182(6):310.

96. Chiu C-C, Chen C-H, Chen B-Y, et al. The time-dependent change of insulin secretion in schizophrenic patients treated with olanzapine. Prog Neuropsychopharmacol Biol Psychiatry 2010;34(6):866–70.

97. van Winkel R, De Hert M, Wampers M, et al. Major changes in glucose metabolism, including new-onset diabetes, within 3 months after initiation of or switch to atypical antipsychotic medication in patients with schizophrenia and schizoaffective disorder. J Clin Psychiatry 2008;69(3):472–9.

98. Nasrallah HA. Atypical antipsychotic-induced metabolic side effects: insights from receptor-binding profiles. Mol Psychiatry 2008;13:27–35.

99. Meltzer H, Massey B. The role of serotonin receptors in the action of atypical antipsychotic drugs. Curr Opin Pharmacol 2011;11:59–67.

100. Kapur S, Mamo D. Half a century of antipsychotics and still a central role for dopamine D2 receptors. Prog Neuropsychopharmacol Biol Psychiatry 2003; 27(7):1081–90.

101. Kroeze WK, Hufeisen SJ, Popadak BA, et al. H1-histamine receptor affinity predicts short-term weight gain for typical and atypical antipsychotic drugs. Neuropsychopharmacology 2003;28(3):519–26.

102. Matsui-Sakata A, Ohtani H, Sawada Y. Receptor occupancy-based analysis of the contributions of various receptors to antipsychotics-induced weight gain and diabetes mellitus. Drug Metab Pharmacokinet 2005;20(5):368–78.

103. Correll CU, Kane JM, Manu P. Obesity and coronary risk in patients treated with second-generation antipsychotics. Eur Arch Psychiatry Clin Neurosci 2011; 261(6):417–23.

104. Lam DD, Garfield AS, Marston OJ, et al. Brain serotonin system in the coordination of food intake and body weight. Pharmacol Biochem Behav 2010;97(1): 84–91.

105. Schreiber R, De Vry J. Role of 5-hT2C receptors in the hypophagic effect of m-CPP, ORG 37684 and CP-94,253 in the rat. Prog Neuropsychopharmacol Biol Psychiatry 2002;26(3):441–9.

106. Kitchener SJ, Dourish CT. An examination of the behavioural specificity of hypophagia induced by 5-HT1B, 5-HT1C and 5-HT2 receptor agonists using the post-prandial satiety sequence in rats. Psychopharmacology (Berl) 1994; 113(3–4):369–77.

107. Kirk SL, Glazebrook J, Grayson B, et al. Olanzapine-induced weight gain in the rat: role of 5-HT2C and histamine H1 receptors. Psychopharmacology (Berl) 2009;207(1):119–25.

108. Kim SH, Ivanova O, Abbasi FA, et al. Metabolic impact of switching antipsychotic therapy to aripiprazole after weight gain: a pilot study. J Clin Psychopharmacol 2007;27(4):365–8.

109. Davoodi N, Kalinichev M, Clifton PG. Comparative effects of olanzapine and ziprasidone on hypophagia induced by enhanced histamine neurotransmission in the rat. Behav Pharmacol 2008;19(2):121–8.

110. Deng C, Lian JM, Pai N, et al. Reducing olanzapine-induced weight gain side effect by using betahistine: a study in the rat model. J Psychopharmacol 2012;26(9):1271–9.

111. Poyurovsky M, Fuchs C, Pashinian A, et al. Reducing antipsychotic-induced weight gain in schizophrenia: a double-blind placebo-controlled study of reboxetine–betahistine combination. Psychopharmacology (Berl) 2013;226(3):615–22.

112. Poyurovsky M, Pashinian A, Levi A, et al. The effect of betahistine, a histamine H1 receptor agonist/H3 antagonist, on olanzapine-induced weight gain in first-episode schizophrenia patients. Int Clin Psychopharmacol 2005;20(2):101–3.

113. Silvestre JS, Prous J. Research on adverse drug events. I. Muscarinic M3 receptor binding affinity could predict the risk of antipsychotics to induce type 2 diabetes. Methods Find Exp Clin Pharmacol 2005;27(5):289–304.

114. Jindal R, Keshavan M. Critical role of M3 muscarinic receptor in insulin secretion: implications for psychopharmacology. J Clin Psychopharmacol 2006; 26(5):449–50 [editorial].

115. Starrenburg FC, Bogers JP. How can antipsychotics cause diabetes mellitus? Insights based on receptor-binding profiles, humoral factors and transporter proteins. Eur Psychiatry 2009;24(3):164–70.

116. Correll CU. From receptor pharmacology to improved outcomes: individualising the selection, dosing, and switching of antipsychotics. Eur Psychiatry 2010; 25(Suppl 2):S12–21.

117. Dockray GJ. The versatility of the vagus. Physiol Behav 2009;97(5):531–6.

118. Hahn M, Chintoh A, Giacca A, et al. Atypical antipsychotics and effects of muscarinic, serotonergic, dopaminergic and histaminergic receptor binding on insulin secretion in vivo: an animal model. Schizophr Res 2011;131(1–3): 90–5.

119. Renuka TR, Ani DV, Paulose CS. Alterations in the muscarinic M1 and M3 receptor gene expression in the brain stem during pancreatic regeneration and insulin secretion in weanling rats. Life Sci 2004;75(19):2269–80.

120. Li Y, Wu X, Zhu J, et al. Hypothalamic regulation of pancreatic secretion is mediated by central cholinergic pathways in the rat. J Physiol 2003;552(2):571–87.

121. Weston-Green K. Alterations in hypothalamic and brainstem neurotransmitter signalling associated with olanzapine-induced metabolic side-effects. Wollongong (Australia): University of Wollongong; 2012.

122. Martins PJF, Haas M, Obici S. Central nervous system delivery of the antipsychotic olanzapine induces hepatic insulin resistance. Diabetes 2010;59(10): 2418–25.

123. Lencz T, Robinson DG, Napolitano B, et al. DRD2 promoter region variation predicts antipsychotic-induced weight gain in first episode schizophrenia. Pharmacogenet Genomics 2010;20(9):569–72.

124. Volkow ND, Wang GJ, Baler RD. Reward, dopamine and the control of food intake: implications for obesity. Trends Cogn Sci 2011;15(1):37–46.

125. Huang X-F, Zavitsanou K, Huang X, et al. Dopamine transporter and D2 receptor binding densities in mice prone or resistant to chronic high fat diet-induced obesity. Behav Brain Res 2006;175(2):415–9.

126. Stahl S. Describing an atypical antipsychotic: receptor binding and its role in pathophysiology. Prim Care Companion J Clin Psychiatry 2003;5:9–13.

127. Elman I, Borsook D, Lukas SE. Food intake and reward mechanisms in patients with schizophrenia: implications for metabolic disturbances and treatment with second-generation antipsychotic agents. Neuropsychopharmacology 2006; 31(10):2091–120.

128. Grimm O, Vollstadt-Klein S, Krebs L, et al. Reduced striatal activation during reward anticipation due to appetite-provoking cues in chronic schizophrenia: a fMRI study. Schizophr Res 2012;134(2–3):151–7.

129. Rubi B, Ljubicic S, Pournourmohammadi S, et al. Dopamine D2-like receptors are expressed in pancreatic beta cells and mediate inhibition of insulin secretion. J Biol Chem 2005;280(44):36824–32.

130. Garcia-Tornadu I, Ornstein AM, Chamson-Reig A, et al. Disruption of the dopamine D2 receptor impairs insulin secretion and causes glucose intolerance. Endocrinology 2010;151(4):1441–50.

131. Haddad P. Weight change with atypical antipsychotics in the treatment of schizophrenia. J Psychopharmacol 2005;19(Suppl 6):16–27.
132. Lane H-Y, Liu Y-C, Huang C-L, et al. Risperidone-related weight gain: genetic and nongenetic predictors. J Clin Psychopharmacol 2006;26(2):128–34.
133. Gebhardt S, Haberhausen M, Heinzel-Gutenbrunner M, et al. Antipsychotic-induced body weight gain: predictors and a systematic categorization of the long-term weight course. J Psychiatr Res 2009;43(6):620–6.
134. Seeman MV. Secondary effects of antipsychotics: women at greater risk than men. Schizophr Bull 2009;35(5):937–48.
135. Treuer T, Pendlebury J, Lockman H, et al. Weight gain risk factor assessment checklist: overview and recommendation for use. Neuroendocrinol Lett 2011; 32(2):199–205.
136. Saddichha S, Ameen S, Akhtar S. Predictors of antipsychotic-induced weight gain in first-episode psychosis: conclusions from a randomized, double-blind, controlled prospective study of olanzapine, risperidone, and haloperidol. J Clin Psychopharmacol 2008;28(1):27–31.

Diabetes and Cancer

Zara Zelenko, BA, PhD(c), Emily Jane Gallagher, MD*

KEYWORDS

- Diabetes mellitus • Obesity • Metabolic syndrome • Cancer • Hyperinsulinemia
- Hyperglycemia • Inflammation

KEY POINTS

- Type 2 diabetes, obesity, and the metabolic syndrome are associated with an increased risk of cancer development.
- Proposed mechanisms to link type 2 diabetes and cancer include insulin resistance, hyperinsulinemia, insulin-like growth factor-1, hyperglycemia and dyslipidemia, inflammatory cytokines, and adipokines.
- Hyperinsulinemia, insulin receptor expression, and insulin receptor signaling are associated with increased tumor growth and metastasis.
- Hyperglycemia can contribute to the development and progression of cancers by promoting transformation of cancer cells, providing an energy source and allowing for cell survival and resistance to chemotherapy.
- Chronic inflammation leads to increased levels of circulating interleukin (IL)-1β, IL-6, and tumor necrosis factor-α that can promote invasion of tumor cells.

INTRODUCTION

Type 2 diabetes (T2D) and obesity are both associated with reduced life expectancy and have been correlated with an increased risk of cancer development. Obesity, the metabolic syndrome, and T2D are also associated with more advanced stage of certain cancers at presentation, resistance to therapy, and recurrence; factors that contribute to greater cancer mortality.[1–4] There are many biologic factors common to obesity and T2D that may contribute to cancer risk. In this review, we discuss the links between T2D and cancer and the various biologic mechanisms associated with T2D, the metabolic syndrome, and obesity that may be promote cancer development, growth, and metastases.

This article originally appeared in Endocrinology and Metabolism Clinics of North America, Volume 43, Issue 1, March 2014.
Disclosure: Authors have nothing to disclose.
Division of Endocrinology, Diabetes and Bone Diseases, Icahn School of Medicine at Mount Sinai, One Gustave L. Levy Place, Box 1055, New York, NY 10029, USA
* Corresponding author.
E-mail address: emily.gallagher@mssm.edu

Clinics Collections 1 (2014) 385–403
http://dx.doi.org/10.1016/j.ccol.2014.08.020
2352-7986/14/$ – see front matter

EPIDEMIOLOGY OF DIABETES AND CANCER
Diabetes, Obesity, and the Metabolic Syndrome

The prevalence of T2D has been growing steadily over the past decade. In 2004, it was predicted that the number of people diagnosed with T2D would rise to 366 million by 2030; however, the numbers are rising more rapidly than predicted. Current estimates from the International Diabetes Federation (IDF), report that 366 million people worldwide had diabetes in 2011, and the projected number of people with diabetes by 2030 is 552 million. Many years before the development of hyperglycemia, the hallmark of diabetes, insulin resistance develops in metabolic tissues and consequently hyperinsulinemia occurs, due to beta cell compensation.[5,6] Eventually, beta cell failure occurs and patients develop hyperglycemia.[7] At this point, diabetes may be diagnosed, although the individual has most likely had insulin resistance and hyperinsulinemia for many preceding years.

Type 1 diabetes mellitus (T1D) results from the autoimmune destruction of the insulin-producing beta cells, which leads to severe insulin deficiency. T1D accounts for about 5% to 10% of diabetes. Various epidemiologic studies have been conducted to investigate the link between T1D and overall cancer incidence.[8] A study conducted in Denmark found that there was no overall increase in cancer cases among individuals with T1D,[8] whereas a Swedish study found a 17% increase in cancer risk in individuals with T1D.[9] This study reported an increased risk of leukemia and skin and stomach cancers.[9] A follow-up study by the same group observed an association between early-onset leukemia and T1D.[10] The highest incidence of acute myeloid leukemia and acute lymphoblastic leukemia in patients with T1D was observed in patients diagnosed with T1D between the ages of 10 and 20 years.[10] Whether the increase in cancer in these patients with T1D is due to a viral etiology or insulin therapy remains to be determined.[10]

The metabolic syndrome is a syndrome of insulin resistance that is associated with a greater risk of developing T2D. The metabolic syndrome is diagnosed by dyslipidemia and hypertension, in addition to abdominal obesity and abnormal glucose homeostasis.[11] The dyslipidemia and hypertension associated with the metabolic syndrome are thought to occur as a consequence of insulin resistance.[11] The Metabolic Syndrome and Cancer (Me-Can) Project in Austria, Sweden, and Norway has examined the association between the syndrome as a whole and its components with cancer risk. The investigators have reported that a higher composite metabolic syndrome score is associated with increased risk of liver cancer as well as bladder cancer in men and postmenopausal breast cancer in women.[12–14] They have also reported an increase in the risk of certain cancers associated with higher glucose levels, hypertriglyceridemia, and hypertension.[15–17]

Obesity, whether defined as a body mass index (BMI) of 30 kg/m^2 or higher or by increased waist circumference ($\geq$102 cm in men or $\geq$ 88 cm in women),[18] also is associated with an increased risk of certain cancers.[19] In 2008, the World Health Organization (WHO) reported that 10% of men and 14% of women worldwide were obese. In the WHO Region of the Americas, 26% of individuals were obese (www.who.int). Obesity is associated with many comorbid conditions, including the metabolic syndrome and T2D. The risk of developing T2D increases with higher BMI levels and with longer duration of obesity. Abdominal obesity is specifically associated with insulin resistance and the metabolic syndrome.[11] A meta-analysis of 221 datasets found that a 5 kg/m^2 increase in BMI was associated with an increased risk of developing esophageal, thyroid, colon, and renal carcinoma and multiple myeloma in men and women, in addition to hepatocellular and rectal cancer, and malignant melanoma in men, and endometrial, gallbladder, postmenopausal breast, and pancreatic cancer and leukemia in women.[19]

The Cancer Prevention Study II reported that obesity was associated with a significant increase in mortality from many similar cancers, including esophageal, colorectal, liver, gallbladder, pancreatic, breast, endometrial, cervical, ovarian, renal, brain, kidney and prostate cancer, non-Hodgkin's lymphoma, and multiple myeloma.[4] Obesity is usually defined by BMI in these epidemiologic studies; however, in certain ethnic groups, such as in individuals from Southeast Asia, insulin resistance may occur at a lower BMI, and waist circumference with race-specific cutoff values is considered to be a better measure of obesity.[11] There is a relative lack of prospective cohort studies examining the association between waist circumference and cancer risk; therefore, BMI is currently used to assess cancer risk associated with obesity.

Diabetes and Cancer Incidence

As for obesity and the metabolic syndrome, T2D has been associated with an increase in the incidence of many cancers and greater cancer mortality.[7,20–23] The association between diabetes and cancer risk is independent of BMI (**Table 1**). Many case-control and cohort studies have been performed in different populations examining the relative risk (RR) of different cancers in individuals with diabetes. Meta-analyses of these studies have reported an increased risk of liver, pancreatic, renal, endometrial, colorectal, bladder, and breast cancer, as well as an increase in the incidence of non-Hodgkin lymphoma.[7,21–24] For those with T2D compared with those without diabetes, the greatest increase in risk is for hepatocellular carcinoma (RR 2.5, 95% confidence interval [CI] 1.8–3.5), with the RR of cancer at other sites being between 1.18 (95% CI 1.05–1.32) for breast cancer and 2.22 (95% CI 1.8–2.74) for endometrial cancer in those with diabetes.[24] Some meta-analyses have addressed whether diabetes increases the risk of specific cancers after adjustment for other factors. Boyle and colleagues[25] examined 39 independent studies investigating women with and without T2D and found that postmenopausal women with T2D had an elevated risk of developing breast cancer compared with women without diabetes, but no increased risk in premenopausal breast cancer was observed in this study. Other cancers, such as hepatocellular cancer, have major risk factors, including infection with hepatitis B or hepatitis C virus.[26] Hepatitis C infection is found in 90% of patients with hepatocellular carcinoma in Japan, and although those with hepatitis C are 15 to 20 times more likely to develop hepatocellular carcinoma than those without, in a recent study of approximately 4000 individuals with treated hepatitis C, T2D was associated with a further 1.7-fold increased risk of developing hepatocellular carcinoma.[27] Notably, the risk

Table 1		
Cancer incidence in type 2 diabetes		
Cancer Type	**RR**	**(95% CI)**
Liver	2.5	(1.8–3.5)
Pancreas	1.9	(1.7–2.3)
Colorectal	1.3	(1.2–1.4)
Endometrium	2.2	(1.8–2.7)
Breast	1.2	(1.1–1.3)
Bladder	1.2	(1.1–1.4)
Prostate	0.9	(0.7–1.2)
All cancer	1.1	(1.0–1.2)

Abbreviations: CI, confidence interval; RR, relative risk.
  Data from Refs.[7,20–23]

of developing prostate cancer has been found to be lower in individuals with diabetes (RR 0.89, 95% CI 0.72–1.11).

Most studies examining the association between T2D and cancer have been performed in individuals of European descent. Fewer studies have been conducted in populations from different ethnic/racial groups and in different countries, where the incidence of certain cancers differ. For example, squamous cell cancer of the esophagus has a higher prevalence in East Asia, and African American men have a higher incidence of prostate cancer than men from European populations.[28,29] A study using Taiwan's Longitudinal Health Insurance Database found a positive association between T2D and the incidence of colorectal cancer.[30] However, in a case-control study in Taiwan, no association between esophageal carcinoma was found.[29] Another retrospective study examined a population of Chinese individuals with T2D and a mean BMI of 23.6 kg/m^2.[22] The study included men and women from a Chinese registry database. The investigators found that both men and women with T2D had increased risks of pancreatic cancers. Furthermore, men had an elevated risk of liver and kidney cancers, whereas women had an elevated risk of breast cancer and leukemia.[22] Although Asian and Western cultures traditionally differ in lifestyles and diets, many developing and industrializing countries are undergoing major changes in diet and lifestyle patterns and adopting a more Western lifestyle.[31] This entails reduced intake of vegetables and whole grains, and increasing the intake of fast foods and processed meats, as well as decreased physical activity.[31] This shift has contributed to the increasing rate of obesity and diabetes worldwide.[32] Therefore, further epidemiologic studies should be conducted in different populations worldwide to determine whether T2D increases the risk of site-specific cancers in individuals of different ethnic/racial background.

Diabetes and Cancer Mortality

Diabetes is associated with a greater mortality from many cancers (**Table 2**). Analysis of prospective data from more than 1 million US men and women followed for 26 years in the prospective Cancer Prevention Study II revealed that after adjustment for age, BMI, and other variables, diabetes was associated with a higher risk of mortality from hepatocellular, pancreatic, endometrial, colon, and breast cancer in women and breast, liver, oral cavity and pharynx, pancreas, and bladder cancer in men.[3] A large meta-analysis performed by the Emerging Risk Factors Collaboration examined the risk of death from cancer in individuals with and without diabetes in 97 prospective studies.[33] They reported that diabetes was associated with death from cancers of

Table 2 Cancer mortality in type 2 diabetes		
Cancer Type	**HR**	**(95% CI)**
Liver	2.2	(1.6–2.9)
Pancreas	1.2	(1.0–1.3)
Colorectal	1.4	(1.1–1.7)
Endometrium	1.4	(1.0–1.8)
Breast	1.4	(1.2–1.6)
Bladder	1.4	(1.0–2.0)
Prostate	1.6	(1.1–1.2)
All cancer	1.4	(1.0–1.8)

Abbreviations: CI, confidence interval; HR, hazard ratio.
  Data from Refs.[7,31,32,36,37]

the liver, pancreas, ovary, colon/rectum, lung, bladder, and breast.[33] Other studies have had similar findings. A retrospective study found that the 5-year overall survival rate of patients with endometrial cancer with T2D was significantly lower than for patients with endometrial cancer without T2D.[34] The patients with endometrial cancer with diabetes were older, had a more advanced stage at diagnosis, and had other complications compared with the patients with endometrial cancer without diabetes.[34] Even after the adjustments for these confounding factors, there was a significant effect of T2D affecting the mortality rate in the patients with endometrial cancer.[34] The study concluded that patients with endometrial cancer with T2D have worse survival rates than patients with endometrial cancer without T2D, 84% versus 68% mortality, respectively.[34] Another retrospective study found similar results between T2D and pancreatic cancer.[35] Patients with pancreatic adenocarcinoma and T2D had greater mortality rates than patients with pancreatic cancer without T2D.[35] Pancreatic cancer has long been associated with diabetes, and a new diagnosis of diabetes may be the first sign of undiagnosed pancreatic cancer. Therefore, many studies on individuals with pancreatic cancer exclude those who are diagnosed with pancreatic cancer within the 5 years of the diagnosis of diabetes. A study by Redaniel and colleagues[36] used the UK General Practice Research Database to investigate the link between T2D and treatment, with breast cancer risk and mortality. They found that women with T2D had a 49% increased mortality rate than women with breast cancer without T2D.[36] Diabetes has been associated with a more advanced stage at diagnosis and an increased risk of breast cancer recurrence after treatment.[1,37] Although men with diabetes have a lower incidence of prostate cancer, those with diabetes are more likely to have high-grade prostate cancer at presentation,[38] and studies have reported more advanced stage in men with diabetes.[2] Some studies also have reported a greater prostate cancer–specific mortality for individuals with diabetes and prostate cancer.[2,39] Others, however, have reported an increase in all-cause mortality in men with prostate cancer and diabetes, but not cancer-specific mortality,[40] and certain studies have shown a decrease in mortality in individuals with diabetes and prostate cancer.[3] A meta-analysis performed in 2010 of 4 studies reported a hazard ratio of 1.57 (95% CI 1.12–1.20) for prostate cancer mortality in men with preexisting diabetes.[41] Differences in study design, different populations, and time of diagnosis of diabetes relative to prostate cancer diagnosis and treatment and possibly diabetes treatments likely account the different results of these studies. Some of the increased cancer mortality associated with diabetes has been attributed to lower rates of cancer screening and more advanced stage at diagnosis.[7] Additionally, some studies have not distinguished cancer-specific mortality from all-cause mortality. These issues have been addressed in some recent studies that have reported greater cancer-specific mortality in individuals with diabetes and a number of different cancers.[2] However, further well-designed prospective epidemiologic studies need to be performed to clarify these issues and to determine the risks of cancer mortality associated with T2D. Many biologic mechanisms may account for the increased cancer incidence and mortality associated with obesity, the metabolic syndrome, and T2D.

BIOLOGIC MECHANISMS LINKING DIABETES AND CANCER

Various aspects of T2D have been suggested as potential mechanisms to promote cancer development (**Fig. 1**).[42–44] The increased risk of cancer with obesity, T2D, and the metabolic syndrome and their relationship to each other suggests common factors may explain the increased risk of cancer in these conditions. Potential

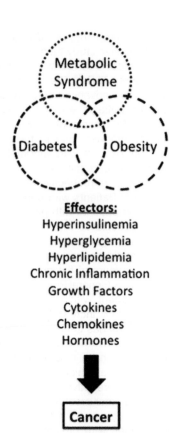

Fig. 1. Aspects of T2D, obesity, and the metabolic syndrome affecting cancer development. The effectors through which T2D, obesity, and the metabolic syndrome may promote cancer development.

mechanisms to explain the relationship between T2D and cancers include insulin resistance, hyperinsulinemia, insulin-like growth factor-1 (IGF-1), hyperglycemia, and dyslipidemia (**Fig. 2**).[36,42,45] Inflammatory cytokines and adipokines also may contribute to metabolic dysfunction and promote cancer development.[34,43] Normal cells have to undergo morphologic changes before tumor growth, invasion, and metastasis occur. T2D can influence these changes either through IGF-1, hyperinsulinemia, hyperglycemia, or chronic inflammation.[44] It is thought that normal cells that have obtained oncogenic mutations are susceptible to the effects of T2D, the metabolic syndrome, and obesity, enabling cancer progression. The various mechanisms through which T2D, the metabolic syndrome, and obesity can promote tumorigenesis will be described in the following sections.

IGF-1, INSULIN, AND GLUCOSE
IGF-1

IGF-1 plays an important role in regulating cell proliferation, differentiation, and apoptosis. Many studies have reported that individuals with higher serum levels of IGF-1 are at an increased risk of developing cancers, such as prostate, colon, cervical, ovarian, and breast.[46] In addition, IGF-1 is expressed in stromal cells adjacent to normal breast epithelial cells.[47] The liver primarily produces IGF-1 and its production

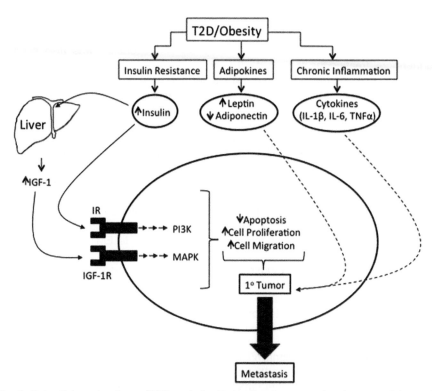

Fig. 2. Potential mechanisms of T2D and obesity leading to cancer development. Schematic representation of aspects of T2D and obesity that suggests insulin resistance and inflammation may promote primary tumor growth. Binding of insulin and IGF-1 to the IR/IGF-1R receptors leads to the activation of the PI3K and MAPK pathways. These signaling pathways promote cell proliferation and cell migration, and inhibit apoptosis, thus enhancing primary tumor progression. Chronic inflammation is associated with increased production of inflammatory cytokines that can directly act on the primary tumor. Furthermore, increased leptin and decreased adiponectin also can promote the development of the primary tumor.

is stimulated by growth hormone (GH) and insulin. IGF-1 binds to the extracellular subunit domain of the IGF-1 receptor (IGF-1R), which is a receptor tyrosine kinase (RTK).[48] The binding of IGF-1 to the receptor activates this RTK, which transduces a series of signaling cascades that activate mitogen-activated protein kinase (MAPK) and the phosphoinositide-3-kinase (PI3K)/Akt pathway.[48] MAPK activation leads to increased cell proliferation, whereas Akt activation leads to increased cell survival and migration.[49] This activation of the IGF-1R receptor has been linked to increased disease progression and poor prognosis in breast cancer.[50]

IGF-1 has been associated with breast cancer progression due to its mitogenic and antiapoptotic effects on mammary epithelial cells.[51] In vitro studies showed that it was possible to induce a transformed phenotype in human immortalized but untransformed mammary epithelial cells (MCF-10A cells), by overexpressing the IGF-1R in these cell lines. The cells adopted a more transformed phenotype, exhibiting growth factor–independent proliferation, lack of contact inhibition, anchorage-independent growth, and tumorigenesis in vivo.[52] The cells also demonstrated characteristics of epithelial-to-mesenchymal transition (EMT). They exhibited downregulation of epithelial markers, such as E-cadherin, β-catenin, and α-catenin, and upregulation of mesenchymal markers, such as vimentin, N-cadherin, and fibronectin. An increase of *snail* mRNA, which represses the transcription of *E-cadherin*, was also seen.[53] Furthermore, treating the malignant estrogen receptor–positive MCF-7 breast cancer cells, with IGF-1 and transforming growth factor β (TGF-β), it is possible to shift these cells from their epithelial nature to a more mesenchymal morphology.[51] Moreover, the gene expression of epithelial markers, *E-cadherin* and *Occludin*, became downregulated and upregulation of the expression of mesenchymal markers, *N-cadherin* and *vimentin* was observed.[51] These in vitro studies demonstrate that IGF-1 and IGF-1R signaling contribute to EMT. EMT is a biologic process in which polarized epithelial cells undergo various changes to take on a mesenchymal phenotype. This phenotype includes increased migratory capacity, invasiveness, resistance to apoptosis, and elevated production of extracellular matrix components.[54] Typically, EMT occurs during implantation, embryogenesis, and organ development. There is increasing evidence that suggests that EMT is associated with cancer progression (metastasis), suggesting that epithelial cancer cells activate EMT while becoming more malignant.[54]

Hepatic IGF-1 production is under the control of GH, other hormones, including insulin, and nutritional status.[55] Mice with higher circulating levels of IGF-1 demonstrate morphologic changes to the mammary epithelial cells and have a higher frequency of breast cancers.[55] Overexpression of IGF-1 under the control of the bovine keratin 5 promoter allowed for the expression of the IGF-1 transgene in the myoepithelial cells of the mouse mammary gland.[56] The mammary epithelial cells were exposed to high levels of IGF-1 by paracrine signaling, which is believed to model the local production of IGF-1 and paracrine signaling that occurs in human breast cancers.[56] Local IGF-1 production in this model promoted mammary gland hyperplasia, spontaneous mammary tumorigenesis, and increased susceptibility to chemical carcinogens.[56] A reduction of circulating IGF-1 levels can prolong tumor latency and reduce tumor size.[57] However, studies inhibiting IGF-1R signaling have not shown the predicted beneficial effects on tumor growth. A study by Konijeti and colleagues[58] combined dietary fat reduction with an IGF-1R blocking antibody to examine the effects on prostate cancer progression in a mouse model. Although, previous in vitro studies by this group and others found that blocking the IGF-1R inhibited cell growth and induced apoptosis, neither the dietary fat reduction nor the IGF-1R blocking therapy separately, or in combination, affected the tumor weight or volume.[58] These results suggest that in prostate cancer there may be other pathways that support tumor growth and progression. Furthermore, clinical trials using specific anti-IGF-1R antibodies have been relatively unsuccessful in reducing cancer growth.[59–61] Phase II studies on patients with squamous cell carcinoma of the head and neck (SCCHN) found that there was no clinically significant benefit of the anti-IGF-1R antibody.[60] The treatment was tolerated but resulted in hyperglycemia in 41% of the patients.[60] This may have been through the resultant increase of circulating GH that is known to have anti-insulin activity through the suppression of glucose uptake in tissues and enhancement of glucose synthesis in the liver. The trial also showed that the anti-IGF-1R antibody was unable to significantly inhibit the PI3K/Akt and MAPK signaling pathways in patients with SCCHN.[60] A phase I/II trial in patients with advanced non–small cell lung cancer also demonstrated little benefit.[61] Moreover, a similar negative result was seen in patients with metastatic refractory colorectal cancer.[59] These clinical trials, as well as other unsuccessful lung, hepatocellular carcinoma, and colorectal cancer trials, indicate that blocking the IGF-1R is not enough to achieve clinical response. Therefore, it is possible that only a specific subset of cancers are responsive to IGF-1R targeted therapy or that other receptors and signaling pathways, such as the insulin receptor signaling pathway, may be compensating for the inhibition of IGF-1R signaling.

Insulin Resistance and Hyperinsulinemia

Insulin resistance and hyperinsulinemia characterize prediabetes and early T2D. Insulin is a well-recognized growth factor. Various meta-analyses have shown that high levels of serum insulin and C-Peptide (a marker of insulin secretion) have correlated with increased risks of colorectal, pancreas, breast, and endometrial cancers in individuals without diabetes.[62] Hyperinsulinemia has also been associated with decreased breast cancer survival and recurrence-free survival.[63,64] Therefore, it is possible that hyperinsulinemia can promote the progression of breast cancer in patients, especially because it has been reported that insulin receptor (IR) expression is elevated in various breast cancer tissues and cancer cell lines.[65] The IR receptor is an RTK that typically signals through the PI3K/Akt pathway.[48] Active phosphorylated forms of the IR, along with phosphorylated insulin receptor substrate-1, trigger phosphorylation and activation of the PI3K catalytic subunit.[66] Downstream of PI3K is a serine/threonine kinase, Akt. It has been noted that Akt activation promotes cell-cycle progression, cell survival, and tumor cell invasion.[67] Furthermore, Akt can induce EMT by repressing the transcription of E-cadherin.[67,68] It is possible that in hyperinsulinemic patients, insulin may act through the IR on breast cancer cells and may promote downstream signaling and more growth of these cells. There are 2 isoforms of the insulin receptor: IR-A and IR-B. IR-B has 22 exons and is mostly expressed in metabolic tissues, including adipose tissue, muscle, and liver.[69] IR-A, which lacks exon 11, is believed to lead to more mitogenic signaling and is expressed normally in the placenta and fetal tissues, as well as cancer tissues.[69] Studies on human breast cancer have shown that greater IR-A to IR-B expression in breast cancer specimens correlated with resistance to hormone-targeted therapy.[70] Insulin may signal through IR-B or IR-A and, thus, in the setting of endogenous hyperinsulinemia, increased mitogenic signaling may occur via IR-A on the cancer cells. Hyperinsulinemia may also exert indirect effects on tumor growth through IGF-1. As noted previously, insulin increases circulating IGF-1 levels.[71] Additionally, insulin decreases insulin-like growth factor binding protein-1 (IGFBP-1), which may lead to an increase in local "free" IGF-1 in the tissues.[62] Through this potential mechanism, hyperinsulinemia may be able to drive tumor growth by acting directly on its cognate IR, likely the IR-A isoform, or by acting indirectly on the IGF-1R or the hybrid IR/IGF-1Rs.[62]

Hyperinsulinemia in a nonobese mouse model (MKR mouse) has been linked to an increase in mammary tumor growth.[72] These MKR mice were generated by the overexpression of the kinase dead IGF-1R, through a point mutation of a lysine-to-arginine residue introduced in the ATP-binding domain, in skeletal muscle under control of the creatine kinase promoter.[73] The overexpression of this dominant negative IGF-1R inhibited both the IGF-1R and IR in skeletal muscle through hybrids formed with the endogenous receptors. The MKR mice showed significant insulin resistance, hyperinsulinemia, and the male mice became hyperglycemic, however the female mice demonstrated only insulin resistance, hyperinsulinemia, and reduced body fat without hyperglycemia and hyperlipidemia, representing a prediabetic condition.[72] The female MKR mice had increased tumor growth following carcinogen, transgenic, or orthotopic induction of mammary tumors.[72] Ferguson and colleagues[74] found an increase in tumor metastases from c-Myc/VEGF overexpressing tumors in MKR mice, the increase in pulmonary metastases was observed even after intravenous injection of tumor cells. These findings suggest that hyperinsulinemia promotes increased survival and/or proliferation of circulating tumor cells that arrest in the lung. The study also demonstrated elevated levels of c-Myc, matrix metalloproteinase 9, IR, IGF-1R, and vascular endothelial growth factor (VEGF) in tumors from the hyperinsulinemic mice.[74] Reducing insulin levels in the MKR mice using an insulin-sensitizing agent resulted in reduced primary tumor growth and metastasis.[74]

Downregulation of the IR has been shown to inhibit anchorage-independent growth in the metastatic human estrogen receptor–negative LCC6 breast cancer cells, and the estrogen receptor–positive human T47D breast cancer cells.[75] In the LCC6, downregulation of the IR inhibited xenograft tumor growth in athymic mice.[75] In this study, Zhang and colleagues[75] investigated the proliferative, angiogenic, lymphangiogenic, and metastatic properties of these 2 breast cancer cells lines during IR downregulation. The reduction of IR expression led to a decrease of VEGF-A production, which is associated with angiogenesis. The group studied lymphangiogenic markers and found that xenografts with decreased IR expression had significantly reduced lymphatic and blood vessel development.[75] Furthermore, they noted that tail vein injections of IR-downregulated tumor cells caused significantly fewer lung metastases.[75] This suggests that by blocking insulin signaling, it is possible to inhibit or reduce the metastatic characteristics of malignant cancer cells.

Therefore, from human and animal studies, hyperinsulinemia, IR expression, and IR signaling are associated with increased tumor growth and metastasis. Potential targets for therapy could be aimed at reducing insulin levels, or blocking IR signaling alone or in addition to blocking IGF-1R signaling.

Hyperglycemia

Chronic hyperglycemia is a characteristic of diabetes. Studies have linked hyperglycemia to promoting tumor cell proliferation and metastasis in cancers associated with T2D.[76] Various epidemiologic studies have shown that elevated blood glucose has a direct association with an increase in breast cancer risk.[77]

Hyperglycemia has been linked to the Warburg Effect, where cancer cells shift to obtaining energy from glycolysis rather than the TCA cycle.[78] Cancer cells have been characterized by high rates of glucose uptake and glucose metabolism. Therefore, a hyperglycemic environment may provide the necessary conditions for these cancer cells to survive and proliferate. Glucose is also a substrate for fatty acid synthase (FAS), an enzyme that allows for the synthesis of fatty acids.[79] The increase of FAS in malignant breast cancer cell lines promoted survival in these cells.[79] Furthermore, FAS also conferred resistance to chemotherapeutic agents in MCF-7 and T47D cells, by preventing apoptosis.[79] This link between hyperglycemia and chemotherapy resistance may contribute to the poor prognosis and increase in cancer mortality that is seen in patients with T2D and breast cancer.[37]

Studies have also found that hyperglycemia induces EMT in various cell lines.[80] In rat renal proximal tubular epithelial (NRK-52E) cells, expressions of alpha-smooth muscle actin and vimentin, which are mesenchymal markers, were increased, whereas these cells lost the expression of the epithelial cell marker E-cadherin after exposure to high glucose.[80] Furthermore, TGF-β levels were also increased in cells exposed to high glucose levels.[80] In many carcinomas, growth factors, such as TGF-β or epidermal growth factor, can lead to the induction of EMT by increasing the expression various EMT-inducing transcription factors, most commonly Snail, Slug, zinc finger E-box binding homeobox 1 (ZEB1), and Twist.[81–83] Hyperglycemia may also promote metastatic spread by increasing angiogenesis. An increase of microRNA 467 (miRNA467) has been found with hyperglycemia. miR467 inhibits thrombospondin-1, an important antiangiogenic protein.[84] This mechanism of silencing thrombospondin-1 can provide insight into how exposure to hyperglycemia can induce angiogenesis and promote tumor progression.

These studies suggest that the hyperglycemia of T2D can contribute to the development and progression of cancers by promoting transformation of cancer cells, providing the necessary energy source and allowing for cell survival and resistance to chemotherapy.

CYTOKINES AND ADIPOKINES
Inflammation

T2D is strongly associated with obesity, which can promote systemic inflammation and insulin resistance in adipose tissues. Epidemiologic studies have linked elevated levels of the inflammatory markers C-reactive protein (CRP) and interleukin 6 (IL-6) with the development of T2D.[85] It has been noted that overeating can result in cytokine hypersecretion, which can promote the development of insulin resistance.[85] Cytokines are signaling molecules, within the immune response system, that are secreted in response to injury from infection, inflammation, and chemicals.[86] Cytokines are known to regulate growth, signaling, and differentiation in stromal and tumor cells. Prolonged exposure and production of these cytokines has been associated with tumor formation and progression. Various cytokines have been associated with tumor development, however IL-1β, IL-6, and tumor necrosis factor-alpha (TNF-α) have been cited as the major cytokines linking T2D to cancer progression.[85]

TNF-α activates the TNF receptors (TNFR) that promote a series of signal transduction pathways and regulate genes involved in inflammation, cell survival and cell death. TNFR activation can lead to the activation of pathways, such as the FAS-associated signal via death domain/caspase 8/caspase 3, MAPK, Jun Kinase, and nuclear factor (NF)-kB pathway.[86] NF-kB activation is known to have antiapoptotic effects through negative regulation of proapoptotic factors.[86] Animal models have shown that constitutive production of TNF-α promotes the growth and metastasis of tumors.[87]

TNF-α homozygous knockout mice on a high-fat, high-caloric diet demonstrated better sensitivity to insulin when compared with the TNF-α wild-type mice on the same diet.[88] Furthermore, these TNF-α–deficient obese mice had lower levels of circulating free fatty acids and higher levels of Glut4 protein in muscle, and mice lacking TNF-α or TNFR demonstrated improved insulin sensitivity.[88] This suggests that TNF-α can promote obesity-related insulin resistance. Furthermore, TNF-α production has been associated with poor prognosis in human cancers.[89] TNF-α has been shown to upregulate the expression of C-X-C chemokine receptor type 4.[86] This chemokine receptor has been associated with an increase in metastasis and tumor cell survival in various cancers.[86] These studies demonstrate that TNF-α can promote the progression of cancer in the setting of inflammation. These studies also suggest that TNF-α/TNFR signaling may be important for therapeutics.

Another group of cytokines important in T2D and cancer are the interleukins, such as IL-1β and IL-6. Studies have shown that patients with high IL-1β–producing tumors generally have a worse prognosis than patients with tumors that do not produce high levels of IL-1β.[86] IL-1β is known to upregulate the inflammatory response and is overexpressed in breast carcinoma cells.[90] Human breast carcinoma samples were assayed for IL-1β levels and the higher levels of IL-1β were correlated with an increased invasion and a more aggressive phenotype of the breast carcinoma cells.[91] Local IL-1β production by cancer cells can, through autocrine signaling, stimulate the tumor cells to proliferate and invade. MCF-7 cells treated with IL-1β showed significantly increased cell proliferation.[92] Furthermore, studies have found that IL-1β can induce the expression of matrix metalloproteinases and stimulate neighboring cells to produce VEGF, IL-6, TNF-α, and TGF-β.[93] This suggests that in the setting of chronic inflammation, such as in obesity, increased levels of circulating IL-1β can promote the proliferation and invasion of tumor cells. Furthermore, autocrine and paracrine IL-1β can provide the tumor with the necessary environment to grow.

IL-6 is also negatively correlated with cancer survival, with high IL-6 levels being associated with worse progression-free and overall survival.[94] IL-6 has pro-tumorigenic effects on cancer cells by increasing the survival and the proliferation of the cells.[95] IL-6 binds to the IL-6R on the cell surface and activates Janus Kinase 1 (JAK1), which has tyrosine kinase activity.[95] JAK1 activates signal transducer and activator of transcription 3 (STAT3), a transcription factor that can lead to the increase of cell growth, differentiation, and inhibition of apoptosis.[95] Constitutive STAT3 expression enhanced breast cancer cell migration. It was shown that constitutive activation of STAT3 in mice did not induce tumor growth alone.[96] However, constitutive activation of STAT3 in a transgenic MMTV-Neu oncogene mouse model of breast cancer showed that there was cooperation between the Neu oncogene and STAT3 to promote tumorigenesis.[96] This suggests that IL-6 does not drive the formation of the tumors, but instead provides an environment in which these malignant cancer cells can grow. In human malignant kidney cells, a short hairpin RNA knockdown of IL-6 resulted in a reduction of tumor growth.[97] Furthermore, IL-6 knockout mice were resistant to carcinogen-induced tumors.[97]

Epidemiologic data indicated that many cancers are related to chronic infections or inflammation.[98] It is believed that obesity is associated with an accumulation of macrophages that aggregate and surround the mammary gland.[99] In obese mice, the macrophages were associated with increased levels of TNF-α and IL-1β.[99] Moreover, the proinflammatory cytokines have been associated with increasing the transcription of aromatase, which converts androgens to estrogens.[99] Obese mice produced higher levels of TNF-α and IL-1β, and had more induction of aromatase activity than lean mice.[99] This is also consistent with the findings that aromatase levels are increased in the breast tissue of obese women compared with healthy individuals.[100] This suggests that inflammation caused by obesity produces an environment that is rich in the proinflammatory markers that allow for increased aromatase expression. This in turn can contribute to the increased risk of cancer in obese patients.

Inflammation is now considered to be one of the key hallmarks of cancer that allows for a permissive tumor-growing microenvironment.[101] These studies show that there is clearly interplay between the inflammatory markers and cancer cell progression. In patients with obesity, the metabolic syndrome, and T2D, these cytokines are increased and can contribute to deregulation of the cell cycle and in turn promote tumorigenesis. In the setting of obesity, the metabolic syndrome, and T2D, decreasing inflammatory cytokines, such as TNF-α, IL-1β, and IL-6, may improve insulin sensitivity and reduce tumor progression.

Adipokines

The adipose tissue produces hormones and cytokine-like factors. Two such adipokines (cytokines produced by the adipose tissue), leptin and adiponectin, are related to obesity, T2D, and breast cancer.

Leptin is a proinflammatory adipokine that is expressed by the Ob gene and regulates food intake, inflammation, immunity, cell proliferation, and differentiation of different cell types.[102] Leptin has been shown to increase proliferation, migration, and invasion of cancer cells. In some cases, it has been reported to increase levels of VEGF.[43] Leptin receptor expression has been reported to be higher in many human breast cancers compared with normal breast epithelial cells.[103] Furthermore, patients who demonstrated higher leptin and leptin receptor levels showed an increase in metastases.[43] In MCF-7 cells, a knockdown of the leptin receptor resulted in a decrease of tumor volume in a mouse xenograft model.[102] About 60% of ovarian cancers have an overexpression of the leptin receptor.[102] In a cell culture model of human ovarian cancer, it was discovered that leptin stimulated the expression of an antiapoptotic protein.[104] Furthermore, leptin was able to induce growth in the ovarian cancer cell line by activating JAK, MAPK, and PI3K/Akt pathways.[104] In a mouse MMTV-TGF-α model with leptin receptor deficiency, mammary tumors failed to form.[105]

Adiponectin is an anti-inflammatory adipokine secreted by adipose tissues. It has been found to possess a protective role against obesity and T2D.[106] Adiponectin binds to its adiponectin receptors 1 and 2 (AdipoR1 and AdipoR2).[106] These receptors then activate various signaling pathways, such as adenosine monophosphate-activated kinase (AMPK) and p38 MAPK.[106] There is an inverse relationship between adiponectin plasma concentrations and BMI.[107] A prospective study found that patients with high adiponectin levels had a 40% lower risk of developing T2D than patients with low adiponectin concentrations.[108] Furthermore, epidemiologic studies have found that low adiponectin levels are associated with an increased risk of breast cancer.[107] In women, low serum adiponectin concentrations correlated with larger tumors and a worse prognosis.[109] Obese and diabetic mice administered adiponectin had a reduction in hyperglycemia, improved insulin sensitivity, and increased fatty acid oxidation in muscle tissue.[43] Therefore, adiponectin may reduce tumor growth by reducing insulin and glucose levels. Moreover, in MDA-MB-231 breast cancer cells, it was discovered that adiponectin activated AMPK, leading to reduced invasion of the cells.[110] Activated AMPK promoted the increase of protein phosphatase 2A (PP2A), a tumor suppressor typically lost or decreased in patients with breast cancer, which dephosphorylates AKT.[110] Furthermore, the reduction of tumor growth and volume in mice with increased adiponectin concentrations demonstrated the protective effect of adiponectin in vivo.[111] These data suggest that adiponectin levels may be used as an additional screen to predict the risk of breast cancer, especially in patients with T2D and obesity. Furthermore, increasing adiponectin concentrations and adiponectin-induced reactivation of PP2A may be a therapeutic target for breast cancer.

This section focused on the potential roles of adipokines and cytokines in promoting cancer growth and metastases in the setting of obesity, the metabolic syndrome, and T2D. Reducing inflammatory cytokines, decreasing leptin levels, or increasing adiponectin may have beneficial effects on tumors by directly influencing the signaling pathways in tumors and by indirectly improving glycemia and insulin resistance.

SUMMARY

There have been numerous epidemiologic studies connecting T2D, the metabolic syndrome, and obesity with increased risk of developing and dying from many different cancers. As discussed in this review, there are various mechanisms that may contribute to the progression of cancer in insulin-resistant, diabetic, or obese individuals. It is hypothesized that normal cells obtain oncogenic mutations that transform the cells into cancer cells, the growth and metastases of which are then propagated in the setting of T2D. Studies are currently ongoing to uncover the precise mechanisms that link T2D, obesity, and the metabolic syndrome with cancer. By understanding the mechanisms that are involved in the link between T2D and cancer, targeted screening could be performed to prevent tumor development, and better therapeutic strategies could be designed to target specific pathways and reduce mortality in individuals with T2D and cancer.

REFERENCES

1. Kaplan MA, Pekkolay Z, Kucukoner M, et al. Type 2 diabetes mellitus and prognosis in early stage breast cancer women. Med Oncol 2012;29(3):1576–80.
2. Liu X, Ji J, Sundquist K, et al. The impact of type 2 diabetes mellitus on cancer-specific survival: a follow-up study in Sweden. Cancer 2012;118(5):1353–61.
3. Campbell PT, Newton CC, Patel AV, et al. Diabetes and cause-specific mortality in a prospective cohort of one million U.S adults. Diabetes Care 2012;35(9): 1835–44.
4. Calle EE, Rodriguez C, Walker-Thurmond K, et al. Overweight, obesity, and mortality from cancer in a prospectively studied cohort of U.S adults. N Engl J Med 2003;348(17):1625–38.
5. DeFronzo RA. Pathogenesis of type 2 diabetes mellitus. Med Clin North Am 2004;88(4):787–835, ix.
6. LeRoith D, Gavrilova O. Mouse models created to study the pathophysiology of type 2 diabetes. Int J Biochem Cell Biol 2006;38(5–6):904–12.
7. Onitilo AA, Engel JM, Glurich I, et al. Diabetes and cancer I: risk, survival, and implications for screening. Cancer Causes Control 2012;23(6):967–81.
8. Gordon-Dseagu VL, Shelton N, Mindell JS. Epidemiological evidence of a relationship between type-1 diabetes mellitus and cancer: a review of the existing literature. Int J Cancer 2013;132(3):501–8.
9. Shu X, Ji J, Li X, et al. Cancer risk among patients hospitalized for Type 1 diabetes mellitus: a population-based cohort study in Sweden. Diabet Med 2010; 27(7):791–7.
10. Hemminki K, Houlston R, Sundquist J, et al. Co-morbidity between early-onset leukemia and type 1 diabetes—suggestive of a shared viral etiology? PLoS One 2012;7(6):e39523.
11. Gallagher EJ, Leroith D, Karnieli E. The metabolic syndrome—from insulin resistance to obesity and diabetes. Med Clin North Am 2011;95(5):855–73.
12. Haggstrom C, Stocks T, Rapp K, et al. Metabolic syndrome and risk of bladder cancer: prospective cohort study in the metabolic syndrome and cancer project (Me-Can). Int J Cancer 2011;128(8):1890–8.
13. Bjorge T, Lukanova A, Jonsson H, et al. Metabolic syndrome and breast cancer in the me-can (metabolic syndrome and cancer) project. Cancer Epidemiol Biomarkers Prev 2010;19(7):1737–45.
14. Borena W, Strohmaier S, Lukanova A, et al. Metabolic risk factors and primary liver cancer in a prospective study of 578,700 adults. Int J Cancer 2012; 131(1):193–200.
15. Stocks T, Rapp K, Bjorge T, et al. Blood glucose and risk of incident and fatal cancer in the metabolic syndrome and cancer project (me-can): analysis of six prospective cohorts. PLoS Med 2009;6(12):e1000201.
16. Borena W, Stocks T, Jonsson H, et al. Serum triglycerides and cancer risk in the metabolic syndrome and cancer (Me-Can) collaborative study. Cancer Causes Control 2011;22(2):291–9.
17. Stocks T, Van Hemelrijck M, Manjer J, et al. Blood pressure and risk of cancer incidence and mortality in the metabolic syndrome and cancer project. Hypertension 2012;59(4):802–10.

18. Grundy SM, Cleeman JI, Daniels SR, et al. Diagnosis and management of the metabolic syndrome: an American Heart Association/National Heart, Lung, and Blood Institute Scientific Statement. Circulation 2005;112(17):2735–52.

19. Renehan AG, Tyson M, Egger M, et al. Body-mass index and incidence of cancer: a systematic review and meta-analysis of prospective observational studies. Lancet 2008;371(9612):569–78.

20. Adami HO, McLaughlin J, Ekbom A, et al. Cancer risk in patients with diabetes mellitus. Cancer Causes Control 1991;2(5):307–14.

21. Chari ST, Leibson CL, Rabe KG, et al. Probability of pancreatic cancer following diabetes: a population-based study. Gastroenterology 2005;129(2):504–11.

22. Zhang PH, Chen ZW, Lv D, et al. Increased risk of cancer in patients with type 2 diabetes mellitus: a retrospective cohort study in China. BMC Public Health 2012;12(1):567.

23. Haslam DW, James WP. Obesity. Lancet 2005;366(9492):1197–209.

24. Vigneri P, Frasca F, Sciacca L, et al. Diabetes and cancer. Endocr Relat Cancer 2009;16(4):1103–23.

25. Boyle P, Boniol M, Koechlin A, et al. Diabetes and breast cancer risk: a meta-analysis. Br J Cancer 2012;107(9):1608–17.

26. El-Serag HB. Hepatocellular carcinoma. N Engl J Med 2011;365(12):1118–27.

27. Arase Y, Kobayashi M, Suzuki F, et al. Effect of type 2 diabetes on risk for malignancies includes hepatocellular carcinoma in chronic hepatitis C. Hepatology 2013;57(3):964–73.

28. Hsing AW, Tsao L, Devesa SS. International trends and patterns of prostate cancer incidence and mortality. Int J Cancer 2000;85(1):60–7.

29. Cheng KC, Chen YL, Lai SW, et al. Risk of esophagus cancer in diabetes mellitus: a population-based case-control study in Taiwan. BMC Gastroenterol 2012; 12:177.

30. Wang JY, Chao TT, Lai CC, et al. Risk of colorectal cancer in type 2 diabetic patients: a population-based cohort study. Jpn J Clin Oncol 2013;43(3):258–63.

31. Pan A, Malik VS, Hu FB. Exporting diabetes mellitus to Asia: the impact of western-style fast food. Circulation 2012;126(2):163–5.

32. Zimmet P, Alberti KG, Shaw J. Global and societal implications of the diabetes epidemic. Nature 2001;414(6865):782–7.

33. Seshasai SR, Kaptoge S, Thompson A, et al. Diabetes mellitus, fasting glucose, and risk of cause-specific death. N Engl J Med 2011;364(9):829–41.

34. Zanders MM, Boll D, van Steenbergen LN, et al. Effect of diabetes on endometrial cancer recurrence and survival. Maturitas 2013;74(1):37–43.

35. Hwang A, Narayan V, Yang YX. Type 2 diabetes mellitus and survival in pancreatic adenocarcinoma: a retrospective cohort study. Cancer 2013; 119(2):404–10.

36. Redaniel MT, Jeffreys M, May MT, et al. Associations of type 2 diabetes and diabetes treatment with breast cancer risk and mortality: a population-based cohort study among British women. Cancer Causes Control 2012;23(11):1785–95.

37. Peairs KS, Barone BB, Snyder CF, et al. Diabetes mellitus and breast cancer outcomes: a systematic review and meta-analysis. J Clin Oncol 2011;29(1): 40–6.

38. Mitin T, Chen MH, Zhang Y, et al. Diabetes mellitus, race and the odds of high grade prostate cancer in men treated with radiation therapy. J Urol 2011;186(6): 2233–7.

39. Yeh HC, Platz EA, Wang NY, et al. A prospective study of the associations between treated diabetes and cancer outcomes. Diabetes Care 2012;35(1):113–8.

40. D'Amico AV, Braccioforte MH, Moran BJ, et al. Causes of death in men with prevalent diabetes and newly diagnosed high- versus favorable-risk prostate cancer. Int J Radiat Oncol Biol Phys 2010;77(5):1329–37.

41. Snyder CF, Stein KB, Barone BB, et al. Does pre-existing diabetes affect prostate cancer prognosis? A systematic review. Prostate Cancer Prostatic Dis 2010; 13(1):58–64.

42. Lawlor DA, Smith GD, Ebrahim S. Hyperinsulinaemia and increased risk of breast cancer: findings from the British Women's Heart and Health Study. Cancer Causes Control 2004;15(3):267–75.

43. Ouchi N, Parker JL, Lugus JJ, et al. Adipokines in inflammation and metabolic disease. Nat Rev Immunol 2011;11(2):85–97.

44. Giovannucci E, Harlan DM, Archer MC, et al. Diabetes and cancer: a consensus report. Diabetes Care 2010;33(7):1674–85.

45. Yang Y, Mauldin PD, Ebeling M, et al. Effect of metabolic syndrome and its components on recurrence and survival in colon cancer patients. Cancer 2012; 119(8):1512–20.

46. Hankinson SE, Willett WC, Colditz GA, et al. Circulating concentrations of insulin-like growth factor-I and risk of breast cancer. Lancet 1998;351(9113):1393–6.

47. Yee D, Paik S, Lebovic GS, et al. Analysis of insulin-like growth factor I gene expression in malignancy: evidence for a paracrine role in human breast cancer. Mol Endocrinol 1989;3(3):509–17.

48. Ikushima H, Miyazono K. TGFbeta signalling: a complex web in cancer progression. Nat Rev Cancer 2010;10(6):415–24.

49. Samani AA, Yakar S, LeRoith D, et al. The role of the IGF system in cancer growth and metastasis: overview and recent insights. Endocr Rev 2007;28(1): 20–47.

50. Creighton CJ, Casa A, Lazard Z, et al. Insulin-like growth factor-I activates gene transcription programs strongly associated with poor breast cancer prognosis. J Clin Oncol 2008;26(25):4078–85.

51. Walsh LA, Damjanovski S. IGF-1 increases invasive potential of MCF 7 breast cancer cells and induces activation of latent TGF-beta1 resulting in epithelial to mesenchymal transition. Cell Commun Signal 2011;9(1):10.

52. Kim HJ, Litzenburger BC, Cui X, et al. Constitutively active type I insulin-like growth factor receptor causes transformation and xenograft growth of immortalized mammary epithelial cells and is accompanied by an epithelial-to-mesenchymal transition mediated by NF-kappaB and snail. Mol Cell Biol 2007;27(8):3165–75.

53. Huber MA, Kraut N, Beug H. Molecular requirements for epithelial-mesenchymal transition during tumor progression. Curr Opin Cell Biol 2005;17(5):548–58.

54. Kalluri R, Weinberg RA. The basics of epithelial-mesenchymal transition. J Clin Invest 2009;119(6):1420–8.

55. Tornell J, Carlsson B, Pohjanen P, et al. High frequency of mammary adenocarcinomas in metallothionein promoter-human growth hormone transgenic mice created from two different strains of mice. J Steroid Biochem Mol Biol 1992; 43(1–3):237–42.

56. de Ostrovich KK, Lambertz I, Colby JK, et al. Paracrine overexpression of insulin-like growth factor-1 enhances mammary tumorigenesis in vivo. Am J Pathol 2008;173(3):824–34.

57. Wu Y, Cui K, Miyoshi K, et al. Reduced circulating insulin-like growth factor I levels delay the onset of chemically and genetically induced mammary tumors. Cancer Res 2003;63(15):4384–8.

58. Konijeti R, Koyama S, Gray A, et al. Effect of a low-fat diet combined with IGF-1 receptor blockade on 22Rv1 prostate cancer xenografts. Mol Cancer Ther 2012; 11(7):1539–46.
59. Reidy DL, Vakiani E, Fakih MG, et al. Randomized, phase II study of the insulin-like growth factor-1 receptor inhibitor IMC-A12, with or without cetuximab, in patients with cetuximab- or panitumumab-refractory metastatic colorectal cancer. J Clin Oncol 2010;28(27):4240–6.
60. Schmitz S, Kaminsky-Forrett MC, Henry S, et al. Phase II study of figitumumab in patients with recurrent and/or metastatic squamous cell carcinoma of the head and neck: clinical activity and molecular response (GORTEC 2008-02). Ann Oncol 2012;23(8):2153–61.
61. Weickhardt A, Doebele R, Oton A, et al. A phase I/II study of erlotinib in combination with the anti-insulin-like growth factor-1 receptor monoclonal antibody IMC-A12 (cixutumumab) in patients with advanced non-small cell lung cancer. J Thorac Oncol 2012;7(2):419–26.
62. Becker S, Dossus L, Kaaks R. Obesity related hyperinsulinaemia and hyperglycaemia and cancer development. Arch Physiol Biochem 2009;115(2):86–96.
63. Goodwin PJ, Ennis M, Pritchard KI, et al. Fasting insulin and outcome in early-stage breast cancer: results of a prospective cohort study. J Clin Oncol 2002; 20(1):42–51.
64. Lipscombe LL, Goodwin PJ, Zinman B, et al. The impact of diabetes on survival following breast cancer. Breast Cancer Res Treat 2008;109(2):389–95.
65. Mauro L, Bartucci M, Morelli C, et al. IGF-I receptor-induced cell-cell adhesion of MCF-7 breast cancer cells requires the expression of junction protein ZO-1. J Biol Chem 2001;276(43):39892–7.
66. Rodriguez-Viciana P, Warne PH, Vanhaesebroeck B, et al. Activation of phosphoinositide 3-kinase by interaction with Ras and by point mutation. EMBO J 1996;15(10):2442–51.
67. Larue L, Bellacosa A. Epithelial-mesenchymal transition in development and cancer: role of phosphatidylinositol 3' kinase/AKT pathways. Oncogene 2005; 24(50):7443–54.
68. Grille SJ, Bellacosa A, Upson J, et al. The protein kinase Akt induces epithelial mesenchymal transition and promotes enhanced motility and invasiveness of squamous cell carcinoma lines. Cancer Res 2003;63(9):2172–8.
69. Frasca F, Pandini G, Scalia P, et al. Insulin receptor isoform A, a newly recognized, high-affinity insulin-like growth factor II receptor in fetal and cancer cells. Mol Cell Biol 1999;19(5):3278–88.
70. Harrington SC, Weroha SJ, Reynolds C, et al. Quantifying insulin receptor isoform expression in FFPE breast tumors. Growth Horm IGF Res 2012;22(3–4): 108–15.
71. Thissen JP, Ketelslegers JM, Underwood LE. Nutritional regulation of the insulin-like growth factors. Endocr Rev 1994;15(1):80–101.
72. Novosyadlyy R, Lann DE, Vijayakumar A, et al. Insulin-mediated acceleration of breast cancer development and progression in a nonobese model of type 2 diabetes. Cancer Res 2010;70(2):741–51.
73. Fernandez AM, Kim JK, Yakar S, et al. Functional inactivation of the IGF-I and insulin receptors in skeletal muscle causes type 2 diabetes. Genes Dev 2001; 15(15):1926–34.
74. Ferguson RD, Novosyadlyy R, Fierz Y, et al. Hyperinsulinemia enhances c-Myc-mediated mammary tumor development and advances metastatic progression to the lung in a mouse model of type 2 diabetes. Breast Cancer Res 2012;14(1):R8.

75. Zhang H, Fagan DH, Zeng X, et al. Inhibition of cancer cell proliferation and metastasis by insulin receptor downregulation. Oncogene 2010;29(17): 2517–27.
76. Shikata K, Ninomiya T, Kiyohara Y. Diabetes mellitus and cancer risk: review of the epidemiological evidence. Cancer Sci 2013;104(1):9–14.
77. Sieri S, Muti P, Claudia A, et al. Prospective study on the role of glucose metabolism in breast cancer occurrence. Int J Cancer 2012;130(4):921–9.
78. Garber K. Energy boost: the Warburg effect returns in a new theory of cancer. J Natl Cancer Inst 2004;96(24):1805–6.
79. Zeng L, Biernacka KM, Holly JM, et al. Hyperglycaemia confers resistance to chemotherapy on breast cancer cells: the role of fatty acid synthase. Endocr Relat Cancer 2010;17(2):539–51.
80. Zhou L, Xue H, Yuan P, et al. Angiotensin AT1 receptor activation mediates high glucose-induced epithelial-mesenchymal transition in renal proximal tubular cells. Clin Exp Pharmacol Physiol 2010;37(9):e152–7.
81. Pan B, Ren H, He Y, et al. HDL of patients with type 2 diabetes mellitus elevates the capability of promoting breast cancer metastasis. Clin Cancer Res 2012; 18(5):1246–56.
82. Shi Y, Massague J. Mechanisms of TGF-beta signaling from cell membrane to the nucleus. Cell 2003;113(6):685–700.
83. Al Moustafa AE, Achkhar A. Yasmeen A: EGF-receptor signaling and epithelial-mesenchymal transition in human carcinomas. Front Biosci (Schol Ed) 2012;4: 671–84.
84. Bhattacharyya S, Sul K, Krukovets I, et al. Novel tissue-specific mechanism of regulation of angiogenesis and cancer growth in response to hyperglycemia. J Am Heart Assoc 2012;1(6):e005967.
85. Haffner SM. Insulin resistance, inflammation, and the prediabetic state. Am J Cardiol 2003;92(4A):18J–26J.
86. Vendramini-Costa DB, Carvalho JE. Molecular link mechanisms between inflammation and cancer. Curr Pharm Des 2012;18(26):3831–52.
87. Hotamisligil GS, Shargill NS, Spiegelman BM. Adipose expression of tumor necrosis factor-alpha: direct role in obesity-linked insulin resistance. Science 1993; 259(5091):87–91.
88. Uysal KT, Wiesbrock SM, Marino MW, et al. Protection from obesity-induced insulin resistance in mice lacking TNF-alpha function. Nature 1997;389(6651): 610–4.
89. Aggarwal BB, Shishodia S, Sandur SK, et al. Inflammation and cancer: how hot is the link? Biochem Pharmacol 2006;72(11):1605–21.
90. Chavey C, Bibeau F, Gourgou-Bourgade S, et al. Oestrogen receptor negative breast cancers exhibit high cytokine content. Breast Cancer Res 2007;9(1):R15.
91. Jin L, Yuan RQ, Fuchs A, et al. Expression of interleukin-1beta in human breast carcinoma. Cancer 1997;80(3):421–34.
92. Honma S, Shimodaira K, Shimizu Y, et al. The influence of inflammatory cytokines on estrogen production and cell proliferation in human breast cancer cells. Endocr J 2002;49(3):371–7.
93. Lewis AM, Varghese S, Xu H, et al. Interleukin-1 and cancer progression: the emerging role of interleukin-1 receptor antagonist as a novel therapeutic agent in cancer treatment. J Transl Med 2006;4:48.
94. Bozcuk H, Uslu G, Samur M, et al. Tumour necrosis factor-alpha, interleukin-6, and fasting serum insulin correlate with clinical outcome in metastatic breast cancer patients treated with chemotherapy. Cytokine 2004;27(2–3):58–65.

95. Ghosh S, Ashcraft K. An IL-6 link between obesity and cancer. Front Biosci (Elite Ed) 2013;5:461–78.
96. Barbieri I, Pensa S, Pannellini T, et al. Constitutively active Stat3 enhances neu-mediated migration and metastasis in mammary tumors via upregulation of Cten. Cancer Res 2010;70(6):2558–67.
97. Ancrile B, Lim KH, Counter CM. Oncogenic Ras-induced secretion of IL6 is required for tumorigenesis. Genes Dev 2007;21(14):1714–9.
98. Schetter AJ, Heegaard NH, Harris CC. Inflammation and cancer: interweaving microRNA, free radical, cytokine and p53 pathways. Carcinogenesis 2010; 31(1):37–49.
99. Subbaramaiah K, Howe LR, Bhardwaj P, et al. Obesity is associated with inflammation and elevated aromatase expression in the mouse mammary gland. Cancer Prev Res (Phila) 2011;4(3):329–46.
100. Morris PG, Hudis CA, Giri D, et al. Inflammation and increased aromatase expression occur in the breast tissue of obese women with breast cancer. Cancer Prev Res (Phila) 2011;4(7):1021–9.
101. Hanahan D, Weinberg RA. Hallmarks of cancer: the next generation. Cell 2011; 144(5):646–74.
102. Vansaun MN. Molecular pathways: adiponectin and leptin signaling in cancer. Clin Cancer Res 2013;19(8):1926–32.
103. Giordano C, Vizza D, Panza S, et al. Leptin increases HER2 protein levels through a STAT3-mediated up-regulation of Hsp90 in breast cancer cells. Mol Oncol 2012;7(3):379–91.
104. Chen C, Chang YC, Lan MS, et al. Leptin stimulates ovarian cancer cell growth and inhibits apoptosis by increasing cyclin D1 and Mcl-1 expression via the activation of the MEK/ERK1/2 and PI3K/Akt signaling pathways. Int J Oncol 2013; 42(3):1113–9.
105. Cleary MP, Juneja SC, Phillips FC, et al. Leptin receptor-deficient MMTV-TGF-alpha/Lepr(db)Lepr(db) female mice do not develop oncogene-induced mammary tumors. Exp Biol Med (Maywood) 2004;229(2):182–93.
106. Duan XF, Tang P, Li Q, et al. Obesity, adipokines, and hepatocellular carcinoma. Int J Cancer 2013;133(8):1776–83.
107. Vona-Davis L, Howard-McNatt M, Rose DP. Adiposity, type 2 diabetes and the metabolic syndrome in breast cancer. Obes Rev 2007;8(5):395–408.
108. Duncan BB, Schmidt MI, Pankow JS, et al. Adiponectin and the development of type 2 diabetes: the atherosclerosis risk in communities study. Diabetes 2004; 53(9):2473–8.
109. Miyoshi Y, Funahashi T, Kihara S, et al. Association of serum adiponectin levels with breast cancer risk. Clin Cancer Res 2003;9(15):5699–704.
110. Kim KY, Baek A, Hwang JE, et al. Adiponectin-activated AMPK stimulates dephosphorylation of AKT through protein phosphatase 2A activation. Cancer Res 2009;69(9):4018–26.
111. Wang Y, Lam JB, Lam KS, et al. Adiponectin modulates the glycogen synthase kinase-3beta/beta-catenin signaling pathway and attenuates mammary tumorigenesis of MDA-MB-231 cells in nude mice. Cancer Res 2006;66(23): 11462–70.

Update on Gestational Diabetes Mellitus

Ann E. Evensen, MD

KEYWORDS

- Gestational diabetes mellitus • Pregnancy • Prenatal care • Obstetrics
- Pregnancy complications • Glyburide • Insulin

DEFINITION

Gestational diabetes mellitus (GDM) is defined as carbohydrate intolerance that begins or is first recognized in pregnancy.[1] Historically, GDM has been labeled as classes A1 (non–insulin requiring) and A2 (insulin requiring).[2] Management of other classes such as diabetes diagnosed before conception (pregestational diabetes) or gestational diabetes insipidus is not covered in this review.

PATHOPHYSIOLOGY

All pregnant women develop some insulin resistance, which likely evolved to facilitate energy delivery to the fetus. Insulin resistance is proposed to occur in response to placental hormones. The role of placental hormones is consistent with the observed worsening of GDM throughout pregnancy (increasing placental size), the increased risk of GDM in pregnancies with multiple fetuses (larger total placental weight), and the rapid resolution of GDM with delivery of the placenta.[3] Insulin resistance may progress to GDM by revealing autoimmune-mediated or genetic abnormalities in pancreatic beta-cell function and/or worsening of chronic insulin resistance. Pregnant women with autoimmune beta-cell dysfunction may have more rapid escalation of blood glucose levels than women with chronic insulin resistance.[4]

PREVALENCE

The estimated prevalence of GDM varies widely depending on the population studied and screening methods used, ranging from 1% to 25%.[5,6] The prevalence is increasing as rates of obesity increase.[4,7] One-third of women with GDM have a

This article originally appeared in Primary Care: Clinics in Office Practice, Volume 39, Issue 1, March 2012.
This work received no grant funding.
The author has nothing to disclose.
Department of Family Medicine, University of Wisconsin School of Medicine and Public Health, 100 North Nine Mound Road, Verona, WI 53593, USA
E-mail address: ann.evensen@uwmf.wisc.edu

Clinics Collections 1 (2014) 405–416
http://dx.doi.org/10.1016/j.ccol.2014.08.021

recurrence in subsequent pregnancies. Risk factors for recurrence are weight gain between pregnancies, older maternal age, and greater parity.[8,9]

SCREENING

Women may have diabetes that existed but was undiagnosed before pregnancy. Patients at very high risk for preexisting diabetes (strong family history of type 2 diabetes, personal history of GDM, delivery of a large-for-gestational-age [LGA] infant, polycystic ovary syndrome, severe obesity, or glucosuria) should undergo a glucose tolerance test early in prenatal care.[9]

For patients not at high risk, there is debate about the need for universal screening. Although there is consensus that treating GDM is beneficial, systematic reviews of the available evidence have not found sufficient evidence to support screening for GDM.[10,11]

Despite the lack of strong evidence for universal screening, it is recommended by the United States Preventative Services Task Force (USPSTF) after 24 weeks gestation (grade B recommendation) and is routinely done in US obstetric practice at 24 to 28 weeks' gestation.[6] Screening before 24 weeks may miss cases of GDM, whereas screening later in pregnancy may delay treatment (although the benefits of early treatment have not been documented).

Selective screening is an alternative to universal screening. Selective screening uses certain criteria (**Box 1**) to avoid screening low-risk women. Selective screening is estimated to have very high sensitivity but only exempts a small percentage (3.5%) of the population from screening.[12] Because glucose intolerance occurs across a continuum, no cutoff identifies all persons with GDM, whether universal or selective screening is chosen.

A 2-step testing procedure is recommended for screening and diagnosis of GDM by the American College of Obstetricians and Gynecologists (ACOG). The most recent ACOG Practice Bulletin, published in August, 2013, recommends screening with the O'Sullivan test—a 1-hour, nonfasting, 50-g glucose challenge.[1] A blood glucose level cutoff of either 130 or 140 mg/dL can be used to diagnose GDM. Using a cutoff of 130 mg/dL increases sensitivity and decreases specificity of the screening tool; the opposite is true for a cutoff of 140 mg/dL. The use of either cutoff is acceptable because the risks and benefits of each cutoff are unknown.[1] If the 1-hour screening test is abnormal, a 3-hour, fasting, 100-g glucose tolerance test is performed to diagnose

---

Box 1
Criteria for selective screening of women at low risk for GDM

You may choose not to screen low-risk women who meet ALL the following criteria:

1. Younger than 25 years

2. Not a member of an ethnic group at an increased risk for the development of type 2 diabetes mellitus (Hispanic, African, Native American, South or East Asian, or Pacific Islands ancestry)

3. Normal weight before pregnancy

4. No history of abnormal glucose tolerance

5. No history of adverse obstetric outcomes usually associated with GDM

6. No known diabetes in first-degree relatives

Data from American Diabetes Association. Standards of medical care in diabetes—2010. Diabetes Care 2010;33(Suppl 1):S11–61.

GDM. Either the Carpenter/Coustan or the National Diabetes Data Group criteria can be used for interpreting the 3-hour test results. As with the 1-hour challenge, there are no data from clinical trials demonstrating superiority of either criterion.[12]

In 2010, the International Association of Diabetes and Pregnancy Study Group (IADPSG) recommended abandoning the 2-step screening process and adopting a 2-hour, fasting, 75-g glucose tolerance test for all women.[13] This method would allow for screening and diagnosis with a single glucose tolerance test. The cutoffs recommended by the IADPSG are much more stringent than the 2-hour, fasting, 75-g glucose tolerance test previously endorsed by the World Health Organization. The IADPSG reported that the new cutoffs were chosen based on the landmark Hyperglycemia and Adverse Pregnancy Outcomes (HAPO) study but acknowledged that no trial has been performed to document benefit to mothers or infants if this method of screening were to be adopted.[14] At this time, the ACOG recommends the 2-step testing because of the costs of treatment and monitoring for an estimated 18% of all pregnancies (more than double the incidence of GDM based on the 2-step testing) without documented benefits and improvements in maternal or neonatal outcomes.[1,15] **Table 1** compares testing methods and cutoffs for screening and diagnosis of GDM.

Regardless of the choice of test, venous samples are recommended over capillary measurements (point-of-care "fingerstick"). Capillary samples overestimate blood glucose levels compared with venous samples.[16] The use of food (such as jelly beans) instead of a standard glucose solution is not recommended because of the decreased test sensitivity.[17]

MATERNAL, FETAL, AND NEONATAL RISKS OF GDM

The risks of GDM are numerous for both the mother and the infant (**Box 2**). The HAPO study, which adjusted results for variables such as age, body mass index, and maternal hypertension, found a linear relationship between complications (fetal

Table 1
Comparison of glucose tolerance tests used for screening and diagnosis of GDM

Test or Criterion Name	Glucose Challenge (g)	Fasting	Time Measurement	Cutoffs (mg/dL)	Number of Abnormal Results Required for a Positive Test Result
O'Sullivan	50	No	At 1 h	>140 or >130	1
IADPSG	75	Yes	Fasting At 1 h At 2 h	≥92 ≥180 ≥153	1
World Health Organization	75	Yes	Fasting At 2 h	>126 >140	1
National Diabetes Data Group	100	Yes	Fasting At 1 h At 2 h At 3 h	≥105 ≥190 ≥165 ≥145	2
Carpenter/ Coustan criteria	100	Yes	Fasting At 1 h At 2 h At 3 h	≥95 ≥180 ≥155 ≥140	2

Data from Refs.[1,55]

Box 2
Maternal, fetal, and neonatal complications of GDM

Maternal

Gestational hypertension and preeclampsia

Polyhydramnios

Risks associated with increased rates of induction (operative delivery, chorioamnionitis, tachysystole, uterine rupture, cord prolapse, and hemorrhage)

Need for cesarean delivery

Maternal trauma from operative delivery

Preterm labor

Fetal

Macrosomia: birthweight exceeding 4000 to 4500 g

Shoulder dystocia

Preterm delivery

Fetal cardiomyopathy

Stillbirth

Congenital malformations (if diabetes was not diagnosed before pregnancy)

Risks of operative delivery (shoulder dystocia, brachial plexus injury, and birth trauma)

Neonatal

Respiratory distress syndrome and lung immaturity

Cardiomyopathy

Small-for-gestational-age (SGA)

Increased lifetime risk of developing diabetes mellitus and obesity

Changes in neurodevelopment including attention and motor skills

Hyperbilirubinemia

Hypoglycemia

Hypocalcemia and hypomagnesemia

Erythremia (increased red blood cells)

Poor feeding

Data from Refs.[1,4,19–23]

---

macrosomia and the need for primary cesarean delivery) and glucose intolerance.[18] This linear relationship was seen even at levels of glucose intolerance that did not meet the criteria for GDM.[14]

Elevated maternal blood glucose levels clearly result in some increased risk. Glucose crosses the placenta but insulin does not, and the fetus produces its own insulin in response to the glucose entering the placental circulation. Fetal insulin allows for the storage of excess glucose as fetal fat deposits. In addition, fetal insulin acts as a growth factor, causing macrosomia. Macrosomia, in turn, increases the risk of an operative delivery and incidence of shoulder dystocia. These delivery complications increase the risk of maternal and fetal trauma, including injury to maternal internal organs, maternal hemorrhage and infection, perineal laceration, brachial plexus injury, and cephalohematoma.

Other risks are less obviously related to hyperglycemia but are found at increased rates in pregnancies complicated by GDM (eg, preeclampsia, fetal cardiomyopathy, delayed fetal lung maturation, and abnormal pediatric psychomotor development).[19–22]

Two potential iatrogenic risks of managing pregnancies complicated by GDM are respiratory distress syndrome and SGA neonates. Aggressive lowering of maternal blood glucose levels during pregnancy increases the risk of SGA infants.[4] Inducing labor before 38 to 39 weeks increases the already-elevated risk of neonatal lung immaturity in infants of mothers with GDM.

ANTEPARTUM MANAGEMENT OF GDM

Although there is debate about the ideal method of screening for GDM, there is agreement that once diagnosed, patients with GDM should be treated with diet and, if needed, medication. The authors of a systematic review of the benefits of treating GDM with diet and insulin (added to diet if needed) found that treatment reduced risk of shoulder dystocia, preeclampsia, and macrosomia. More intensive treatment was more effective than less-intensive treatment in reducing the risk of shoulder dystocia. Treatment of GDM had no effect on the rates of SGA infants and perinatal or neonatal mortality.[7,12,21]

The 3 primary goals in antenatal management of GDM are to prevent macrosomia, avoid ketosis, and detect pregnancy complications (eg, hypertension, intrauterine growth restriction, and fetal distress). Despite agreement on these goals, there is no evidence to support specific management recommendations. Diet, exercise, oral hypoglycemic medications, and insulin may be used to treat GDM.

The goals of diet therapy in GDM are to avoid ketosis, achieve normal blood glucose levels, obtain proper nutrition, and gain weight appropriately. The American Diabetes Association recommends nutrition counseling, preferably with a registered dietician.[24] Counseling should be individualized, combined with recommendations for exercise, and culturally appropriate. The amount and distribution of carbohydrate should be based on clinical outcome measures (eg, hunger, blood glucose levels, weight gain, and [rarely used] ketone levels), but a minimum of 175 g of carbohydrate per day should be provided.[24] Carbohydrate should be distributed throughout the day in 5 to 7 meals and snacks. Carbohydrate is generally less well tolerated at breakfast than at other meals. Use of a low–glycemic index diet decreases the need for insulin to maintain euglycemia.[25,26] Fiber supplementation is not known to benefit patients with GDM.[24]

Experts recommend that women with GDM should exercise regularly to control blood glucose levels, but an improvement in clinical outcomes has not been demonstrated from compliance with this recommendation.[1,4,27]

Weight loss during pregnancy is not recommended, but the ideal weight gain for patients with GDM is unknown.[4,24] The Institute of Medicine (IOM) has published recommendations for weight gain in pregnancy, but the guidelines are the same for patients with and without GDM.[28] A cohort study showed that women with GDM who gained more weight than was recommended by the IOM had an increased risk of preterm delivery, macrosomic neonates, and cesarean delivery. Women with GDM who gained less weight than was recommended had an increased rate of SGA infants.[29]

TREATMENT WITH INSULIN

Traditionally, insulin is used if dietary management does not maintain fasting blood glucose level measurements less than 96 mg/dL, 1-hour measurements less than 130 to 140 mg/dL, and 2-hour measurements less than 120 mg/dL.[4] Another gauge that is used to determine the need for insulin is the fetal abdominal circumference measured at 29 to 33 weeks. If this measurement exceeds the 75th percentile, adding insulin to a management regimen will decrease the incidence of LGA infants.[30]

Insulin does not cross the placenta. Humalog, neutral protamine Hagedorn (NPH), and insulin lispro are used because of their rapid action and documented safety.[31] Long-acting glargine and detemir may be more convenient to use but may not adequately manage postprandial hyperglycemia. A recent systematic review and meta-analysis of retrospective cohort studies evaluating the use of glargine in the treatment of GDM found no adverse fetal outcomes.[4,31,32] However, no prospective studies of glargine or detemir have been carried out.

Two large randomized controlled trials of GDM treatment using diet and insulin (if needed) showed benefits including decreased incidence of fetal overgrowth, shoulder dystocia, cesarean delivery, hypertensive disorders, and serious perinatal complications (defined as death, shoulder dystocia, bone fracture, and nerve palsy).[7,21]

Insulin may be initiated at 0.7 U/kg actual body weight/d given in divided dosages: two-thirds of the daily dosage before breakfast (given as two-thirds NPH and one-third regular insulin) and the remainder of the dosage before dinner (given as half regular insulin and half NPH). It is also acceptable to use rapid-acting insulin with each meal instead of the twice-daily regular insulin. All regimens require close monitoring and adjustment based on blood glucose levels, meal choices, and activity levels.[33]

TREATMENT WITH ORAL HYPOGLYCEMIC AGENTS

OHA therapy was initially rejected when early-generation sulfonylureas were found to cross the placenta and cause fetal hyperinsulinemia.[1] There was also concern that OHAs would not be sufficient to manage postprandial hyperglycemia. However, glyburide was subsequently found to be safe and effective in randomized, prospective, cohort studies.[34–36] Metformin has also been evaluated in randomized prospective studies comparing it with insulin and glyburide. These studies have found no difference in perinatal complications.[37–40] A 2010 systematic review and meta-analysis of OHAs compared with insulin showed no significant difference in maternal fasting or postprandial glycemic control. The use of OHAs was not associated with the risk of neonatal hypoglycemia, increased birth weight, incidence of cesarean section, or incidence of LGA infants.[39]

An appropriate starting dosage of glyburide is 1.25 to 2.5 mg/d, which can be gradually increased as needed to 10 mg twice a day (rarely 15 mg twice a day).[1,18] Metformin can be started at 500 mg/d and increased to a maximum of 2000 mg/d. Long-acting formulations of both glyburide and metformin are available but were not used in the trials evaluating safety and effectiveness. OHAs should be initiated only if there is a willingness to abandon them. Failure of OHAs occurs more often in pregnancies complicated by early diagnosis of GDM, older age, higher parity, and higher fasting blood glucose levels and is more common in pregnancies managed with metformin (25%–46%) than in those managed with glyburide (16%–24%).[37,38,41]

It is unclear whether the use of OHAs during the first trimester of pregnancy is safe. In Dhulkotia's systematic review, none of the trials evaluated women who required treatment before 11 weeks.[39] A Cochrane study group attempted to review the safety of OHA use in the treatment of women with diabetes and glucose intolerance diagnosed before pregnancy. However, no well-designed trial could be identified for analysis.[35] The use of OHAs other than glyburide and metformin (such as thiazolidinediones, alpha-glucosidase inhibitors, meglitinides, and peptide analogs) is untested and not recommended at this time. **Table 2** shows the safety of GDM medications in pregnant and lactating women.

WHEN TO TEST?

The growth and well-being of a fetus is more sensitive to hyperglycemia than hypoglycemia. To detect and avoid postprandial hyperglycemia, it is recommended that patients test blood glucose levels after meals. A study of patients with insulin-requiring GDM documented improved outcomes (improved glycemic control and decreased risk of neonatal hypoglycemia, macrosomia, and cesarean delivery) with postprandial testing rather than with testing when fasting.[42]

HOW OFTEN TO TEST?

Since treatment of GDM is beneficial and more intensive treatment results in better perinatal outcomes, it is assumed that frequent self-monitoring of blood glucose levels is necessary.[7,12,21] Studies of high-frequency testing (self-testing 7 times a day for insulin-requiring patients and once a day for diet-controlled patients) found better maternal and fetal outcomes when compared to low-frequency testing.[42–44] The optimal frequency of testing for patients on OHAs is unknown, but a reasonable frequency may be 4 to 6 times daily.[3]

Laboratory studies, ultrasonographies, and assessments of fetal well-being are used to monitor pregnancies complicated by GDM. Patients should undergo baseline urine protein (because of the increased risk of preeclampsia) and baseline hemoglobin A1c (HbA1c) assessments.[4] An initial HbA1c level of more than 7 or an initial fasting blood glucose level of more than 120 should be assumed to be undiagnosed,

Table 2
Safety of GDM medications in pregnancy and breastfeeding

Drug	Pregnancy Class	Breastfeeding Class
Insulin	B (regular, lispro, NPH) C (glargine, detemir)	All forms safe in breastfeeding (infants cannot absorb insulin intact through their gastrointestinal tracts)
Glyburide	B/C (manufacturer dependent)	Does not enter breast milk, but breastfeeding is not recommended by the manufacturer
Glipizide	C	Does not enter breast milk, but breastfeeding is not recommended by the manufacturer
Metformin	B	Small amount (<1% weight-adjusted maternal dose) enters breast milk, but breastfeeding is not recommended by the manufacturer

Experts consider insulin, glyburide, glipizide, and metformin safe to use in women who are breastfeeding despite the manufacturers' cautions.

Data from Metzger BE, Buchanan TA, Coustan DR, et al. Summary and recommendations of the Fifth International Workshop—Conference on Gestational Diabetes Mellitus. Diabetes Care 2007;30(Suppl 2):S251–60; and Lexi-Comp [Internet]. Ohio: Lexi-Comp, Inc.; 2011. Available at: http://www.lexi.com/. Accessed July 7, 2014.

preexisting diabetes mellitus rather than GDM. Preexisting diabetes increases the risk of many congenital malformations, especially in the cardiovascular and central nervous systems. A sonogram that includes careful assessment of fetal cardiac structures and screening for other anomalies should be offered to these patients.

Measurement of ketones in the blood or urine may aid in the management of a pregnancy complicated by severe hyperglycemia or weight loss, but there is no evidence that this monitoring improves outcomes in less-complicated pregnancies.[4]

Ultrasonography is commonly performed early in the second trimester and repeated to evaluate for excessive or inadequate growth.[4] Ultrasonography may be performed more frequently for patients treated with insulin or OHAs. A study showed that having 2 second- or third-trimester ultrasounds demonstrating fetal abdominal circumference below the 90th percentile reliably excluded the risk of having an LGA newborn.[45]

In contrast, ruling in the diagnosis of macrosomia is difficult. A systematic review reported ultrasonography underestimating or overestimating the fetal weight by no better than 14%.[46] In pregnancies not complicated by diabetes, suspected fetal macrosomia is not an indication for cesarean delivery.[23] However, suspected fetal macrosomia is taken into consideration in the management of pregnancies complicated by GDM. When comparing deliveries of fetuses of similar weights, a woman with diabetes has an increased risk of shoulder dystocia, even if the fetus is not macrosomic.[47] If fetal weight is estimated to be more than 4500 g, a trial of labor is not recommended; instead, a cesarean delivery should be offered. If the fetal weight is estimated to be 4000 to 4500 g, a clinician should consider the patient's delivery history, clinical pelvimetry, and progress of labor in determining the best delivery method. A cesarean delivery should be offered to a patient with GDM who has a prolonged second stage or arrest of descent in the second stage of labor.

The frequency of assessments of maternal and fetal well-being such as office visits (including discussion of blood glucose level management), nonstress testing (NST), fetal kick counts, contraction stress testing (CST), amniotic fluid index (AFI) measurements, and biophysical profiles (BPPs) may be decided according to local obstetric practice. There is no evidence of better outcomes with any particular monitoring pattern. Patients who require medication to control GDM are seen every 1 to 2 weeks in the office. Assessments of fetal well-being (NSTs, AFIs, and BPPs, or CSTs when interpretation of NST or BPP is unclear) begin at 32 weeks' gestation and are scheduled 2 times per week. Monitoring of very high–risk patients can be started at 26 to 28 weeks' gestation.[1,4,48] Patients with GDM who control blood glucose levels with diet alone and have no other complications should have antenatal testing beginning at 40 weeks or consider induction of labor (see Decision to deliver, below).[3]

DECISION TO DELIVER

The goal of intrapartum GDM management is to avoid operative delivery, shoulder dystocia, birth trauma, and neonatal hypoglycemia. For patients who have maintained excellent control of blood glucose levels with diet and exercise, delivery is recommended at 40 weeks (or antenatal testing should begin at that time). For patients with medication-requiring GDM, induction at 39 weeks' gestation is recommended based on consensus opinion and the results of a single trial of patients with insulin-requiring diabetes who were randomized to induction at 38 to 39 weeks versus expectant management.[1] There was no difference in cesarean delivery between the 2 groups, and fewer shoulder dystocias occurred in the induction group.[49] A clinician may choose to assess fetal lung maturity before induction at 39 weeks.

INTRAPARTUM MANAGEMENT OF GDM

For patients with diet-controlled GDM, a random blood glucose level may be measured on admission to the labor ward.[33] If the blood glucose levels are normal, routine glucose measurements are not required. If a patient with GDM was treated with OHAs or insulin before admission, intrapartum blood glucose level monitoring and dextrose and/or insulin intravenous infusions may be required. Long-acting and subcutaneous insulins are not used in labor because of the slower onset of action and risk of hypoglycemia. Maintaining maternal euglycemia may prevent fetal hypoxia and neonatal hypoglycemia. The ideal intrapartum glucose target is unknown.[4] Intrapartum insulin, dextrose, and monitoring regimens are reviewed elsewhere.[3,50]

POSTPARTUM MANAGEMENT OF GDM AND INTERCONCEPTION CARE

In most women with GDM, hyperglycemia rapidly resolves shortly after delivery. It is reasonable to measure a single random (normal level <200 mg/dL) or fasting (normal level <126 mg/dL) blood glucose level before discharge from the hospital.

With few exceptions, women with GDM should be encouraged to exclusively breast-feed their infants. In addition to the many advantages of breastfeeding to mothers and infants, breastfeeding decreases the risk of obesity in children of mothers with GDM and lowers the rates of postpartum diabetes and fasting blood glucose levels in mothers with prior GDM.[4,51,52] Experts consider insulin, glyburide, glipizide, and metformin safe to use in women who are breastfeeding despite the manufacturers' cautions (see **Table 2**).[4]

Contraception choices for women with GDM are not limited unless the patient is determined to be at an increased risk for cardiovascular diseases (in this situation, estrogen-containing contraceptives should be avoided). Hormonal contraception does not increase blood glucose levels.[53] However, patients should be counseled about the risk of weight gain with injectable medroxyprogesterone (DepoProvera).[4] Patients should also be counseled about the risk of miscarriage and congenital malformations because of maternal hyperglycemia and encouraged to be evaluated for hyperglycemia before their next conception.

Postpartum glucose tolerance testing is exceptionally important for women who had GDM. Women with GDM have a 7-fold increased risk of developing type 2 diabetes mellitus compared with those who had a normoglycemic pregnancy.[54] At 6 to 12 weeks postpartum, only one-third of women with persistent glucose intolerance have an abnormal fasting blood glucose level.[4] Therefore, to detect all women with glucose intolerance, a 75-g, fasting, 2-hour, oral glucose tolerance test is recommended.[13] Blood glucose norms for nonpregnant patients should be used to interpret the results. If the 6 to 12 weeks' postpartum test findings are normal, repeating an assessment (oral glucose tolerance test, fasting blood glucose level, or HbA1c) every 3 years is recommended.[1] A clinician should evaluate other cardiovascular risk factors (lipid disorders, blood pressure, tobacco use, etc) based on the standard population screening guidelines.[13]

TREATMENT OF THE NEWBORN

Children born to mothers with GDM are at an increased risk for immediate and long-term complications. Management of GDM-exposed neonates in the immediate newborn period is reviewed elsewhere. After discharge from the hospital, the newborn's physician should be aware of the mother's diagnosis of GDM, which allows for family counseling about weight gain, screening for diabetes and lipid disorders, and monitoring for abnormalities in neurodevelopment including attention and motor skills.[19,20]

REFERENCES

1. American College of Obstetricians and Gynecologists Committee on Practice Bulletins—Obstetrics. ACOG Practice Bulletin. Clinical management guidelines for obstetrician-gynecologists. Number 137, August 2013 (replaces Practice Bulletin Number 30, September 2001, Committee Opinion Number 435, June 2009, and Committee Opinion Number 504, September 2011). Gestational diabetes mellitus. Obstet Gynecol 2013;122:406–16.
2. White P. Pregnancy complicating diabetes. Am J Med 1949;7:609–16.
3. Cheng YW, Caughey AB. Gestational diabetes: diagnosis and management. J Perinatol 2008;28:657–64.
4. Metzger BE, Buchanan TA, Coustan DR, et al. Summary and recommendations of the Fifth International Workshop—Conference on Gestational Diabetes Mellitus. Diabetes Care 2007;30(Suppl 2):S251–60.
5. National Diabetes Information Clearinghouse [Internet]. Maryland: National Institutes of Health 2011. Available at: http://diabetes.niddk.nih.gov/dm/pubs/statistics/#Gestational. Accessed November 3, 2011.
6. Moyer V. Screening for gestational diabetes mellitus: U.S. Preventive Services Task Force Recommendation Statement. Ann Intern Med 2014;160:414–20.
7. Landon MB, Spong CY, Thom E, et al. A multicenter, randomized trial of treatment for mild gestational diabetes. N Engl J Med 2009;361:1339–48.
8. Moses RG. The recurrence rate of gestational diabetes in subsequent pregnancies. Diabetes Care 1996;19:1348–50.
9. American Diabetes Association. Standards of medical care in diabetes—2010. Diabetes Care 2010;33(Suppl 1):S11–61.
10. Tieu J, McPhee AJ, Crowther CA, et al. Screening and subsequent management for gestational diabetes for improving maternal and infant health. Cochrane Database Syst Rev 2014;(2):CD007222.
11. Horvath K, Koch K, Jeitler K, et al. Effects of treatment in women with gestational diabetes mellitus: systematic review and meta-analysis. BMJ 2010;340:c1395.
12. Teh WT, Teede HJ, Paul E, et al. Risk factors for gestational diabetes mellitus: implications for the application of screening guidelines. Aust N Z J Obstet Gynaecol 2011;51:26–30.
13. American Diabetes Association. Standards of medical care in diabetes—2011. Diabetes Care 2011;34(Suppl 1):S11–61.
14. HAPO Study Cooperative Research Group, Metzger BE, Lowe LP, et al. Hyperglycemia and adverse pregnancy outcomes. N Engl J Med 2008;358:1991–2002.
15. Meltzer SJ, Snyder J, Penrod JR, et al. Gestational diabetes mellitus screening and diagnosis: a prospective randomised controlled trial comparing costs of one-step and two-step methods. BJOG 2010;117(4):407–15.
16. Carr SR, Slocum J, Tefft L, et al. Precision of office-based blood glucose meters in screening for gestational diabetes. Am J Obstet Gynecol 1995;173:1267–72.
17. Lamar ME, Kuehl TJ, Cooney AT, et al. Jelly beans as an alternative to a fifty-gram glucose beverage for gestational diabetes screening. Am J Obstet Gynecol 1999;181:1154–7.
18. Landon MB, Gabbe SG. Gestational diabetes mellitus. Obstet Gynecol 2011;118(6):1379–93.

19. Weintrob N, Karp M, Hod M. Short- and long-range complications in offspring of diabetic mothers. J Diabetes Complications 1996;10:294–301.
20. Rizzo TA, Dooley SL, Metzger BE, et al. Prenatal and perinatal influences on long-term psychomotor development in offspring of diabetic mothers. Am J Obstet Gynecol 1995;173:1753–8.
21. Crowther CA, Hiller JE, Moss JR, et al. Effect of treatment of gestational diabetes mellitus on pregnancy outcomes. N Engl J Med 2005;352:2477–86.
22. Mitanchez D. Foetal and neonatal complications in gestational diabetes: perinatal mortality, congenital malformations, macrosomia, shoulder dystocia, birth injuries, neonatal complications. Diabetes Metab 2010;36:617–27.
23. ACOG Committee on Practice Bulletins—Obstetrics. ACOG Practice Bulletin No. 107: induction of labor. Obstet Gynecol 2009;114:386–97.
24. American Diabetes Association, Bantle JP, Wylie-Rosett J, et al. Nutrition recommendations and interventions for diabetes: a position statement of the American Diabetes Association. Diabetes Care 2008;31(Suppl 1):S61–78.
25. Tieu J, Crowther CA, Middleton P. Dietary advice in pregnancy for preventing gestational diabetes mellitus. Cochrane Database Syst Rev 2008;2:CD006674.
26. Moses RG, Barker M, Winter M, et al. Can a low-glycemic index diet reduce the need for insulin in gestational diabetes mellitus? A randomized trial. Diabetes Care 2009;32:996–1000.
27. Ceysens G, Rouiller D, Boulvain M. Exercise for diabetic pregnant women. Cochrane Database Syst Rev 2006;3:CD004225.
28. Rasmussen KM, Yaktine AN. Weight Gain During Pregnancy: Reexamining the Guidelines. Committee to Reexamine IOM Pregnancy Weight Guidelines; Institute of Medicine; National Resource Council. The National Academies Press 2009. Available at: http://books.nap.edu/openbook.php?record_id=12584. Accessed November 3, 2011.
29. Cheng YW, Chung JH, Kurbisch-Block I, et al. Gestational weight gain and gestational diabetes mellitus: perinatal outcomes. Obstet Gynecol 2008;112:1015–22.
30. Buchanan TA, Kjos SL, Montoro MN, et al. Use of fetal ultrasound to select metabolic therapy for pregnancies complicated by mild gestational diabetes. Diabetes Care 1994;17:275–83.
31. Torlone E, Di Cianni G, Mannino D, et al. Insulin analogs and pregnancy: an update. Acta Diabetol 2009;46:163–72.
32. Pollex E, Moretti ME, Koren G, et al. Safety of insulin glargine use in pregnancy: a systematic review and meta-analysis. Ann Pharmacother 2011;45:9–16.
33. Patel P, Macerollo A. Diabetes mellitus: diagnosis and screening. Am Fam Physician 2010;81:863–70.
34. Alwan N, Tuffnell DJ, West J. Treatments for gestational diabetes. Cochrane Database Syst Rev 2009;3:CD003395.
35. Tieu J, Coat S, Hague W, et al. Oral anti-diabetic agents for women with pre-existing diabetes mellitus/impaired glucose tolerance or previous gestational diabetes mellitus. Cochrane Database Syst Rev 2010;10:CD007724.
36. Rosenn BM. The glyburide report card. J Matern Fetal Neonatal Med 2010;23:219–23.
37. Moore LE, Clokey D, Rappaport VJ, et al. Metformin compared with glyburide in gestational diabetes: a randomized controlled trial. Obstet Gynecol 2010;115:55–9.
38. Silva JC, Pacheco C, Bizato J, et al. Metformin compared with glyburide for the management of gestational diabetes. Int J Gynaecol Obstet 2010;111:37–40.

39. Dhulkotia JS, Ola B, Fraser R, et al. Oral hypoglycemic agents vs insulin in management of gestational diabetes: a systematic review and metaanalysis. Am J Obstet Gynecol 2010;203:457.e1–9.
40. Nicholson W, Bolen S, Witkop CT, et al. Benefits and risks of oral diabetes agents compared with insulin in women with gestational diabetes: a systematic review. Obstet Gynecol 2009;113:193–205.
41. Rowan JA, Hague WM, Gao W, et al, MiG Trial Investigators. Metformin versus insulin for the treatment of gestational diabetes. N Engl J Med 2008;358:2003–15.
42. de Veciana M, Major CA, Morgan MA, et al. Postprandial versus preprandial blood glucose monitoring in women with gestational diabetes mellitus requiring insulin therapy. N Engl J Med 1995;333:1237–41.
43. Jovanovic LG. Using meal-based self-monitoring of blood glucose as a tool to improve outcomes in pregnancy complicated by diabetes. Endocr Pract 2008;14:239–47.
44. Hawkins JS, Casey BM, Lo JY, et al. Weekly compared with daily blood glucose monitoring in women with diet-treated gestational diabetes. Obstet Gynecol 2009;113:1307–12.
45. Schaefer-Graf UM, Wendt L, Sacks DA, et al. How many sonograms are needed to reliably predict the absence of fetal overgrowth in gestational diabetes mellitus pregnancies? Diabetes Care 2011;34:39–43.
46. Dudley NJ. A systematic review of the ultrasound estimation of fetal weight. Ultrasound Obstet Gynecol 2005;25:80–9.
47. Acker DB, Sachs BP, Friedman EA. Risk factors for shoulder dystocia. Obstet Gynecol 1985;66:762–8.
48. ACOG Practice Bulletin. Antepartum fetal surveillance. Number 145, July 2014 (replaces Practice Bulletin Number 9, October 1999). Clinical management guidelines for obstetrician-gynecologists. Obstet Gynecol 2014;124:182–92.
49. Kjos SL, Henry OA, Montoro M, et al. Insulin-requiring diabetes in pregnancy: a randomized trial of active induction of labor and expectant management. Am J Obstet Gynecol 1993;169:611–5.
50. Caplan RH, Pagliara AS, Beguin EA, et al. Constant intravenous insulin infusion during labor and delivery in diabetes mellitus. Diabetes Care 1982;5:6–10.
51. Schaefer-Graf UM, Hartmann R, Pawliczak J, et al. Association of breast-feeding and early childhood overweight in children from mothers with gestational diabetes mellitus. Diabetes Care 2006;29:1105–7.
52. Horta BL, Bahl R, Martines JC, et al. Evidence on the long-term effects of breast-feeding: systematic reviews and meta-analyses. Geneva (Switzerland): World Health Organization, Department of Child and Adolescent Health and Development; 2007.
53. Kerlan V. Postpartum and contraception in women after gestational diabetes. Diabetes Metab 2010;36:566–74.
54. Bellamy L, Casas JP, Hingorani AD, et al. Type 2 diabetes mellitus after gestational diabetes: a systematic review and meta-analysis. Lancet 2009;373:1773–9.
55. National Institutes of Health consensus development conference statement: diagnosing gestational diabetes mellitus, March 4–6, 2013. Obstet Gynecol 2013;122:358–69.

Osteoporosis-associated Fracture and Diabetes

Salila Kurra, MD[a],*, Dorothy A. Fink, MD[b], Ethel S. Siris, MD[c]

KEYWORDS

- Bone • Osteoporosis • Diabetes • Diabetes complications • Fracture
- Skeletal disorder

KEY POINTS

- Because osteoporosis and diabetes mellitus are chronic diseases that are increasing in prevalence, understanding their complex interaction is integral to providing optimal care for patients.
- Osteoporosis-associated fracture is an important complication of diabetes to consider when evaluating patients with diabetes.
- Given the different causes of type 1 and type 2 diabetes, they have a unique relationship with bone but also have similar effects on bone when not treated adequately.
- Osteoporosis treatment options for diabetic patients are the same as for nondiabetic patients, including ensuring normal renal function before starting a bisphosphonate.

INTRODUCTION

Osteoporosis and diabetes mellitus (DM) are chronic diseases with increasing prevalence. Both have significant associated morbidity and mortality and may lead to severe debilitation if not treated adequately. Osteoporosis is a skeletal disorder characterized by reduced bone quantity and quality, which predisposes to fracture.[1,2] Fragility fractures, or low-trauma fractures, are common, affecting almost 1 in 2 older women and 1 in 3 older men.[3] The global burden of osteoporosis is significant, with

This article originally appeared in Endocrinology and Metabolism Clinics of North America, Volume 43, Issue 1, March 2014.

Disclosures: Dr E.S. Siris is a consultant for Amgen, Eli Lilly, Merck, Novartis, and Pfizer, and a speaker for Amgen, Eli Lilly.

[a] Metabolic Bone Diseases Unit, Department of Medicine, Toni Stabile Osteoporosis Center, Columbia University Medical Center, 180 Fort Washington Avenue, 9-904, New York, NY 10032, USA; [b] Division of Endocrinology, Department of Medicine, Columbia University Medical Center, 630 West 168th Street, PH8, New York, NY 10032, USA; [c] Metabolic Bone Diseases Unit, Department of Medicine, Toni Stabile Osteoporosis Center, Columbia University Medical Center, New York-Presbyterian Hospital, 180 Fort Washington Avenue, 9-904, New York, NY 10032, USA
* Corresponding author.
E-mail address: sk850@columbia.edu

approximately 9 million new osteoporotic fractures worldwide in the year 2000.[4] Diabetes is also increasing in prevalence. Prevalence of diabetes for all age groups is estimated to be 4.4% of the worldwide population by the year 2030.[5]

Recent evidence shows that both type 1 and type 2 DM are associated with an increased fracture risk.[6] Although microvascular and macrovascular complications are the complications most commonly associated with diabetes, osteoporosis and risk of fracture must also be considered when treating patients with diabetes. Type 1 diabetes (T1D) is defined as a state of insulin deficiency, whereas type 2 diabetes (T2D) is characterized by insulin resistance with increased insulin levels. Given the different causes of T1D and T2D, they have unique interactions with bone. Skeletal disorders often associated with diabetes include osteoporosis-associated fracture, Charcot arthropathy, and renal osteodystrophy secondary to end-stage renal disease as a complication of diabetes.[7,8] Like others in the past,[9,10] this article focuses on osteoporosis-associated fracture as a metabolic complication of diabetes.

In recent years, osteoporosis-associated fracture has come to the forefront of complications associated with diabetes. Controversy exists over the exact mechanisms of bone loss in the setting of diabetes, but there is significant evidence to support that diabetes affects bone health. The meta-analysis by Vestergaard[11] showed that adults with T1D have a 6.9 relative risk of hip fracture and adults with T2D have a 1.3 relative risk of hip fracture. In addition, a meta-analysis by Janghorbani and colleagues[12] showed similar results with a 6.3 relative risk of hip fracture in adults with T1D and a 2.8 relative risk of hip fracture in adults with T2D. In the Vestergaard[11] study, patients with T1D had decreased bone mineral density (BMD) and increased fracture risk, but although the study noted a 6.9 relative risk of hip fracture, the BMD expected relative risk was only 1.4, suggesting that there are additional factors contributing to fracture risk. Another finding of the Vestergaard[11] study was that, despite an increased fracture risk, patients with T2D had higher than expected BMD. With data from the Health, Aging, and Body Composition (Health ABC) Study, Schwartz and colleagues[13] showed increased incidence of vertebral fracture in T2D despite increased BMD. The interaction between diabetes and bone health is complex and requires further exploration.

T1D VERSUS T2D AND BONE: SIMILARITIES

Despite their different underlying causes, without proper treatment or compliance with treatment both T1D and T2D can be complicated by hyperglycemia. Hyperglycemia in turn can be detrimental to bone; it has been shown that glucose can be toxic to osteoblasts, the cells associated with bone formation. High glucose concentrations impair the ability of osteoblastic cells to synthesize osteocalcin, which is a protein integral to bone formation.[14] Also serum osteocalcin levels seem to be suppressed by hyperglycemia in diabetic patients.[15] Bone biopsies done on individuals with diabetes have shown low bone formation on histomorphometry.[16] For a given BMD, diabetic bone seems to be less strong and therefore more likely to fracture.[17,18]

Chronic hyperglycemia also promotes advanced glycation and accumulation of advanced glycation end products (AGEs), which contribute to diabetes complications. Impaired renal function is also thought to lead to accumulation of AGEs. They are formed through a nonenzymatic reaction between reducing sugars and amine residues. AGEs act directly to induce cross-linking of long-lived proteins, resulting in alteration of vascular structure and function.[19] Accumulation of AGEs in bone collagen likely contributes to the reduction in bone strength for a given BMD.[20] The prime targets of AGE accumulation are the structural components of the connective tissue matrix. This accumulation can alter collagen function and thereby alter the function of bone.

Pentosidine is the most commonly measured AGE because of its intrinsic fluorescence.[19] Complications of diabetes including nephropathy, retinopathy, neuropathy, atherosclerotic disease, cardiomyopathy, and peripheral arterial disease have been studied extensively with regard to AGEs, and diabetes-associated bone disease has also come to the forefront of AGE-related complications.[13,21–23] Katayama and colleagues[24] showed that AGE modification of type 1 collagen impaired osteoblast cell differentiation and function in rodent models. AGEs may exert their effects on the receptor for advanced glycation end products (RAGE). Zhou and colleagues[25] showed that RAGE knockout mice had increased bone mass with decreased resorption ability, leading the investigators to conclude that RAGE enhances bone resorption through osteoclasts, the cells associated with bone resorption. In postmenopausal women with T2D and vertebral fractures, Yamamoto and colleagues[21] found that there were higher serum pentosidine levels compared with controls independently of BMD and osteoporosis risk factors and even after adjusting for diabetes duration, complications, and treatment with insulin or pioglitazone.

Studies examining glycemic control and its implications on the skeleton have not shown that tight control limits osteoporosis-related fracture.[26,27] However, in most studies, a single hemoglobin A_{1c} (HbA_{1c}) is the only measure of diabetes control and only represents glycemic control over a short period of time. Most postmenopausal women and men with T1D and T2D who develop fractures have had diabetes for decades and it is challenging to adequately assess an individual's lifetime diabetes control. Regardless, several studies have documented increased fracture rates associated with longer duration of diabetes in patients with both T1D and T2D.[28,29] Challenges to many of these studies include confounding factors such as other complications of diabetes, which may increase fracture risk as well. For example, the aforementioned study by Ivers and colleagues[29] showed that patients with both T1D and T2D who develop the visual complications of diabetes such as diabetic retinopathy and advanced cortical cataract are also at increased risk for fracture.

Based on prospective data on falls from the Study of Osteoporotic Fractures, Schwartz and colleagues[30] found an increased risk of falls in women older than 65 years with diabetes with a further increased risk in the setting of insulin use. This increased risk of falls likely contributes to the increased risk of fracture noted in this population. Although this increased fall risk is multifactorial, the complications commonly seen with diabetes, such as poor vision, peripheral neuropathy, reduced balance, and treatment-associated hypoglycemia, are themselves risk factors for falls. However, a case-control study by Vestergaard and colleagues[31] showed that both T1D and T2D confer an increased risk of fracture, but, except for diabetic kidney disease, the other complications associated with diabetes added little to the overall risk of fracture. The investigators concluded that the hyperglycemia likely contributes to decreases in bone strength.

Low states of bone turnover have been documented in both T1D and T2D, which may lead to lower mechanical strength and an increased risk of fracture.[16,32,33] Gennari and colleagues[33] recently showed that sclerostin, which is a protein that inhibits osteoblastic bone formation, is higher in T2D compared with T1D and controls, even after adjusting for age and body mass index (BMI). However, the negative association between sclerostin and parathyroid hormone (PTH) that is normally seen was not documented in patients with T1D or T2D, leading the investigators to conclude that PTH suppression of sclerostin may be impaired in both T1D and T2D. This mechanism may be another reason for bone loss in patients with diabetes.

T1D VERSUS T2D AND BONE: DIFFERENCES

Although T1D and T2D both result in states of chronic hyperglycemia, the underlying pathophysiology of T1D and T2D is different. The anabolic hormone insulin is absent in T1D and present (often increased) in T2D. However, given the changing milieu of diabetes, many patients with T1D who are insulin deficient have a BMI in the obese range and develop an insulin-resistant phenotype. In addition, many patients with T2D require insulin as their disease progresses, further complicating the effects that diabetes has on bone health.

Literature describing bone disease in patients with T1D dates to the 1920s.[34] Although there is controversy in the literature over the mechanisms of increased fracture risk, the occurrence of low BMD and fractures is well documented in patients with T1D.[35,36] Several studies have postulated that patients with T1D do not achieve peak bone mass during adolescence, which leads to a lower lifetime BMD and may ultimately increase risk of fracture.[37,38] Although T1D may be diagnosed after puberty, peak bone mass accrual continues into the early 20s and thus may be affected by hyperglycemia as well.

Insulinlike growth factor 1 (IGF-1), which is also a marker of bone formation, has been noted to be low in patients with uncomplicated insulin-dependent DM.[39] Kemink and colleagues[39] showed that, in diabetic patients with femoral neck osteopenia, the mean plasma IGF-I level was significantly lower ($P<.05$) than in those without osteopenia at this site. When they assessed only the male diabetic patients, significantly lower mean plasma IGF-I (−26%), serum alkaline phosphatase (−24%), and serum osteocalcin (−38%) levels were present in the patients with femoral neck osteopenia than in those without osteopenia at this site, suggesting reduced bone formation. They concluded that their data showed that, at least in male patients with insulin-dependent DM, osteopenia is the consequence of a reduced bone formation with a predominance of bone resorption rather than formation. This uncoupling of bone formation and resorption resembles the effects that glucocorticoids have on bone.

The most striking difference in patients with T2D compared with patients with T1D is not only their insulin resistance but that they paradoxically have an increased BMD compared with patients with T1D.[17,40–42] Despite this increased BMD, which seems to protect against fracture, patients with T2D have an increased risk of fracture, suggesting a bone quality defect given that they have a greater quantity of bone based on BMD. Lipscombe and colleagues[43] showed an increased risk of hip fracture in patients with T2D despite an increased BMD (hazard ratio [HR], 1.18 for men and 1.11 for women).

In the Women's Health Initiative Observational Study, postmenopausal women with diabetes were at increased risk of hip, foot, and spine fractures, and fractures overall, even after adjusting for falls.[41] Other studies that accounted for falls but still found an association of T2D with fracture risk are the Study of Osteoporotic Fractures; the Rotterdam Study; and the Health, Aging, and Body Composition Study.[17,42,44]

de Liefde and colleagues[42] showed that in the Rotterdam Study there was an increased nonvertebral fracture risk in patients with T2D even though they had higher BMDs in the femoral neck and lumbar spine (HR, 1.33 [1.00–1.77]). The study also performed a subset analysis comparing patients with treated T2D with patients with impaired glucose tolerance (IGT). The patients with treated T2D had an increased nonvertebral fracture risk compared with the patients with IGT, leading the investigators to conclude that duration of diabetes affects fracture risk. Using the Study of Osteoporotic Fractures, the Osteoporotic Fractures in Men Study, and the Health ABC study, Schwartz and colleagues[45] showed that patients with T2D had a higher risk of fracture for a given T score and age or fracture risk assessment tool (FRAX) score. The mean T-score difference for hip fracture was 0.59 and 0.38 for women and men, respectively.

Another difference between patients with T1D and T2D is that patients with T2D may be treated with thiazolidinediones. Using the data from A Diabetes Outcome Progression Trial, Kahn and colleagues[46,47] found that women randomized to rosiglitazone had an increased fracture risk. In addition, the Takeda Pharmaceutical Company issued a letter in 2007 that described an increased fracture risk in women receiving pioglitazone.[48]

Most recently, in a randomized, double-blind study in postmenopausal women with T2D, Bilezikian and colleagues[49] showed reductions in femoral neck, total hip, and lumbar spine BMD with daily use of rosiglitazone for 52 weeks compared with metformin. During the 24-week open-label phase when all patients received metformin, the BMD loss associated with rosiglitazone use was attenuated. In addition, both serum c-telopeptide, which is a marker of bone resorption, and procollagen type 1 N-terminal propeptide (P1NP), which is a marker of bone formation, increased in the patients randomized to rosiglitazone. In contrast, bone-specific alkaline phosphatase (BSAP), another marker of bone formation, decreased after treatment with rosiglitazone, which was similar to the results of the study by Berberoglu and colleagues.[50] The discordance between the bone turnover markers P1NP and BSAP is not fully understood, and Bilezikian and colleagues[49] postulated that impairment in mineralization processes may be required to increase BSAP.

QUANTIFYING RISK OF FRACTURE ASSOCIATED WITH DIABETES AND OSTEOPOROSIS

As detailed earlier, there is strong evidence to suggest that diabetes, regardless of the cause, and its associated complications can lead to bone loss and increased risk of fracture. Although both T1D and T2D are listed in the National Osteoporosis Foundation (NOF) guidelines as endocrine disorders that may cause or contribute to osteoporosis and fractures, there are currently no specific guidelines for screening for fracture risk in patients with diabetes.[51] It is also not currently part of the World Health Organization FRAX algorithm for assessing fracture risk.

Age, sex, BMI, prolonged glucocorticoid use, current smoking, 3 or more units per day of alcohol, secondary osteoporosis, rheumatoid arthritis, prior fragility fracture, parental history of hip fracture, and femoral neck BMD or T score are all included in the FRAX algorithm.[52] T1D is listed as a secondary cause of osteoporosis in FRAX, but is not included in the FRAX risk calculation if the femoral neck BMD is known. T2D is not formally part of FRAX. Schwartz and colleagues[45] estimated that the mean differences in T score for women and men with diabetes were 0.59 and 0.38, respectively. Giangregorio and colleagues[6] showed that, after adjusting for confounding factors, diabetes was a significant predictor of major osteoporotic fracture (HR, 1.61).

Apart from the inclusion of T1D as a secondary risk factor for osteoporosis in the FRAX algorithm, there are no guidelines that address screening for fracture risk for patients with T1D or T2D. The 2013 NOF Clinician's Guide to Prevention and Treatment of Osteoporosis recommends that women aged 65 years and older, and men aged 70 years and older, have BMD testing with dual-energy x-ray absorptiometry (DXA).[51] They also recommend that postmenopausal women and men aged 50 to 69 years have an osteoporosis evaluation based on risk factor profile, which includes T1D and T2D. The United States Preventive Service Task Force recommendations are in agreement with the NOF guidelines.[53]

MANAGEMENT

In the Ontario population-based study, Lipscombe and colleagues[43] found that, compared with individuals without diabetes, individuals with diabetes were less likely to have had a BMD test, and were more likely to be taking medications that increase risk of falling and decrease BMD. This finding underscores the importance of education regarding diabetes and associated osteoporosis and fractures. Health care providers must include bone health as part of routine clinical care for patients with diabetes in addition to addressing microvascular and macrovascular complications. Diabetes is associated with delayed fracture healing and therefore prevention is essential.[54,55] During clinical evaluations, dairy intake should be addressed. Given the concern of calcium deposition in blood vessels instead of bones in osteoporosis,[56] patients should be questioned regarding the amount of both dairy intake and calcium supplementation to ensure adequate, but not excessive, daily calcium intake.[51] In accordance with The Institute of Medicine (IOM), the NOF recommends that women older than 50 years and men older than 70 years have a calcium intake of 1200 mg per day. Men aged 50 to 70 years are recommended to take 1000 mg per day of calcium. In addition, for adults older than 50 years, the NOF recommends 800 to 1000 international units (IU) of vitamin D per day. They recommend that 25-hydroxy (OH) vitamin D levels be measured in patients at risk for deficiency with a goal 25-OH vitamin D level of 30 ng/mL.

Given the data showing a higher risk of fracture in women with T1D, it is reasonable to order a DXA scan on these patients at menopause instead of waiting until age 65 years. Although patients with T2D are also at increased risk of fracture, their BMD results may underestimate their relative risk for fracture, as discussed earlier. A diabetic patient compared with a nondiabetic patient with the same BMD and the same osteoporosis risk factors (other than diabetes) is at a higher risk of fracture. To account for this higher risk, using evidence from Schwartz and colleagues,[45] it may be prudent to adjust T scores in women with T2D by −0.6 and men with T2D by −0.4 to have a T score that more accurately identifies the level of fracture risk. Leslie and colleagues[9] concluded that it is also prudent to consider treating patients with T2D even if they are slightly below FRAX-based intervention thresholds given the challenges of interpreting BMD results and correctly determining fracture risk in patients with T2D. In the future, T2D may be included in fracture risk algorithms.

The Action to Control Cardiovascular Risk in Diabetes (ACCORD) randomized trial did not show any differences in fracture or fall risk between the intensive and standard glycemia groups.[26] However, the median HbA_{1c} in the intensive glycemic group was 6.4% and the median HbA_{1c} in the standard glycemic strategy was 7.5%. Most patients with uncontrolled diabetes do not have HbA_{1c} in the 7% range and thus more studies need to be completed to address uncontrolled, chronic hyperglycemia with fracture and fall risk. Regardless of the ACCORD data, patients with diabetes and osteoporosis need to have personalized diabetes plans to achieve glycemic control safely. Schwartz and colleagues[27] also showed in a substudy of the ACCORD trial using peripheral quantitative computed tomographic scans that bone strength at the radius and tibia was not improved with intensive glycemic control. When interpreting these data, it is important to take into account that the standard HbA_{1c} group is not representative of many patients who have chronic, uncontrolled hyperglycemia. It is well documented that achieving adequate glycemic control in patients with diabetes decreases the incidence of microvascular complications, such as retinopathy and neuropathy, which may lead to falls and subsequent fractures. Therefore, it is important to address fall prevention as well.[30]

The NOF recommends that postmenopausal women and men older than 50 years be considered for pharmacologic treatment in addition to calcium and vitamin D if they present with one of the following[51]:

1. A hip or vertebral fracture, which is a clinical diagnosis of osteoporosis
2. A T score of ≤2.5 at the femoral neck, total hip, or lumbar spine, which is the BMD-based diagnosis of osteoporosis
3. Low bone mass (T score between −1.0 and −2.5 at the hip or spine) and a 10-year absolute probability of fracture as assessed by FRAX of greater than or equal to 3% for hip fracture or greater than or equal to 20% for major osteoporotic fracture

TREATMENT

Osteoporosis treatment options for diabetic patients are the same as for nondiabetic patients. When a patient meets guidelines for treatment, there are several options including antiresorptive medications such as bisphosphonates and the anabolic agent teriparatide.

Diabetic nephropathy may limit use of bisphosphonates because they are contra-indicated if estimated glomerular filtration rate is less than 30 to 35 mL/min because they are renally cleared. Potent antiresorptives such as bisphosphonates or denosumab are also a concern if patients have renal osteodystrophy in which potent antire-sorptive treatment is contraindicated. The nature of the patient's bone disorder needs to be characterized before any pharmacologic treatment of osteoporosis can be initiated.

In postmenopausal women and older men with DM who do not have severe renal failure or renal bone disease and in whom there is an increase in bone resorption exceeding that of bone formation, an antiresorptive agent may be appropriate. Vester-gaard and colleagues[57] showed that bisphosphonates and raloxifene exert bone-protective effects even in diabetic patients with states of low bone turnover. Keegan and colleagues[58] also showed that BMD in patients with T2D increased after treatment with alendronate. However, in both the Vestergaard and colleagues[57] and Giangre-gorio and colleagues[6] studies, patients with diabetes were less likely to receive oste-oporosis treatment despite having a higher prevalence of fracture.

The uncoupling of bone resorption and bone formation that is seen in patients with DM resembles the effect of glucocorticoids on bone (namely some increase in bone resorption with a decrease in bone formation) so it is possible that the agents used to treat glucocorticoid-induced osteoporosis may be effective in the reduction in frac-ture risk in patients with DM. Both bisphosphonates and teriparatide are approved for the treatment of glucocorticoid-induced osteoporosis. One study in patients with glucocorticoid-induced osteoporosis found that the anabolic agent teriparatide led to a greater increase in total hip BMD and fewer vertebral fractures than alendronate.[59] Following a 2-year course of teriparatide, an antiresorptive is needed to preserve the increase in bone mass from the anabolic agent. Thus, until more data are available regarding the effectiveness and safety of antiresorptives such as bisphosphonates, raloxifene or denosumab, or the anabolic agent teriparatide in patients with diabetes, it is important to base decisions regarding treatment on the individual characteristics of patients and their absolute risk for fractures.

In conclusion, diabetes and osteoporosis are both chronic diseases that may lead to severe morbidity and mortality if not treated. Diabetes-associated osteoporosis and fracture are now at the forefront of diabetes complications and must be considered in evaluating, counseling, and treating patients with diabetes.

REFERENCES

1. NIH Consensus Development Panel on Osteoporosis Prevention, Diagnosis, and Therapy. Osteoporosis prevention, diagnosis, and therapy. JAMA 2001; 285(6):785–95 Epub 2001/02/15.
2. Bone health and osteoporosis: a report of the surgeon general. Rockville (MD): U.S. Department of Health and Human Services, Office of the Surgeon General; 2004.
3. Eisman JA, Bogoch ER, Dell R, et al. Making the first fracture the last fracture: ASBMR task force report on secondary fracture prevention. J Bone Miner Res 2012;27(10):2039–46 Epub 2012/07/28.
4. Johnell O, Kanis JA. An estimate of the worldwide prevalence and disability associated with osteoporotic fractures. Osteoporos Int 2006;17(12):1726–33 Epub 2006/09/20.
5. Wild S, Roglic G, Green A, et al. Global prevalence of diabetes: estimates for the year 2000 and projections for 2030. Diabetes Care 2004;27(5):1047–53 Epub 2004/04/28.
6. Giangregorio LM, Leslie WD, Lix LM, et al. FRAX underestimates fracture risk in patients with diabetes. J Bone Miner Res 2012;27(2):301–8 Epub 2011/11/05.
7. Pei Y, Hercz G, Greenwood C, et al. Renal osteodystrophy in diabetic patients. Kidney Int 1993;44(1):159–64 Epub 1993/07/01.
8. Schwartz AV. Diabetes mellitus: does it affect bone? Calcif Tissue Int 2003;73(6): 515–9 Epub 2003/10/01.
9. Leslie WD, Rubin MR, Schwartz AV, et al. Type 2 diabetes and bone. J Bone Miner Res 2012;27(11):2231–7 Epub 2012/10/02.
10. Kurra S, Siris E. Diabetes and bone health: the relationship between diabetes and osteoporosis-associated fractures. Diabetes Metab Res Rev 2011;27(5): 430–5 Epub 2011/03/25.
11. Vestergaard P. Discrepancies in bone mineral density and fracture risk in patients with type 1 and type 2 diabetes–a meta-analysis. Osteoporos Int 2007; 18(4):427–44 Epub 2006/10/28.
12. Janghorbani M, Van Dam RM, Willett WC, et al. Systematic review of type 1 and type 2 diabetes mellitus and risk of fracture. Am J Epidemiol 2007;166(5): 495–505 Epub 2007/06/19.
13. Schwartz AV, Garnero P, Hillier TA, et al. Pentosidine and increased fracture risk in older adults with type 2 diabetes. J Clin Endocrinol Metab 2009;94(7):2380–6 Epub 2009/04/23.
14. Inaba M, Terada M, Koyama H, et al. Influence of high glucose on 1,25-dihydroxyvitamin D3-induced effect on human osteoblast-like MG-63 cells. J Bone Miner Res 1995;10(7):1050–6 Epub 1995/07/01.
15. Kanazawa I, Yamaguchi T, Yamamoto M, et al. Serum osteocalcin level is associated with glucose metabolism and atherosclerosis parameters in type 2 diabetes mellitus. J Clin Endocrinol Metab 2009;94(1):45–9 Epub 2008/11/06.
16. Krakauer JC, McKenna MJ, Buderer NF, et al. Bone loss and bone turnover in diabetes. Diabetes 1995;44(7):775–82 Epub 1995/07/01.
17. Schwartz AV, Sellmeyer DE, Ensrud KE, et al. Older women with diabetes have an increased risk of fracture: a prospective study. J Clin Endocrinol Metab 2001; 86(1):32–8 Epub 2001/03/07.
18. Verhaeghe J, Suiker AM, Einhorn TA, et al. Brittle bones in spontaneously diabetic female rats cannot be predicted by bone mineral measurements: studies in diabetic and ovariectomized rats. J Bone Miner Res 1994;9(10):1657–67 Epub 1994/10/01.

19. Goh SY, Cooper ME. Clinical review: the role of advanced glycation end products in progression and complications of diabetes. J Clin Endocrinol Metab 2008;93(4):1143–52 Epub 2008/01/10.
20. Saito M, Fujii K, Mori Y, et al. Role of collagen enzymatic and glycation induced cross-links as a determinant of bone quality in spontaneously diabetic WBN/Kob rats. Osteoporos Int 2006;17(10):1514–23 Epub 2006/06/14.
21. Yamamoto M, Yamaguchi T, Yamauchi M, et al. Serum pentosidine levels are positively associated with the presence of vertebral fractures in postmenopausal women with type 2 diabetes. J Clin Endocrinol Metab 2008;93(3): 1013–9 Epub 2007/12/28.
22. Tanaka S, Kuroda T, Saito M, et al. Urinary pentosidine improves risk classification using fracture risk assessment tools for postmenopausal women. J Bone Miner Res 2011;26(11):2778–84 Epub 2011/07/21.
23. Gineyts E, Munoz F, Bertholon C, et al. Urinary levels of pentosidine and the risk of fracture in postmenopausal women: the OFELY study. Osteoporos Int 2010; 21(2):243–50 Epub 2009/05/08.
24. Katayama Y, Akatsu T, Yamamoto M, et al. Role of nonenzymatic glycosylation of type I collagen in diabetic osteopenia. J Bone Miner Res 1996;11(7):931–7 Epub 1996/07/01.
25. Zhou Z, Immel D, Xi CX, et al. Regulation of osteoclast function and bone mass by RAGE. J Exp Med 2006;203(4):1067–80 Epub 2006/04/12.
26. Schwartz AV, Margolis KL, Sellmeyer DE, et al. Intensive glycemic control is not associated with fractures or falls in the ACCORD randomized trial. Diabetes Care 2012;35(7):1525–31 Epub 2012/06/23.
27. Schwartz AV, Vittinghoff E, Margolis KL, et al. Intensive glycemic control and thiazolidinedione use: effects on cortical and trabecular bone at the radius and tibia. Calcif Tissue Int 2013;92(5):477–86 Epub 2013/02/05.
28. Forsen L, Meyer HE, Midthjell K, et al. Diabetes mellitus and the incidence of hip fracture: results from the Nord-Trondelag Health Survey. Diabetologia 1999; 42(8):920–5 Epub 1999/09/24.
29. Ivers RQ, Cumming RG, Mitchell P, et al. Diabetes and risk of fracture: the Blue Mountains Eye Study. Diabetes Care 2001;24(7):1198–203 Epub 2001/06/26.
30. Schwartz AV, Hillier TA, Sellmeyer DE, et al. Older women with diabetes have a higher risk of falls: a prospective study. Diabetes Care 2002;25(10):1749–54 Epub 2002/09/28.
31. Vestergaard P, Rejnmark L, Mosekilde L. Diabetes and its complications and their relationship with risk of fractures in type 1 and 2 diabetes. Calcif Tissue Int 2009;84(1):45–55 Epub 2008/12/11.
32. Shu A, Yin MT, Stein E, et al. Bone structure and turnover in type 2 diabetes mellitus. Osteoporos Int 2012;23(2):635–41 Epub 2011/03/23.
33. Gennari L, Merlotti D, Valenti R, et al. Circulating sclerostin levels and bone turnover in type 1 and type 2 diabetes. J Clin Endocrinol Metab 2012;97(5):1737–44 Epub 2012/03/09.
34. Bouillon R. Diabetic bone disease. Calcif Tissue Int 1991;49(3):155–60 Epub 1991/09/01.
35. Miao J, Brismar K, Nyren O, et al. Elevated hip fracture risk in type 1 diabetic patients: a population-based cohort study in Sweden. Diabetes Care 2005; 28(12):2850–5 Epub 2005/11/25.
36. Hadjidakis DJ, Raptis AE, Sfakianakis M, et al. Bone mineral density of both genders in type 1 diabetes according to bone composition. J Diabetes Complications 2006;20(5):302–7 Epub 2006/09/05.

37. Mastrandrea LD, Wactawski-Wende J, Donahue RP, et al. Young women with type 1 diabetes have lower bone mineral density that persists over time. Diabetes Care 2008;31(9):1729–35 Epub 2008/07/02.
38. Liu EY, Wactawski-Wende J, Donahue RP, et al. Does low bone mineral density start in post-teenage years in women with type 1 diabetes? Diabetes Care 2003; 26(8):2365–9 Epub 2003/07/29.
39. Kemink SA, Hermus AR, Swinkels LM, et al. Osteopenia in insulin-dependent diabetes mellitus; prevalence and aspects of pathophysiology. J Endocrinol Invest 2000;23(5):295–303 Epub 2000/07/06.
40. Melton LJ 3rd, Riggs BL, Leibson CL, et al. A bone structural basis for fracture risk in diabetes. J Clin Endocrinol Metab 2008;93(12):4804–9 Epub 2008/09/18.
41. Bonds DE, Larson JC, Schwartz AV, et al. Risk of fracture in women with type 2 diabetes: the Women's Health Initiative Observational Study. J Clin Endocrinol Metab 2006;91(9):3404–10 Epub 2006/06/29.
42. de Liefde II, van der Klift M, de Laet CE, et al. Bone mineral density and fracture risk in type-2 diabetes mellitus: the Rotterdam Study. Osteoporos Int 2005; 16(12):1713–20 Epub 2005/06/09.
43. Lipscombe LL, Jamal SA, Booth GL, et al. The risk of hip fractures in older individuals with diabetes: a population-based study. Diabetes Care 2007;30(4): 835–41 Epub 2007/03/30.
44. Strotmeyer ES, Cauley JA, Schwartz AV, et al. Nontraumatic fracture risk with diabetes mellitus and impaired fasting glucose in older white and black adults: the health, aging, and body composition study. Ann Intern Med 2005;165(14): 1612–7 Epub 2005/07/27.
45. Schwartz AV, Vittinghoff E, Bauer DC, et al. Association of BMD and FRAX score with risk of fracture in older adults with type 2 diabetes. JAMA 2011;305(21): 2184–92 Epub 2011/06/03.
46. Kahn SE, Zinman B, Lachin JM, et al. Rosiglitazone-associated fractures in type 2 diabetes: an Analysis from A Diabetes Outcome Progression Trial (ADOPT). Diabetes Care 2008;31(5):845–51 Epub 2008/01/29.
47. Kahn SE, Haffner SM, Heise MA, et al. Glycemic durability of rosiglitazone, metformin, or glyburide monotherapy. N Engl J Med 2006;355(23):2427–43 Epub 2006/12/06.
48. Takeda Pharmaceutical Company. Observation of an increased incidence of fractures in female patients who received long-term treatment with ACTOS (pioglitazone HCl) tablets for type 2 diabetes mellitus (letter to health care providers). Osaka (Japan): Takeda Pharmaceutical Company; 2007.
49. Bilezikian JP, Josse RG, Eastell R, et al. Rosiglitazone decreases bone mineral density and increases bone turnover in postmenopausal women with type 2 diabetes mellitus. J Clin Endocrinol Metab 2013;98(4):1519–28 Epub 2013/03/02.
50. Berberoglu Z, Gursoy A, Bayraktar N, et al. Rosiglitazone decreases serum bone-specific alkaline phosphatase activity in postmenopausal diabetic women. J Clin Endocrinol Metab 2007;92(9):3523–30 Epub 2007/06/28.
51. Cosman F, Lindsay R, LeBeur MS, et al. Clinician's guide to prevention and treatment of osteoporosis. Washington, DC: National Osteoporosis Foundation; 2013. p. 1–53.
52. Kanis JA, Johnell O, Oden A, et al. FRAX and the assessment of fracture probability in men and women from the UK. Osteoporos Int 2008;19(4):385–97 Epub 2008/02/23.

53. Nelson HD, Haney EM, Dana T, et al. Screening for osteoporosis: an update for the U.S. Preventive Services Task Force. Ann Intern Med 2010;153(2):99–111 Epub 2010/07/14.
54. Cozen L. Does diabetes delay fracture healing? Clin Orthop Relat Res 1972;82: 134–40 Epub 1972/01/01.
55. Chaudhary SB, Liporace FA, Gandhi A, et al. Complications of ankle fracture in patients with diabetes. J Am Acad Orthop Surg 2008;16(3):159–70 Epub 2008/03/05.
56. Vestergaard P. Acute myocardial infarction and atherosclerosis of the coronary arteries in patients treated with drugs against osteoporosis: calcium in the vessels and not the bones? Calcif Tissue Int 2012;90(1):22–9 Epub 2011/11/29.
57. Vestergaard P, Schwartz F, Rejnmark L, et al. Risk of femoral shaft and subtrochanteric fractures among users of bisphosphonates and raloxifene. Osteoporos Int 2011;22(3):993–1001 Epub 2010/12/18.
58. Keegan TH, Schwartz AV, Bauer DC, et al. Effect of alendronate on bone mineral density and biochemical markers of bone turnover in type 2 diabetic women: the fracture intervention trial. Diabetes Care 2004;27(7):1547–53 Epub 2004/06/29.
59. Saag KG, Shane E, Boonen S, et al. Teriparatide or alendronate in glucocorticoid-induced osteoporosis. N Engl J Med 2007;357(20):2028–39 Epub 2007/11/16.

Guidelines for Care of the Hospitalized Patient with Hyperglycemia and Diabetes

Kate Crawford, RN, MSN, ANP-C, BC-ADM

KEYWORDS

- Diabetes • Hyperglycemia • Diabetes medications • Insulin • Hypoglycemia

KEY POINTS

- Hyperglycemia and diabetes place hospitalized patients at greater risk for serious complications such as infections, diabetic ketoacidosis, hyperosmolar hyperglycemic state, dehydration, electrolyte imbalances, greater antibiotic use, and lengthened hospitalization.
- Identification and proper treatment of hyperglycemia and diabetes are essential for prevention of significant morbidity and mortality to the patient and to conserve ever-shrinking health care resources.
- It important for the nurse to understand current recommendations for diabetes treatment in the non–critically ill hospitalized patient.

HYPERGLYCEMIA AND DIABETES IN THE HOSPITAL

It is well known that the number of persons with diabetes in the United States is reaching epidemic levels and is expected to grow. In 2011, the Centers for Disease Control and Prevention reported that 8.3% of the US population had diabetes.[1] As the number of persons with diabetes is growing, it is expected that the percentage of hospitalized persons with diabetes will continue to grow. In 2009, diabetes was the second most frequent primary diagnosis noted on hospital discharge in patients aged 18 years and older.[2] The prevalence of diabetes in community hospitals has been reported to range from 32% to 38%.[2] The estimate is dramatically higher, 70% to 80%, in patients with acute coronary syndrome or those undergoing cardiovascular surgery.[3]

Much research has been focused on the best practice for the management of hyperglycemia in specific subgroups of inpatients such as those in perioperative, cardiovascular postsurgical, and intensive care.[4] Numerous studies report reduced rates of

This article originally appeared in Critical Care Nursing Clinics of North America, Vol. 25, Issue 1, March 2013.

Disclosure: The author has no relationship with a commercial company that has a direct financial interest in the subject matter or materials discussed in the article or with a company making a competing product.

Department of Endocrine Neoplasia and Hormonal Disorders, The University of Texas MD Anderson Cancer Center, 1515 Holcombe Boulevard, Unit 1461, Houston, TX 77030, USA

E-mail address: kcrawford@mdanderson.org

Clinics Collections 1 (2014) 429–434
http://dx.doi.org/10.1016/j.ccol.2014.08.023
2352-7986/14/$ – see front matter Published by Elsevier Inc.

infection, length of hospitalization, and mortality with tight glycemic control in these specific populations. As with critically ill patients, hyperglycemia in non–critically ill hospitalized patients has also been associated with lengthened hospital stay, more infections, and increased mortality.[4] Unfortunately, less data are available for hospitalized patients with hyperglycemia who are not in intensive care. Guidelines for the treatment of inpatient hyperglycemia can be found from numerous expert sources such as the American Diabetes Association (ADA), the American Association of Clinical Endocrinologists (AACE), and the Endocrine Society. In 2009, the ADA and the AACE published a consensus statement on inpatient glycemic control, which will serve as the main reference for this article. This article will discuss the identification of hyperglycemia, assessment of the patient with hyperglycemia, glycemic targets, treatment of hyperglycemia and hypoglycemia, and transition to outpatient care of non–critically ill hospitalized patients.

IDENTIFICATION OF HYPERGLYCEMIA AND DIABETES IN THE HOSPITAL

Hyperglycemia and diabetes are associated with longer hospitalizations, more antibiotic use, more time spent in critical care, and worse overall mortality.[4,5] Unfortunately, for many patients, if diabetes is not the primary diagnosis on admission, the management of hyperglycemia and diabetes is often viewed as less important than the illness that precipitated admission to the hospital. Hyperglycemia in the hospital is not limited to those patients with a known diagnosis of diabetes. In patients without diabetes, transient elevations in glucose can result from numerous factors such as increased catecholamine production, medications such as glucocorticoids, treatments such as parenteral or enteral nutrition, or surgical procedures. In patients being treated for cancer, one study noted worse overall outcomes for those patients with no formal diagnosis of diabetes than for those patients with diagnosed diabetes (P. Shah, MD Anderson Cancer Center, unpublished data, 2009). Because nearly one third of persons with diabetes in the United States are undiagnosed, a significant number of patients may have unrecognized hyperglycemia on hospital admission.[1] Hyperglycemia, regardless of the cause, is an independent predictor of increased morbidity in hospitalized patients.[5] Therefore, to prevent serious complications, it is necessary to identify and treat not only patients with known diabetes but also patients with previously undetected or newly developed hyperglycemia. Hyperglycemia in the hospital is defined as any glucose value greater than140 mg/dL or a hemoglobin A_{1c} value of 5.7% to 6.4%, indicating impaired glucose tolerance, whereas hemoglobin A_{1c} values greater than 6.5% are diagnostic for overt diabetes.[6]

ASSESSING FOR HYPERGLYCEMIA

Patients at high risk for hyperglycemia need to be assessed on admission and throughout their hospitalization for elevated glucose values. For patients with a known diagnosis of diabetes, it is imperative that this diagnosis is noted in the medical record and that glucose monitoring be initiated on admission.[6] Initial assessment of the patient should include at minimum a description of the outpatient medication regimen, level of glycemic control, and frequency of hypoglycemia.

For patients without a history of diabetes or hyperglycemia, glucose monitoring should be initiated in those patients receiving glucocorticoids, enteral or parenteral nutrition, or other medications known to cause hyperglycemia such as octreotide or immunosuppressants.[6]

Patients who are tolerating a diet should have their glucose level monitored before meals and bedtime. Of note, if meals are provided on demand, monitoring should be performed based on the patient's actual meal schedule instead of at fixed intervals. For patients taking nothing by mouth or receiving continuous enteral or parenteral nutrition, monitoring every 6 hours is sufficient. A hemoglobin A_{1c} level can be checked on admission if not previously measured within the past 3 months, however, a hemoglobin A_{1c} may not indict usual glycemic control in those patients with red blood cell pathologies, those receiving frequent transfusions, or patients with anemia.

GLYCEMIC TARGETS

There are little data to support specific glucose goals outside of critical care.[6] The ADA/AACE consensus statement recommends a preprandial glucose range from 100 to no greater than 140 mg/dL, with random glucose values no greater than 180 mg/dL.[4] They recommend treatment of any glucose value of greater than 180 mg/dL. Glucose values less than 70 mg/dL represent hypoglycemia and should be avoided. In stable patients with previously well-controlled diabetes, lower glucose targets may be appropriate. Less stringent targets are appropriate in patients at high risk for hypoglycemia such as those with hepatic or renal dysfunction, the elderly, patients with altered mental status, or patients for whom tight glycemic control is not clinically beneficial such as those in palliative care.

TREATMENT OF HYPERGLYCEMIA

The ADA/AACE consensus statement recommends treatment of any glucose level greater than 180 mg/dL.[4] The preferred regimen for the treatment of hyperglycemia is with scheduled subcutaneous injections of insulin, which includes 3 components: basal, bolus, and correctional.[6] Basal insulin is provided to control glucose elevations from hepatic glucose output between meals and during sleep. Basal insulin is long-acting and is administered only once or twice daily. Because patients with type 1 diabetes are absolutely insulin deficient, it is critical that they receive basal insulin daily, regardless of nutritional status, to prevent diabetic ketoacidosis. Bolus insulin is provided to control glucose elevations that result from food intake. Bolus insulin is typically rapid or short-acting and is administered before meals only. It is important to administer bolus insulin based on the actual timing of the patient's meal instead of on standardized or predetermined hospital administration times. Correctional insulin is a dose of rapid or short-acting insulin, usually administered with a bolus dose to correct for high glucose before a meal. Correctional doses of insulin without regard to meals or at bedtime should be avoided to prevent hypoglycemia. Insulin regimens should be reassessed if glucose values are less than 100, as the patient is at risk for hypoglycemia.[4] Insulin regimens need to be adjusted if glucose values decrease to less than 70 mg/dL.[4] Patients who use continuous subcutaneous infusions of insulin via insulin pumps can continue to manage their diabetes while in the hospital only if they are willing and cognitively capable of independently managing the insulin pump. Nursing staff must document patient-administered basal and bolus insulin doses administered via the insulin pump. Infusion sites should be changed at a minimum every 72 hours.

"Sliding scale" insulin should not be used for hyperglycemia lasting longer than 24 hours.[7] If patients experience persistent elevations in glucose, a physiologic insulin program using basal, bolus, and correction insulin should be instituted.[8] Sliding scale protocols do not deliver insulin in a physiologic fashion, resulting in wide glucose variability. In addition, sliding scale insulin places the patient at greater risk for hypoglycemia because it is usually administered without regard to meals.[7] Patients with type 1 diabetes require scheduled injections of basal insulin, despite nutritional status, and therefore should never be prescribed sliding scale insulin alone as treatment of their diabetes. The use of noninsulin treatments for hyperglycemia in the hospital is discouraged.[4] Hospitalized patients can have rapidly deteriorating hepatic and renal function, widely variable nutrition intake, and frequent medication changes. They often undergo unscheduled testing with contrast media that is contraindicated for use with some oral diabetes medications. **Table 1** provides a list of noninsulin diabetes medications and their indications for use in hospitalized patients. For a detailed discussion of insulin and oral regimens, please refer to the articles by Levesque and Martin in this issue.

TREATMENT OF HYPOGLYCEMIA

Hypoglycemia is the central limiting factor in the treatment of hyperglycemia and is a critical component of hyperglycemia management.[6] Hypoglycemia is defined as a

Table 1
Noninsulin diabetes medications and indications for use in hospitalized patients

Medication Names, Generic (Brand)	Use in Hospital
Oral Diabetes Medications	
Sulfonylureas: Glimepiride (Amaryl) Glipizide (Glucotrol, Glucotrol XL) Glyburide (Diabeta, Glynase PresTab, Micronase)	Discontinue: high risk for hypoglycemia due to unpredictable PO intake, fasting, elevated creatinine
Meglitinides: Nateglinide (Starlix) Repaglinide (Prandin)	Discontinue: high risk for hypoglycemia because of unpredictable oral intake or fasting
Thiazolidinediones: Pioglitazone (Actos) Rosiglitizone (Avandia)	Can continue in stable patients because they do not cause hypoglycemia. Do not initiate in patients with congestive heart failure or edema
Biguanides: Metformin (Glucophage, Glucophage XR, Fortamet, Riomet)	Hold: for creatinine >1.4 mg/dL women, >1.5 mg/dL in men. Hold after contrast until renal function is verified. Do not initiate in patient with nausea, vomiting, or diarrhea
α-Glucosidase inhibitors: Acarbose (Precose) Miglitol (Glyset)	Discontinue: high risk for hypoglycemia because of unpredictable oral intake, fasting Do not initiate in patient with nausea, vomiting, or diarrhea
Dipeptidyl peptidase-4 inhibitors: Sitagliptin phosphate (Januvia) Saxagliptin (Onglyza), Linagliptin (Tradjenta)	Do not cause hypoglycemia; OK for stable patients or those ready for discharge
Noninsulin Injectable Diabetes Medications	
Incretin mimetics: Exenatide (Byetta) Exenatide extended release (Bydureon) Liraglutide (Victoza)	Do not produce hypoglycemia Caution in gastrointestinal/surgical patients; cause delayed gastric emptying and can cause nausea
Amylin agonists: Pramlintide (Symlin)	Given immediately before meals with rapid-acting insulin; would not be given unless the patient is eating a meal

glucose value of less than 70 mg/dL, with severe hypoglycemia defined as a glucose value of less than 40 mg/dL.[6] Hospitalized patients are at high risk for hypoglycemia because of rapidly changing clinical circumstances such as changes in nutrition status, reduction in glucocorticoids, reduction in dextrose content in intravenous fluids, cessation of total parenteral nutrition or tube feeding, prolonged use of sliding scale insulin therapy, sulfonylurea use, and improper administration of insulin.[6,9] Patients at greatest risk for hypoglycemia include the elderly; the undernourished; those with a history of severe hypoglycemia; patients with hepatic, renal, or cardiac failure; and patients with sepsis. Hypoglycemia can result in serious injury to the patient if not corrected. Standardized hypoglycemia protocols should be implemented for all patients receiving treatment of hyperglycemia.[4] For patients who are alert and able to swallow, 15 g of oral glucose is the preferred treatment.[6] The use of intravenous dextrose 50% should be limited to those patients who are unable to take carbohydrates by mouth. Glucagon can be administered intramuscularly or subcutaneously to revive an unconscious patient in whom intravenous access cannot be established. In patients receiving insulin therapy, care needs to be paid to any change in oral status; the development of nausea, vomiting, or sepsis; and avoidance of nonphysiologic insulin administration to avoid hypoglycemia.

TRANSITION TO OUTPATIENT CARE

Transition from acute care to home can be a stressful time for patients and caregivers. Patients with hyperglycemia have several skills they must master, usually in a short duration of time. This necessitates the need to begin discharge planning and education either on admission or as soon as hyperglycemia is detected to facilitate a smooth transition from hospital to home. At a minimum, patients with hyperglycemia need education on the following areas before discharge[6]:

- Understanding of the diagnosis of diabetes/hyperglycemia, glucose monitoring, and home glucose goals
- Signs, symptoms, and treatment of hypoglycemia
- Signs, symptoms, and treatment of hyperglycemia
- Diet recommendations
- Medication instructions
- Sick day management
- Insulin injection and needle disposal instruction
- Plan for follow up after discharge

Providers must ensure the patient has the appropriate supplies for discharge, including medications, syringes or needles, lancets, test strips, and a glucometer. A certified diabetes educator is an invaluable resource for educating patients and families and should be utilized if available.

SUMMARY

Although there are limited randomized trials supporting a single approach to the management of inpatient hyperglycemia, the ADA/AACE consensus statement provides guidelines. Clinicians need to conduct a thorough admission assessment to screen for diabetes and should be vigilant for hyperglycemia that develops during hospitalization. Treatment of hyperglycemia should focus on physiologic insulin replacement using a basal/bolus/correction regimen rather than sliding scale coverage. Glucose values should be controlled, minimizing acute complications such as hypoglycemia, infections, and increased length of stay.

REFERENCES

1. Centers for Disease Control and Prevention. 2011 National Diabetes Fact Sheet. 2011. Available at: http://www.dcd.gov/diabetes/pubs/estimates11htm. Accessed August 20, 2012.
2. Centers for Disease Control and Prevention. Distribution of first-listed diagnoses among hospital discharges with diabetes as any listed diagnosis, adults aged 18 years and older, United States. 2009. Available at: http://www.cdc.gov/diabetes/statistics/hosp/adulttable1.htm. Accessed August 20, 2012.
3. Smiley D, Umpierrez GE. Management of hyperglycemia in the hospitalized patient. Ann N Y Acad Sci 2010;1212:1–11. http://dx.doi.org/10.1111/j.1749-6632.2010.05805.
4. Moghissi E, Korytkowsi M, DiNardo M, et al. American Association of Clinical Endocrinologists and American Diabetes Association consensus statement on inpatient glycemic control. Diabetes Care 2009;32:1119–31.
5. Lieva RR, Inzucchi SE. Hospital management of hyperglycemia. Curr Opin Endocrinol Diabetes Obes 2011;18:110–8. http://dx.doi.org/10.1097/MED.0b013e3283447a6d.
6. American Diabetes Association. Standards of medical care in diabetes: 2012. Diabetes Care 2012;35(Suppl 1):S11–63.
7. Kitabchi AE, Nyenue E. Sliding scale insulin: more evidence needed before the final exit? Diabetes Care 2007;30:2409–10.
8. Umpierrez GE, Smiley D, Jacobs S, et al. Randomized study of basal-bolus insulin therapy in the inpatient management of patients with type 2 diabetes undergoing general surgery (RABBIT 2 surgery). Diabetes Care 2011;34:256–61.
9. Umpierrez GE, Palacio A, Smiley D. Sliding scale insulin use: myth or insanity? Am J Med 2007;120:563–7.

Printed and bound by CPI Group (UK) Ltd, Croydon, CR0 4YY

03/10/2024

01040496-0013